Surgery of the Cerebellopontine Angle

Nicholas C. Bambakidis • Cliff A. Megerian
Robert F. Spetzler
Editors

Surgery of the Cerebellopontine Angle

Second Edition

Springer

Editors
Nicholas C. Bambakidis, MD
Chair of Neurological Surgery
Vice President and Director
The Neurological Institute
University Hospitals of Cleveland
Cleveland, OH, USA

Harvey Huntington Brown Jr.
Endowed Chair of Neurological Surgery
Professor, Neurological Surgery
Case Western Reserve University
School of Medicine
Cleveland, OH, USA

Robert F. Spetzler, MD, FACS
Emeritus President and CEO, Emeritus Chair
Department of Neurosurgery
Barrow Neurological Institute
Phoenix, AZ, USA

Cliff A. Megerian, MD, FACS
Chief Executive Officer
University Hospitals Health System
Jane and Henry Meyer Distinguished CEO
Endowed Chair, Professor of Otolaryngology
Head and Neck Surgery
Professor of Neurological Surgery
Case Western Reserve University
School of Medicine
Cleveland, OH, USA

Videos in Cases 1–10, 12, and 13 are used with permission from the Congress of Neurological Surgeons, CNS Nexus Cases. 2018. https://www.cns.org/nexus/cases

ISBN 978-3-031-12506-5 ISBN 978-3-031-12507-2 (eBook)
https://doi.org/10.1007/978-3-031-12507-2

This Springer imprint is published by the registered company Springer Nature Switzerland AG
The registered company address is: Gewerbestrasse 11, 6330 Cham, Switzerland

This book is dedicated to educators in the subspecialties of neurosurgery and neurotology who have labored so hard to unlock the secrets of the skull base in the interest of our patients whom we ultimately serve.

To my amazing wife, Kim, and our children, Eva and Peter, of whom I am so proud. And to the memory of my mother and father for cultivating my curiosity in science, teaching me patience, and inspiring me to discover.

Nicholas C. Bambakidis

To my lovely wife, Lynne, and our wonderful children, Andrew (Drew), Mark, and Caroline, for their love and encouragement.

Cliff A. Megerian

To my grandchildren, Olivia, Charlotte, and Abigail, whose wonder at the world rekindles my own delight.

Robert F. Spetzler

Preface

Assembling this text would not have been possible without the generous participation of the contributing authors, each of whom is a worldwide expert in this subspecialty. We have carried forward from the first edition the invaluable contribution of the illustrators (Mark Schornak, MS, and Kristen Larson, MS), animator (Michael Hickman), and interactive multimedia specialist (Marie Clarkson) whose illustrations and digital media have eased the tasks of understanding and visualizing the complex anatomic relationships ubiquitous to the cerebellopontine angle. We are grateful to Brian Decker for his support of the first edition and to Linda Mehta for her leadership and dedication to both the first and second editions. We thank Kim Sender Duvall, MA, for her editorial expertise and commitment to producing a clear, cohesive, first-rate publication. Finally, we offer thanks to our friends at Springer Publishing for their belief in this long-awaited second edition and for sharing our determination to make it happen.

Cleveland, OH, USA	Nicholas C. Bambakidis
Cleveland, OH, USA	Cliff A. Megerian
Phoenix, AZ, USA	Robert F. Spetzler

Contents

Contributors

Dunia Abdul-Aziz, MD Massachusetts Eye and Ear, Boston, MA, USA
Otolaryngology—Head and Neck Surgery, Harvard Medical School, Boston, MA, USA

Rami Almefty, MD Department of Neurosurgery, Temple University, Lewis Katz School of Medicine, Philadelphia, PA, USA

João Paulo Almeida, MD Department of Neurosurgery, Cleveland Clinic, Cleveland, OH, USA

Biji Bahuleyan, MBBS, MCh Lisie Hospital, Kaloor, Ernakulam, Kerala, India

Nicholas C. Bambakidis, MD Neurological Surgery, The Neurological Institute, University Hospitals of Cleveland, Case Western Reserve University School of Medicine, Cleveland, OH, USA

Eric M. Bershad, MD Neurology, Baylor College of Medicine, Houston, TX, USA
Neurosurgery, Baylor College of Medicine, Houston, TX, USA
Space Medicine, Baylor College of Medicine, Houston, TX, USA

Kristine A. Blackham, MD Universitätsspital, Klinik für Radiologie und Nuklearmedizin, Basel, Switzerland

Derald E. Brackmann, MD Neurotology and Otolaryngology, House Clinic, Inc., Los Angeles, CA, USA

Craig A. Buchman, MD, FACS Department of Otolaryngology—Head and Neck Surgery, Washington University School of Medicine, St. Louis, MO, USA

Steven B. Carr, MD Division of Neurological Surgery, Department of Neurosurgery, University of Missouri School of Medicine, Columbia, MO, USA

Steve W. Chang, MD Department of Neurosurgery, Barrow Neurological Institute, St. Joseph's Hospital and Medical Center, Phoenix, AZ, USA

Jacob Cherian, MD University of Maryland School of Medicine, Baltimore, MD, USA

Shakeel A. Chowdhry, MD NorthShore Neurological Institute, Evanston, IL, USA

Patrick J. Codd, MD Duke Cancer Center, Duke University Medical Center, Durham, NC, USA

Simone E. Dekker, MD, PhD Department of Neurological Surgery, The Neurological Institute, University Hospitals Cleveland Medical Center, Case Western Reserve University, Cleveland, OH, USA

Nicholas A. Dewyer, MD Department of Otolaryngology—Head and Neck Surgery, Department of Otology, Neurotology, and Skull Base Surgery, Department of Audiology, University of Arizona College of Medicine, Tucson, AZ, USA

Colin L. W. Driscoll, MD Department of Otolaryngology—Head and Neck Surgery, Mayo Clinic, Rochester, MN, USA

Nedim Durakovic, MD Department of Otolaryngology—Head and Neck Surgery, Washington University School of Medicine, St. Louis, MO, USA

Allan H. Friedman, MD The Preston Robert Tisch Brain Tumor Center, Duke Health, Durham, NC, USA

David Fusco, MD Inpatient Neurosurgical Care, Chandler Regional Hospital, Phoenix, AZ, USA

Bruce J. Gantz, MD Department of Otolaryngology—Head and Neck Surgery, University of Iowa Hospitals and Clinics, Iowa City, IA, USA

Anisha Garg, MA, MD Yale New Haven Hospital, New Haven, CT, USA

Chad A. Glenn, MD Comprehensive Brain Tumor Program, Neurosurgery, Stephenson Cancer Center, University of Oklahoma School of Medicine, Oklahoma City, OK, USA

L. Fernando Gonzalez, MD Neurosurgery, Cerebrovascular and Endovascular Neurosurgery, Duke University, Durham, NC, USA

Pankaj A. Gore, MD Division of Neurological Surgery, The Oregon Clinic, Providence Brain and Spine Institute, Portland, OR, USA

Tessa A. Hadlock, MD Department of Otolaryngology—Head and Neck Surgery, Massachusetts Eye and Ear Infirmary, Harvard Medical School, Boston, MA, USA

Griffith R. Harsh IV, MD, MBA Department of Neurological Surgery, UC Davis Health and School of Medicine, UC Davis Comprehensive Cancer Center, Center for Skull Base Surgery, Sacramento, CA, USA

Christian Herold, MD Department of Biomedical Imaging and Image-Guided Therapy Medical, Medical University of Vienna, Vienna General Hospital, Vienna, Austria

Department of Radiology, Johns Hopkins Medical Institutions, Baltimore, MD, USA

Jacques A. Herzog, MD Department of Otolaryngology—Head and Neck Surgery, Washington University School of Medicine, St. Louis, MO, USA

Jacob B. Hunter, MD Department of Otolaryngology—Head and Neck Surgery, University of Texas Southwestern Medical Center, Dallas, TX, USA

Robert K. Jackler, MD Department of Otolaryngology—Head and Neck Surgery, Department of Neurosurgery, Department of Surgery, Stanford University School of Medicine, Stanford, CA, USA

Daniel Jethanamest, MD Division of Otology and Neurotology, Department of Otolaryngology—Head and Neck Surgery, New York University School of Medicine, New York, NY, USA

Nate Jowett, MD, FSCRC Department of Otolaryngology—Head and Neck Surgery, Massachusetts Eye and Ear Infirmary, Harvard Medical School, Boston, MA, USA

Yashar Kalani, MS, MD, PhD Department of Surgery, University of Oklahoma School of Medicine, Tulsa, OK, USA

Panagiotis Kerezoudis, MD, MS Department of Neurologic Surgery, Mayo Clinic, Rochester, MN, USA

Wesley A. King, MD Center for Minimally Invasive Brain Pituitary and Skull Base Surgery, Department of Neurosurgery, Cedars Sinai Medical Center, Los Angeles, CA, USA

Orofacial Pain Program, School of Dentistry at UCLA, Los Angeles, CA, USA

Wenceslas Krakowiecki, MD School of Medicine and Dentistry, University of Rochester, Rochester, NY, USA

Max O. Krucoff, MD Neurosurgery, Neurosurgical Oncology, Medical College of Wisconsin, Milwaukee, WI, USA

Biomedical Engineering, Marquette University and Medical College of Wisconsin, Milwaukee, WI, USA

Shekar N. Kurpad, MD, PhD Department of Neurosurgery, Froedtert & Medical College of Wisconsin, Milwaukee, WI, USA

Michaela Lee, MD University of Arizona College of Medicine, Banner—University Medical Center Phoenix, Phoenix, AZ, USA

Gregory P. Lekovic, MD, PhD, JD Division of Neurosurgery, House Clinic, House Ear Institute, Los Angeles, CA, USA

Brandon Liebelt, MD Larner College of Medicine, University of Vermont Medical Center, Burlington, VT, USA

Michael J. Link, MD Department of Neurologic Surgery, Mayo Clinic, Rochester, MN, USA

Department of Otorhinolaryngology, Mayo Clinic, Rochester, MN, USA

Nauman F. Manzoor, MD Department of Otolaryngology—Head and Neck Surgery and Neurological Surgery, University Hospitals Cleveland Medical Center, Case Western University School of Medicine, Cleveland, OH, USA

Nikolay Martirosyan, MD, PhD Unity Point Health, Allen Memorial Hospital, Waterloo, IA, USA

Cliff A. Megerian, MD, FACS University Hospitals Health System, Department of Otolaryngology-Head and Neck Surgery, Department of Neurological Surgery, Case Western Reserve University School of Medicine, Cleveland, OH, USA

Justin M. Moore, MD, PhD, MPH, LLB Neurosurgery, Skull-Base Neuro-Oncology, Beth Israel Deaconess Medical Center, Harvard Medical School, Boston, MA, USA

Sarah Mowry, MD, FACS Division of Otology/Neurotology, Department of Otolaryngology—Head and Neck Surgery, University Hospitals Cleveland Medical Center, Case Western Reserve University, Cleveland, OH, USA

Peter Nakaji, MD Department of Neurosurgery, University of Arizona College of Medicine—Banner, Phoenix, AZ, USA

Surgery, University of Arizona College of Medicine—Phoenix, Phoenix, AZ, USA

Neurosurgery, Neuroscience Institute, Phoenix, AZ, USA

Anil Nanda, MD Department of Neurosurgery, Rutgers—New Jersey Medical School, New Brunswick, NJ, USA

Neurosurgical Services, Robert Wood Johnson Barnabas Health, New Brunswick, NJ, USA

Ameya Nayate, MD Department of Radiology, Neuroradiology, University Hospitals Cleveland Medical Center, Cleveland, OH, USA

Jeffrey T. Nelson, MD Neurological Surgery, Case Western Reserve University School of Medicine, University Hospitals Cleveland Medical Center, Cleveland, OH, USA

Sacit B. Omay, MD Department of Neurosurgery, Yale School of Medicine, New Haven, CT, USA

Thomas Ostergard, MD, MS Carolina Neurosurgery and Spine Associates, Greensboro, NC, USA

Akash J. Patel, MD Baylor College of Medicine, Houston, TX, USA

David Peace, MS Department of Neurosurgery, University of Florida School of Medicine, Gainesville, FL, USA

Kevin A. Peng, MD House Clinic Foundation, Los Angeles, CA, USA

Shervin Rahimpour, MD Department of Neurosurgery, University of Utah, Salt Lake City, UT, USA

Rohan Ramakrishna, MD Department of Neurological Surgery and Neuro-oncology, New York–Presbyterian Brooklyn Methodist Hospital, Weill Cornell Medicine, New York, NY, USA

Albert L. Rhoton Jr., MD Lillian S. Wells Department of Neurosurgery, University of Florida College of Medicine, Gainesville, FL, USA

Guilherme Carvalhal Ribas, PhD, MD Department of Surgery, University of São Paulo Medical School, São Paulo, Brazil

Albert Einstein Medical School, Hospital Israelita Albert Einstein, São Paulo, Brazil

Department of Neurosurgery, University of Virginia School of Medicine, Charlottesville, VA, USA

J. Thomas Roland Jr., MD Department of Otolaryngology—Head and Neck Surgery, Department of Neurosurgery, New York University School of Medicine, New York, NY, USA

Sam Safavi-Abbasi, MD, PhD Flagstaff Neurosurgery, Flagstaff, AZ, USA

Amir Samii, MD International Neuroscience Institute—Hannover, Hannover, Germany

Madjid Samii, MD International Neuroscience Institute—Hannover, Hannover, Germany

Theodore H. Schwartz, MD, FACS Departments of Neurological Surgery, Otolaryngology and Neuroscience, Weill Cornell Medicine, New York, NY, USA

Warren R. Selman, MD Department of Neurological Surgery, The Neurological Institute, University Hospitals Cleveland Medical Center, Case Western Reserve University, Cleveland, OH, USA

Maroun T. Semaan, MD Otolaryngology—Otology, University Hospitals Cleveland Medical Center, Cleveland, OH, USA

Vasu Sidagam, MD University Hospitals Cleveland Medical Center, Cleveland, OH, USA

Robert F. Spetzler, MD, FACS Neurosurgery, Barrow Neurological Institute, Phoenix, AZ, USA

Jose I. Suarez, MD Division of Neurosciences Critical Care, Neurology, Johns Hopkins School of Medicine, Baltimore, MD, USA

Daniel Q. Sun, MD Department of Otorhinolaryngology—Head and Neck Surgery, University of Iowa Hospitals and Clinics, Iowa City, IA, USA

Alex D. Sweeney, MD Baylor College of Medicine, Houston, TX, USA

Robert W. Tarr, MD Radiology, Neurology, Neurological Surgery, University Hospitals Cleveland Medical Center, Case Western Reserve University School of Medicine, Cleveland, OH, USA

Charles Teo, AM Centre for Minimally Invasive Neurosurgery, Prince of Wales Private Hospital, Randwick, NSW, Australia

Marte Van Keulen, MD Neurological Surgery, Case Western Reserve University School of Medicine, University Hospitals Cleveland Medical Center, Cleveland, OH, USA

P. Ashley Wackym, MD Department of Otolaryngology—Head and Neck Surgery, Rutgers Robert Wood Johnson Medical School, New Brunswick, NJ, USA

George B. Wanna, MD Department of Otolaryngology—Head and Neck Surgery, Icahn School of Medicine of Mount Sinai, New York, NY, USA

Neurology, Icahn School of Medicine of Mount Sinai, New York, NY, USA

Department of Otolaryngology, New York Eye and Ear Infirmary of Mount Sinai and Mount Sinai Beth Israel, New York, NY, USA

Audiology, Hearing and Balance Center, Mount Sinai Health System, New York, NY, USA

Peter A. Weisskopf, MD Department of Surgery, Department of Neurosurgery, Department of Otolaryngology, Head and Neck Cancer Center, Mayo Clinic, Phoenix, AZ, USA

D. Bradley Welling, MD, PhD, FACS Massachusetts Eye and Ear, Boston, MA, USA

Otolaryngology—Head and Neck Surgery, Harvard Medical School, Boston, MA, USA

Cameron C. Wick, MD Department of Otolaryngology—Head and Neck Surgery, Washington University School of Medicine, St. Louis, MO, USA

Alexandre Yasuda, MD, PhD Hospital Israelita Albert Einstein, São Paulo, Brazil

Kevin K. Yoo, MD Alvarado Hospital Medical Center and Paradise Valley Hospital, Scripps Memorial Hospital Encinitas, San Diego, CA, USA

Xiaochun Zhao, MD Department of Neurosurgery, University of Oklahoma Health Sciences Center, Oklahoma City, OK, USA

Ali R. Zomorodi, MD Neurosurgery, Duke Health, Duke University School of Medicine, Durham, NC, USA

Part I

Foundations for Treatment

Historical Perspectives

1

Nicholas C. Bambakidis, Thomas Ostergard, and Cliff A. Megerian

The study of the historical development of surgical treatment of lesions of the cerebellopontine angle (CPA) provides a dynamic view of the evolution of neurosurgery as a distinct medical specialty in its own right. The unique challenges posed by the dense anatomical structures located in this region of the posterior fossa led Harvey Cushing to describe it as "the bloody angle" [1]. Improvements in technique and advances in technology have diminished the risks associated with surgical treatment of lesions in the CPA. Even so, surgery in this area can still be daunting and can challenge the surgical skills of even the most experienced surgeon. Advances in surgery of the CPA occurred across multiple specialties for a variety of pathologies. But the history of surgical treatment of the CPA is best described by recounting the history of surgical treatment of vestibular schwannomas (VSs).

History of Vestibular Schwannoma Surgery

As Pirsig and colleagues discuss [2], evidence for the presence of vestibular schwannomas dates as far back as 2500 BCE, based on changes in the internal auditory meatus of temporal bones consistent with the diagnosis of neurofibromatosis type 2 (NF2). In 1771, Sandifort provided the first reliable postmortem description of a vestibular schwannoma [3]. He described a firm, encapsulated, yet internally soft tumor "clinging to the right auditory nerve of such toughness that it was supposed surely to be of cartilage … insinuating itself into the foramen as an obstruction in the inferior of the petrous portion of the temporal bone which said nerve enters" (Fig. 1.1). Vestibular schwannomas were subsequently described by Leveque-Lasource in 1810 and, as reported by Bell, by Whiting in 1830 [4, 5]. The latter also described the progression of symptoms, including the involvement of multiple cranial nerves in a patient who finally died "at length with difficult respiration and want of the power of swallowing." Based on postmortem dissection, Whiting described a tumor filling the CPA, indenting the pons, and extending into the internal meatus.

In the late nineteenth century, direct surgical approaches to the CPA were significantly limited by the resources available at the time. From a diagnostic perspective, it was only during the last 20 years of the nineteenth century that localization became accurate enough to justify the recommendation of surgery. Despite the introduction of the tuning fork by Weber in 1825, it was not until 1938 that Lempert, by introducing the one-stage fenestration operation, made the distinction between sensorineural and conductive hearing loss clinically worthwhile for otologists. He thereby facilitated the accurate diagnosis of unilateral sensorineural hearing loss, an important symptom associated with CPA lesions [6]. Accurate temporal bone X-rays were unavailable until the 1920s.

The absence of antibiotic therapy, consistent anesthetic technique, and adequate hemostatic agents or cauterization increased the difficulty of attempting surgery at the time. Some remarkable successes were reported, but these were unfortunately tempered by a larger number of failures. In 1892, Sir Charles Ballance described the resection of a dural-based lesion in its entirety by which the "finger had to be

N. C. Bambakidis (✉)
Neurological Surgery, The Neurological Institute, University Hospitals of Cleveland, Case Western Reserve University School of Medicine, Cleveland, OH, USA
e-mail: Nicholas.Bambakidis2@UHhospitals.org

T. Ostergard
Carolina Neurosurgery and Spine Associates, Greensboro, NC, USA

C. A. Megerian
University Hospitals Health System, Department of Otolaryngology-Head and Neck Surgery, Department of Neurological Surgery, Case Western Reserve University School of Medicine, Cleveland, OH, USA

N. C. Bambakidis et al. (eds.), *Surgery of the Cerebellopontine Angle*, https://doi.org/10.1007/978-3-031-12507-2_1

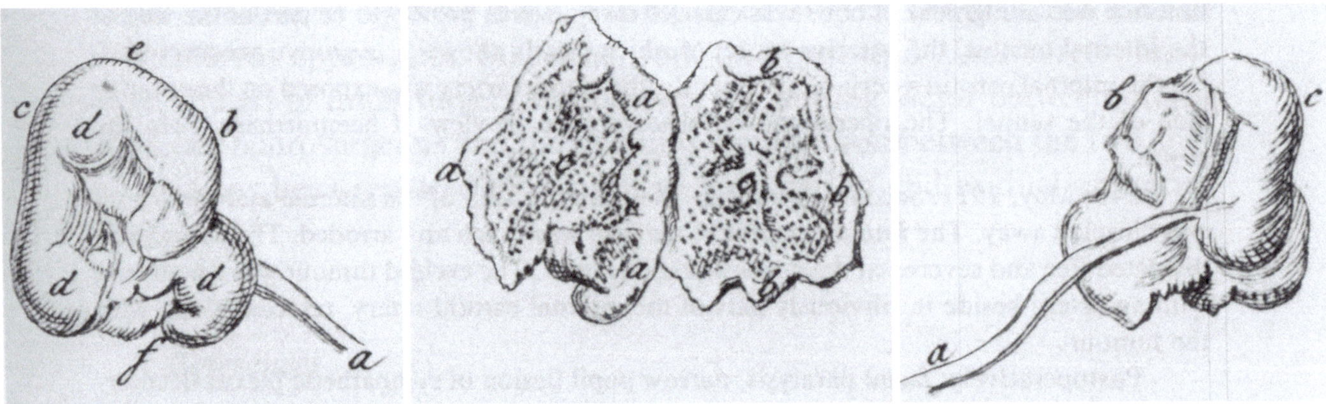

Fig. 1.1 Drawing from the first postmortem description of a vestibular schwannoma. (Reproduced from Pirsig W et al. [2]. With permission from Karger-Basel)

insinuated between the pons and tumor to get it away" [7]. As later pointed out by Cushing, this tumor was likely a meningioma. In fact, Cushing credited Thomas Annandale from Edinburgh with the first successful resection of a vestibular schwannoma in a young pregnant woman [8, 9]. Other than her preexisting deafness, she recovered with no neurological deficits. Such results were encouraging but proved to be the exception and not the rule at the time.

Curative resection was seldom possible before Dandy. The early era of vestibular schwannoma surgery was still characterized by what Cushing called "shocking" mortality. This was best exemplified at the International Congress of Medicine in 1913. Three of the most experienced vestibular schwannoma surgeons reported their surgical experience to date. The largest series was reported by Krause with a mortality rate of 84% [8, 10]. The lowest mortality of the three was Horsley's series of 15 patients, which still had a mortality of 67% [6]. Nevertheless, such high rates of operative mortality were considered justifiable, given the dismal prognosis associated with vestibular schwannomas at the time. A major factor contributing to these high rates of morbidity and mortality was the use of relatively blind digital removal of the tumor. This inevitably led to a complete facial nerve paralysis. A common reason for mortality was the inadvertent avulsion of the anterior inferior cerebellar artery. It was not until 1949 that Atkinson demonstrated the importance of this maneuver as a cause of death [11]. It should also be remembered that these operations were being performed without modern anesthetic techniques, light amplification, or cerebrospinal diversion. Due to poor diagnostic modalities, the patients also presented very late with large tumors, which carry significantly greater morbidity.

Harvey Cushing introduced a new era in CPA surgery in 1917 when he published *Tumors of the Nervus Acusticus and the Syndrome of the Cerebellopontine Angle*. By accepting the technological limitations of that time, he was able to reduce the operative mortality from 80% to 20% (Fig. 1.2) [8]. Cushing embraced the idea of subtotal resection and focused on internal debulking of the tumor. He performed a large craniectomy that allowed access to the CPA as well as early access to drainage of cerebrospinal fluid (CSF) in the cerebellomedullary cistern. This report marks an important evolution in philosophy. Early surgeons emphasized speed to minimize mortality. Cushing performed a slower, more meticulous surgical approach that emphasized hemostasis. Cushing also accurately associated the development of tinnitus followed by unilateral deafness with these tumors. While these results were impressive, long-term follow-up proved disappointing, with a high rate of tumor recurrence and a 5-year mortality of 54%.

As described in 1917 [8], Cushing's own surgical approach entailed a large bilateral suboccipital craniectomy made through a crossbow incision. The advantages of the bilateral procedure were to allow access to both CPAs in case localization was incorrect, to allow drainage of CSF from the cisterna magna, and to provide the possibility of C1 laminectomy, if needed (to prevent medullary compression).

In sharp contrast to Cushing's methods were those of his erstwhile pupil and rival, Walter Dandy. Similar to many other areas of disagreement, Dandy preferred a more aggressive approach with complete tumor removal with upfront morbidity in exchange for long-term survival. He described his unilateral approach for vestibular schwannomas in 1934 [12], on which the contemporary suboccipital or retrosigmoid approach is based (Fig. 1.3). His technique was an important progression of Cushing's. Following internal debulking, he took the additional step of then removing the tumor capsule.

In the time since Cushing's original description in 1917, Stenvers and then Towne had described the diagnosis of ves-

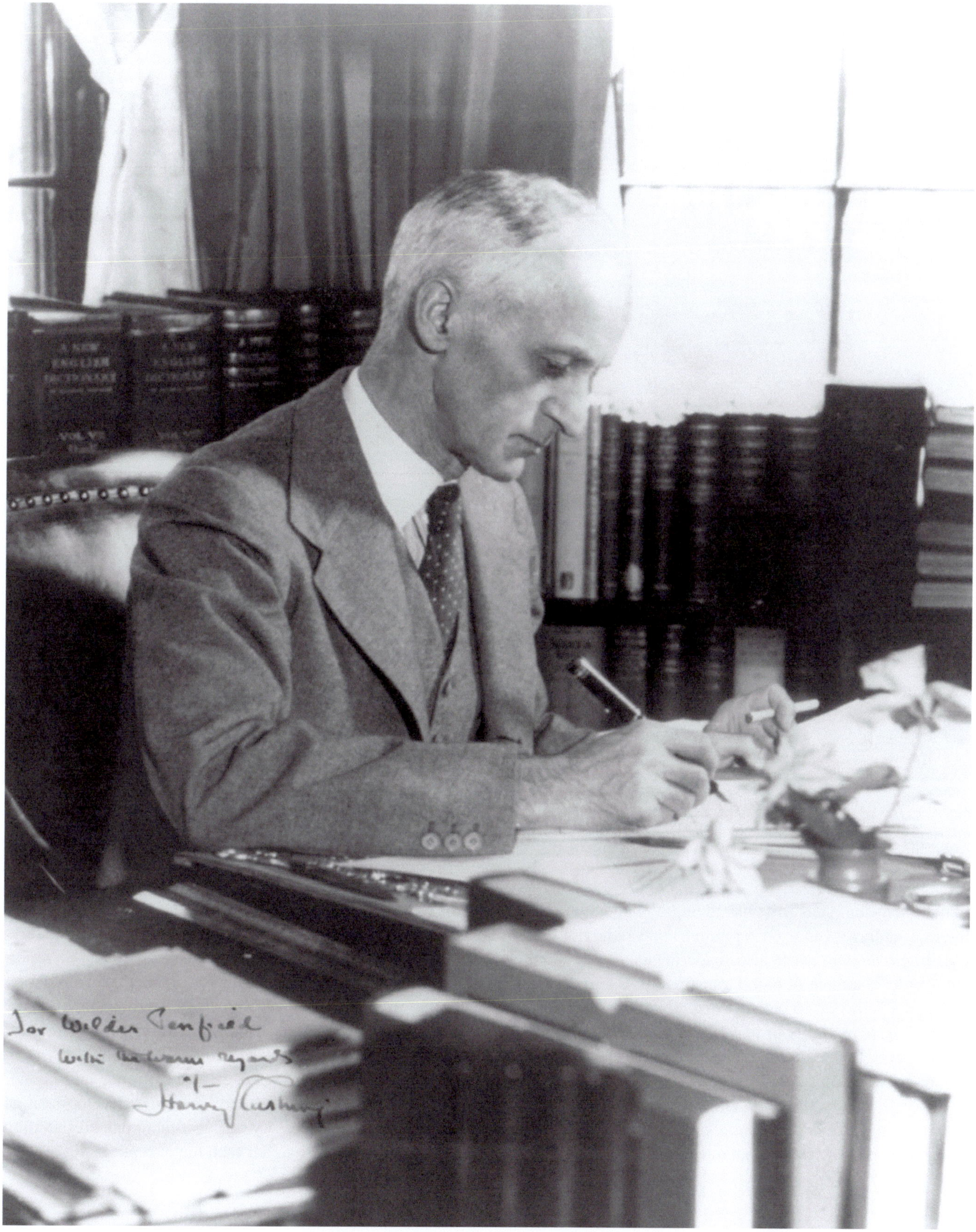

Fig. 1.2 The photograph of Harvey Cushing, fountain pen in one hand, unlit cigarette in the other, was signed "For Wilder Penfield with the warm regards of Harvey Cushing" and received by Penfield in December 1924. (Reproduced with permission from the Wilder Penfield Archive, Osler Library, McGill University)

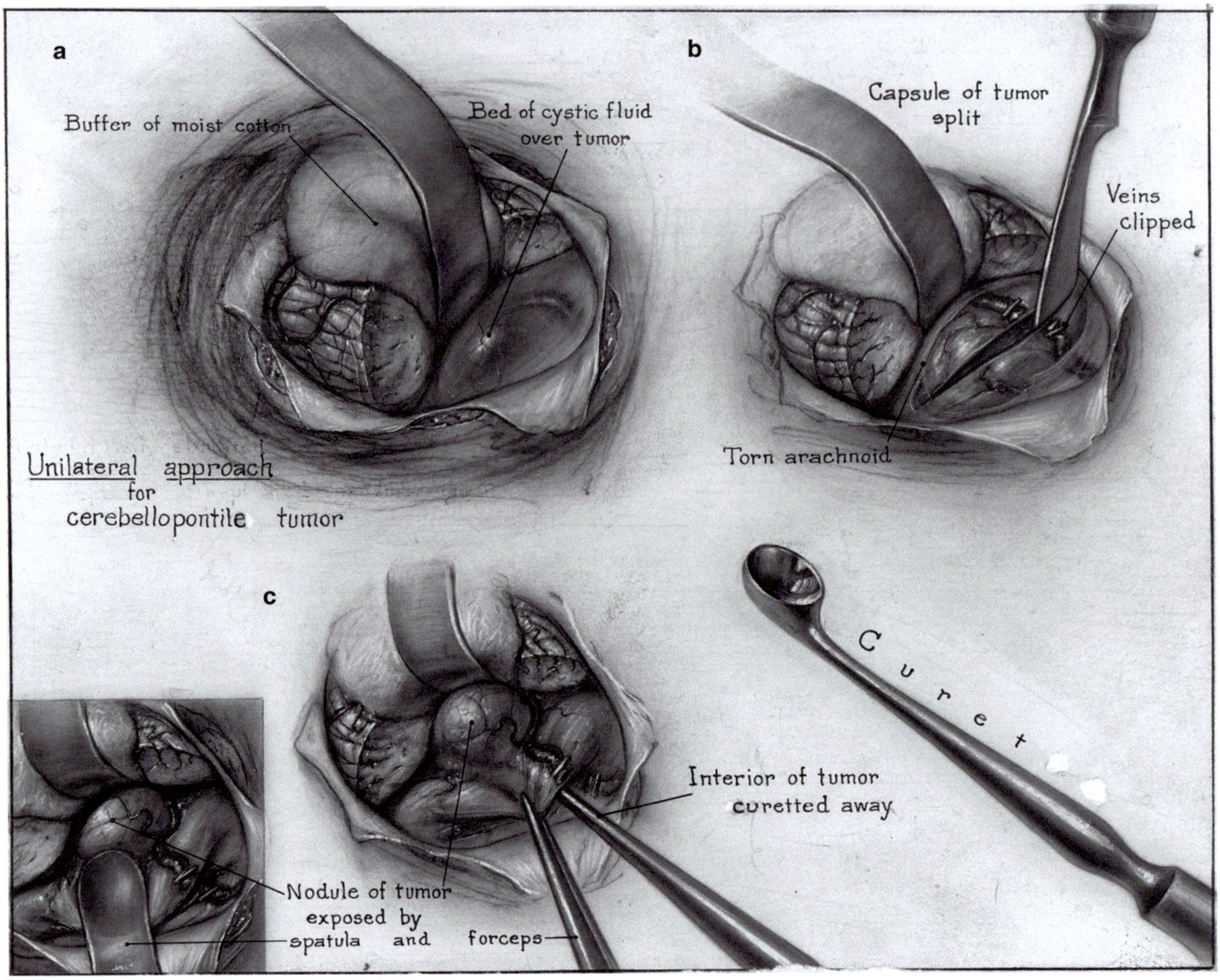

Fig. 1.3 The method of attacking the tumor after the reduction of the intracranial pressure: (**a**) exposure of the tumor, (**b**) splitting the capsule of the tumor preparatory to intracapsular enucleation, and (**c**) the gradual withdrawal of the capsule from its bed. (Reproduced from Dandy WE [12]. Original art in the Max Brödel Archives, Department of Art as Applied to Medicine, The John Hopkins University School of Medicine)

tibular schwannomas by visualizing enlargement of the internal auditory canal on temporal bone radiographs [13, 14]. Improvements were also made in hemostatic adjuncts and the development of blood transfusions. By 1941, Dandy reported a series of 46 patients with complete resection and an impressive mortality of just 10%. Interestingly, it appears that Cushing did perform some complete resections of vestibular schwannomas, but, presumably due to his increasing rivalry with Dandy, did not publish his results.

These improvements in surgical mortality were impressive, but it should be noted that intact facial nerve function or hearing preservation were extremely rare in this era. One of Dandy's many famous quotes stated that facial nerve paralysis was "a necessary sequel of the operation." The first report of complete tumor removal with intact facial nerve function occurred in 1931, by Sir Hugh Cairns. Elliot and McKissick were the first to report hearing preservation after complete resection of a vestibular schwannoma in 1954. Reports of functional preservation increased as experience and knowledge of the CPA increased. However, the development of microsurgery was necessary before functional preservation would become the rule rather than the exception.

Otology and the Operating Microscope

The translabyrinthine approach was first conceived by Rudolf Panse in a manuscript regarding the pathology of vestibular schwannomas. Impressively, this potential approach was described in 1904, just 1 year after Krause described the suboccipital approach. He described the possibility of using a chisel to perform a transcochlear approach (using modern terminology), which included facial nerve mobilization. There are a few reports of attempted translabyrinthine approaches in the early twentieth century. Not surprisingly, given the technology of the time, they included facial nerve sacrifice and almost always reported fatal results.

Without the operating microscope, it was difficult to get proper magnification and illumination into the depths of the surgical field. There were also no motorized drills; the labyrinthectomy was performed with a hammer and chisel. Given the complex three-dimensional anatomy of the temporal bone and associated neurovascular structures, the difficulty and risk of this approach was significantly increased. Because facial nerve preservation was not considered possible at the time, the goal of the operation was to decompress the brainstem, which was then technically difficult. Finally, the approach increased the risk of patients developing CSF fistulas and meningitis. In the era before permanent CSF diversion and antibiotics, these complications were often fatal.

In contrast to the modern, team-based approach to skull-base surgery, some neurosurgeons provided significant opposition to otolaryngologists performing cranial surgery. Cushing went as far as to publish some of his more inflammatory comments in *Laryngoscope*. The translabyrinthine approach would have to wait nearly half a century for William House.

House popularized the use of the microscope for the treatment of vestibular schwannomas, describing his experience practicing on cadavers in the Los Angeles County morgue [15]. The introduction of the operating microscope in the 1950s revolutionized the field of neurosurgery and allowed tremendous advances in the surgical treatment of lesions of the CPA. Interestingly, his use of a suction-irrigator and high-speed drill was inspired by his experience as a dentist.

Due to multiple poor outcomes that he witnessed during suboccipital approaches, he began working on alternative approaches. He developed the subtemporal approach to the internal auditory canal for vestibular neurectomy and later adapted it to tumor removal. He also resurrected the translabyrinthine approach and perfected it. He has been quoted as saying that he did not know of the original descriptions of the procedure until he started writing the manuscript.

Table 1.1 Representative mortality rates from historical series of vestibular schwannoma surgery[a]

Surgeon	Year	No. of cases	Operative mortality (%)	Facial nerve preservation (%)
Krause	1912	30	87	Unknown
Cushing	1917	29	20	Unknown
Olivecrona	1967	Unknown	22	21
House	1968	200	7	88
Yasargil	1976	164	2.4	81.6

[a]Before the advent of microneurosurgery, the facial nerve could not be preserved

There had previously been rare reports of facial nerve preservation, but routinely preserving it was not considered possible. This was an era without facial nerve monitoring, using primitive versions of the surgical adjuncts that modern surgeons take for granted. While the translabyrinthine and subtemporal approaches had been described in the past, they had never been used safely and routinely. In 1963, he reported his use of the middle fossa approach for VS with a mortality of 5% and facial nerve preservation of 95%. In 1964 [16], they published results of the first 53 cases (Table 1.1) with 88% facial nerve preservation. These were some of the first results in what can be called the modern, function-preserving era of vestibular schwannoma surgery.

Modern Surgery in the Cerebellopontine Angle

Continued improvements in technique and technology led to the modern era of surgical approaches to the CPA. In 1973, Hounsfield developed computed tomography (CT), allowing for detection of much smaller tumors. Also in 1973, Emile-Rioux developed bipolar electrocautery, specifically designed to create hemostasis without current spreading to and injuring adjacent tissues. Delgado introduced facial nerve monitoring in 1979, significantly improving the safety of all surgical approaches to vestibular schwannomas.

Along the same timeline, surgeons from both otology and neurosurgery advanced the field of vestibular schwannoma surgery. In 1965, Rand and Kurze reported their results with the suboccipital transmeatal approach, with anatomic preservation of the facial nerve [17]. In the same year, Rand and Kurze introduced variations that popularized removal of the posterior aspect of the meatal wall with a high-speed drill. This maneuver provides ideal exposure of an intracanalicular tumor at its origin on the vestibular nerve. Retraction of the tumor after section of the vestibular nerve allows early visualization of the facial and cochlear nerves. As evidenced by the early microsurgical results of Yasargil and Koos [18, 19], this strategy maximizes the chances of preserving these nerves [20, 21].

Surgeons started the twentieth century by celebrating mere survival as a success. Due to the sacrifice of numerous determined physicians (and, unfortunately, many of their patients), they closed the twentieth century with results that would have astounded the field's pioneers. Technique began as digital delivery of a tumor with avulsion of the facial nerve and, frequently, a fatal hemorrhage from avulsion of the anterior inferior cerebellar artery. By the 1970s, surgeons were operating in a manner that is best described by Dr. Rhoton as "accurate, gentle, and safe."

In the modern era of surgery for vestibular schwannomas, mortality has decreased to roughly 0.5% [22, 23]. The incidence of permanent facial nerve dysfunction is roughly 15%. This number still is significantly influenced by tumor size. Smaller tumors are often treated with radiosurgery or monitored, and large tumors often require surgical resection. In tumors measuring less than 1 cm, the rate of facial nerve dysfunction is nearly zero in modern surgical series. Additionally, in contrast to prior eras, most of these are incomplete injuries that carry much less morbidity. The rate of CSF leak is still significant, affecting almost 10% of patients. However, with modern antibiotics and CSF diversion techniques, this complication does not result in the high morbidity of years past. Surgical treatment is frequently curative, with only 1.5% of patients requiring additional treatment.

At the majority of high-volume centers, the treatment team consists of otologists and neurosurgeons working in conjunction to maximize safety and efficacy. In the modern era, vestibular schwannomas are frequently treated at a smaller size, yet the technical difficulty of these surgical procedures remains high. The care of patients with vestibular schwannomas requires significant experience, technical ability, and judgment. While modern results are far from perfect, our patients continue to benefit from improvements in the treatment of these difficult tumors.

Neurovascular Decompression

In a discussion of the historical development of treatment modalities for the CPA, treatment of trigeminal neuralgia deserves special consideration. As described by Spiller and Frazier [24], for many years this painful affliction was treated through an extradural approach that involved division of the sensory root of the gasserian ganglion [25]. Although relatively safe, such approaches were associated with high rates of corneal anesthetic complications and motor weakness. In 1929, Dandy proposed an alternative route of attack through the CPA [26]. In this unilateral cerebellar approach, the sensory root of the trigeminal nerve is divided at the pons (Fig. 1.4). As noted by Gardner [27], Dandy later presented his series of 215 cases explored via the suboccipital approach. In 60% of his cases, compression from abnormalities distorted the nerve to some degree. The abnormalities encompassed a variety of pathologies that included tumors, aneurysms, angiomas, and direct arterial or venous compression.

Dandy's landmark findings were later expanded by Gardner, who first proposed that the painful syndrome of trigeminal neuralgia was a direct result of focal demyelination caused by abnormal compression [27, 28]. From 1955 to 1961, he used Dandy's approach to treat 18 patients with recurrent trigeminal neuralgia after neurolysis; he discovered abnormal compressive lesions in 66% of these cases [29, 30]. His method of treatment consisted of freeing the nerve from the source of compression and sectioning the sensory root if decompression proved impossible. Jannetta further developed and popularized this operation, a variant of which has been used successfully to treat patients with hemifacial spasm [31–34]. Use of microvascular decompression with or without rhizotomy has since expanded to treat tinnitus [35–38].

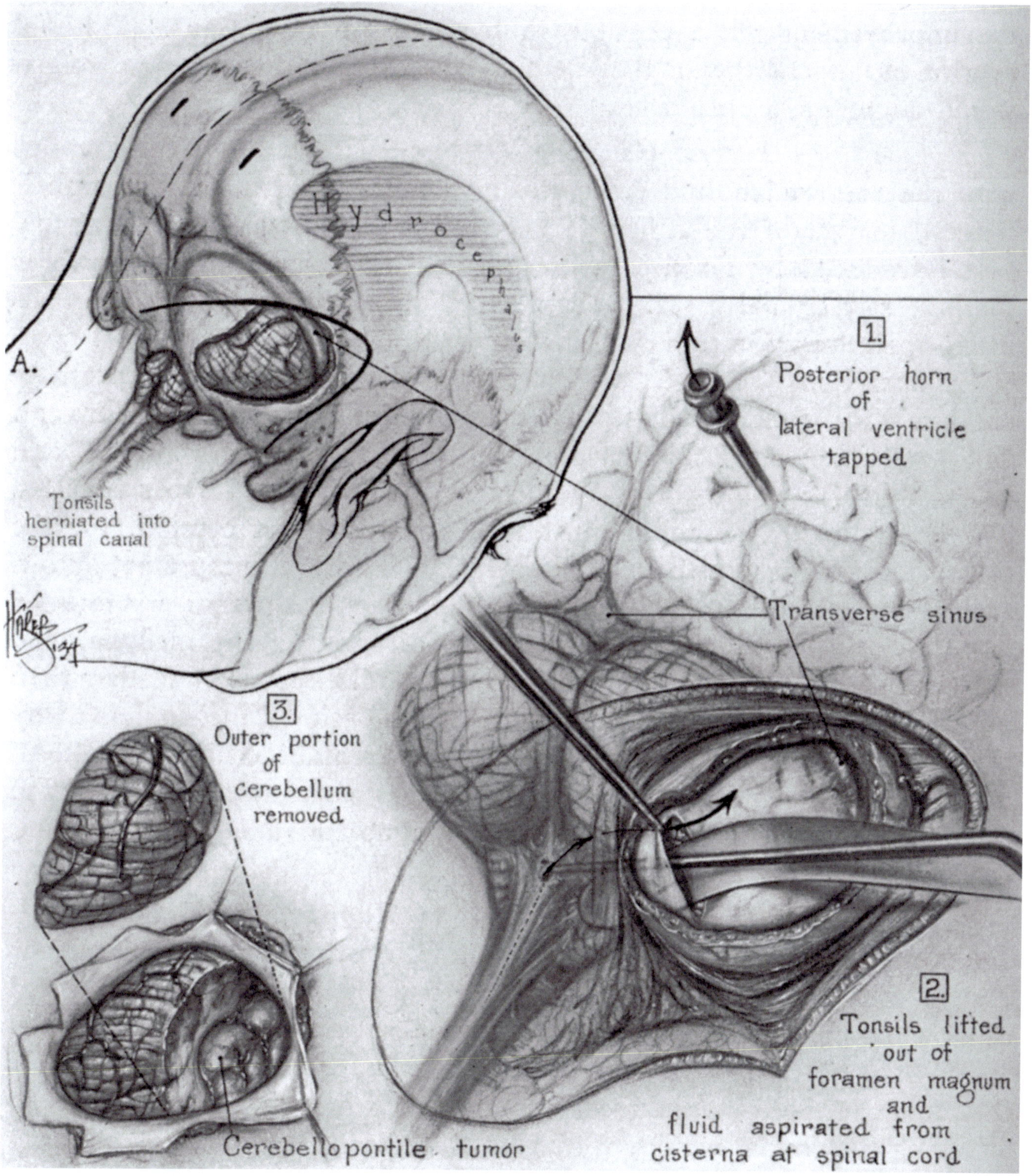

Fig. 1.4 The relative exposure used in the removal of cerebellopontine tumors by the unilateral approach: (**1**) the method of releasing the supratentorial pressure by puncture of the posterior horn of the lateral ventricle, (**2**) further release of pressure in the posterior cranial fossa by evacuation of the cisterna magna in the spinal canal, and (**3**) final stage by the resection of the outer cap of the cerebellum. (Reproduced from Dandy WE [12]. Original art in the Max Brödel Archives, Department of Art as Applied to Medicine, The John Hopkins University School of Medicine)

Radiosurgery

No historical perspective on the surgical treatment of the CPA would be complete without a brief review of the role of radiosurgery. The development of radiosurgical techniques for the treatment of lesions in the CPA dates to 1971. In that year, as Kondziolka and colleagues noted [39], Lars Leksell applied radiosurgery to the treatment of a vestibular schwannoma based on the concept of radiosurgical therapy reported 20 years earlier [40]. Those involved with Leksell's initial development of radiosurgical techniques believe that his primary motivation was to develop an alternative treatment to open surgery for pathology within the CPA and for vestibular schwannomas in particular [41, 42]. The first patient to undergo Gamma Knife radiosurgery was a young woman with NF2. At that time localization of the target was based on nonstereotactic pneumoencephalography and stereotactic skull X-rays. This patient's initial treatment resulted in tumor control for 12 years. Subsequent computed CT showed medial growth of her tumor, which was then resected.

In the 1970s, advances in CT led to increasingly accurate localization and dosimetry associated with a concomitant improvement in the control of tumor growth and a reduction in radiation-induced morbidity. Nonetheless, the rate of complications remained high. During the early years of Gamma Knife treatment, the rate of new facial weakness approached 45% [39, 41, 43]. Subsequent modifications to the prescription dose administered and the advent of high-resolution magnetic resonance imaging ushered in the contemporary era of radiosurgical treatment of CPA lesions. Excellent long-term control of tumor growth and low complication rates are now associated with the radiosurgical treatment of tumors of the CPA.

Conclusions

In the past 100 years, surgical options for the treatment of lesions of the CPA have undergone revolutionary changes. These changes mirror the developments that spurred the emergence of neurosurgery as a distinct medical subspecialty. The work of pioneers such as Cushing and Dandy was modified and refined as the development of the operating microscope led to dramatic reductions in surgical rates of morbidity and mortality. The complexity of the anatomic region of the posterior fossa encompassing the CPA led to the cooperative endeavors of neurosurgeons and otologists to refine surgical treatment of lesions involving the CPA. Innovators such as House and Hitselberger refused to be bound by the traditional limitations of their specialties. Instead, they collaborated to develop cooperative treatments to the great benefit of their patients. Likewise, the continuing evolution of technological advances in alternative treatment modalities, such as radiosurgery, further expands the therapeutic options for patients with lesions involving the CPA.

References

1. Ramsden RT. The bloody angle: 100 years of vestibular schwannoma surgery. J R Soc Med. 1985;88:464–8.
2. Pirsig W, Ziemann-Becker B, Teschler-Nicola M. Vestibular schwannoma: four thousand years ago. In: Tos M, Thomsen J, editors. Vestibular schwannoma. Proceedings of the first international conference on vestibular schwannoma, Copenhagen, Denmark, August 25–29, 1991. Amsterdam/New York: Kugler Publications; 1992. p. 7–12.
3. Sandifort E. Observationes anatomico-pathologicae, 1742–1814. Lugduni Batavorum; 1777–1781.
4. Leveque-Lasource AL. Observation sur un amaurosis et un cophosis, avec perte ou diminution de la voix, des mouvemens, etc, par suite de lesion organique apparente de plusieurs parties du cerveau. J Gen Med Chir Pharm. 1810;37:386–73.
5. Bell C. The nervous system of the human body, embracing the papers delivered to the Royal Society on the subject of nerves. London: Longman, Rees, Orme, Brown & Green; 1830.
6. Glasscock ME III. History of the diagnosis and treatment of vestibular schwannoma. Arch Otolaryngol. 1968;88:578–85.
7. Ballance CA. Some points in the surgery of the brain and its membranes. London: Macmillan and Co.; 1907.
8. Cushing H. Tumors of the nervus acusticus and the syndrome of the cerebellopontine angle, reprinted in 1963. New York: Haffner Publishing Company; 1917.
9. Gibson GA. Remarks on the results of surgical measures in a series of cerebral cases. Edinb Med J. 1896;41:689–700.
10. Krause F. Zur Freilegung der hinteren Felsenbeinflache und des Kleinhirns. Beitr Klin Chir. 1903;37:728–64.
11. Atkinson WJ. The anterior inferior cerebellar artery. Its variations, pontine distribution, and significance in the surgery of cerebello-pontine angle tumors. J Neurol Neurosurg Psychiatry. 1949;12:137–51.
12. Dandy WE. Removal of cerebellopontine (acoustic) tumors through a unilateral approach. Arch Surg. 1934;29:337–44.
13. Stenvers HW. Roentgenology of the os petrosum. Arch Radiol Electrother. 1917;22:97–112.
14. Towne EB. Erosion of the petrous bone by acoustic nerve tumor: Demonstration by roentgen ray. Arch Otolaryngol. 1926;4(6): 515–9.
15. House WF. Surgical exposure of the internal auditory canal and its contents through the middle, cranial fossa. Laryngoscope. 1961;71:1363–85.
16. Nguyen-Huynh AT, Jackler RK, Pfister M, Tseng J. The aborted early history of the translabyrinthine approach: a victim of suppression or technical prematurity? Otol Neurotol. 2007;28:269–79.
17. Rand RW, Kurze TL. Facial nerve preservation by posterior fossa transmeatal microdissection in total removal of vestibular schwannomas. J Neurol Neurosurg Psychiatry. 1965;28:311–6.
18. Yasargil MG. Mikrochirurgie der kleinhirnbruckenwinkeltumoren. In: Pleaster D, Wende S, Nakayama N, editors. Kleinhirnbrücken-winkel-tumoren, diagnostik und therapie. Berlin: Springer-Verlag; 1978. p. 215–57.
19. Koos W. [Microsurgery as a condition for progress in the treatment of acoustic nerve neurinoma] [German]. Wien Med Wochenschr. 1977;127:246–9.

20. Penzholz H. Development and present state of cerebellopontine angle surgery from the neuroand otosurgical point of view. Arch Otorhinolaryngol. 1984;240:167–74.
21. Spiller WG, Frazier CH. Tic douloreux; anatomic and clinical basis for subtotal section of sensory root of trigeminal nerve. Arch Neurol Psychiatr. 1933;29:50–5.
22. Yamakami I, et al. Conservative management, gamma-knife radiosurgery, and microsurgery for acoustic neurinomas: a systematic review of outcome and risk of three therapeutic options. Neurol Res. 2003;25:682–90.
23. Kaylie DM, et al. A meta-analysis comparing outcomes of microsurgery and gamma knife radiosurgery. Laryngoscope. 2000;110:1850–6.
24. Spiller WG, Frazier CH. The division of the sensory root of the trigeminus for relief of tic douloureux; an experimental, pathologic and clinical study with a preliminary report of one surgically successful case. Philadelphia Med J. 1901;8:1039–49.
25. Dandy WE. Concerning the cause of trigeminal neuralgia. Am J Surg. 1934;24:447–55.
26. Dandy WE. An operation for the cure of tic douloreux. Partial section of the sensory root at the pons. Arch Surg. 1929;18:687–734.
27. Gardner WJ. The mechanism of tic doulоureux. Trans Am Neurol Assoc. 1953;78:168–73.
28. Gardner WJ. Concerning the mechanism of trigeminal neuralgia and hemifacial spasm. J Neurosurg. 1962;19:947–58.
29. Gardner G, Robertson JT, Cocke EW. Glomus jugulare tumors. In: Schmidek HH, Sweet WH, editors. Operative neurosurgical techniques: indications, methods, and results. New York: Grune & Stratton; 1982. p. 649–70.
30. Rand RW. The Gardner neurovascular decompression operation for trigeminal neuralgia. Acta Neurochir (Wien). 1981;58:161–6.
31. Jannetta PJ. Arterial compression of the trigeminal nerve at the pons in patients with trigeminal neuralgia. J Neurosurg. 1967;26: 159–62.
32. Jannetta PJ. Cranial rhizopathies. In: Youmans JR, editor. Neurological surgery: a comprehensive reference guide to the diagnosis and management of neurosurgical problems. Philadelphia: W.B. Saunders; 1982. p. 3771–84.
33. Jannetta PH. Hemifacial spasm. In: Samii M, Jannetta PJ, editors. The cranial nerves: anatomy, pathology, pathophysiology, diagnosis, treatment. Berlin: Springer-Verlag; 1981. p. 4840–93.
34. Jannetta PJ. Hemifacial spasm: microvascular decompression of the VIIth nerve intracranially. In: Symon L, editor. Neurosurgery. London: Butterworths; 1979. p. 374–81.
35. Nash B, Carlson ML, Van Gompel JJ. Microvascular decompression for tinnitus: systematic review. J Neurosurg. 2017;126: 1148–57.
36. Patel A, Kassam A, Horowitz M, Chang YF. Microvascular decompression in the management of glossopharyngeal neuralgia: analysis of 217 cases. Neurosurgery. 2002;50:705–11.
37. Laha RK, Jannetta PJ. Glossopharyngeal neuralgia. J Neurosurg. 1977;47:316–20.
38. Brackmann DE, Kesser BW, Day JD. Microvascular decompression of the vestibulocochlear nerve for disabling positional vertigo: the House Ear Clinic experience. Otol Neurotol. 2001;22: 882–7.
39. Kondziolka D, Lunsford LD, Flickinger JC. Vestibular schwannoma radiosurgery. Origins, contemporary use and future expectations. Neurochirurgie. 2004;50:427–35.
40. Leksell L. A note on the treatment of acoustic tumours. Acta Chir Scand. 1971;137:763–5.
41. Leksell L. The stereotaxic method and radiosurgery of the brain. Acta Chir Scand. 1951;102:316–9.
42. Noren G, Arndt J, Hindmarsh T. Stereotactic radiosurgery in cases of acoustic neurinoma: further experiences. Neurosurgery. 1983;13:12–22.
43. Olivecrona H. Acoustic Tumors. J Neurosurg. 1967;26:6–13.

Microsurgical Anatomy of the Cerebellopontine Angle and Its Suboccipital Retromastoid Approaches

2

Guilherme Carvalhal Ribas, Alexandre Yasuda, David Peace, and Albert L. Rhoton Jr.

When dealing with cerebellopontine angle (CPA) approaches, surgeons initially confront the occipital and temporal bones and their related structures. In the CPA itself, identification of the cranial nerves at the brainstem and of their vascular relationships within the upper, middle, and lower aspects of the CPA cisternal space is mandatory. This chapter describes the anatomy related to these topics and stresses practical surgical issues. The different suboccipital retromastoid exposures of the CPA required by common surgical conditions are then described.

Relationships Between the Cranial Surface and the CPA

The occipital bone surrounds the foramen magnum and is divided into a squamosal portion located above and behind the foramen magnum, a basal portion situated in front of the foramen magnum, and paired condylar portions located lateral to the foramen magnum (Fig. 2.1) [2]. The squamous portion is an internally concave plate, and its upper margins articulate with the parietal bones at the lambdoid sutures. Its lower margins articulate with the mastoid portion of the temporal bones at the occipitomastoid sutures. The convex external surface has several prominences on which the muscles of the neck attach. The largest prominence, the external occipital protuberance, or inion, is situated at the central portion of the external surface and is located over the inferior margin of the confluence of the sagittal and transverse sinuses. Two parallel ridges radiate laterally from the protuberance. The highest nuchal line is the upper and thinner ridge; the superior nuchal line is lower and more prominent. The rough and irregular area below the nuchal lines serves as the site of attachment of numerous muscles. A vertical ridge, the external occipital crest, descends from the external occipital protuberance to the midpoint of the posterior margin of the foramen magnum. The inferior nuchal lines run laterally from the midpoint of the crest.

The basilar portion of the occipital bone, which is also referred to as the clivus, is a thick quadrangular plate of bone that extends anteriorly and superiorly, at about a 45° angle from the foramen magnum. It joins the sphenoid bone at the spheno-occipital synchondrosis just below the dorsum sellae [3]. The superior surface of the clivus is concave from side to side and is separated on each side from the petrous portion of the temporal bone by the petroclival fissure. This fissure has the inferior petrosal sinus on its upper surface and ends posteriorly at the jugular foramen. On the inferior surface of the basilar part, in front of the foramen magnum, a small elevation, the pharyngeal tubercle, attaches to the fibrous raphe of the pharynx.

The paired lateral or condylar portions are situated at the sides of the foramen magnum. The occipital condyles, which articulate with the atlas, protrude from the external surface of this part. These condyles are located lateral to the anterior half of the foramen magnum. They are oval, convex downward, and face downward and laterally. Their long axes are directed anteriorly and medially. A tubercle that attaches to the alar ligament of the odontoid process is situated on the medial side of each condyle. The hypoglossal canal, which transmits the hypoglossal nerve, is situated above the condyle, and is directed anteriorly and laterally from the

G. C. Ribas (✉)
Department of Surgery, University of São Paulo Medical School, São Paulo, Brazil

Albert Einstein Medical School, Hospital Israelita Albert Einstein, São Paulo, Brazil

Department of Neurosurgery, University of Virginia School of Medicine, Charlottesville, VA, USA
e-mail: guilherme@ribas.med.br

A. Yasuda
Hospital Israelita Albert Einstein, São Paulo, Brazil

D. Peace
Department of Neurosurgery, University of Florida School of Medicine, Gainesville, FL, USA

A. L. RhotonJr.
Lillian S. Wells Department of Neurosurgery, University of Florida College of Medicine, Gainesville, FL, USA

N. C. Bambakidis et al. (eds.), *Surgery of the Cerebellopontine Angle*, https://doi.org/10.1007/978-3-031-12507-2_2

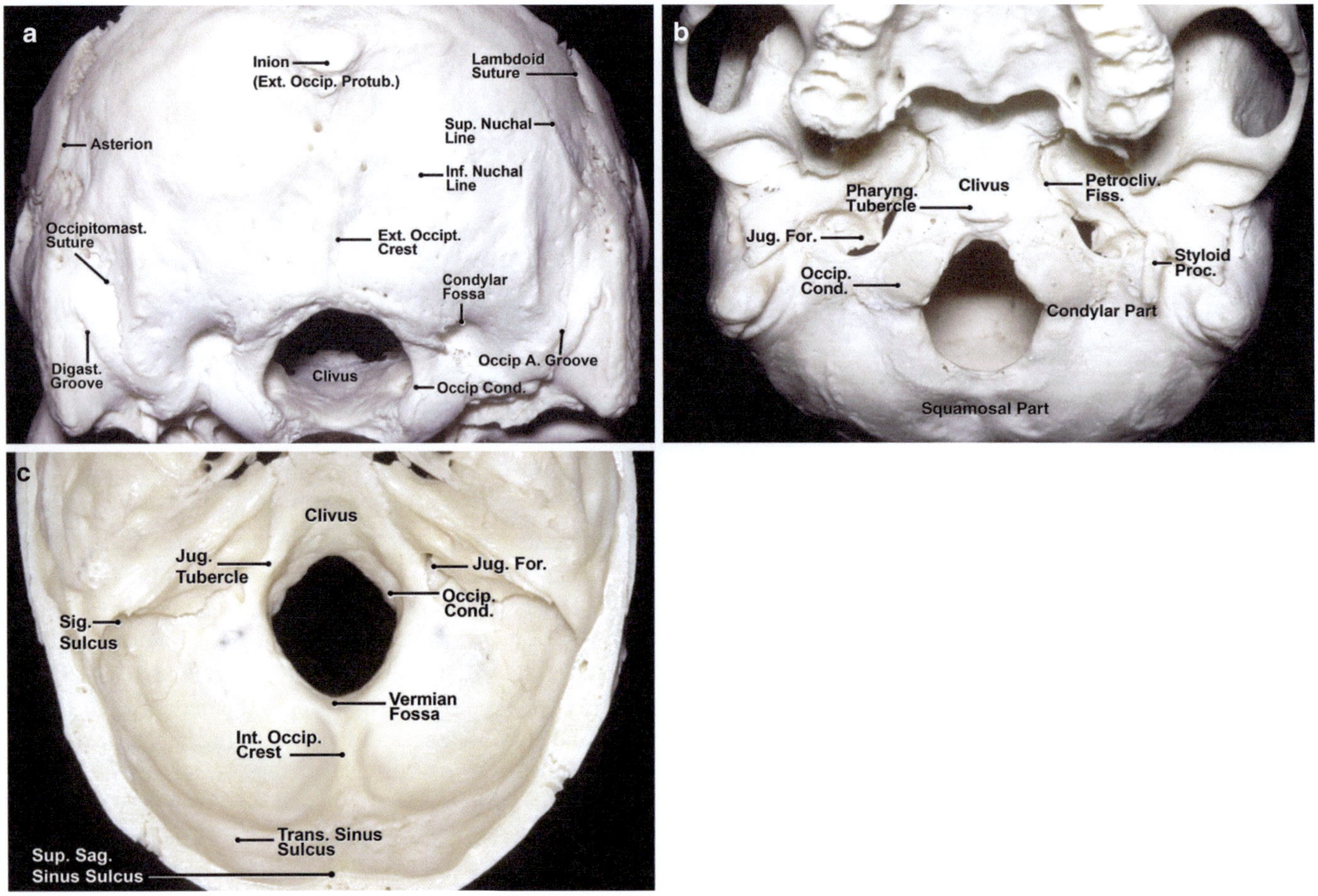

Fig. 2.1 The occipital bone and foramen magnum: (**a**) external posteroinferior view, (**b**) external anteroinferior view, and (**c**) internal superior view. A. = artery; Cond. = condyle; Digast. = digastric; Ext. = external; Fiss. = fissure; For. = foramen; Int. = internal; Jug. = jugular; Occip. = occipital; Occipitomast. = occipitomastoid; Petrocliv. = petroclival; Pharyng. = pharyngeal; Proc. = process; Protub. = probuterance; Sag. = sagittal; Sig. = sigmoid; Sup. = superior; Trans. = transverse. (From Rhoton AL Jr. [1]. Reproduced with permission from Lippincott Williams & Wilkins)

posterior cranial fossa. The canal may be partially or completely divided by a bony septum [4].

The anatomical relationships of the temporal bone are also critical to understanding the various challenges involved in surgical approaches to the CPA. This topic is covered in detail elsewhere in this text.

Osseous and Muscular Relationships, Transverse and Sigmoid Sinuses, and External Surgical Landmarks

Careful exposure, particularly of bony sutures and other osseous prominences and depressions, enables these sites to be used as important landmarks for surgical orientation and for more restricted and appropriate CPA approaches.

The superior nuchal lines, which extend laterally and horizontally from the external occipital protuberance, are the boundary between the scalp and neck. These lines are often sharp [5]. Each line is located at the level of an imaginary line formed by the inion and external acoustic meatus [6]. Along this imaginary line, the trapezius inserts medially. The sternocleidomastoid muscle, which covers the semispinalis and splenius capitis muscles, inserts laterally (Fig. 2.2). The highest nuchal lines, which are more arched than the superior nuchal lines, are eventually identified. Medially, the galea aponeurotica inserts, and laterally the occipitofrontalis muscle inserts. The slightly arched inferior nuchal lines are located below the external occipital protuberance. The semispinalis capitis and the superior oblique muscles are inserted medially and laterally between the inferior and superior nuchal lines. The rectus capitis posterior minor and major muscles are inserted medially and laterally, respectively, below each inferior nuchal line.

The suboccipital triangle is a region bounded superiorly and medially by the rectus capitis posterior major muscle, superiorly and laterally by the superior oblique muscle, and inferiorly and laterally by the inferior oblique muscle. It is

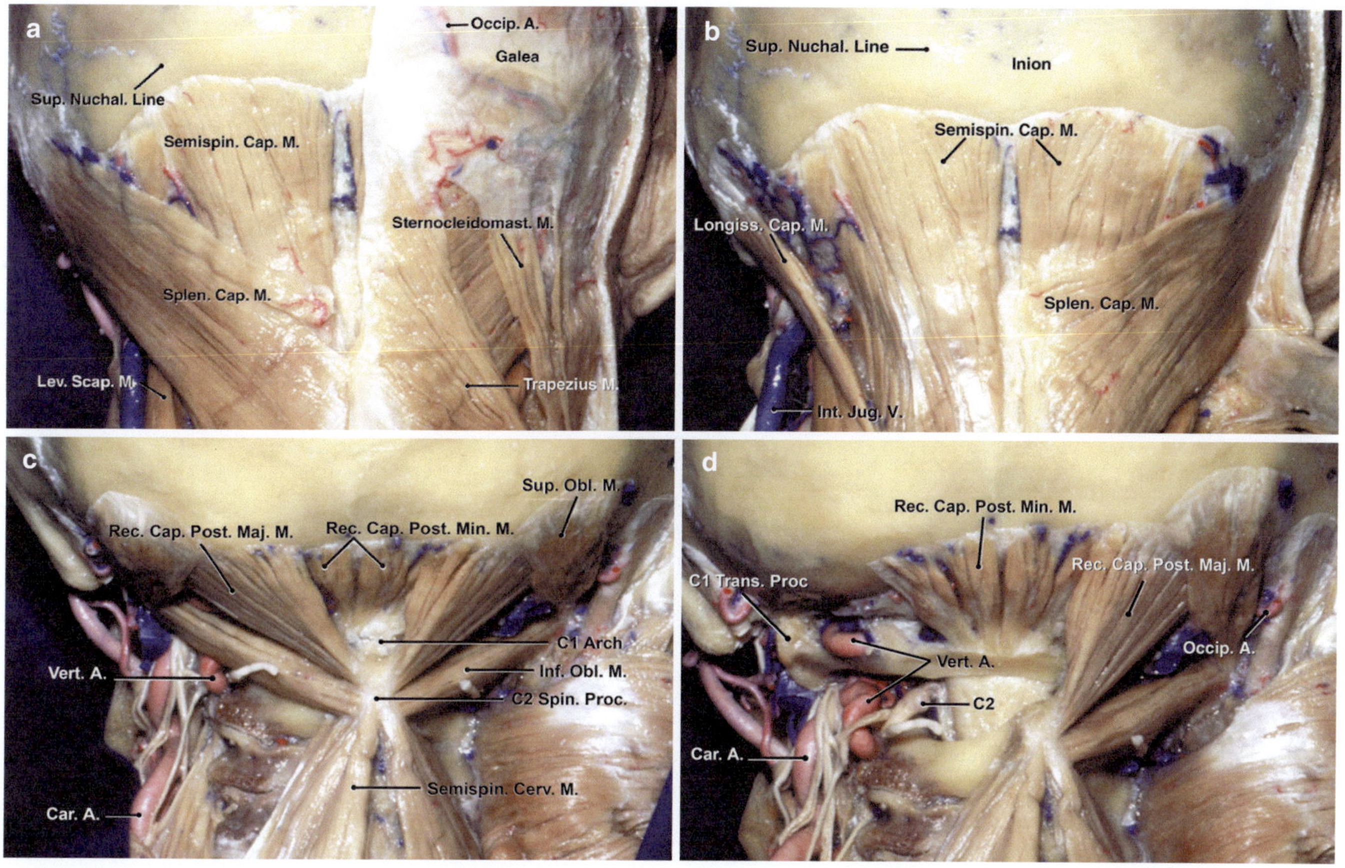

Fig. 2.2 The suboccipital muscles. (**a**) The right trapezius and sternocleidomastoid muscles have been preserved. The left trapezius and sternocleidomastoid muscles have been reflected with the galea aponeurotica to expose the underlying semispinalis capitis, splenius capitis, and levator scapulae muscles. (**b**) The right sternocleidomastoid and trapezius muscles have been reflected to expose the splenius capitis muscles. The left splenius capitis has been removed to expose the underlying semispinalis and longissimus capitis muscles. (**c**) Both semispinalis capitis muscles have been reflected laterally to expose the suboccipital triangles bilaterally. (**d**) The muscles forming the left suboccipital triangle have been removed. The vertebral artery ascends slightly lateral from the transverse process of C2 to reach the transverse process of C1. Behind the superior facet of C1, the artery turns medially to reach the upper surface of the posterior arch of C1. The C2 ganglion is located between the posterior arch of C1 and the lamina of C2. The dorsal ramus of C2 produces a medial branch that forms most of the greater occipital nerve. A. = artery; Cap. = capitis; Car. = carotid; Inf. = inferior; Int. = internal; Jug. = jugular; Lev. = levator; Longiss. = longissimus; M. = muscle; Maj. = major; Min. = minor; Obl. = oblique; Occip. = occipital; Post. = posterior; Proc. = process; Rec. = rectus; Scap. = scapulae; Semispin. = semispinalis; Spin. = spinalis; Splen. = splenius; Sternocleidomast. = sternocleidomastoid; Sup. = superior; Trans. = transverse; V. = vein; Vert. = vertebral. (From Rhoton AL Jr. [1]. Reproduced with permission from Lippincott Williams & Wilkins)

covered by the semispinalis capitis muscle medially and by the splenius capitis muscle laterally. The floor of the triangle is formed by the posterior atlantooccipital membrane and the posterior arch of the atlas. The structures in the triangle are the terminal extradural segment of the vertebral artery and the first cervical nerve [2].

The external occipital crest descends from the external occipital protuberance, with the nuchal ligament attached. The lambdoid, occipitomastoid, and parietomastoid sutures [2, 7–13] are united at the asterion and separate the occipital, parietal, and temporal bones (Fig. 2.3).

The lambdoid suture begins at lambda, where it meets the sagittal suture. Along its oblique course, it separates the squamous portion of the occipital bone from the parietal bone. It is particularly evident superiorly due to its more deep and prominent serrations [13]. Inferior to the asterion, the lambdoid suture continues as the occipitomastoid suture, which separates the lower portion of the occipital squamous from the petromastoid portion of the temporal bone, ending at the jugular foramen. The parietomastoid suture separates the mastoid temporal portion from the posteroinferior portion [13], or mastoid angle, of the parietal bone. The suture is horizontal to the skull base. Occasionally sutural bones are present, usually along the lambdoid suture. An isolated bone at the lambda is named the Inca bone.

Laterally and parallel to the occipitomastoid suture, along and medial to the mastoid process, the deep groove of the mastoid notch is where the posterior belly of the digastric muscle inserts. Also parallel to and between this notch and the occipitomastoid suture, the occipital artery lies in a

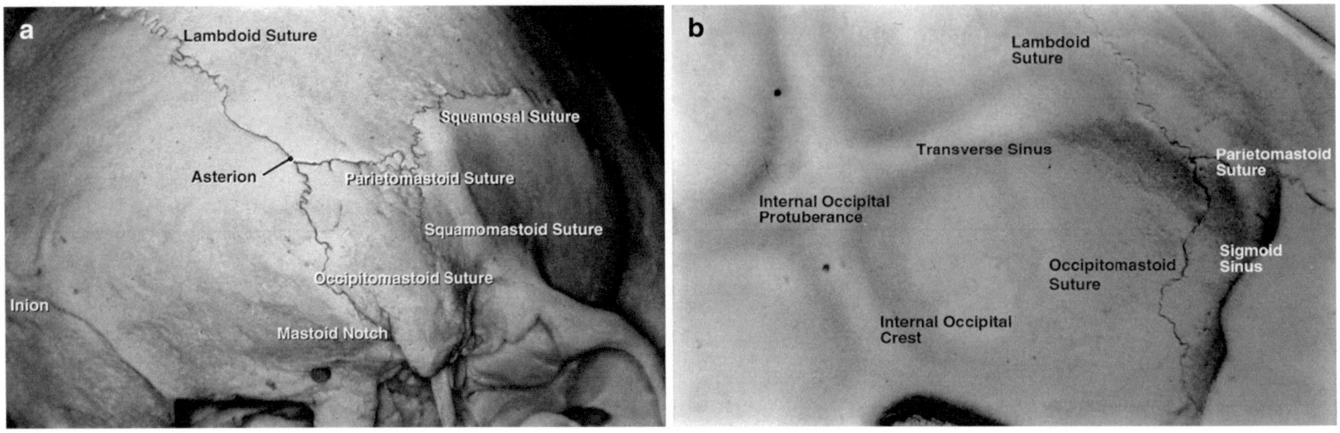

Fig. 2.3 (**a**) External cranial surface with the cranial sutures and (**b**) internal cranial surface with cranial sutures and sinus groove. (From Ribas GC et al. [14]. Reproduced with permission from *Journal of Neurosurgery*)

shallow occipital groove [13]. The sulcus of the transverse sinus extends laterally from the protuberance on each cranial side; the tentorium cerebelli attaches to its margins [15]. Frequently the larger sulcus, usually the right one, is continuous with the sulcus of the superior sagittal sinus. The smaller sulcus is usually more related with the straight sinus [13, 16].

The transverse sinuses are sites of frequent anatomical variations [11, 13, 17–32], but they usually communicate along the confluence of the sinuses, which is indicated by a depression on one side or the other of the internal occipital protuberance [13]. Each transverse sinus is situated posteriorly over the squamous portion of the occipital bone and anteriorly over the posterior and inferior portions of each parietal bone. This sinus ends at the posterolateral extremity of the petrous portion of the temporal bone from where it extends inferiorly as the sigmoid sinus. Along their courses the transverse sinuses can receive occipital, temporal, cerebellar, and tentorial veins [15, 16, 33–39].

The transition of the transverse sinus into the sigmoid sinus occurs at the point where the former receives the superior petrosal sinus, at the level of the so-called sinodural angle of Citelli [17]. The sigmoid sulcus lies over a deep curved groove situated on the inner surface of the mastoid portion of the temporal bone, which is anteriorly separated from the mastoid air cells by a thin lamina of bone. It ends at the jugular fossa, where the sinus enters the jugular foramen [40–43].

The relationship between the cranial sutures and venous sinuses can be used in surgical planning [14, 44, 45]. The asterion corresponds to the meeting point of the lambdoid, occipitomastoid, and parietomastoid sutures. This important anthropological point [46, 47] is usually located over the lower aspect of the transverse sinus at its distal margin (Fig. 2.4). The midpoint of the inion–asterion line is particularly related to the bottom of the transverse sinus. This relationship has led to the observation that the inion–asterion line usually corresponds to the inferior aspect of the transverse sinus (Fig. 2.5) [14, 44, 45].

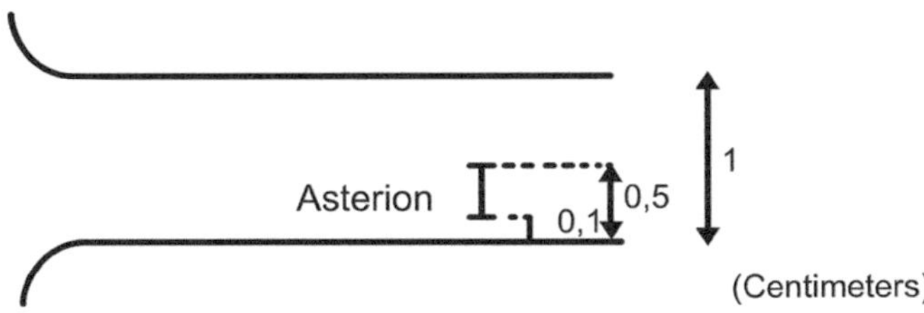

Fig. 2.4 Variation in the position of the asterion in relation to the transverse sinus. (From Ribas GC et al. [14]. Reproduced with permission from *Journal of Neurosurgery*)

The occipitomastoid suture always crosses the posterior margin of the sigmoid sinus at the level of the superior aspect of the mastoid notch. This crossing point also coincides with the intersection of the occipitomastoid suture and an imaginary line between the inion and mastoid tip (Fig. 2.6). The relationships among these external landmarks can be specified relative to the transverse and sigmoid sinuses. In particular, (1) the asterion and the midpoint of the inion–asterion line are related to the inferior half of the transverse sinus; (2) the superior and inferior points of the transverse and sigmoid sinus junction, respectively, are situated above and below the posterior portion of the parietomastoid suture; (3) the intersection of the parietomastoid and squamous sutures is located at the level of the posterior aspect of the superior surface of the petrous bone; and (4) the occipitomastoid suture and the posterior margin of the sigmoid sinus crossing point is situated at the level of the superior and posterior aspects of the mastoid notch. This point also corresponds to the intersection of the occipitomastoid suture with the inion–mastoid tip line (see Fig. 2.6c) [14, 44, 45].

These relationships can be used intraoperatively to plan the placement of burr holes during a retromastoid exposure

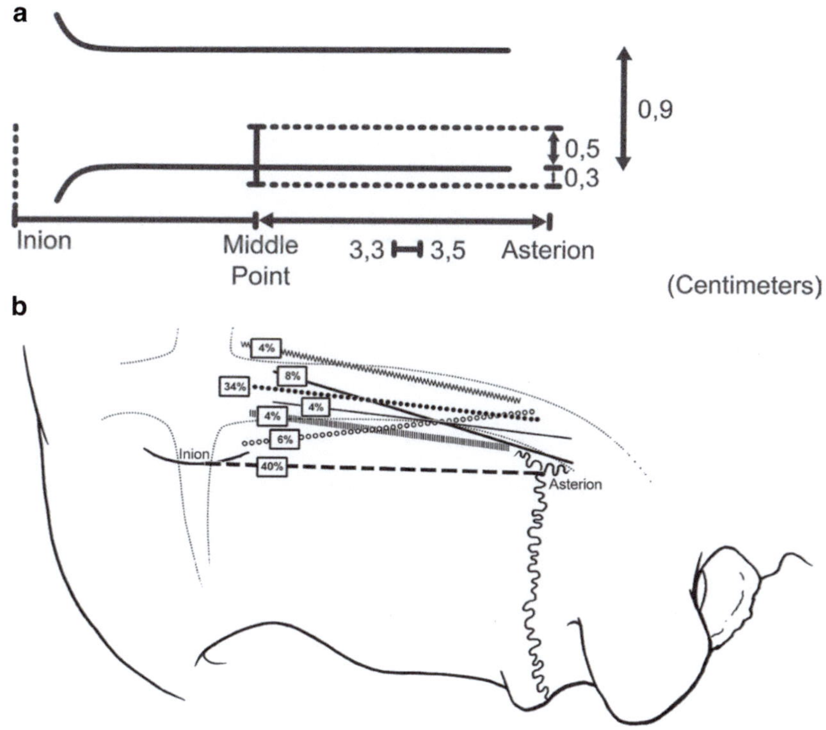

Fig. 2.5 (**a**) Variation in the position of the midpoint of the inion–asterion line in relation to the transverse sinus. (**b**) Disposition of the inion–asterion line in relation to the transverse sinus. (From Ribas GC et al. [14]. Reproduced with permission from *Journal of Neurosurgery*; Figure (**b**) modified, also with permission from *Journal of Neurosurgery*)

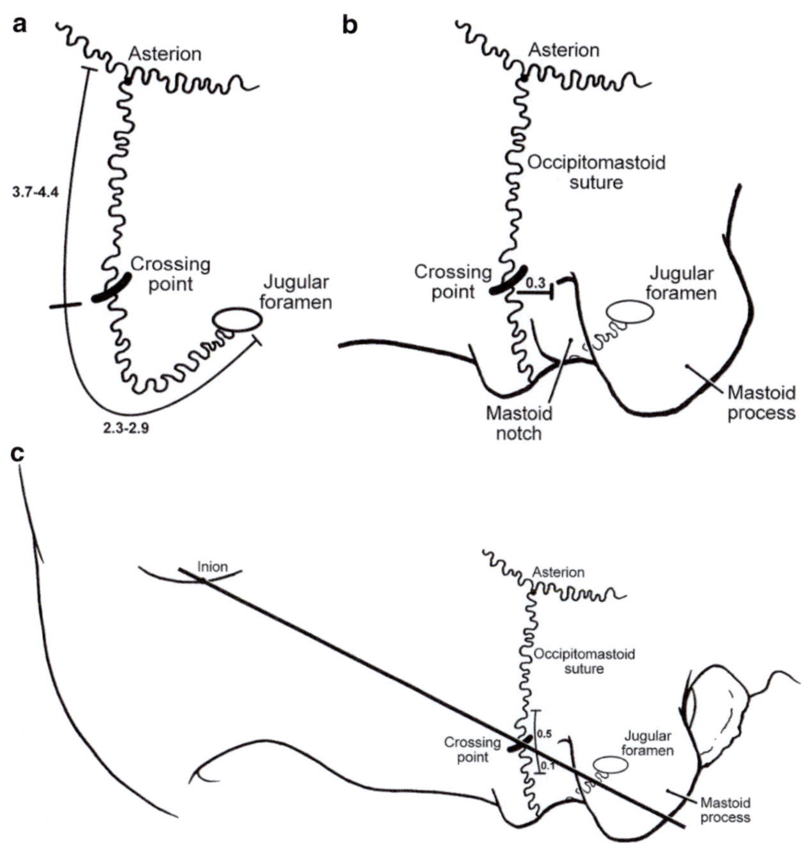

Fig. 2.6 Variations in the position of the crossing point between the occipitomastoid suture and the crossing point at the posterior margin of the sigmoid sinus in relation to: (**a**) the asterion and jugular foramen, (**b**) the superior aspect of the mastoid notch, and (**c**) the lateral aspect of the inion–mastoid tip (imaginary line). (From Ribas GC et al. [14]. Modified with permission from *Journal of Neurosurgery*)

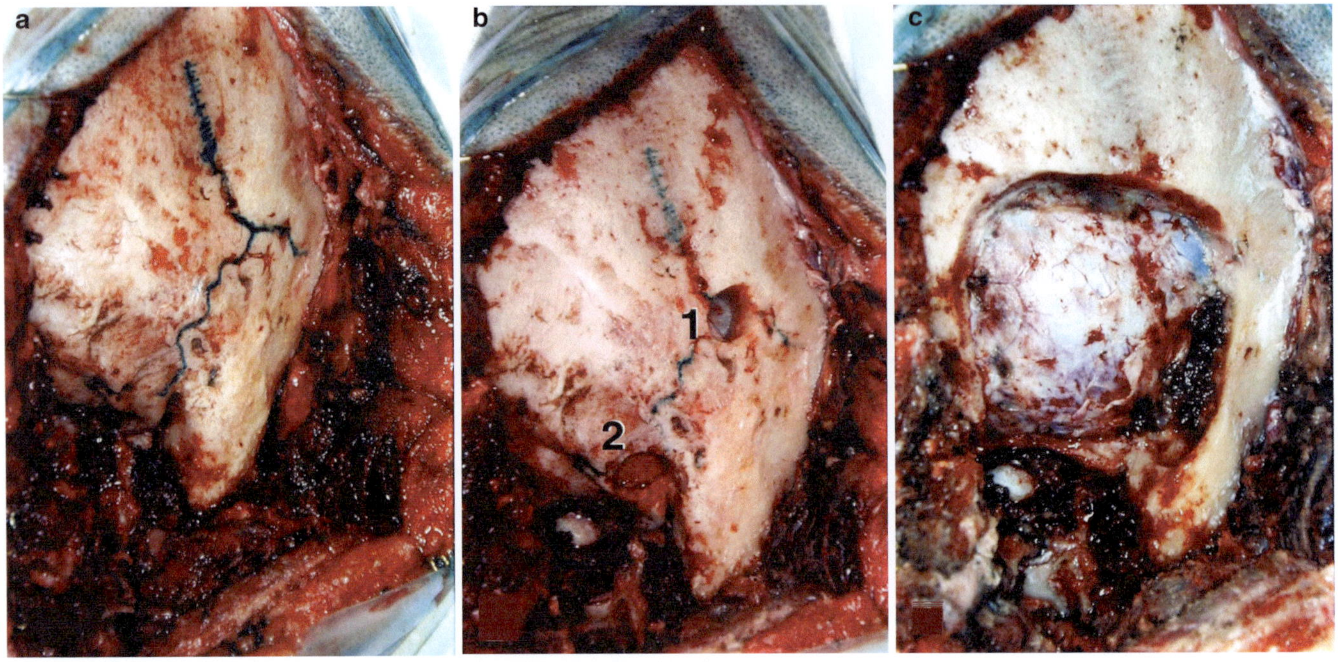

Fig. 2.7 Intraoperative identification of the asterion, lambdoid, occipitomastoid, and parietomastoid sutures (**a**). After the initial burr hole is placed just anterior to the asterion to expose the transition between the transverse and sigmoid sinuses (1), and over the occipitomastoid suture just posterior to the mastoid process at the most posterior level of the mastoid notch (2) and just posterior to the posterior margin of the sigmoid sinus (**b**), a wide suboccipital craniectomy is performed (**c**). (From Ribas GC et al. [14]. Reproduced with permission from *Journal of Neurosurgery*)

(Fig. 2.7). An initial burr hole placed just anterior to the asterion can expose the transition between the transverse and sigmoid sinuses. A second burr hole placed over the occipitomastoid suture posterior to the mastoid process at the most posterior level of the mastoid notch demarcates the posterior margin of the sigmoid sinus.

Relationships Among CPA Nerves and Brainstem

The CPA is located between the superior and inferior limbs of the angular cerebellopontine fissure. This fissure is formed by the petrosal cerebellar surface folding around the pons and the middle cerebellar peduncle. The cerebellopontine fissure opens medially and has superior and inferior limbs that meet at a lateral apex. The 4th through the 11th cranial nerves are located near or within the angular space between the two limbs commonly referred to as the CPA (Fig. 2.8). The trochlear and trigeminal nerves are located near the fissure's superior limb, and the glossopharyngeal, vagus, and accessory nerves are located near the inferior limb. The abducens nerve is located near the base of the fissure, along a line connecting the anterior ends of the superior and inferior limbs [49].

A consistent set of neural, arterial, and venous relationships at the brainstem facilitates the identification of these cranial nerves (Fig. 2.9). The landmarks on the medial or brainstem side of structures that are helpful in guiding the surgeon to the junction of the facial nerve with the brainstem are the pontomedullary sulcus; the junction of the glossopharyngeal, vagus, and spinal accessory nerves with the medulla; the foramen of Luschka and its choroid plexus; and the flocculus. The facial nerve arises from the brainstem near the lateral end of the pontomedullary sulcus, 1–2 mm anterior to the point at which the vestibulocochlear nerve joins the brainstem at the lateral end of the sulcus. The interval between the vestibulocochlear and facial nerves is greatest at the level of the pontomedullary sulcus and decreases as these nerves approach the meatus.

The facial nerve enjoys a consistent relationship to the junction of the glossopharyngeal, vagus, and spinal accessory nerves with the medulla. The facial nerve arises 2–3 mm

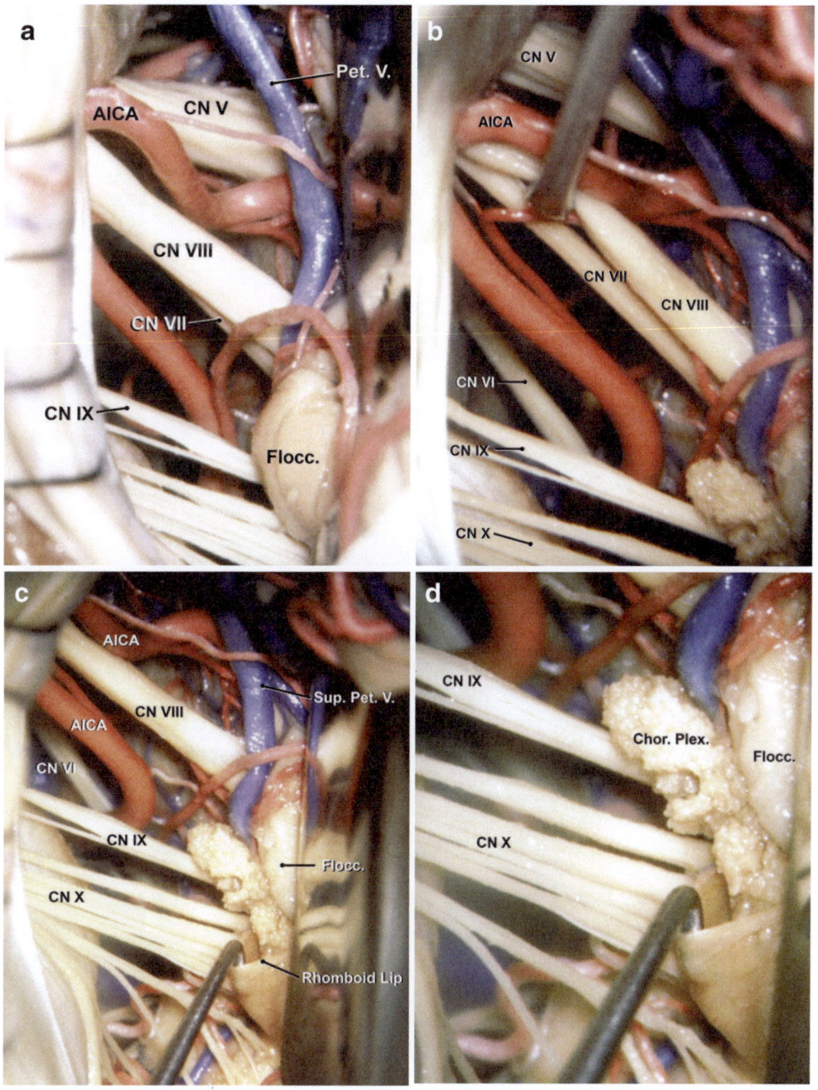

Fig. 2.8 Left side of CPA and brainstem through a retrosigmoid exposure. (**a**) The cerebellum has been elevated. The junction of the facial nerve (CN VII) with the brainstem is located inferior and slightly in front of the vestibulocochlear nerve (CN VIII). (**b**) The vestibulocochlear nerve has been elevated to provide additional exposure of the facial nerve. (**c**) Choroid plexus protrudes from the foramen of Luschka into the CPA behind the glossopharyngeal (CN IX) and vagus nerves (CN X). A nerve hook has been placed inside the rhomboid lip, and a pouch of neural tissue attached along the anterior margin of the lateral recess and extending laterally behind the glossopharyngeal and vagus nerves. (**d**) Enlarged view of the rhomboid lip. A.I.C.A. = anterior inferior cerebellar artery; Chor. Plex. = choroid plexus; CN = cranial nerve; CN V = trigeminal nerve; CN VI = abducens nerve; Flocc. = flocculus; Pet. = petrosal; Sup. = superior; V. = vein. (From Rhoton AL Jr. [48]. Reproduced with permission from Lippincott Williams & Wilkins)

above the most rostral rootlet contributing to these nerves. A helpful way of visualizing the point where the facial nerve exits from the brainstem, even when displaced by a tumor, is to project an imaginary line along the medullary junction of the rootlets forming the glossopharyngeal, vagus, and spinal accessory nerves upward through the pontomedullary junction. This line, at a point 2–3 mm above the junction of the glossopharyngeal nerve with the medulla, passes through the pontomedullary junction at the site where the facial nerve exits the brainstem. The filaments of the nervus intermedius also are stretched around an acoustic neuroma.

Structures related to the lateral recess of the fourth ventricle with a consistent relationship to the facial and vestibulocochlear nerves are the foramen of Luschka and its choroid plexus, and the flocculus (Fig. 2.10) [51, 52]. The foramen of Luschka is situated at the lateral margin of the pontomedullary sulcus, just behind the junction of the glossopharyngeal nerve with the brainstem, and immediately posteroinferior to the junction of the facial and vestibulocochlear nerves with the brainstem. The foramen of Luschka is seldom well visualized. A consistently identifiable tuft of choroid plexus, however, hangs out of the foramen of Luschka and sits on the posterior surface of the glossopharyngeal and vagus nerves just inferior to the junction of the facial and vestibulocochlear nerves with the brainstem. Another structure related to the lateral recess, the flocculus, projects from the margin of the lateral recess and foramen of Luschka into the CPA, just posterior to where the facial and vestibulocochlear nerves join the pontomedullary sulcus.

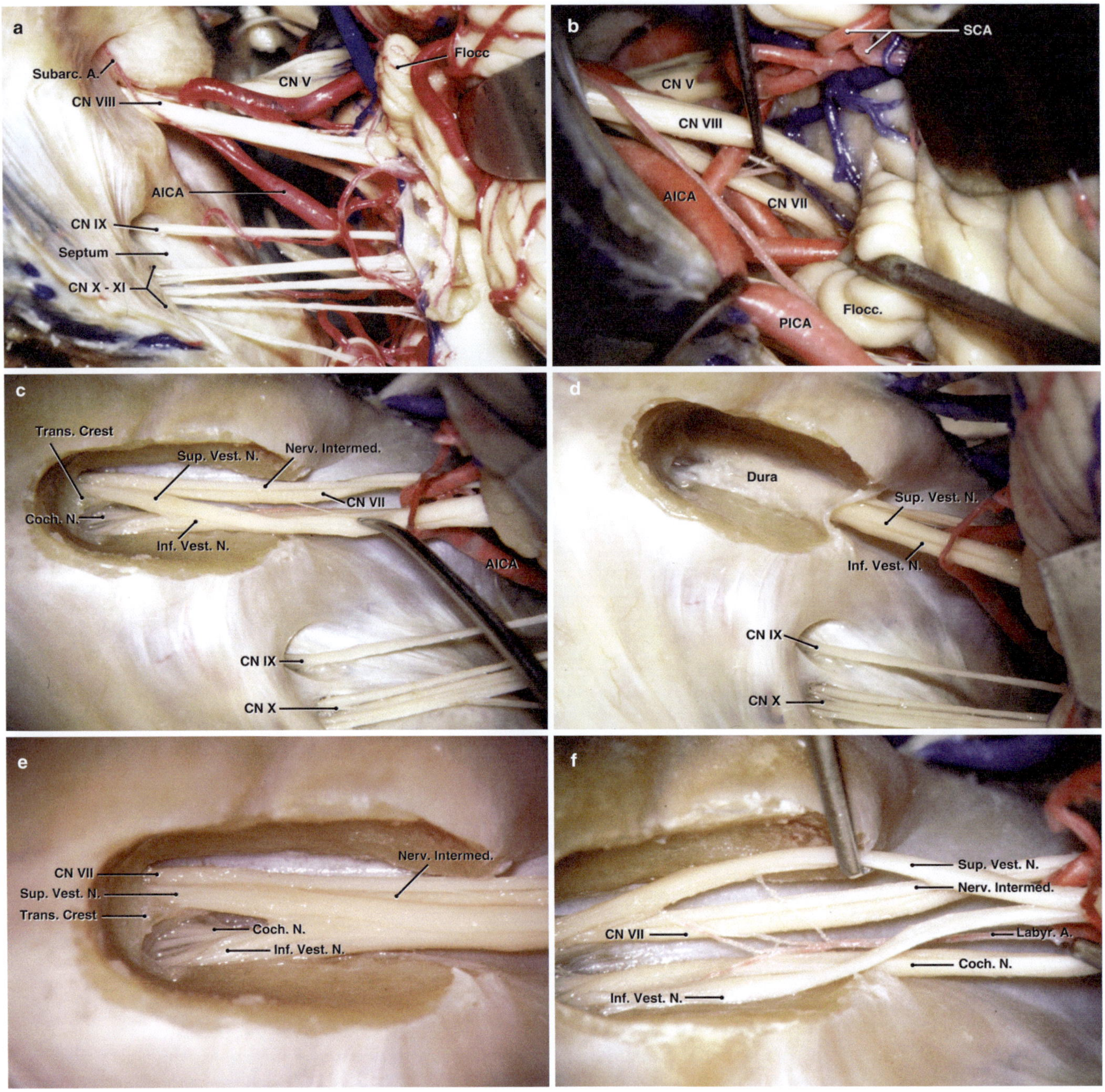

Fig. 2.9 Left side of CPA and skull through a retrosigmoid exposure. (**a**) The AICA passes between the facial and vestibulocochlear nerves (CN VIII). (**b**) The vestibulocochlear nerve and flocculus have been elevated to expose the junction of the facial nerve (CN VII) with the brainstem. In the retrosigmoid approach, the junction of the facial nerve with the brainstem can be exposed below the vestibulocochlear nerve. (**c**) The posterior wall of the internal acoustic meatus has been removed. (**d**) The dura lining the internal acoustic meatus has been opened. The transverse crest separates the superior vestibular and facial nerves above from the inferior vestibular and cochlear nerves below. (**e**) Enlarged view of the nerves within the meatus. The cochlear nerve is partially hidden anterior to the inferior vestibular nerve. (**f**) The cleavage plane between the superior and inferior vestibular and cochlear nerves has been started laterally and extended medially to expose the individual nerve bundles. A. = artery; AICA = anterior inferior cerebellar artery; Arc. = arcuate; CN = cranial nerve; CN V = trigeminal nerve; CN IX = glossopharyngeal nerve; CN X = vagus nerve; CN XI = spinal accessory nerve; Coch. = cochlear; Emin. = eminence; endolymph. = endolymphatic; Flocc. = flocculus; Inf. = inferior; Intermed. = intermedius; Jug. = jugular; Labyr. = labyrinth; N. = nerve; Nerv. = nervus = PICA = posteroinferior cerebellar artery; Post. = posterior; SCA = superior cerebellar artery; Subarc. = subarcuate; Sup. = superior; Trans. = transverse; Vert. = vertebral; Vest. = vestibular. (From Rhoton AL Jr. [48]. Reproduced with permission from Lippincott Williams & Wilkins)

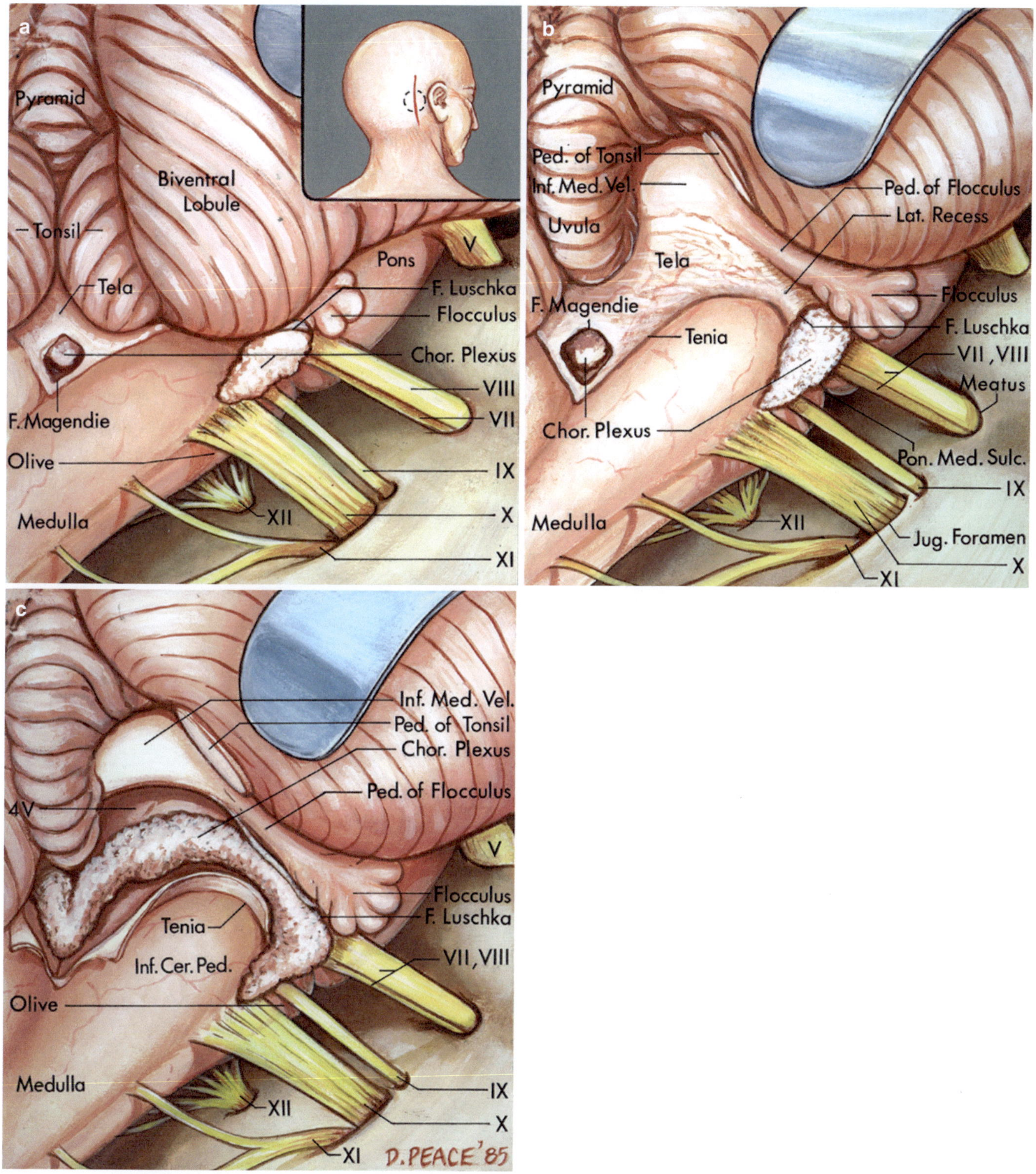

Fig. 2.10 Relationship of the foramen of Luschka and the lateral recess of the fourth ventricle to the junction of the facial (VII) and vestibulocochlear nerves (VIII) with the brainstem, as seen through a suboccipital craniotomy. (**a**) The foramen of Luschka opens into the CPA behind the glossopharyngeal (IX) and vagus nerves (X). The choroid plexus protrudes from the foramen of Luschka, slightly below and behind the facial and vestibulocochlear nerves, and behind the glossopharyngeal and vagus nerves. (**b**) The right cerebellar tonsil has been removed by dividing the tonsillar peduncle to show the relationship of the lateral recess to the facial and vestibulocochlear nerves. (**c**) The tela choroidea has been opened, but the choroid plexus, which arises on the inner surface of the tela in the fourth ventricle, has been preserved. Br. = bridging; Ca. = caudal; Cer. = cerebellar; Cer. Med. = cerebellomedullary; Cer. Pon. = cerebellopontine; Chor. = choroid; F. = foramen; Fiss. = fissure; Inf. inferior; Lat. = lateral; Ped. = peduncle; Pon. Med. = pontomedullary; Ro. = rostral; Subarc. = subarcuate; sulc. = sulcus; Tr. trunk; V. = trigeminal nerve; 4V = fourth ventricle; V. = vein; Vel. = velum; XI = spinal accessory nerve; XII = hypoglossal nerve. (From Rhoton AL Jr. [50]. Reproduced with permission from Elsevier)

CPA Upper Neurovascular Complex

The upper CPA neurovascular complex includes the pons, trigeminal nerve, supracerebellar artery (SCA), and superior petrosal veins.

The posterior trigeminal root joins the brainstem about halfway between the lower and upper borders of the pons. Frequently, a lip of cerebellum projects forward and obscures the junction of the posterior root with the pons. In its intradural course, the trigeminal nerve uniformly runs obliquely upward from the lateral portion of the pons toward the petrous apex. It exits the posterior fossa to enter the middle cranial fossa by passing forward beneath the tentorial attachment to enter Meckel's cave, which sits in the trigeminal impression on the upper surface of the petrous portion of the temporal bone (Fig. 2.11). The most common operation directed to the upper neurovascular complex is exposure and decompression of the posterior root of the trigeminal nerve.

Normally, the SCA encircles the brainstem well above the trigeminal nerve. When a prominent caudally projecting loop is present, the SCA and trigeminal nerve come in contact (Fig. 2.12), usually on the superior or superomedial aspect of the nerve. Often a few fascicles of the nerve are distorted by an SCA that has looped down into the axilla between the medial side of the nerve and pons. From the retrosigmoid view, an arterial loop in the axilla may not be visible behind the trigeminal nerve if the SCA courses around the brainstem directly in front of the nerve. The loop of the SCA also may be difficult to see if the artery passes over the rostral aspect of the nerve close to the brainstem, where it may be hidden by the overhanging lip of the cerebellomesencephalic fissure. The loop of the SCA may be seen dangling below the lower margin of the nerve, even though it is not visible above the nerve. These loops of the SCA, however, always pass rostrally along the medial and superior surfaces of the nerve to reach the cerebellomesencephalic fissure. The trunks do not pass directly from the side

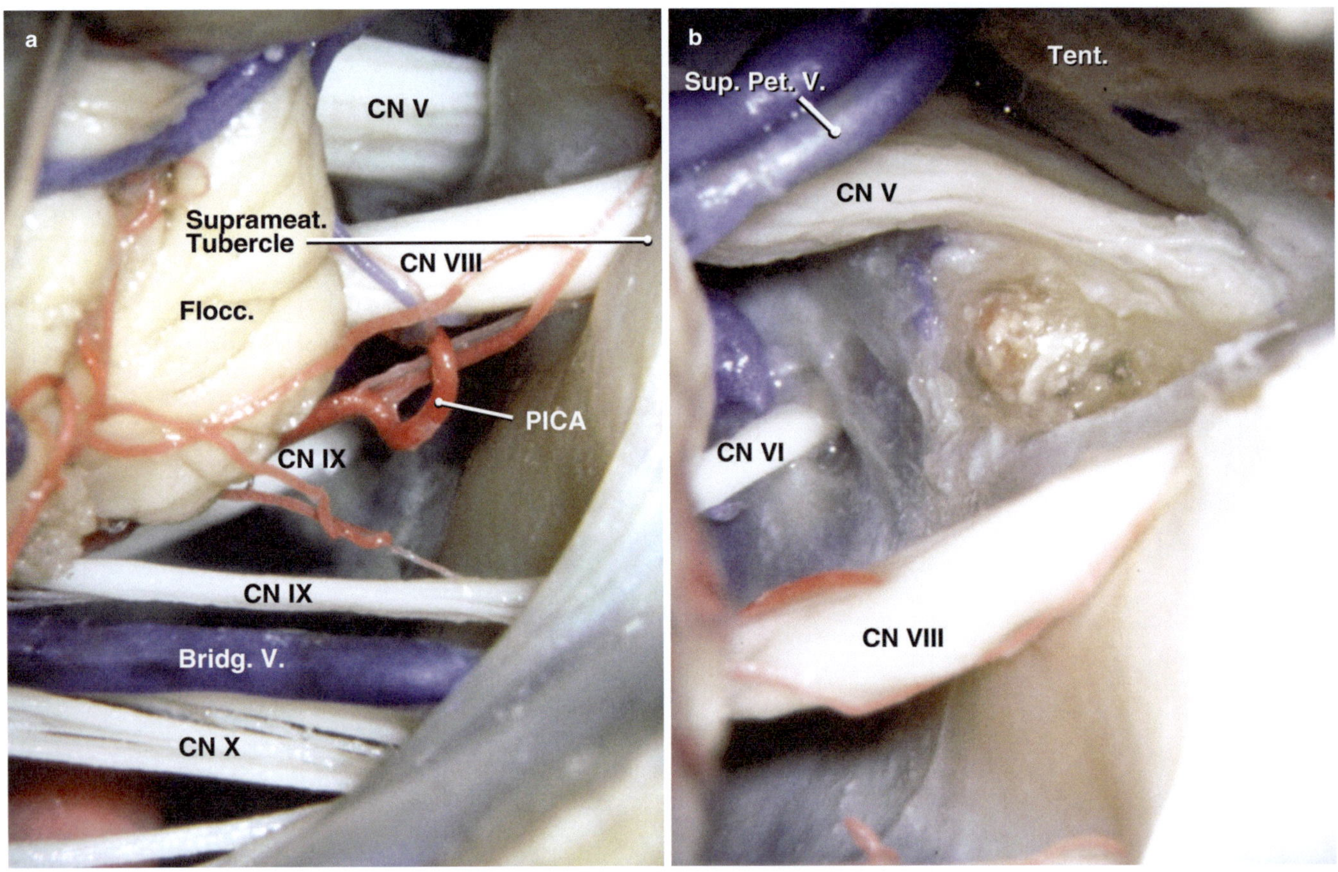

Fig. 2.11 Suprameatal approach to the posterior portion of Meckel's cave. (**a**) Right CPA. The suprameatal tubercle is located above the porus of the internal meatus. A large inferior petrosal vein passes behind the vagus nerve (CN X). (**b**) The suprameatal tubercle has been removed. The dura extending anteriorly toward Meckel's cave has been opened to provide 1 cm of additional exposure along the posterior trigeminal root. In addition, access to the side of the clivus is improved. Bridg. = bridging; CN = cranial nerve; CN V = trigeminal nerve; CN VI = abducens nerve; CN VIII = vestibulocochlear nerve; CN IX = glossopharyngeal nerve; Flocc. = flocculus; Pet. = petrosal; PICA = posterior inferior cerebellar artery; Suprameat. = suprameatal; Tent. = tentorium; V. = vein. (From Rhoton AL Jr. [48]. Reproduced with permission from Lippincott Williams & Wilkins)

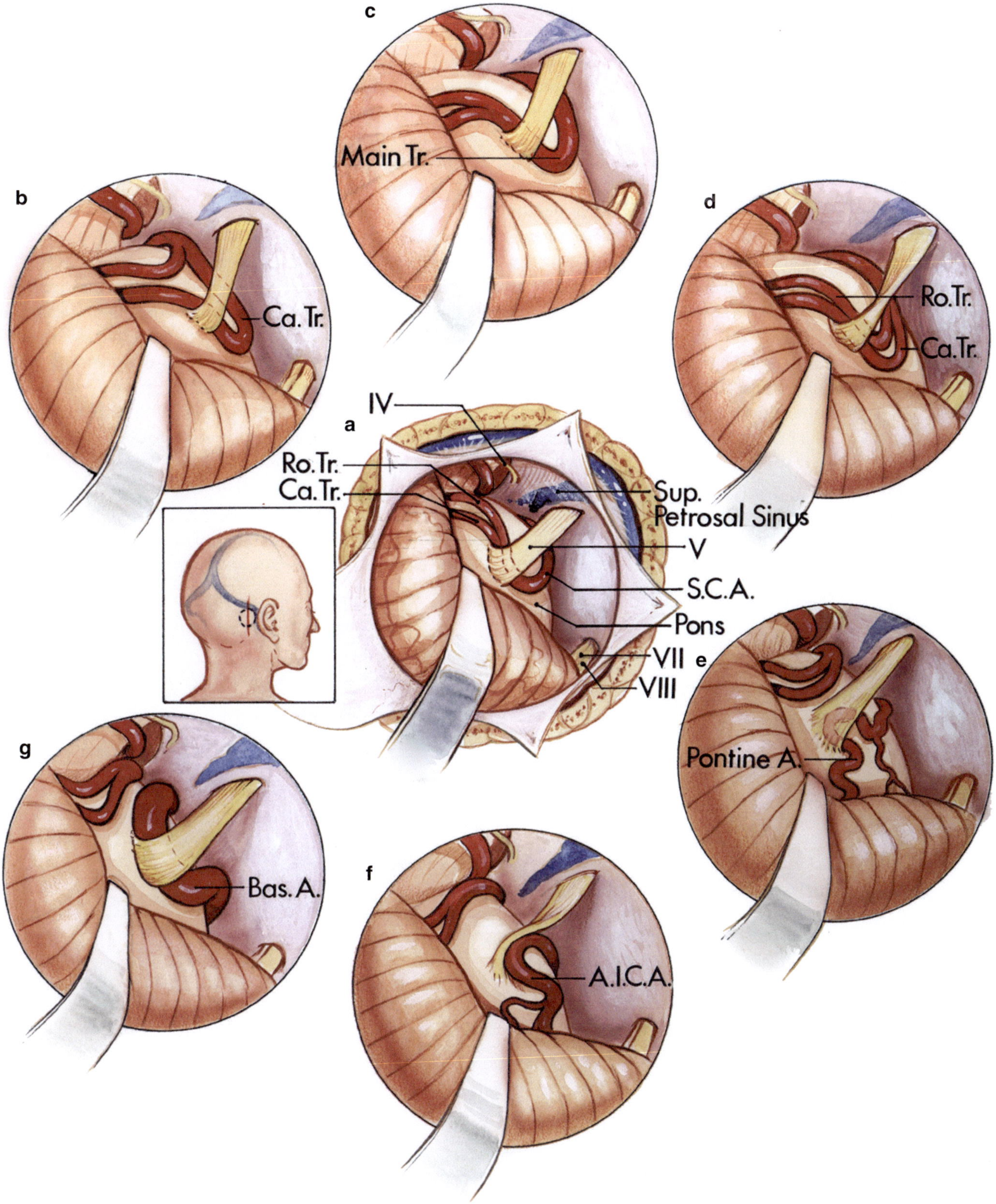

Fig. 2.12 Complex arterial relationships of upper CPA. Sites of arterial compression of the trigeminal nerve as seen through a suboccipital craniotomy. (**a**) Central diagram. The trigeminal nerve is compressed by a loop of the SCA that dangles down into the axilla of the nerve. The site of arterial compression is at the junction of the main trunk with the rostral and caudal trunks. (**b**) The nerve is compressed by the caudal trunk. (**c**) The nerve is compressed by the main trunk. (**d**) The nerve is compressed by both the rostral and caudal trunks. (**e**) The nerve is compressed by a pontine branch of the basilar artery. (**f**) The nerve is compressed by the AICA. (**g**) The nerve is compressed by a tortuous basilar artery. A. = artery; A.I.C.A. = anterior inferior cerebellar artery; Bas. = basilar; Ca. = caudal; Ro. = rostral; S.C.A. = superior cerebellar artery; sup. = superior; Tr. = trunk; V. = vein; VII = facial nerve; VIII = vestibulocochlear nerve. (From Rhoton AL Jr. [53]. Reproduced with permission from Lippincott Williams & Wilkins)

of the brainstem to the superior surface of the cerebellum. Rather, they dip into the deep fissure between the cerebellum and midbrain at the posterior margin of the trigeminal nerve.

Less frequently, the anterior inferior cerebellar artery (AICA) compresses the trigeminal nerve. Normally, the AICA passes around the pons below the trigeminal nerve with the facial and vestibulocochlear nerves. The AICA, however, may have a high origin and loop upward to indent the medial or lower surface of the trigeminal nerve before passing downward to course with the facial and vestibulocochlear nerves. A serpentine basilar artery also may wander laterally and compress the medial side of the trigeminal nerve. In such cases, the basilar artery is often elongated and has a fusiform configuration.

More than one artery can compress the nerve. In a few cases the SCA will compress the rostral surface of the nerve, and the AICA will compress the caudal surface. Infrequently, the posteroinferior cerebellar artery (PICA) may reach the trigeminal nerve from inferiorly.

The superior petrosal veins are among the largest and most frequently encountered veins in the posterior fossa. The superior petrosal veins can be formed by the terminal segment of a single vein or by the common stem formed by the union of several veins. The most common tributaries of the superior petrosal veins are the transverse pontine and pontotrigeminal veins, the veins of the cerebellopontine fissure and middle cerebellar peduncle, and the common stem of the veins draining the lateral part of the cerebellar hemisphere. The transverse pontine veins, which pass near the trigeminal nerve to reach the bridging veins entering the superior petrosal sinus, are the most frequent veins to compress the trigeminal nerve (Fig. 2.13). They can course medially in the axilla of the nerve, or they can pass above, below, or lateral to the nerve and indent any of its surfaces. The vein of the middle cerebellar peduncle can compress the lateral or medial surface of the trigeminal nerve before joining the petrosal veins as it ascends in the pons. The vein of the cerebellopontine fissure can indent the lateral margin of the trigeminal nerve as it ascends toward the superior petrosal sinus, and the pontotrigeminal vein may indent the upper margin of the nerve.

The junction of these veins, which converge and form a single trunk before entering the superior petrosal sinus, is usually lateral to the trigeminal nerve. This junction, however, may be located medial to the trigeminal nerve, in which case the common trunk must pass around the trigeminal nerve before reaching the superior petrosal sinus. These common trunks can also compress the trigeminal nerve.

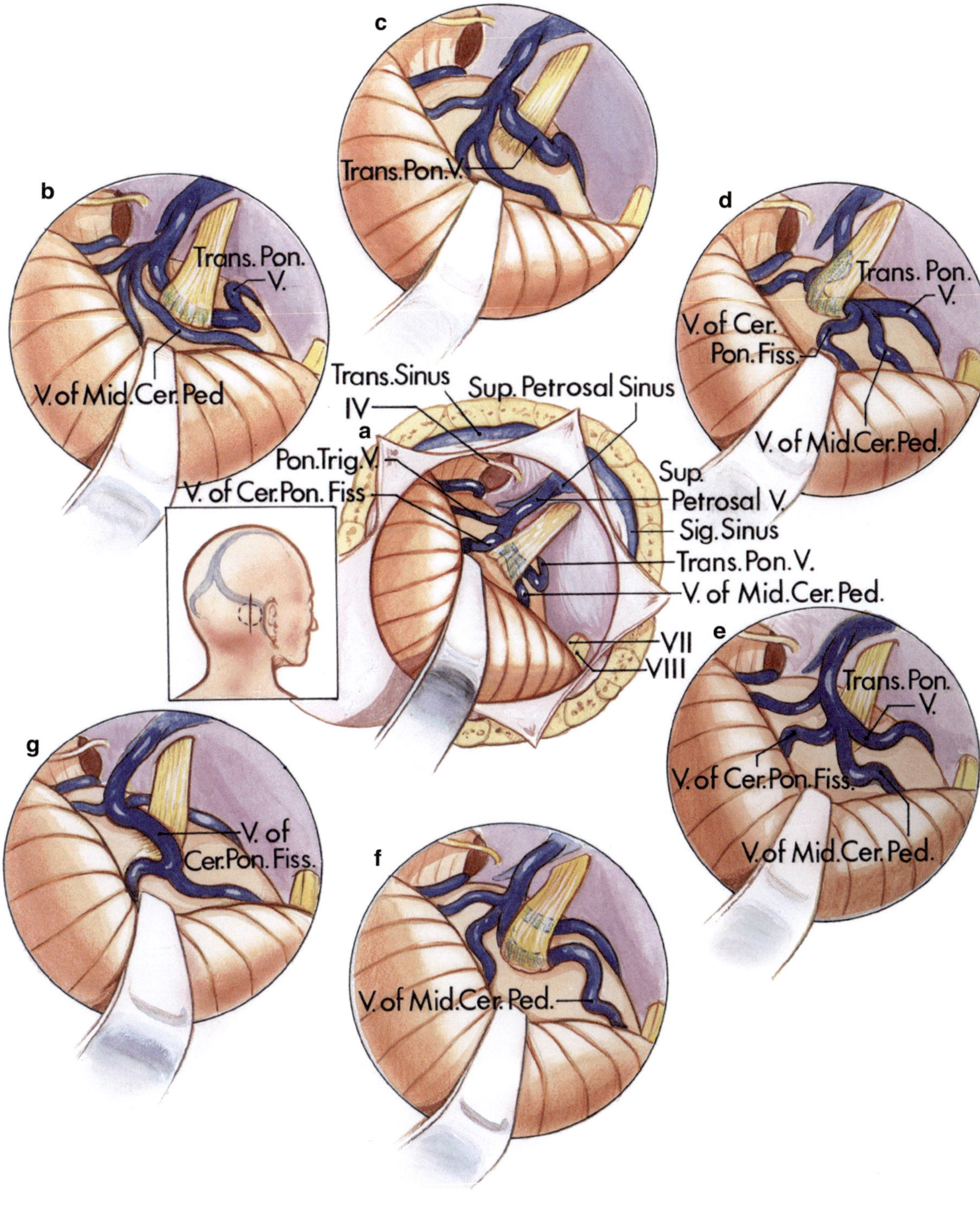

Fig. 2.13 Complex venous relationships of upper CPA. Sites of venous compression of the trigeminal nerve as seen through a retrosigmoid craniotomy. (**a**) The superior petrosal veins empty into the superior petrosal sinus. The trigeminal nerve is compressed by the junction of a transverse pontine vein and the vein of the middle cerebellar peduncle with the superior petrosal vein. (**b**) The trigeminal nerve is compressed on its medial side by a transverse pontine vein and on its lateral side by the vein of the middle cerebellar peduncle. (**c**) The lateral side of the nerve is compressed by a transverse pontine vein. (**d**) The medial side of the nerve is compressed by the junction of a transverse pontine vein with the veins of the middle cerebellar peduncle and cerebellopontine fissure. (**e**) The lateral side of the nerve is compressed by the junction of the transverse pontine vein with the veins of the middle cerebellar peduncle and cerebellopontine fissure. (**f**) The medial side of the nerve is compressed by the vein of the middle cerebellar peduncle. (**g**) The lateral side of the nerve is compressed by the vein of the cerebellopontine fissure. Cer. = cerebellar; Cer. Pon. = cerebellopontine; Fiss. = fissure; Mid. = middle; Ped. = peduncle; Pon. = pontine; Sig. = sigmoid; Sup. = superior; Trans. = transverse; Trig. = trigeminal; V. = vein; IV = trochlear nerve; VII = facial nerve; VIII = vestibulocochlear nerve. (From Rhoton AL Jr. [53]. Reproduced with permission from Lippincott Williams & Wilkins)

Middle Neurovascular Complex of the CPA

The middle complex includes the AICA; pons; middle cerebellar peduncle; cerebellopontine fissure; petrosal surface of the cerebellum; and the abducens, facial, and vestibulocochlear nerves. The AICA arises at the pontine level and courses in relationship to the abducens, facial, and vestibulocochlear nerves to reach the surface of the middle cerebellar peduncle. There it courses along the cerebellopontine fissure and terminates by supplying the petrosal surface of the cerebellum. Operations directed to the middle complex are for the removal of acoustic neuromas and other tumors and for neurovascular decompression to relieve hemifacial spasm (Fig. 2.14).

The arteries crossing the CPA, especially the AICA, enjoy a consistent relationship to the facial and vestibulocochlear nerves, foramen of Luschka, and flocculus (Fig. 2.15) [54–57]. In most cases, the AICA passes below the facial and vestibulocochlear nerves as it encircles the brainstem. However, it also can pass above or between these nerves in its course around the brainstem. The labyrinthine, recurrent perforating, and subarcuate branches arise from the AICA near the facial and vestibulocochlear nerves. When the meatus is opened via the middle fossa, translabyrinthine, or posterior approaches, care is required to avoid injury to the AICA if it is located at or protrudes through the porus.

On the side of the brainstem, the vein of the pontomedullary sulcus and the veins of the cerebellomedullary fissure, middle cerebellar peduncle, and cerebellopontine fissure have a predictable relationship to the facial and vestibulocochlear nerves [52].

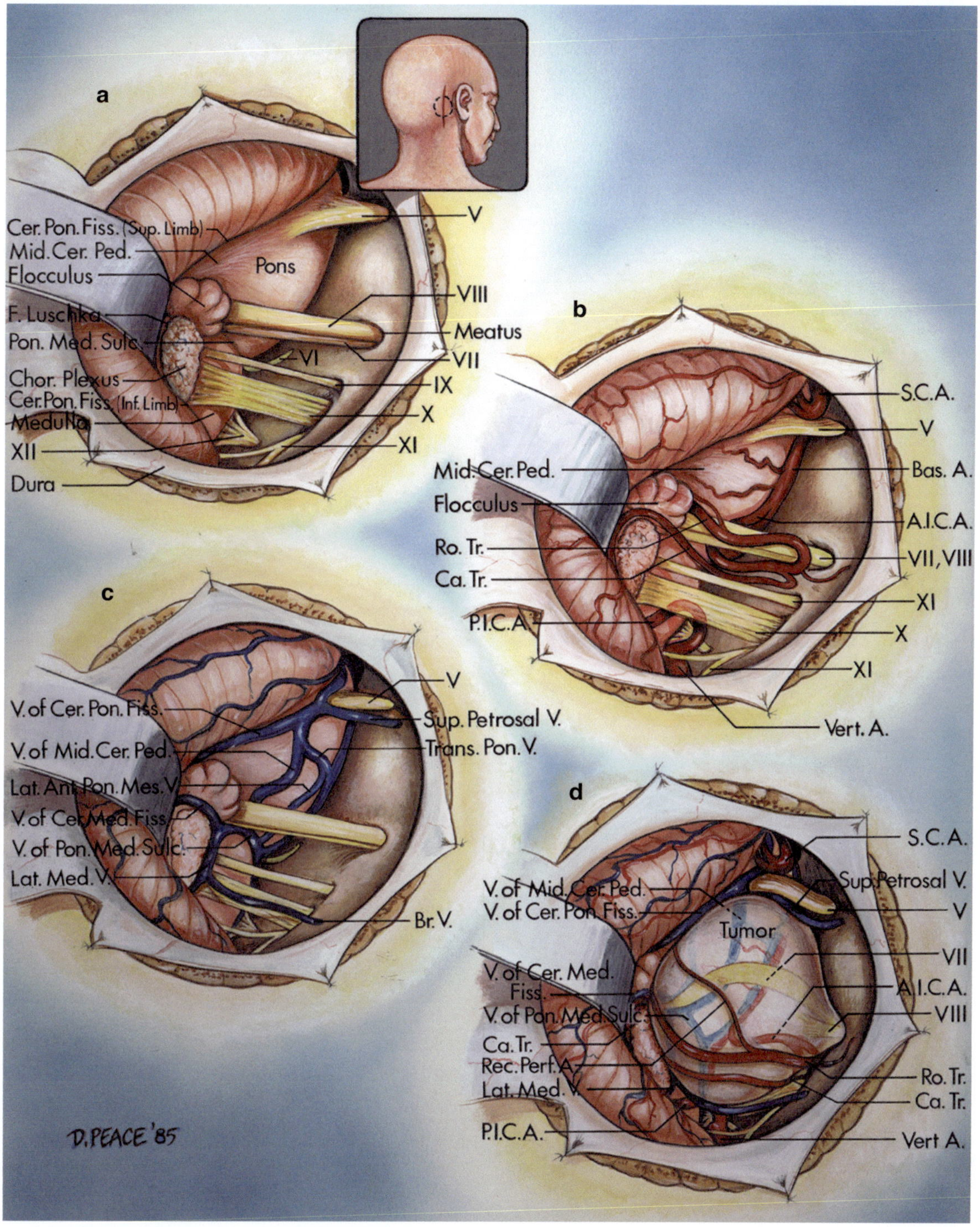

Fig. 2.14 Neurovascular relationships on the brainstem side of an acoustic neuroma. Posterior view through a retrosigmoid craniotomy. (**a**) Neural relationships. (**b**) Arterial relationships. The AICA arises from the basilar artery and divides into a rostral trunk, which passes above the flocculus to reach the surface of the middle cerebellar peduncle, and into a caudal trunk, which supplies the area below the flocculus. The PICA arises from the vertebral artery and passes dorsally between the vagus and accessory nerves. The superior cerebellar artery courses above the trigeminal nerve (V). (**c**) Venous relationships. (**d**) Neurovascular relationships of an acoustic neuroma. The tumor arises from the vestibulocochlear nerve (VIII) and displaces the facial nerve (VII) anteriorly, the trigeminal nerve superiorly, and the glossopharyngeal (IX) and vagus nerves (X) inferiorly. The vestibulocochlear nerve disappears into the tumor. The facial nerve enters the brainstem at the lateral margin of the pontomedullary sulcus anterior to the flocculus and rostral to the choroid plexus protruding from the foramen of Luschka. A recurrent perforating branch of the AICA passes across the tumor and supplies the brainstem. A. = artery; A.I.C.A. = anterior inferior cerebellar artery; Ant. = anterior; Bas. = basilar; Br. = bridging; Ca. = caudal; Cer. = cerebellar; Cer. Pont. = cerebellopontine; Chor. = choroid; F. = foramen; Fiss. = fissure; inf. = inferior; Lat. = lateral; Med. = medulla; Mid. = middle; Ped. = peduncle; Perf. = perforating; P.I.C.A. = posterior inferior cerebellar artery; Pon. = pontine; Pon. Med. = pontomedullary; Rec. = recurrent; Ro. = rostral; S.C.A. = superior cerebellar artery; Sulc. = sulcus; Sup. = superior; Tr. = trunk; V. = vein; Vert. = vertebral; XI = spinal accessory nerve; XII = hypoglossal nerve. (From Rhoton AL Jr. [50]. Reproduced with permission from Elsevier)

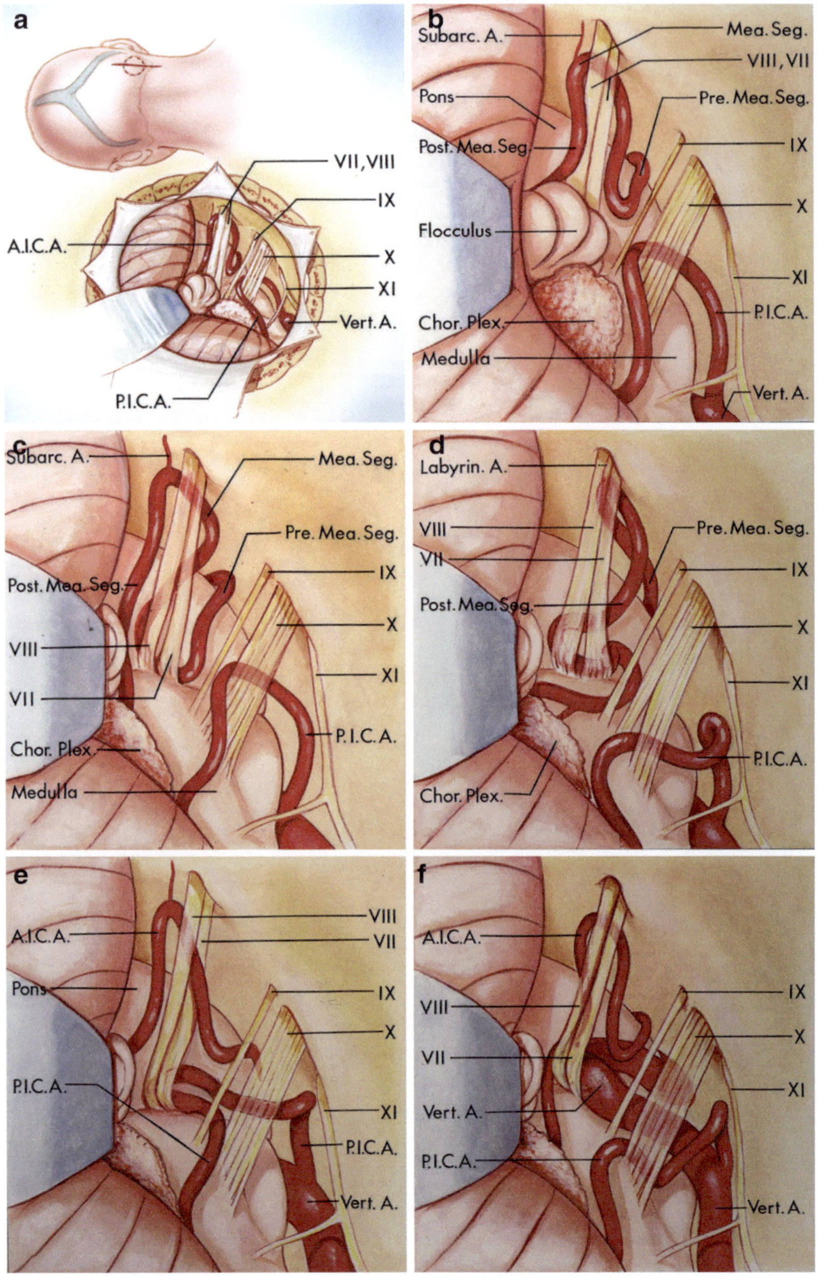

Fig. 2.15 Complex neurovascular relationships of the middle CPA. (**a**) The upper illustration shows the site of the incision (*straight line*) and the location of the craniotomy (*broken line*). The *lower* illustration shows the surgical exposure obtained with this approach. (**b**) The cerebellum is elevated to expose the facial (VII) and vestibulocochlear nerves (VIII) and the premeatal, meatal, and postmeatal segments of the AICA. (**c**) The flocculus and choroid plexus have been elevated to expose the root entry/exit zone of the facial and vestibulocochlear nerves. (**d**) The nerve root entry/exit zone is compressed by the postmeatal segment. (**e**) A tortuous PICA loops upward to compress the nerves at their junction with the brainstem before turning inferiorly to pass between the glossopharyngeal (IX) and vagus nerves (X). (**f**) A tortuous vertebral artery compresses the nerve root entry/exit zone. A. = artery; A.I.C.A. = anterior inferior cerebellar artery; Chor. Plex. = choroid plexus; Labyrin. = labyrinthine; MEA = meatal; P.I.C.A. = posterior inferior cerebellar artery; Post. = posterior; Seg. = segment; Subarc. = subarcuate; Vert. = vertebral; XI = spinal accessory nerve. (From Rhoton AL Jr. [48]. Reproduced with permission from Lippincott Williams & Wilkins)

Lower Neurovascular Complex of the CPA

The lower complex, which is related to the PICA, includes the medulla; inferior cerebellar peduncle; cerebellomedullary fissure; suboccipital surface of the cerebellum; and the glossopharyngeal, vagus, spinal accessory, and hypoglossal nerves. The PICA arises at the medullary level, encircles the medulla, passing in relationship to the glossopharyngeal, vagus, spinal accessory, and hypoglossal nerves, to reach the surface of the inferior cerebellar peduncle. There it dips into the cerebellomedullary fissure and terminates by supplying the suboccipital surface of the cerebellum (Fig. 2.16).

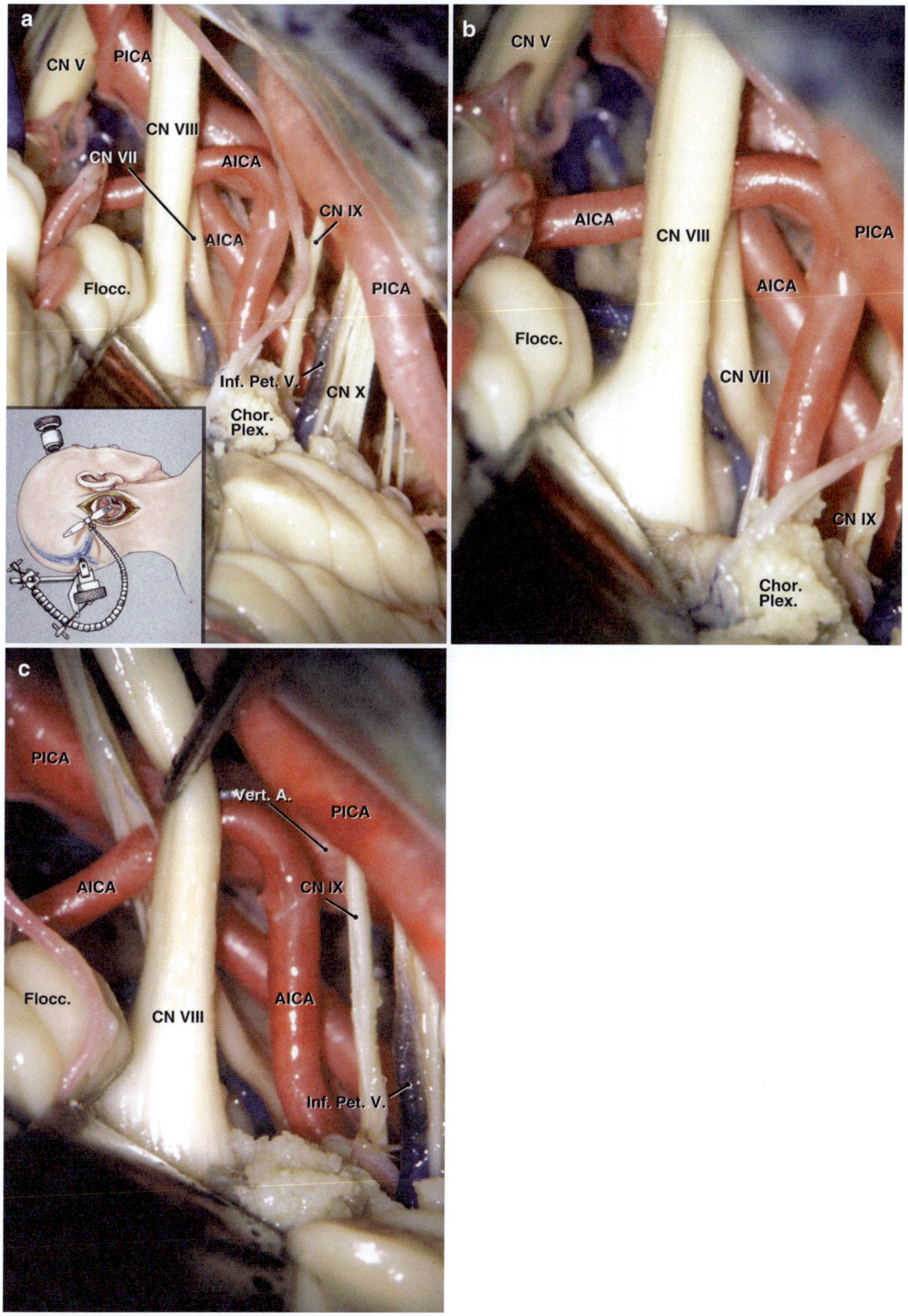

Fig. 2.16 Complex neurovascular relationships of the lower CPA. (**a**) Insert shows the approach along the inferolateral margin of the cerebellum. The AICA passes between the facial (CN VII) and vestibulocochlear (CN VIII) nerves. A large tortuous PICA loops upward anterior to the facial and vestibulocochlear nerves and behind the trigeminal nerve (CN V), before turning downward to reach the medulla. (**b**) Exposing the facial nerve exit zone from the brainstem is facilitated by directing the exposure along the inferolateral margin of the cerebellum in the area above the glossopharyngeal nerve (CN IX) and below the lower edge of the flocculus. (**c**) The vestibulocochlear nerve has been depressed to expose the distal segment of the facial nerve. No access is provided to the junction of the facial nerve with the brainstem, which should be visualized when treating hemifacial spasm. A = artery; AICA = anterior inferior cerebellar artery; Chor. Plex. = choroid plexus; CN = cranial nerve; CN X = vagus nerve; Flocc. = flocculus; Inf. = inferior; Pet. = petrosal; P.I.C.A. = posterior inferior cerebellar artery; V. = vein; Vert. = vertebral. (From Rhoton AL Jr. [48]. Reproduced with permission from Lippincott Williams & Wilkins)

The glossopharyngeal, vagus, spinal accessory, and hypoglossal nerves arise from the medulla along the margin of the inferior olive. The glossopharyngeal, vagus, and spinal accessory nerves arise as a line of rootlets that exit the brainstem along the posterior edge of the olive in the postolivary sulcus, a shallow groove between the olive and posterolateral surface of the medulla. The hypoglossal nerve arises as a line of rootlets that exit the brainstem along the anterior margin of the lower two-thirds of the olive in the preolivary sulcus, a groove between the olive and the medullary pyramid. The glossopharyngeal and vagus nerves arise at the level of the superior third of the olive. The spinal accessory rootlets arise along the posterior margin of the inferior two-thirds of the olive and from the lower medulla and the upper segments of the cervical spinal cord. The glossopharyngeal and vagus nerves arise rostral to the level of the origin of the hypoglossal rootlets.

The glossopharyngeal nerve arises as one or rarely two rootlets from the upper medulla, posterior to the olive, just caudal to the origin of the facial nerve. It courses ventral to the choroid plexus, protruding from the foramen of Luschka on its way to the jugular foramen. Frequently, a larger dorsal and a smaller ventral component is visible at the junction with the brainstem [58, 59]. The smaller ventral rootlets are motor fibers, and the larger main bundle is composed of sensory fibers [60, 61]. The larger dorsal component usually arises from the medulla as one root. In a few cases, however, it originates as two rootlets, which can remain separate throughout their course to the dura.

The vagus nerve arises below the glossopharyngeal nerve as a 2–5.5 mm line of tightly packed rootlets posterior to the superior third of the olive. The most rostral vagal fibers arise adjacent to the glossopharyngeal origin, from which they are sometimes separated by as much as 2 mm. The vagus nerve is composed of multiple combinations of large and small rootlets that pass ventral to the choroid plexus, protruding from the foramen of Luschka on its way to the jugular foramen. Occasionally, several small rootlets originate ventral to the majority of vagal rootlets. These small ventral rootlets are considered to be motor fibers [60].

The accessory nerve arises as a widely separated series of rootlets that originated from the medulla at the level of the lower two-thirds of the olive and from the upper cervical cord. Immediately caudal to the vagal fibers, the cranial rootlets of the accessory nerve arise as a line of rootlets that range from 0.1 to 1 mm in diameter. The cranial rootlets of the accessory nerve are more appropriately regarded as inferior vagal rootlets because they arise from vagal nuclei [58, 59]. It may be difficult to distinguish the lower vagal fibers from the upper accessory rootlets because the vagal and cranial accessory fibers usually enter the vagal meatus as a single bundle.

The upper rootlets of the spinal portion of the accessory nerve originate several millimeters caudal to the lowest cranial accessory fibers. They course to join the cranial accessory bundle or to enter the lower border of the vagal meatus separate from the cranial accessory rootlets. The spinal accessory fibers pass superolaterally from their origin to reach the jugular foramen. Although the cranial and spinal portions of the accessory nerve usually enter the vagal meatus together, they are occasionally separated by a dural septum.

The rootlets forming the hypoglossal nerve arise from the medulla along a line that is continuous inferiorly with the line along which the ventral spinal roots arise. These rootlets arise in a nucleus whose rostral portion sits deep to the hypoglossal triangle in the floor of the fourth ventricle. They exit the medulla along the anterior margin of the caudal two-thirds of the olive. The hypoglossal rootlets course anterolaterally through the subarachnoid space and pass behind the vertebral artery to reach the hypoglossal canal. If the vertebral artery is short and straight, it may not contact or distort the hypoglossal rootlets. If the artery is tortuous, it can stretch the hypoglossal rootlets posteriorly over its dorsal surface [54]. Infrequently, the vertebral artery passes between the rootlets of the hypoglossal nerve [56]. Before entering the hypoglossal canal, the rootlets collect into two bundles. In some cases, this canal is divided by a bony septum that separates the two bundles. After passing through the canal, the bundles unite and the nerve lies medial to the internal jugular vein and to the glossopharyngeal, vagus, and accessory nerves.

The vertebral artery courses anterior to the nerves in the lower neurovascular complex. The hypoglossal rootlets usually pass behind the vertebral artery. However, some hypoglossal rootlets occasionally pass anterior to the artery. If the vertebral artery is elongated or tortuous and courses lateral to the olive, it stretches the hypoglossal rootlets over its posterior surface. Some tortuous vertebral arteries stretch the hypoglossal rootlets so far posteriorly that they intermingle with the glossopharyngeal, vagus, and spinal accessory nerves.

The PICA has a much more complex relationship to these nerves. The proximal portion of the PICA passes around or between and often stretches or distorts the rootlets of the nerves in the lower complex. At the anterolateral medulla, the PICA passes around or between the rootlets of the hypoglossal nerve. At the posterolateral margin of the medulla, it passes between the fila of the glossopharyngeal, vagus, and spinal accessory nerves. The PICA may be ascending, descending, or passing laterally or medially, or it may be involved in a complex loop that stretches and distorts these nerves as it passes between them.

The close relationships of the PICA and vertebral artery to the glossopharyngeal and vagus nerves make it logical to explore these relationships in glossopharyngeal neuralgia [5, 62]. Both the glossopharyngeal and vagus nerves have been found to be compressed at their junction with the brainstem by the PICA or the vertebral artery, or both, and the neuralgia has been relieved after the arteries and nerves have been separated [63]. The adverse cardiovascular effects associated with mobilizing these nerves and the risk of causing swallowing and vocal cord defects have led some to conclude that rhizotomy of the glossopharyngeal nerve and upper vagal rootlets is a reasonable alternative to vascular mobilization along the lateral medulla [53, 64–67].

Summary

The asterion and the most posterior portion of the parietomastoid suture are related with the most lateral aspect of the inferior margin of the transverse sinus and with the transition between the transverse and sigmoid sinuses, respectively. Hence, they constitute appropriate sites to start and delimit exposure of the superior aspect of the CPA. At the level of the mastoid notch, the occipitomastoid suture is particularly associated with the posterior margin of the sigmoid sinus. Hence, it constitutes an appropriate initial site for a burr hole for a basal suboccipital craniectomy to expose the lower portion of the CPA. Once they are already located over the infratentorial lateral limits, both can be used as initial sites for burr holes for wide suboccipital exposures.

References

1. Rhoton AL Jr. The foramen magnum. Neurosurgery. 2003;53:587–625.
2. Oliveira E, Rhoton AL Jr, Peace D. Microsurgical anatomy of the region of the foramen magnum. Surg Neurol. 1985;24:293–352.
3. Di Chiro G, Anderson WB. The clivus. Clin Radiol. 1965;16:211–23.
4. Kirdani MA. The normal hypoglossal canal. Am J Roentgenol Radium Therapy Nucl Med. 1967;99:700–4.
5. Watt JC, McKillop AN. Relation of arteries to roots of nerves in posterior cranial fossa in man. Arch Surg. 1935;30:336–45.
6. Bremond G, Garcin M, Magnan JI. Preservation of hearing in the removal of acoustic neuroma ("minima" posterior approach by retrosigmoidal route). J Laryngol Otol. 1980;94:1199–204.
7. Lang J. Inferior skull base anatomy. In: Sekhar LN, Schramm Jr VL, editors. Tumors of the cranial base: diagnosis and treatment. New York: Futura; 1987. p. 461–529.
8. McMinn RMH, Hutchings RT, Logan BM. Color atlas of head and neck anatomy. Chicago: Year Book Medical Publ; 1981.
9. Pernkoff E. Atlas of topographical and applied human anatomy. Baltimore: Urban & Schwarzenberg; 1980.
10. Testut L, Jacob O. Tratado de anatomía humana. 8th ed. Barcelona: Salvat; 1932.
11. Testut L, Jacob O. Tratado de anatomía topográfica. 5th ed. Barcelona: Salvat; 1932.
12. Waddington M. Atlas of the human skull. Rutland: Academy Books; 1981.
13. Williams PL, Warwik R, editors. Gray's anatomy. 36th ed. Philadelphia: Saunders; 1980.
14. Ribas GC, Rhoton AL Jr, Cruz OR, Peace D. Suboccipital burr holes and craniectomies. Neurosurg Focus. 2005;19:E1.
15. Ono M, Ono M, Rhoton AL Jr, Barry M. Microsurgical anatomy of the region of the tentorial incisura. J Neurosurg. 1984;60:365–99.
16. Oka K, Rhoton AL Jr, Barry M, Rodriguez R. Microsurgical anatomy of the superficial veins of the cerebrum. Neurosurgery. 1985;17:711–48.
17. Baló J. The dural venous sinuses. Anat Rec. 1950;106:319–26.
18. Bisaria KK. Anatomic variations of venous sinuses in the region of the torcular herophili. J Neurosurg. 1985;62:90–5.
19. Hempel KJ, Elmohamed A. Anatomie, Formvarianten und Typisierungen des venösen intrakraniellen Systems beim Menschen. Radiologe. 1971;11:451–6.
20. Johanson C. The central veins and deep dural sinuses of the brain. Stockholm: Serafimer Lasarettet; 1954.
21. Johanson C. The central veins and deep dural sinuses of the brain: an anatomical and angiographic study. Acta Radiol. 1954;107:5–184.
22. Kaplan HA, Browder J. Narrow and atretic transverse dural sinuses: clinical significance. Ann Otol. 1973;82:351–4.
23. Kaplan HA, Browder J. Neurosurgical considerations of some features of the cerebral dural sinuses and their tributaries. Clin Neurosurg. 1976;23:155–69.
24. Kaplan HA, Browder J, Knightly JJ, et al. Variations of the cerebral dural sinuses at the torcular herophili. Am J Surg. 1972;124:456–61.
25. Kimbel WH. Variation in the pattern of cranial venous sinuses and hominid phylogeny. Am J Phys Anthropol. 1984;63:243–63.
26. Paglioli E. Atlas anátomo-radiológico do sistema venoso intracraniano. Porto Algre: Missau; 1978.
27. Saxena RC, Beg MA, Das AC. Double straight sinus. Report of six cases. J Neurosurg. 1973;39:540–2.
28. Waltner JG. Anatomic variations of the lateral and sigmoid sinuses. Arch Otolaryngol. 1944;39:307–12.
29. Wolf-Heidgger G. Atlas de anatomia humana. 2nd ed. Rio de Janeiro: Guanabara Koogan; 1972.
30. Woodhall B. Anatomy of the cranial blood sinuses with particular reference to the lateral. Laryngoscope. 1939;49:966–1109.
31. Woodhall B. Variations of the cranial venous sinuses in the region of the torcular herophili. Arch Surg. 1936;33:297–314.
32. Woodhall B, Seeds AE. Cranial venous sinuses: correlations between skull markings and roentgenograms of the occipital bone. Arch Surg. 1936;33:867–75.
33. Browder J, Kaplan HA, Krieger AJ. Anatomical features of the straight sinus and its tributaries. J Neurosurg. 1976;44:55–61.
34. Browder J, Kaplan HA, Krieger AJ. Venous channels in the tentorium cerebelli: surgical significance. Surg Neurol. 1975;3:37–9.
35. Duwal JM, Latouche X, Mondine P, Robillard D. Sinus de la tente du cervelet. Bull Assoc Anat Nancy. 1975;59:855–62.
36. Kaplan HA, Browder A, Browder J, Krieger AJ. Venous channels within the intracranial dural partitions. Radiology. 1975;115:641–5.
37. Matsushima T, Rhoton AL Jr, Oliveira E, Peace D. Microsurgical anatomy of the veins of the posterior fossa. J Neurosurg. 1983;59:63–105.
38. Ono M, Rhoton AL Jr, Peace D, Rodriguez RJ. Microsurgical anatomy of the deep venous system of the brain. Neurosurgery. 1984;15:621–57.
39. Saxena RC, Beg MA, Das AC. The straight sinus. J Neurosurg. 1974;41:724–7.
40. Di Chiro G, Fischer RS, Nelson KB. The jugular foramen. J Neurosurg. 1964;21:447–60.
41. Haas LL. The posterior condylar fossa, foramen and canal, and the jugular foramen. Radiology. 1957;69:549–52.
42. Rhoton AL Jr, Buza RC. Microsurgical anatomy of the jugular foramen. J Neurosurg. 1975;42:541–50.
43. Rhoton AL Jr, Buza RC. Microsurgical anatomy of the jugular foramen. In: Rand RW, editor. Microneurosurgery. 2nd ed. Saint Louis: Mosby; 1978. p. 252–64.
44. Ribas GC. Estudo das relações topográficas das suturas lambdóide, occiptomastóidea e parietomastóidea com os seios transverso e sig-

móide, e de trepanações da região [tese]. São Paulo: Faculdade de Medicina, Universidade de São Paulo; 1991.
45. Ribas GC, Rhoton AL Jr, Cruz OR, Peace D. Temporoparieto-occipital burrhole sites study and systematized approaches proposal. In: Samii M, editor. Skull base surgery, first int., skull base congr., Hannover 1992. Basel: Karger; 1994. p. 723–30.
46. Broca P. Instructions crâniologiques et crâniométriques de la Sociètè d'Anthropologie. Paris: G. Masson; 1875.
47. Broca P. Sur la topographie crânie-cerébrale ou sur les rapports anatomiques du crâne et du cerveau. Rev d'Anthrop. 1876;5:193–248.
48. Rhoton AL Jr. The cerebellopontine angle and posterior fossa cranial nerves by the retrosigmoid approach. Neurosurgery. 2003;53:525–61.
49. Rhoton AL Jr. The cerebellopontine angle and posterior fossa cranial nerves by the retrosigmoid approach [Chapter 4]. In: Rhoton Jr AL, editor. Cranial anatomy and surgical approaches. Schaumburg: Lippincott Williams & Wilkins; 2003. p. 525–61.
50. Rhoton AL Jr. Microsurgical anatomy of the brainstem surface facing an acoustic neuroma. Surg Neurol. 1986;25:326–39.
51. Fujii K, Lenkey C, Rhoton AL Jr. Microsurgical anatomy of the choroidal arteries: fourth ventricle and cerebellopontine angles. J Neurosurg. 1980;52:504–24.
52. Matsushima T, Rhoton AL Jr, Lenkey C. Microsurgery of the fourth ventricle: part I. Microsurgical anatomy. Neurosurgery. 1982;11:631–67.
53. Rhoton AL Jr. Microsurgical anatomy of decompression operations on the trigeminal nerve. In: Rovit RL, Murali R, Jannetta PJ, editors. Trigeminal neuralgia. Baltimore: Williams & Wilkins; 1990. p. 165–200.
54. Hardy DG, Peace DA, Rhoton AL Jr. Microsurgical anatomy of the superior cerebellar artery. Neurosurgery. 1980;6:10–28.
55. Hardy DG, Rhoton AL Jr. Microsurgical relationships of the superior cerebellar artery and the trigeminal nerve. J Neurosurg. 1978;49:669–78.
56. Lister JR, Rhoton AL Jr, Matsushima T, Peace DA. Microsurgical anatomy of the posterior inferior cerebellar artery. Neurosurgery. 1982;10:170–99.
57. Martin RG, Grant JL, Peace DA, et al. Microsurgical relationships of the anterior inferior cerebellar artery and the facial-vestibulocochlear nerve complex. Neurosurgery. 1980;6:483–507.
58. Katsuta T, Rhoton AL Jr, Matsushima T. The jugular foramen: microsurgical anatomy and operative approaches. Neurosurgery. 1997;41:149–202.
59. DuBois FS, Foley JO. Experimental studies on the vagus and spinal accessory nerves in the cat. Anat Rec. 1936;64:285–307.
60. Tarlov IM. Structure of the nerve root: II. Differentiation of sensory from motor roots: observations on identification of function in roots of mixed cranial nerves. Arch Neurol Psychiatr. 1937;37:1338–55.
61. Rhoton AL Jr. Microsurgical anatomy of posterior fossa cranial nerves. In: Barrow DL, editor. Surgery of the cranial nerves of the posterior fossa: neurosurgical topics. Park Ridge, IL: American Association of Neurological Surgeons Publications; 1993. p. 1–103.
62. Laha RK, Jannetta PJ. Glossopharyngeal neuralgia. J Neurosurg. 1977;47:316–20.
63. Jannetta PJ, Abbasy M, Maroon JC, et al. Etiology and definitive microsurgical treatment of hemifacial spasm: operative techniques and results in 47 patients. J Neurosurg. 1977;47:321–8.
64. Jannetta PJ, Gendell HM. Clinical observations on etiology essential hypertension. Surg Forum. 1979;30:431–2.
65. Jannetta PJ, Møller MB, Møller AR, Sekhar LN. Neurosurgical treatment of vertigo by microvascular decompression of the eighth cranial nerve. Clin Neurosurg. 1986;33:645.
66. Ouaknine GE, Robert F, Molina-Negro P, Hardy J. Geniculate neuralgia and audio-vestibular disturbances due to compression of the intermediate and eighth nerves by the postero-inferior cerebellar artery. Surg Neurol. 1980;13:147–50.
67. Segal R, Gendell HM, Canfield D, et al. Cardiovascular response to pulsatile pressure applied to ventrolateral medulla. Surg Forum. 1979;30:433–5.

Radiology

3

Simone E. Dekker, Kristine A. Blackham, Robert W. Tarr, and Ameya Nayate

When evaluating pathology of the cerebellopontine angle (CPA), imaging is used as a tool to screen, to generate differential diagnoses, and to help plan therapy. The two modalities used most frequently in these endeavors are magnetic resonance imaging (MRI) and computed tomography (CT). Catheter-based digital subtraction angiography (DSA) plays a role in evaluating a lesion previously identified radiographically for quality and location of vascular supply. Angiography can also be used for embolization as a preoperative aid when treating vascular lesions of the CPA.

Technical Considerations

CT is typically used to evaluate the temporal bone and is tailored for bone detail. At our institution, multidetector CT is used for spiral data acquisition in the axial plane with reconstruction using a sharp kernel into images that are 0.8 mm thick at 0.4 mm intervals. These thin slices with overlap are routinely reformatted into the coronal plane. However, with the availability of the initial axial dataset and off-line three-dimensional (3D) workstations, the data can be reformatted into any plane and slice thickness desired.

Vascular CPA pathology can be evaluated with CT angiography (CTA), which utilizes the same principle of thin-slice collimation with overlap. However, a bolus of intravenous contrast is administered, and imaging is performed when vascular opacification peaks in the region of interest. These images can then be reformatted into a multiplanar reconstruction, maximum-intensity projection image, or a 3D-shaded surface display.

The CPA is typically evaluated with thin-slice, axial T1- and T2-weighted MRI followed by postgadolinium administration fat-saturated axial and coronal T1-weighted MRI through the same region. T2-weighted and fluid-attenuated inversion recovery (FLAIR) images are obtained to evaluate for parenchymal reaction or edema in the brainstem and cerebellum. These sequences are the most conventional for screening and for further evaluation of known pathology.

MRI has an inherent advantage over CT for the evaluation of the CPA: cerebrospinal fluid (CSF) acts like a contrast agent on T2-weighted images. Heavily T2-weighted sequences and 3D acquisition can be used to further exploit the contrast between high signal intensity CSF and the intermediate-to-low signal intensity structures of the CPA such as normal cranial nerves, vasculature, and pathology [1, 2]. Constructive interference in steady state (CISS) is one magnetic resonance (MR) sequence that allows acquisition of thin-slice, heavily T2-weighted images with a high signal-to-noise ratio (Fig. 3.1) [3]. These images can be postprocessed into datasets that can be reformatted into 3D images [4, 5].

S. E. Dekker (✉)
Department of Neurological Surgery, The Neurological Institute, University Hospitals Cleveland Medical Center, Case Western Reserve University, Cleveland, OH, USA

K. A. Blackham
Universitätsspital, Klinik für Radiologie und Nuklearmedizin, Basel, Switzerland

R. W. Tarr
Radiology, Neurology, Neurological Surgery, University Hospitals Cleveland Medical Center, Case Western Reserve University School of Medicine, Cleveland, OH, USA

A. Nayate
Department of Radiology, Neuroradiology, University Hospitals Cleveland Medical Center, Cleveland, OH, USA

N. C. Bambakidis et al. (eds.), *Surgery of the Cerebellopontine Angle*, https://doi.org/10.1007/978-3-031-12507-2_3

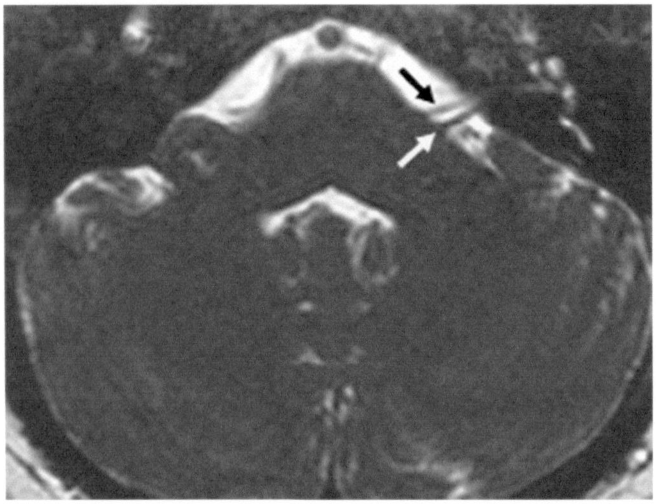

Fig. 3.1 CISS imaging through the CPA with clear delineation of left cranial nerves VII (*black arrow*) and VIII (*white arrow*)

Typical 3D reformation allows a strict 1:1 translation of the acquired data into 3D images and does account for the viewpoints and distortion caused by the lens of the surgical microscope or endoscope. Virtual endoscopy is a method for reformatting datasets into 3D images that mimic the surgeon's view with a divergent field of view. It also accounts for the distortion caused by spatial location; that is, objects closer to the "lens" of the virtual endoscope are larger than objects in the background (Figs. 3.2 and 3.3) [6–8].

Although useful as a potential aid in preoperative planning for lesions of the CPA, virtual endoscopic images are reformatted from a raw dataset. The manipulation of this dataset can change the size of a lesion on reconstructed images. All diagnostic information should be gathered from the source images as well as from the traditional imaging sequences.

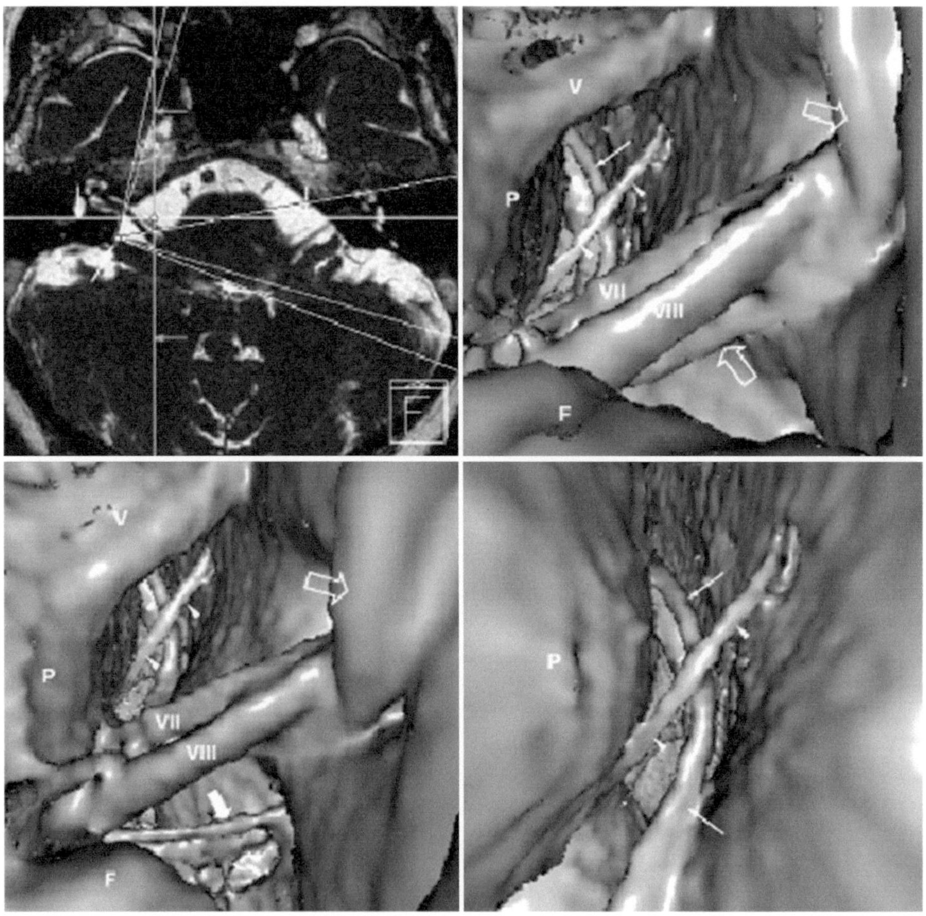

Fig. 3.2 Normal anatomy of the CPA seen on source MRI (top left) and virtual endoscopy (top right, bottom left and right) from surgical approach, mimicking retrosigmoid approach. Virtual MR endoscopy images show posterior aspect of facial nerve (VII), vestibulocochlear nerve (VIII), trigeminal nerve (V), abducens (*arrowhead*), pons (P), flocculus (F), and normal blood vessels (*arrows*). (From Nowe V et al. [103]. Reproduced with permission from *American Journal of Roentgenology.* Photos courtesy of Parizel PM, Nowe V, and Van de Heyning PH)

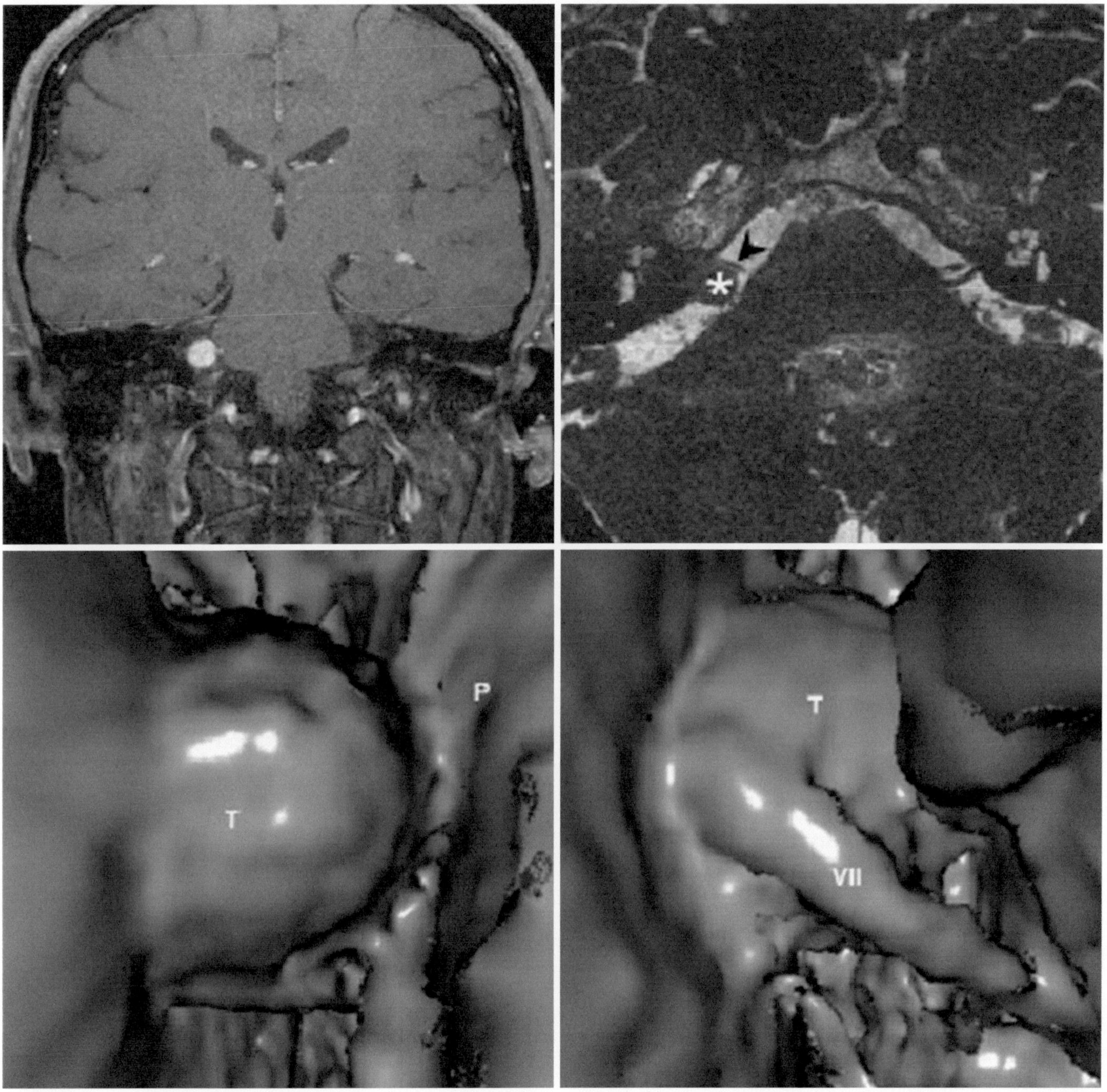

Fig. 3.3 Coronal (top left) gadolinium-enhanced T1-weighted image with fat saturation shows enhancing ovoid lesions in right CPA. Axial (top right) thin-section CISS image shows fusiform mass (*) in right internal auditory canal and CPA. Facial nerve (arrow). Virtual (bottom left) MR endoscopy image of the right CPA seen in cranial-to-caudal projection. Tumor (T) and pons (P). Virtual (bottom right) MR endoscopy image of the right CPA seen in anterior-to-posterior projection reveals facial nerve (VII) is displaced and compressed over anterior surface of the tumor (T). (Reproduced with permission from *American Journal of Roentgenology*. Photos courtesy of Parizel PM, Nowe V, and Van de Heyning PH)

Screening Studies

At present, there are no universally accepted guidelines on screening in patients with asymmetrical sensorineural hearing loss (SNHL), with clinical presentation being used by most otolaryngologists [9]. Clinical concern for a predominant sensory component to hearing loss directs attention to the cochlea and cochlear nerve (CN VIII). When there is concern about a traumatic or congenital cause of sensory or cochlear hearing loss, unenhanced CT of the temporal bones is likely the most useful initial examination [10]. If there is concern about a cochlear lesion or an inflammatory process such as labyrinthitis, MRI of the internal auditory canals with gadolinium would likely be of greater benefit than CT.

In the case of a clinically presumed neural or retrocochlear cause of hearing loss, MRI is the preferred modality for screening [11]. The Congress of Neurological Surgeons (CNS) Systematic Review and Evidence-Based Guideline on Otologic and Audiologic Screening for Patients with Vestibular Schwannomas recommends the following: MRI screening on patients with ≥10 dB of interaural difference at two or more contiguous frequencies or ≥15 dB at one frequency. However, selectively screening patients with ≥15 dB of interaural difference at 3000 Hz alone may minimize the incidence of MRIs performed that do not diagnose a vestibular schwannoma. It is recommended to use MRI to evaluate patients with asymmetric tinnitus and patients with a verified sudden sensorineural hearing loss on an audiogram. However, this practice is low yield in terms of vestibular schwannoma diagnosis (<1% and <3%, respectively) [12].

The best MRI protocol for screening this patient population is debated. The current gold standard for diagnosis and surveillance in patients with suspected vestibular schwannoma is gadolinium-enhanced T1-weighted MRI. However, high-resolution T2-weighted (HRT2) MRI, such as 3D constructive interference in steady state (CISS) or fast imaging employing steady-state acquisition–cycled phases (FIESTA), has been suggested as a lower-cost alternative to T1-weighted MRI for screening of patients with suspected vestibular schwannoma. CISS and FIESTA are fully refocused steady-state gradient echo sequences that combine separate, balanced, steady-state free precession images acquired with different radiofrequency pulses [13, 14]. These HRT2 MR images provide high spatial resolution without the use of contrast agents [15]. Crowson and colleagues showed that a noncontrast vestibular schwannoma screening MRI protocol utilizing HRT2 MRI is more cost-effective than a full MRI with contrast protocol when evaluating for a vestibular schwannoma in adult patients presenting with asymmetric hearing loss. Screening with HRT2 MRI likely also involves shorter exam times.

Yet, further studies are needed to confirm the relative performance of HRT2 screening protocols for vestibular schwannomas [16]. While T2-weighted imaging alone has a high diagnostic accuracy for detection of CPA lesions larger than 2 mm, lesions smaller than 2 mm as well as rare differential diagnoses may be missed on T2-weighted imaging only [17]. Other studies showed no significant differences for sensitivity and specificity when utilizing T2-weighted MRI alone versus conventional gadolinium-enhanced MRI of the CPA [18, 19]. Other investigators have shown that HRT2 is either not superior or should be used as a complementary investigative tool to gadolinium-enhanced MRI [20–23]. We recommend that postcontrast T1-weighted MRI should be considered in patients with a known history of inflammatory, infectious, or malignant disorders, or a broader variety of symptoms [17].

General Classification of Lesions

Extraaxial Lesions

When evaluating lesions of the CPA, it is critical to determine whether they are located extraaxially, extradurally, or intraaxially. At times, it can be difficult to discern the exact origin of a lesion. However, certain imaging findings can be used to suggest an extraaxial rather than an intraaxial location: (1) ipsilateral enlargement of the CPA cistern, (2) CSF or a vascular cleft between the mass and cerebellum, and (3) buckling of the gray–white matter interface adjacent to the mass (Fig. 3.4). Neither simple contiguity to a bony or dural surface nor vasogenic edema in the adjacent parenchyma of the posterior fossa is a reliable predictor of intraaxial versus extraaxial masses [24].

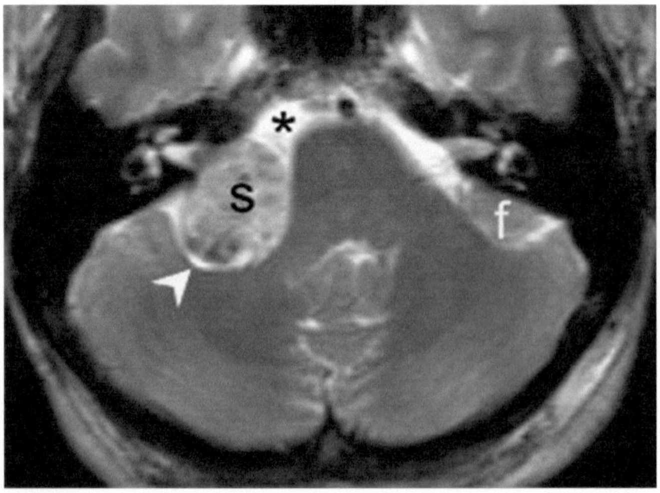

Fig. 3.4 Axial T2-weighted MRI shows a right CPA lesion with classic findings of an extraaxial mass (S). Enlargement of the ipsilateral CPA cistern (*), presence of a CSF cleft between the mass and cerebellum (*arrowhead*), and buckling of the gray–white matter interface. Within the left CPA is a pseudolesion created by the flocculus of the cerebellum (f)

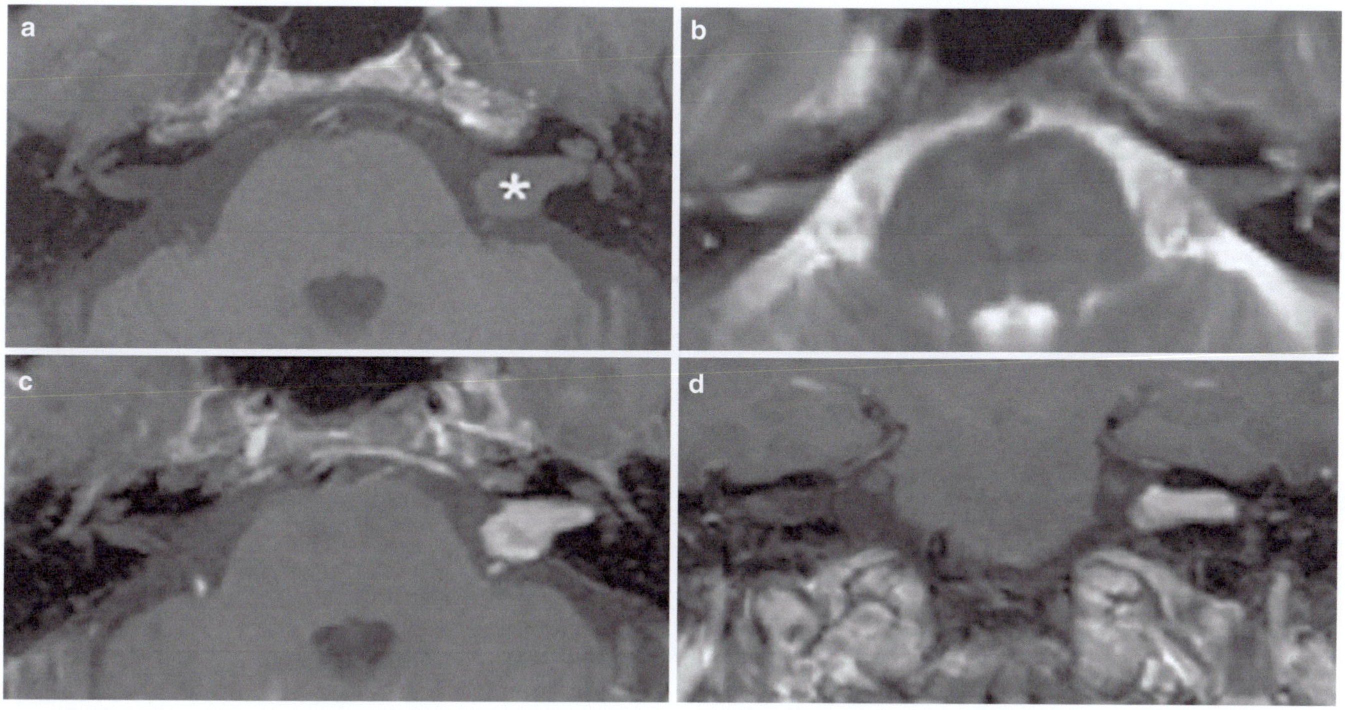

Fig. 3.5 (**a**) T1- and (**b**) T2-weighted MRIs show an extraaxial mass (*) with both intracanalicular and CPA cistern components. This lesion avidly enhances on (**c**) axial and (**d**) coronal images after gadolinium administration and is consistent with schwannoma

Most lesions are extraaxial, and schwannomas and meningiomas are the two most common. Of these two, acoustic schwannomas are by far the most common, accounting for 85–90% of the lesions of the CPA [25–28].

Schwannomas are typically isointense to mildly hypointense to adjacent brainstem parenchyma on T1-weighted MRI and hyperintense on T2-weighted MRI with avid enhancement after gadolinium administration (Fig. 3.5) [29, 30]. The morphology of a lesion depends on its size and origin. Findings range from complete containment within a normal-sized internal auditory canal to expansion of the internal auditory canal, with or without an exophytic component, into the cistern of the CPA [26, 31]. Because these lesions usually grow slowly, the exophytic component involving the CPA can be quite large at presentation. There can be uniform enhancement of schwannomas of any size, but areas of heterogeneity or intratumoral cysts can be seen within lesions [32]. In fact, the presence of intratumoral cysts suggests the diagnosis of acoustic schwannoma rather than meningioma.

Several helpful imaging signs on CT and MRI have been described in the literature to distinguish vestibular schwannomas from CPA meningiomas (Table 3.1). Although meningiomas are the most common nonglial primary brain tumor, only 10% occur in the posterior fossa [33, 34]. Like schwannomas, meningiomas enhance intensely. Their signal intensity on T1- and T2-weighted MRIs can vary, but meningiomas are usually isointense to brainstem parenchyma on T1-weighted images with varied signal intensity on T2-weighted images [35]. Atypical meningiomas arising from and completely contained within the internal auditory canal have been reported [36, 37]. However, meningiomas are usually centered eccentrically to the porus acusticus, whereas typical schwannomas are centered over the porus acusticus when a CPA component is present [38]. Meningiomas tend to have a similar shape with a broad-

Table 3.1 Imaging signs on CT and MRI to distinguish vestibular schwannomas from CPA meningiomas

CPA meningioma	Vestibular schwannoma
Sessile tumor	Globular tumor morphology
Isointense to brainstem parenchyma on T1-weighted MRI with varied signal intensity on T2-weighted MRI	Isointense to mildly hypointense to brainstem parenchyma on T1-weighted MRI and hyperintense on T2-weighted MRI
Broad-base against petrous bone or tentorium	Canalicular component in association with dilation of the internal auditory canal
Formation of an obtuse angle with the petrous temporal bone	Formation of an acute angle by the anterolateral or posterolateral tumor border with the adjacent petrous bone
Homogeneous contrast enhancement	Microhemorrhages on T2-weighted gradient echo
Dural tail	Decreased vestibular signal intensity on 3D-FIESTA [46]
Intratumoral calcification	
Hyperostotic changes	

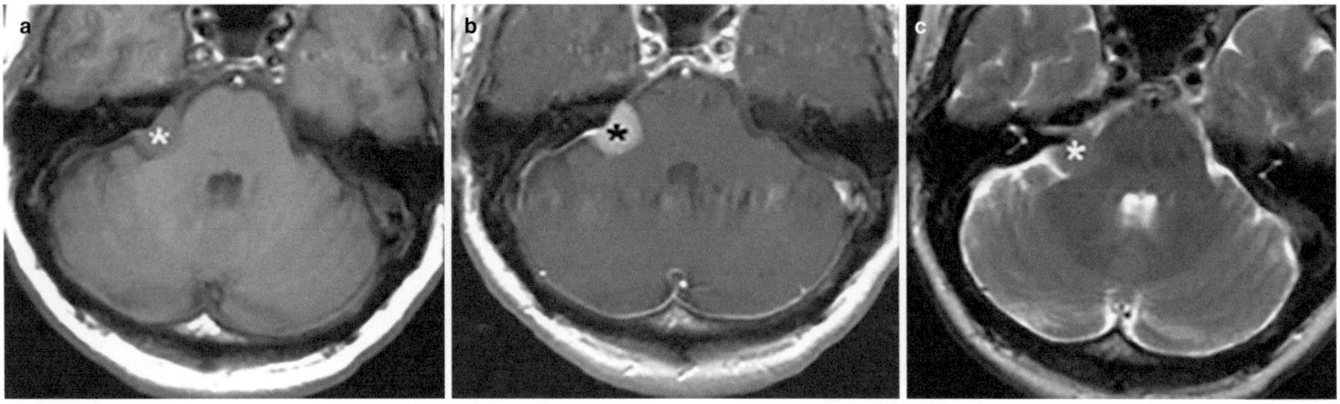

Fig. 3.6 (**a**) Axial T1-weighted, (**b**) T1-weighted postgadolinium, and (**c**) T2-weighted MRIs show a right CPA lesion (*) that is isointense to adjacent gray matter and associated with a broad-based dural attachment that enhances intensely and uniformly

based dural attachment [30, 39]. This "dural tail" is a sign associated with and suggestive of meningioma. However, by no means is it sensitive or specific for meningioma. The dural tail has been described in numerous other entities, including schwannomas (Fig. 3.6) [40, 41]. Thus, it is not surprising that approximately 25% of CPA meningiomas are mistaken for vestibular schwannoma [42].

Differentiation of nonacoustic schwannomas from vestibular schwannomas is largely dependent on the location of the tumor and the associated foraminal widening [43]. Facial nerve schwannomas are rare lesions that account for less than 1% of temporal bone tumors. Such schwannomas are typically multisegmental, that is, involving segments of the facial nerve distal to the meatal segment. This can be a clue to the diagnosis; however, it requires MRI for detailed evaluation. CT can be advantageous for demonstrating osseous changes, but CT can underestimate the number of segments involved [44]. It is challenging to differentiate facial nerve schwannomas involving the internal acoustic canal or cisternal segments from vestibular schwannomas [45].

The two most common nonenhancing lesions of the CPA are arachnoid cysts and epidermoids [25]. Classically, both lesions follow the signal intensity of CSF on T1- and T2-weighted imaging with no intralesional enhancement [47]. FLAIR and diffusion-weighted imaging (DWI) are helpful sequences for differentiating these two lesions [48–52]. FLAIR imaging is a T2-weighted sequence that attenuates the signal from free fluid. Therefore, on FLAIR imaging free fluid such as CSF is hypointense compared with the hyperintensity of CSF seen on conventional T2-weighted spin-echo images. Classically, arachnoid cysts follow the signal intensity of CSF on all pulse sequences, including FLAIR and DWI. On DWI, epidermoid tumors demonstrate diffusion restriction and slight signal hyperintensity on FLAIR sequences (Fig. 3.7) [53].

Although uncommon, lipomas of the CPA have characteristic findings on both CT and MRI and are worth mentioning. On CT, the attenuation of a lipoma is the same as fat [54, 55]. Consequently, the attenuation of lipomas is uniformly markedly decreased. This pattern could be mistaken for pneumocephalus if the diagnosis of lipoma is not considered. Fat content can be verified by placing Hounsfield units (HU) on the area of interest and obtaining values in the expected range of fat (HU: −120 to −90). Lipomas are inherently hyperintense on T1-weighted and T2-weighted MRIs. This finding could lead to confusion if postgadolinium images are viewed in isolation. A seemingly avidly enhancing mass would be seen as actually nonenhancing when compared with noncontrasted images. Techniques such as fat suppression are used to verify the fatty content of a lipoma (Fig. 3.8).

Given this list of imaging characteristics of extraaxial masses, a general algorithm for evaluating tumors of the CPA is presented in Fig. 3.9.

Vascular Lesions

Vascular lesions of the CPA that can cause compressive symptomatology include dolichoectasia of the vertebrobasilar circulation, posterior circulation aneurysms (Fig. 3.10), and vascular loops. Clinically, pure vertebrobasilar dolichoectasia associated with severe compression of the adjacent brainstem is rarely symptomatic but can be associated with subclinical dysfunction [56]. Nonetheless, compression of cranial nerves within the CPA is well described clinically,

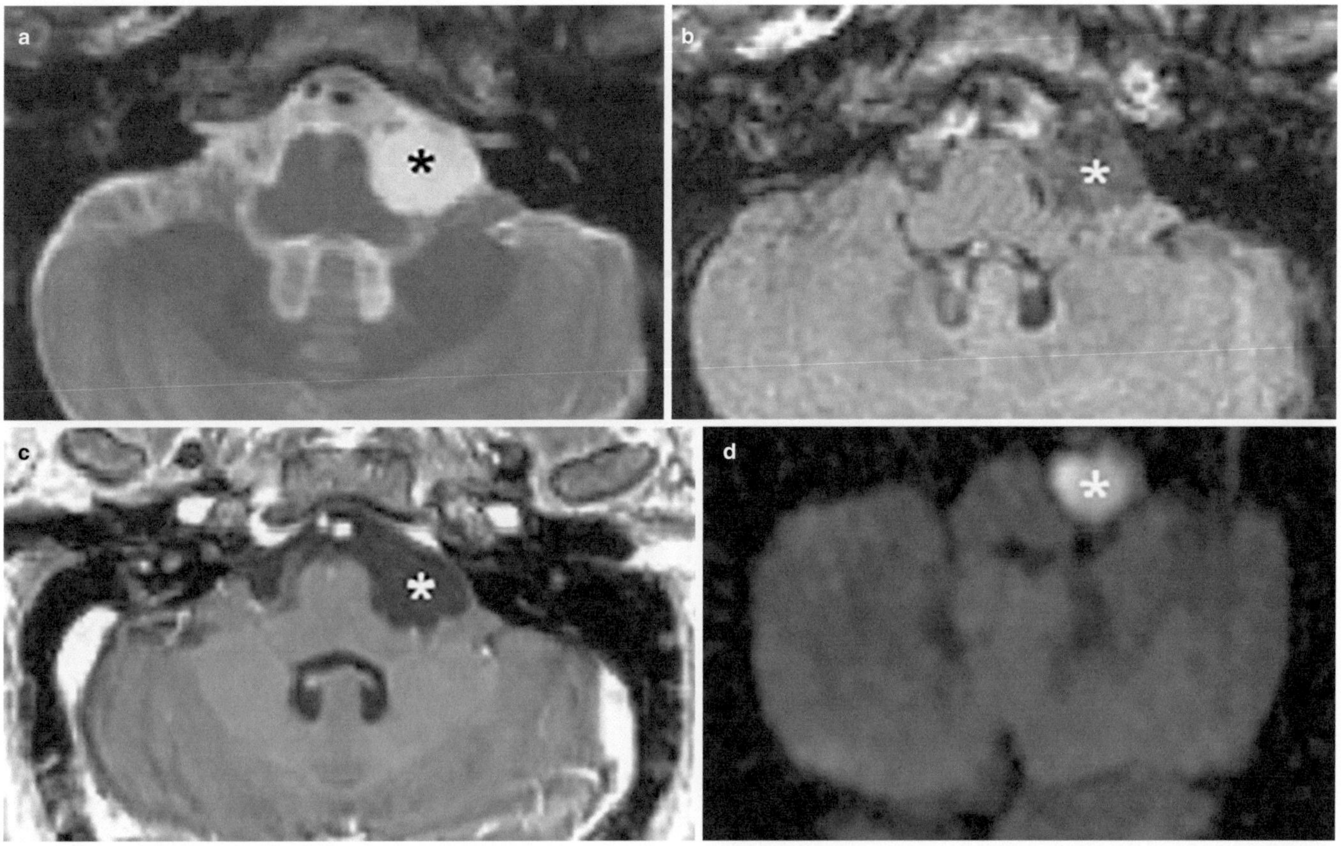

Fig. 3.7 Cystic lesion (*) of the left CPA is isointense to CSF on (**a**) axial T2-weighted, (**b**) FLAIR, and (**c**) T1-weighted postgadolinium images. The lesion could represent either an epidermoid or arachnoid cyst. (**d**) On DWI, the lesion demonstrates increased signal intensity, which is consistent with the diagnosis of epidermoid

surgically, and radiographically [57]. Furthermore, mechanical neurovascular compression can occur from normal branches from a normal basilar artery.

The optimal way to image these patients would be with high-resolution, steady-state T2-weighted MRI. In cases of trigeminal neuralgia, this sequence often correctly identifies the offending vessel contact before intervention [58–60]. A recent double-blinded assessment of surgical and radiographic findings demonstrated 76% sensitivity and 75% specificity for identifying compressive vessels in patients with trigeminal neuralgia when conventional 3D time of flight MR angiography was used in conjunction with 3D gadolinium-enhanced spoiled gradient-recalled sequences [60].

It is crucial for skull-base/CPA surgeons to identify vascular lesions as indeed vascular and not to mistake them for a process such as meningioma. Because both lesions can contain calcium and enhance avidly, pulsation artifact on MRI is helpful to identify aneurysms correctly. Conventional angiography is definitive for differentiating the two types of lesions. A detailed review of vascular lesions of the CPA is available elsewhere in this text (see Chap. 21).

Extradural Lesions

Any lesion centered within the temporal bone can extend into the CPA cistern. The most common lesions growing from the temporal bone into the CPA are temporal paragangliomas [61]. Paragangliomas are of interest to radiologists owing to their striking findings of an avidly enhancing mass that demonstrates areas of hypo- and hyperintensity on T1- and T2-weighted MRI. This appearance has been labeled a salt-and-pepper pattern [62]. It is caused by the hypertrophied vascular supply and multiple flow voids within and adjacent to the lesion.

Combined CT and MRI tend to be helpful in evaluating cholesterol granulomas of the petrous apex. On CT, choles-

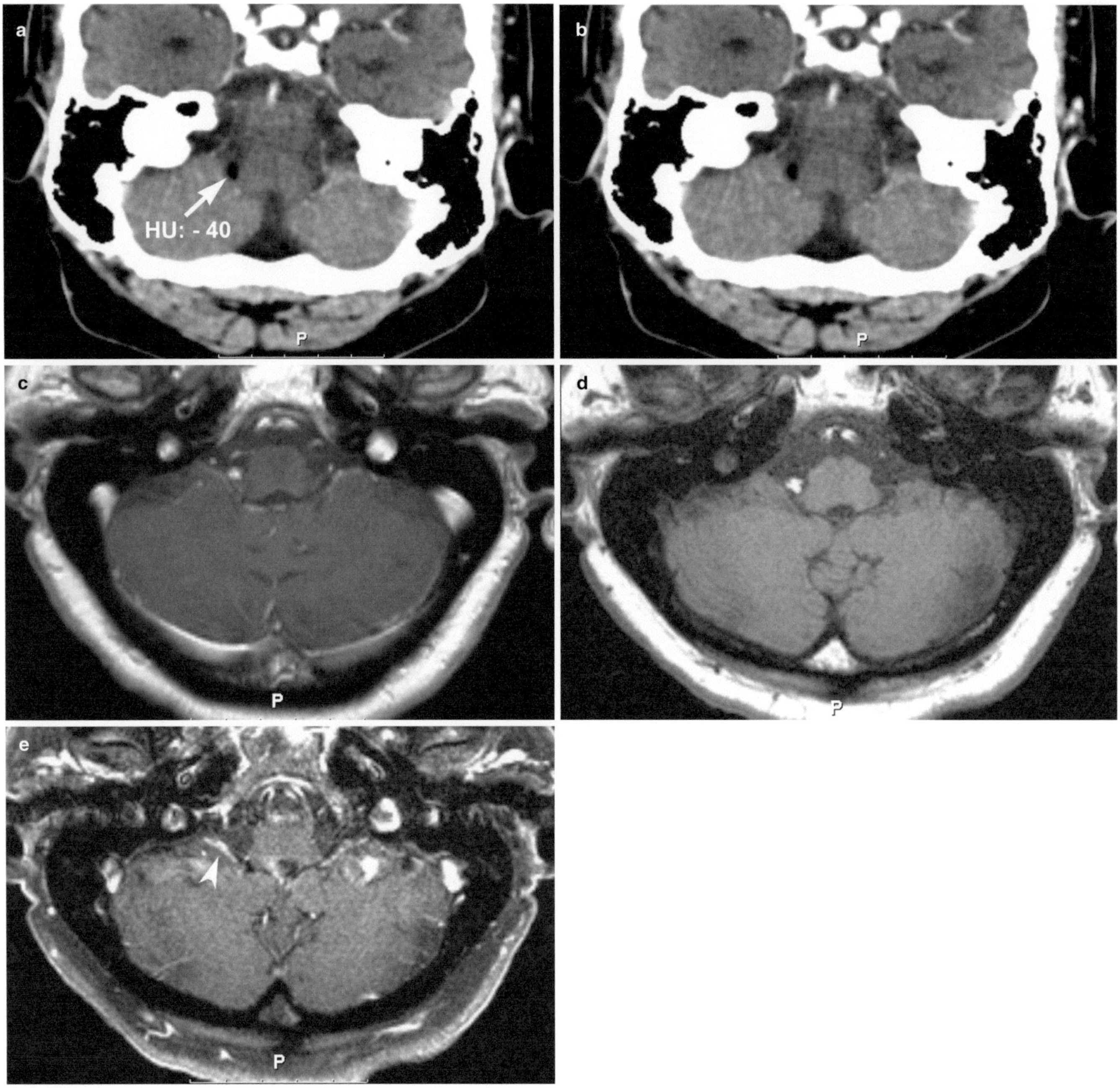

Fig. 3.8 Right CPA lipoma (*arrow*). (**a**, **b**) CTs show a nonenhancing, homogenously low-attenuation lesion with Hounsfield units within the range for fat. (**c**) On contrast-enhanced T1-weighted MRI, the mass appears to enhance in the right CPA. (**d**) Noncontrast-enhanced T1-weighted MRI shows an inherently bright lesion, which is verified on (**e**) fat-saturated T1-weighted MRI with subsequent loss of signal in the region of the known mass. The enhancement posterior to the mass is normal choroid plexus (*arrowhead*) and should not be mistaken for a lesion

terol granulomas are well-defined expansile lesions with smoothly marginated, nonaggressive borders. These lesions are homogenous and lytic compared with native bone [63]. After contrast administration, only thin, rim-like peripheral enhancement can be seen [64]. On MRI, cholesterol granulomas have a characteristic appearance attributed to intralesional hemorrhage that results in a hyperintense signal on T1-weighted and T2-weighted MRIs, explained by cholesterol crystals, multinucleated giant cells, and blood products (Fig. 3.11) [65, 66].

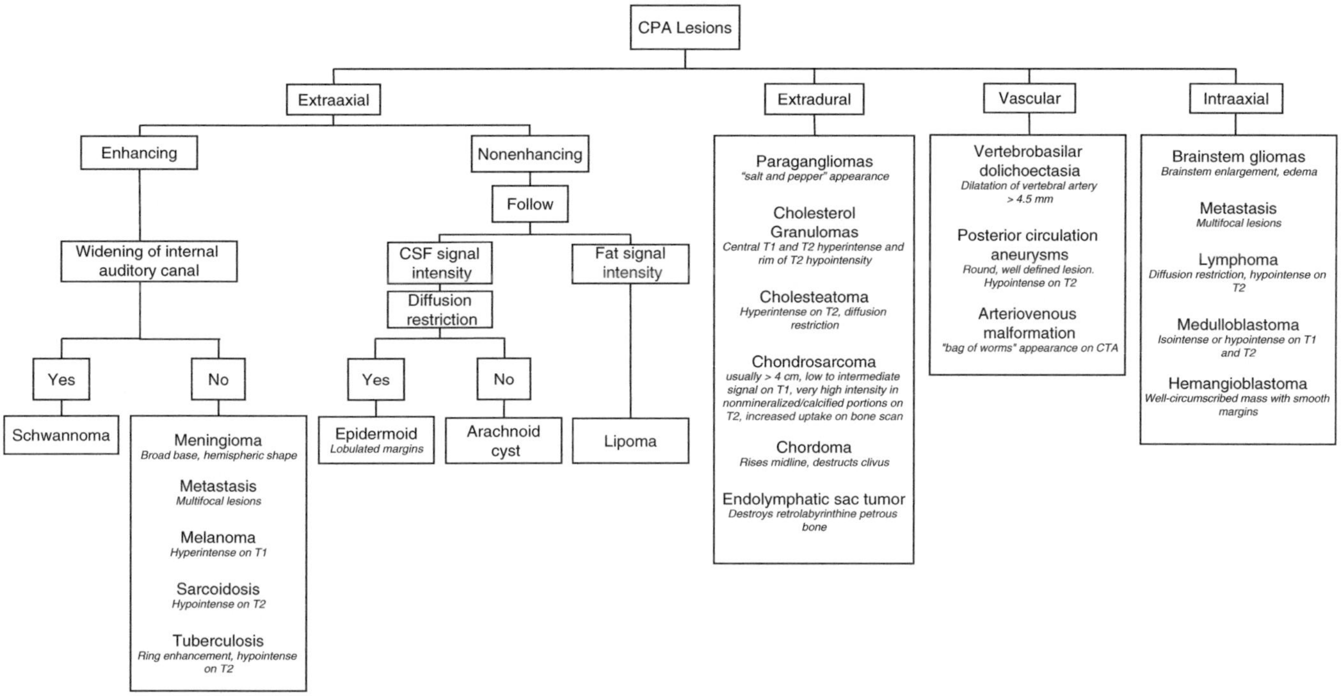

Fig. 3.9 (**a**) Algorithm for evaluating lesions of the CPA. Algorithm shows general MRI characteristics for extraaxial, extradural, vascular, and intraaxial CPA lesions

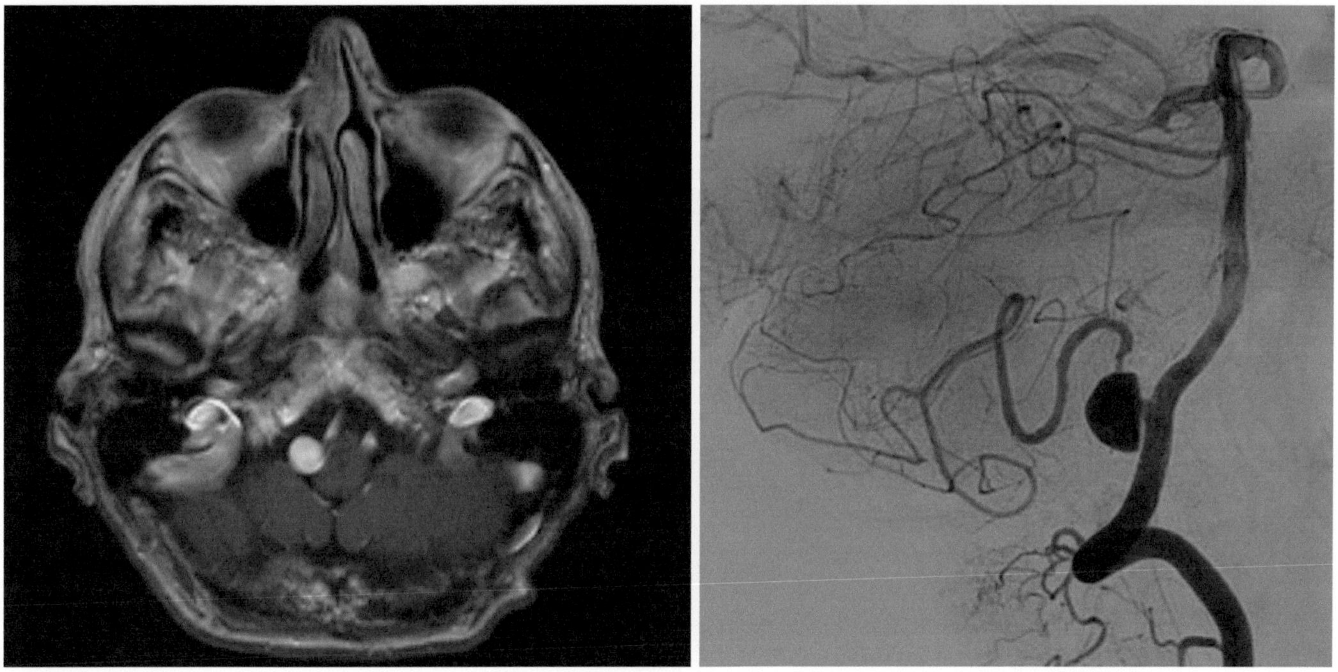

Fig. 3.10 Aneurysm of the right posterior inferior cerebellar artery (PICA). (Left) Axial T1-weighted MR image with gadolinium. (Right) Digital subtraction angiogram showing the PICA aneurysm

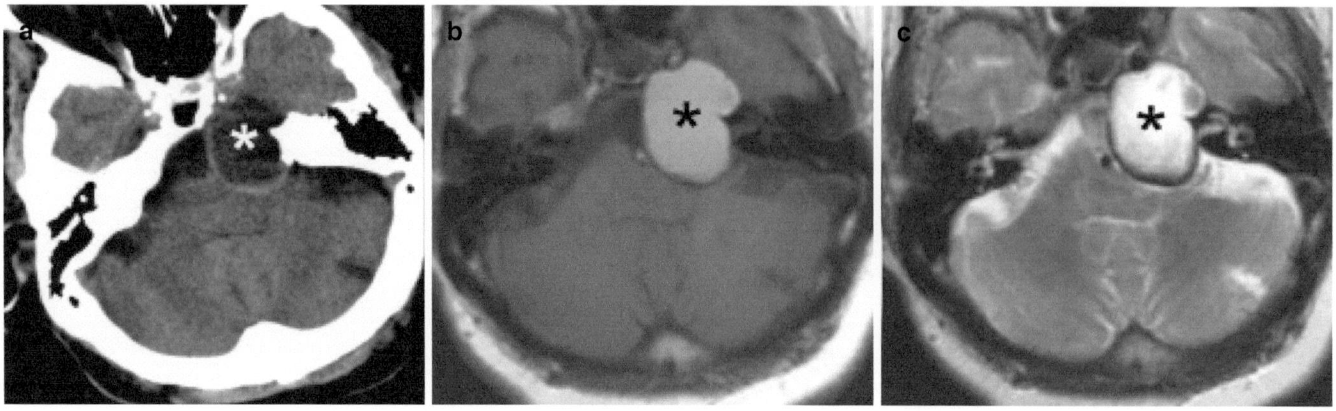

Fig. 3.11 (**a**) Noncontrast-enhanced CT shows an expansile, lytic lesion (*) of the left petrous apex extending into the left CPA. (**b**) Noncontrast-enhanced T1- and (**c**) T2-weighted images show the same lesion with increased signal intensity on both pulse sequences and rim of hypointense signal due to hemosiderin deposition, consistent with a cholesterol granuloma

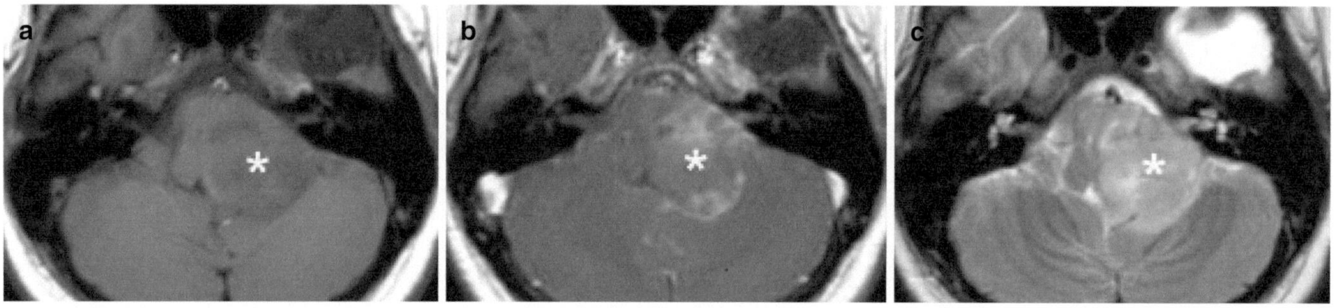

Fig. 3.12 Axial (**a**) T1-weighted, (**b**) T1-weighted postgadolinium, and (**c**) T2-weighted MRI show an exophytic brainstem glioblastoma multiforme (*) growing into the left CPA cistern

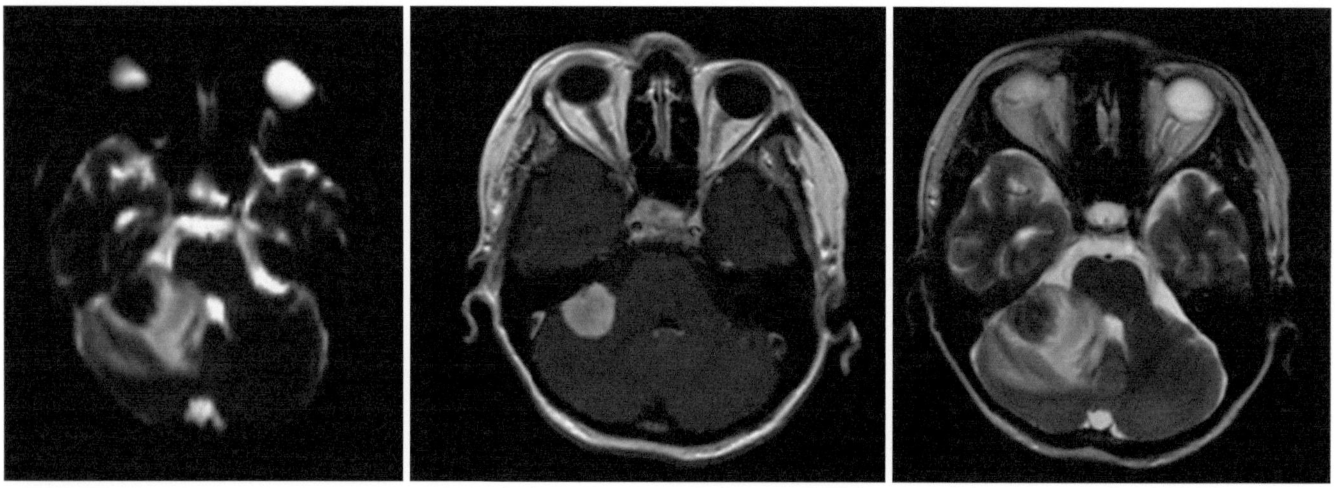

Fig. 3.13 Axial (left) ADC map of DWI sequence, (center) postcontrast T1-weighted, and (right) T2-weighted MR images demonstrate a right CPA lymphoma

Intraaxial Lesions

In adults, lesions less commonly encountered within the CPA are intraaxial posterior fossa masses associated with exophytic growth into the CPA. Brainstem gliomas have been shown to grow into the CPA (Fig. 3.12) [67]. Other possible intraaxial lesions within the CPA are metastasis, lymphoma (Fig. 3.13), medulloblastoma (Fig. 3.14), and hemangioblastoma (Fig. 3.15). However, the most common pathologic entity seen intraaxially in patients with CPA symptomatology, specifically sensorineural hearing loss (SNHL), is demyelination from a process such as multiple sclerosis [68].

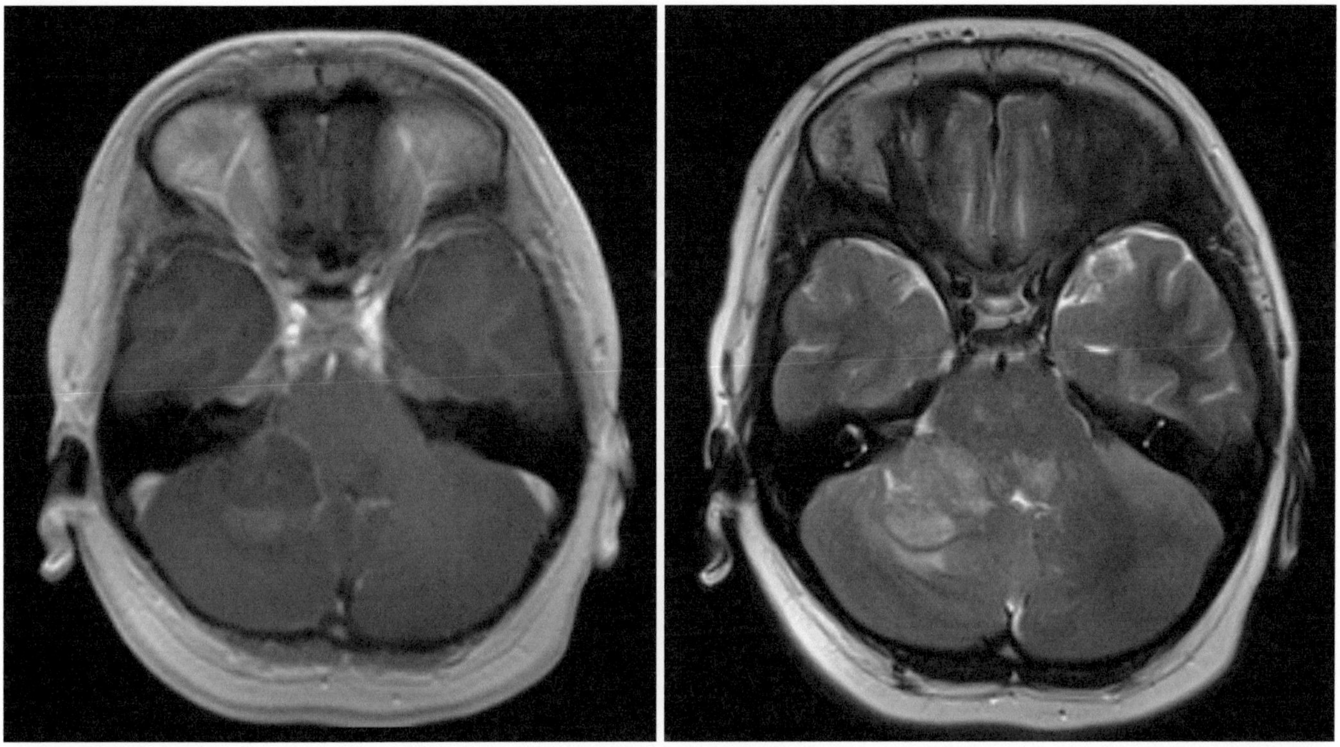

Fig. 3.14 Axial postcontrast (left) T1-weighted and (right) T2-weighted MR images show an intraaxial mass in the right middle cerebellar peduncle/CPA. Pathology confirmed a medulloblastoma

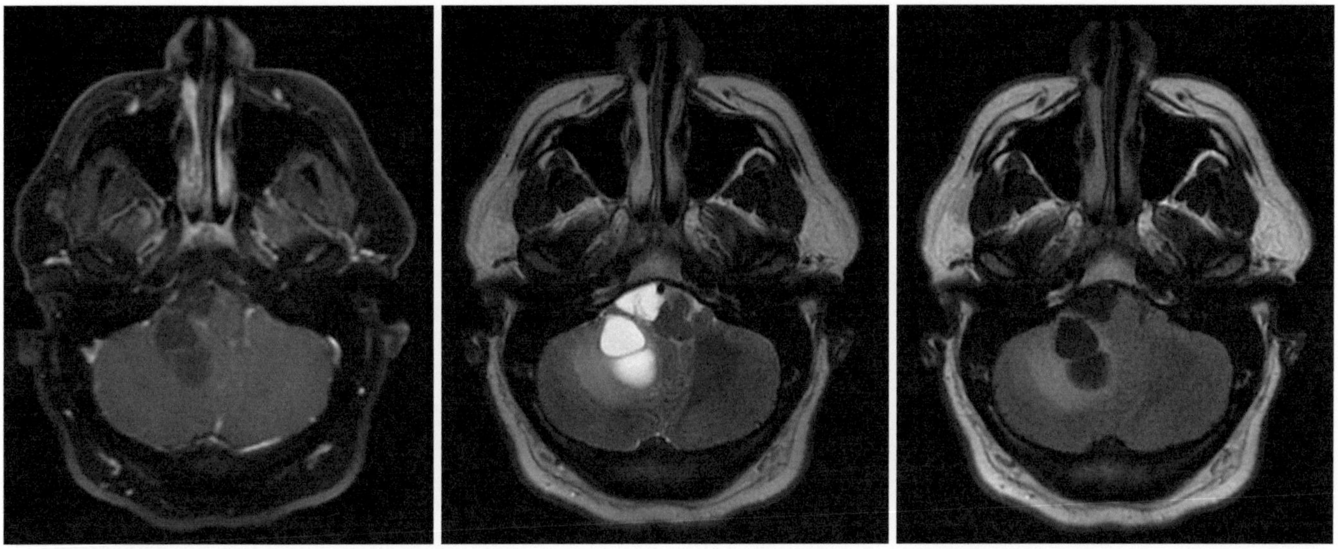

Fig. 3.15 Axial postcontrast (left) T1-weighted, (center) T2-weighted, and FLAIR T2-weighted (right) MR images show a cystic intraaxial mass in the right cerebellum/CPA. Pathology confirmed a hemangioblastoma

Angiography

With continued advances in cross-sectional and multiplanar imaging, the role of angiography in the initial diagnostic evaluation of lesions of the CPA has diminished. Typically, DSA is used to evaluate lesions with a diagnosis known or highly suspected based on prior imaging, patient demographics, and symptomatology. DSA can be used to examine the vascularity of these lesions and to define their anatomy further.

Anatomic delineation is critical when evaluating intracranial aneurysms for treatment. Traditionally, DSA has been the only reasonable tool for the precise definition of aneurysmal anatomy. DSA remains the gold standard in aneurysm evaluation [69, 70]. With the continued ability to decrease slice thickness, and thereby improve resolution, and with improved data-processing capabilities, the quality of CTA is approaching the standard set by catheter-based angiography [71–73]. In some studies, CTA surpassed the capabilities of the latter. In prospective studies, CTA has been used as the primary diagnostic tool; DSA has served to clarify equivocal findings with good result [74, 75].

The obvious advantage of catheter-based angiography is the ability to intervene. The goals of endovascular intervention can be divided into adjuvant therapies and definitive treatments. Definitive endovascular therapies include detachable coil embolization of posterior circulation saccular aneurysms and intentional parent vessel sacrifice to treat fusiform or dissecting aneurysms.

Adjuvant endovascular therapy mainly consists of pre-therapeutic embolization. Lesions well suited to preoperative embolization include paragangliomas that extend from the skull-base into the CPA. Traditionally, surgical resection of paragangliomas has been associated with a high risk of neurovascular injury. Stroke or excessive blood loss results from the hypervascular nature of these lesions and their location adjacent to vital neurovascular structures [76]. Preoperative embolization of paragangliomas with polyvinyl alcohol particles and *N*-butyl-2-cyanoacrylate (NBCA), for example, effectively reduces operative bleeding and reduces the length of the operative procedure [77–79].

Of course, the inherent risk of embolization should be assessed with diagnostic angiography to identify potentially harmful intracranial anastomoses and hence detailed anatomic knowledge is essential [80]. Provocative testing with intraarterial lidocaine can assess the potential for cranial nerve damage and guide embolization technique. Even if no clear dangerous intracranial anastomosis is identified with DSA, the presence of embolic material penetrating the lesion can lead to flow alterations that cause dangerous anastomoses to open. Furthermore, complications can occur from the reflux of embolic material into the parent artery. Nevertheless, percutaneous injections of NBCA into cervical paragangliomas and into jugular paragangliomas have been successful [81].

Meningiomas can also benefit from preoperative embolization with similar goals of reducing operative times and blood loss. Again, there is always a risk of endovascular embolization, including transient or permanent neurological deficits, difficulty with postoperative skin healing, and the potential for excessive radiation exposure [82, 83].

Preoperative and Follow-Up Imaging

Preoperative Imaging of Vestibular Schwannomas

The Congress of Neurological Surgeons Systematic Review and Evidence-Based Guideline on the Role of Imaging in the Diagnosis and Management of Patients with Vestibular Schwannomas recommends that preoperative surveillance for growth of a vestibular schwannoma should be followed with either contrast-enhanced 3D T1 magnetization prepared rapid acquisition gradient echo (MPRAGE) or HRT2 MRI [84]. HRT2 CISS imaging does exhibit equal characterization of tumor size as postcontrast T1-weighted imaging [85, 86]. However, T2 CISS imaging does not appear to supplant postcontrast T1-weighted imaging for identifying regions of necrosis and understanding internal tumor architecture [14].

If a "watch and wait" philosophy is pursued, the Congress of Neurological Surgeons (CNS) Systematic Review and Evidence-Based Guideline recommends that MRI should be obtained annually for 5 years, with interval lengthening thereafter with tumor stability [84]. The cochlear signal on FLAIR images is an additional parameter to evaluate when monitoring the degree of functional impairment during follow-up of patients with small acoustic neuromas confined to the internal auditory canals [87].

Investigators have attempted to identify preoperative radiologic features that may predict tumor consistency and functional results following vestibular schwannoma surgery. The extent of lateral internal auditory canal involvement should be emphasized when interpreting imaging for preoperative planning because the degree of canal involvement adversely affects facial nerve and hearing outcomes [84]. Moreover, widening of the internal auditory canal on bony CT scan may also predict whether the tumor is firm or soft [88]. Some investigators found that firm schwannomas were more likely to be hypointense, while soft schwannomas were more likely to be hyperintense [89]. In contrast, other investigators found no significant correlation between intraoperative vestibular schwannoma consistency and tumor intensity in T2-weighted imaging [88].

Identification of the facial nerve during vestibular schwannoma surgery is imperative. However, in large vestibular schwannomas, the nerve can be morphologically changed and/or displaced by the tumor in an unpredictable manner. Various studies have explored the optimal imaging sequence to augment visualization of the facial nerve and to predict the position of the facial and vestibulocochlear nerves in relation to the vestibular schwannoma. These imaging modalities include T1-weighted with contrast MR sequences as well as specialized T2-weighted sequences, such as CISS and diffusion tensor imaging-based fiber tracking (DTT) [84, 90–92].

T2-based MRI sequences can be used to delineate the course of the facial nerve in small vestibular schwannomas with a sensitivity of 63–90% [20, 93, 94]. However, visualization of the course of the facial nerve is more challenging in tumors larger than 25 mm. In an effort to predict the location of the facial nerve in very large (>50 mm) facial nerve schwannomas, Jung and colleagues integrated contrast-enhanced T1 and T2 sequences and extrapolated the location of the facial nerve based on the appearance of intrameatal and extrameatal portions of the tumor. Using this strategy, the direction of the facial nerve displacement was accurate in 80% of cases [93].

CISS has been shown to successfully identify cisternal and canalicular segments of both the vestibulocochlear and facial nerves in 100% of the cases in a study of 48 normal subjects and 8 patients with facial or vestibulocochlear pathology. Preoperative DTT of the facial nerve has shown 100% congruence between preoperative DTT prediction and intraoperative findings [95, 96]. However, a lower concordance rate of 71.4% was reported in a different study by Taoka and colleagues [97]. A combined approach of both DTT and CISS imaging resulted in a 90.9% concordance between preoperative prediction of the cisternal segment of the facial nerve in relation to the tumor, and intraoperative findings [91].

To conclude, the course of the facial nerve may be determined on preoperative MRI, especially with T2-weighted sequences and with tractography reconstruction. However, the reliability of these predictions remains to be established, and further research is necessary to develop the technology as a standard scheme for facial nerve visualization.

Follow-Up Assessment After Treatment of Vestibular Schwannomas

Regardless of the chosen clinical management path, serial T1-weighted MRI is the mainstay for monitoring tumor growth (or regrowth) in observation or postprimary intervention. The exact surveillance algorithm varies, but most reports suggest a role for postoperative imaging at 1 and 5 years [84]. Objectives for follow-up imaging include identification of residual or recurrent tumor, assessment of tumor size, response to radiation therapy, and the presence of post-therapeutic complications such as infarcts, hemorrhage, or sinus thrombosis (Fig. 3.16).

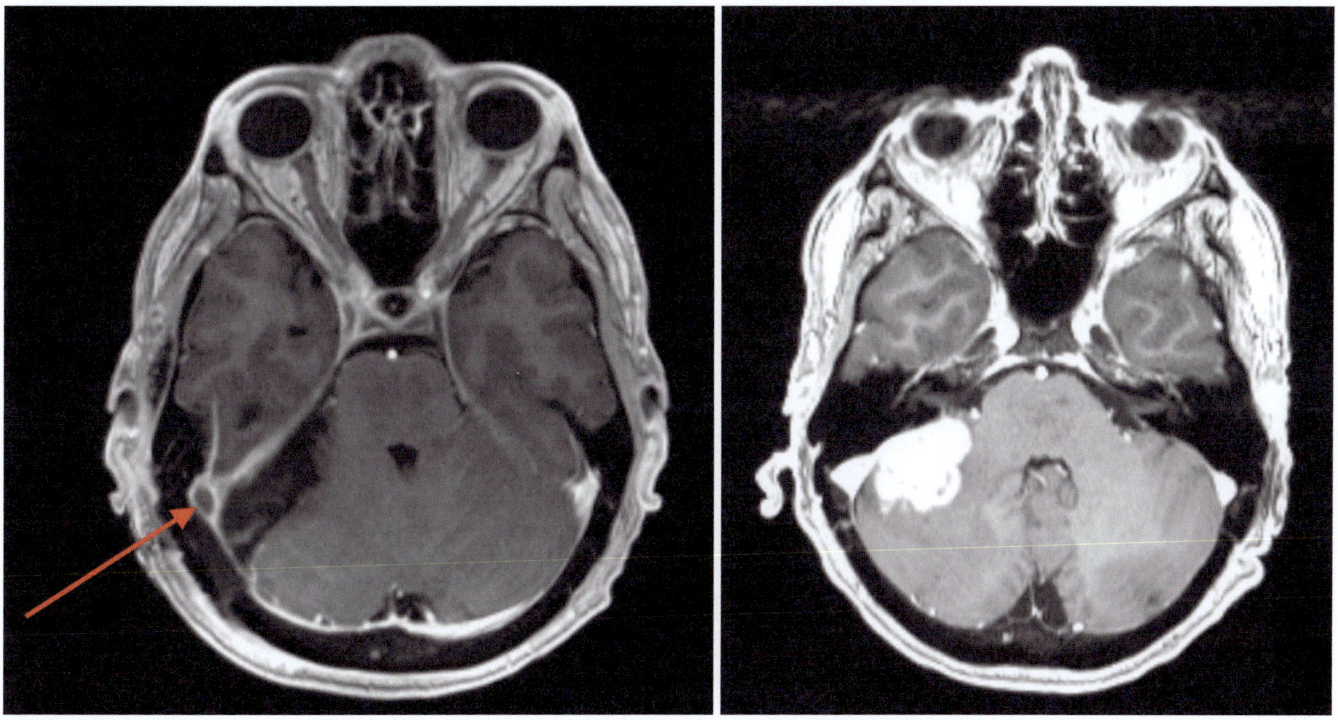

Fig. 3.16 (Left) Axial postcontrast T1-weighted MR image shows postoperative sinus thrombosis in the right transverse sinus after a retrosigmoid approach for removal of a metastatic adenocarcinoma. (Right) Preoperative axial postcontrast T1-weighted MR image shows no thrombus

Patients receiving gross total resection should undergo a postoperative MRI to document the surgical impression, but this may occur as late as 1 year after surgery. More frequent surveillance scans are suggested for patients not receiving gross total resection, such as annual MRI scans for a period of 5 years. Nodular enhancement on postcontrast imaging is suspicious for recurrence, and continued surveillance is necessary if any change in nodular enhancement is demonstrated [84]. If muscle is used to close the surgical defect, postoperative changes may mimic enhancing tumor and should therefore be correlated clinically [98]. Postoperative imaging of the facial nerve may vary, making the evaluation of patients with postoperative facial nerve paralysis challenging. The facial nerve may be stretched and displaced in large tumors. However, poor or absent visualization of the facial nerve does not necessarily indicate injury or transection [98].

In general, vestibular schwannomas associated with neurofibromatosis type-2 should be imaged more frequently due to a more variable growth rate for these lesions. When one of two bilateral schwannomas is resected, the rate of growth of the remaining vestibular schwannoma may increase, and therefore more frequent imaging may be indicated [99, 100]. One study demonstrated an almost doubling of the contralateral tumor growth rate following resection of one of the bilateral tumors (2.5 ± 2.2 vs 4.4 ± 3.4 mm/year) [100].

Following stereotactic radiosurgery (SRS), follow-up imaging had been performed at 6-month intervals for less than 2 years, annually for the next 3 years, and biannually thereafter [101]. Of note, the tumor size may temporarily increase after SRS due to intralesional edema [102].

Imaging Pitfalls and Pseudomasses

Artifact from CSF flow and normal structures located within the CPA can mimic pathology (pseudolesions). These structures include the flocculus of the cerebellum, the jugular tubercle, and enhancing choroid plexus extending through the foramen of Luschka.

The flocculus of the cerebellum juts into the CPA cistern. On T2-weighted MRIs, it is made conspicuous by surrounding bright CSF. This tissue is isointense to the adjacent cerebellum on all pulse sequences and fails to demonstrate enhancement after gadolinium administration, which are clues that this structure is normal. On contiguous images, this apparent mass can be connected directly to the cerebellum (Fig. 3.4).

In contrast to the nonenhancing pseudomass caused by the flocculus, the choroid plexus extending through the foramen of Luschka from the fourth ventricle enhances avidly after gadolinium administration. It can be connected to the enhancing choroid plexus from the fourth ventricle (Fig. 3.8).

Similarly, the jugular tubercle of the occipital bone can extend into the CPA cistern. This configuration is most readily seen on CT and can be mistaken for a calcified meningioma. Examination of bone windows will show this apparent exophytic calcified mass to be in direct continuity with the occipital bone (Fig. 3.17).

CSF flow artifact is most readily identified on conventional spin echo (nonvolumetrically acquired or nonsteady state) T2-weighted MRIs [2]. The presence of flow artifact can be determined by the absence of signal abnormality on other sequences of routine imaging and by the absolute absence of an enhancing mass in the CPA (Fig. 3.18).

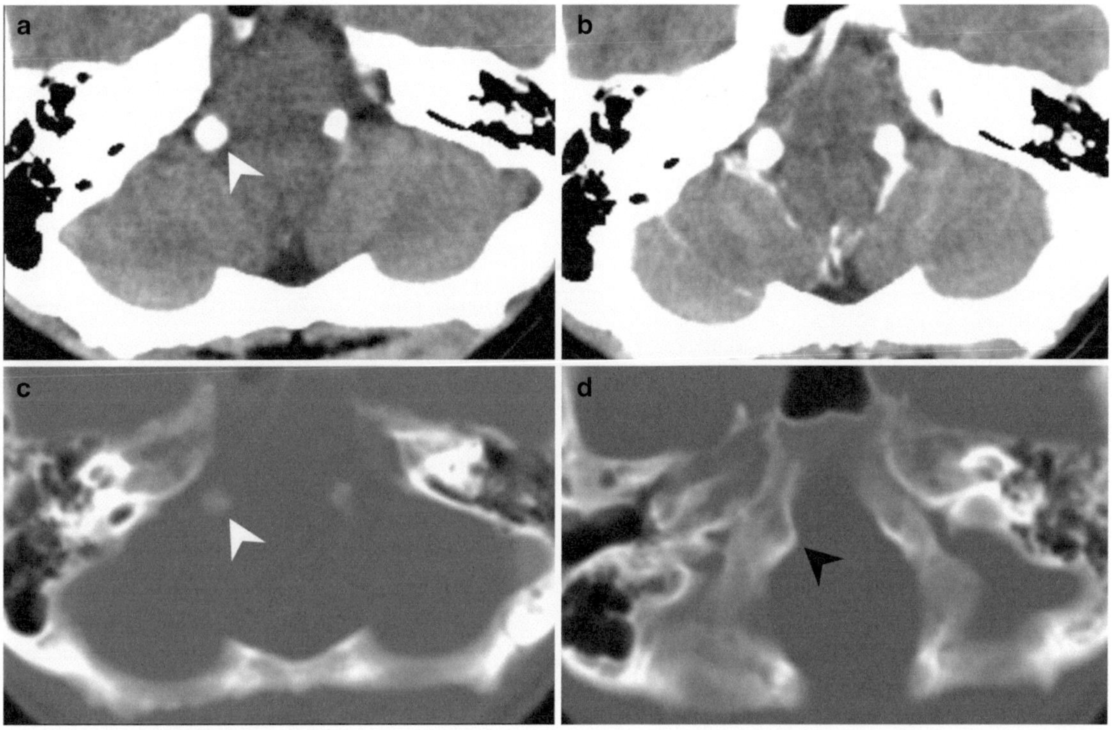

Fig. 3.17 CT (**a**) with and (**b**) without contrast shows a hyperdense lesion in the bilateral CPA (*white arrowhead*). (**c**) Bone window through the same level and (**d**) a contiguous, inferior slice showing continuity with jugular tubercle (*black arrowhead*)

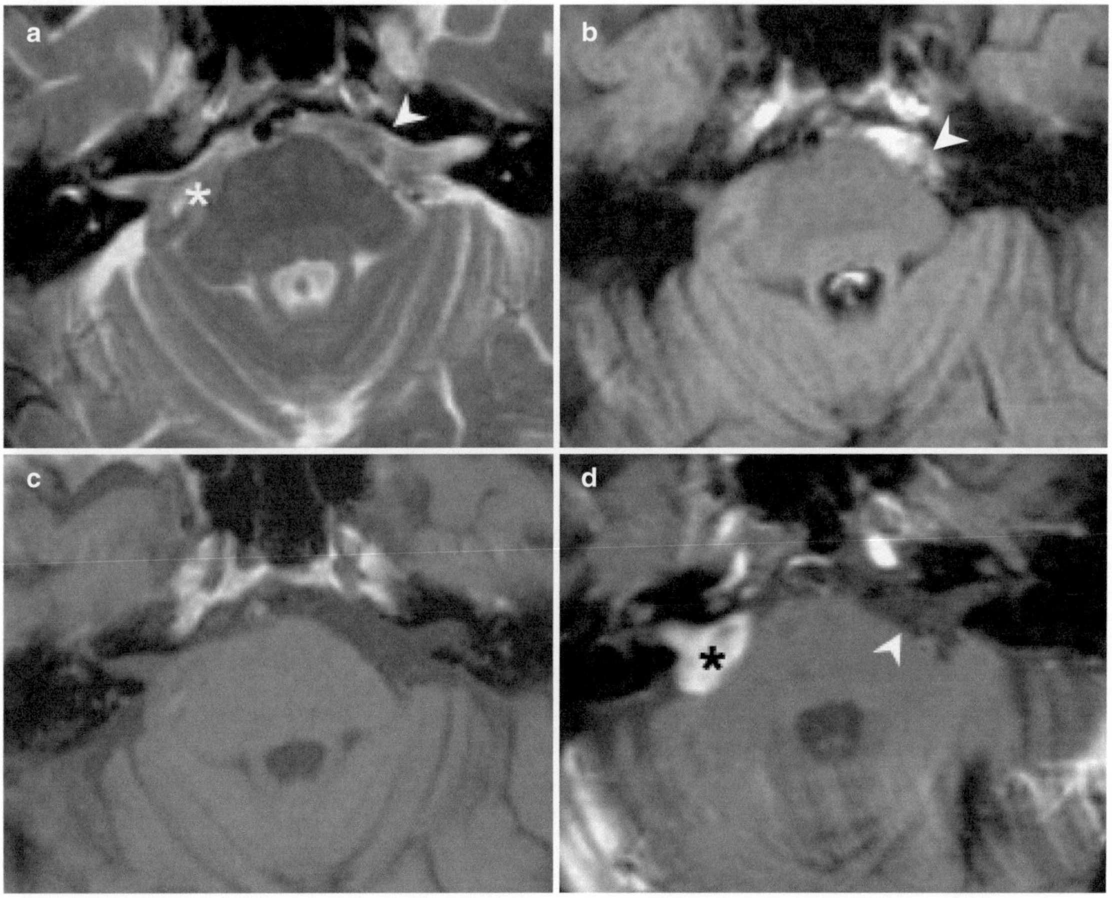

Fig. 3.18 (**a**) T2-weighted and (**b**) FLAIR images show abnormal signal in the left CPA cistern (*arrowhead* and *). T1-weighted (**c**) precontrast and (**d**) postcontrast administration showing no abnormality in the left CPA cistern consistent with flow artifact (*arrowhead*). A schwannoma (Asterisk) is seen in the right CPA cistern

References

1. Schmalbrock P, Brogan MA, Chakeres DW, et al. Optimization of submillimeter-resolution MR imaging methods for the inner ear. J Magn Reson Imaging. 1993;3:451–9.
2. Iwayama E, Naganawa S, Ito T, et al. High-resolution MR cisternography of the cerebellopontine angle: 2D versus 3D fast spin-echo sequences. AJNR Am J Neuroradiol. 1999;20:889–95.
3. Casselman JW, Kuhweide R, Deimling M, et al. Constructive interference in steady state-3DFT MR imaging of the inner ear and cerebellopontine angle. AJNR Am J Neuroradiol. 1993;14:47–57.
4. Guirado CR, Martinez P, Roig R, et al. Three-dimensional MR of the inner ear with steady-state free precession. AJNR Am J Neuroradiol. 1995;16:1909–13.
5. Brogan M, Chakeres DW, Schmalbrock P. High-resolution 3DFT MR imaging of the endolymphatic duct and soft tissues of the otic capsule. AJNR Am J Neuroradiol. 1991;12:1–11.
6. Boor S, Maurer J, Mann W, Stoeter P. Virtual endoscopy of the inner ear and the auditory canal. Neuroradiology. 2000;42:543–7.
7. Diamantopoulos II, Ludman CN, Martel AL, O'Donoghue GM. Magnetic resonance imaging virtual endoscopy of the labyrinth. Am J Otol. 1999;20:748–51.
8. Rabinov JD, Barker FG, McKenna MJ, Curtin HD. Virtual cisternoscopy: 3D MRI models of the cerebellopontine angle for lesions related to the cranial nerves. Skull Base. 2004;14:93–9.
9. Newton JR, Shakeel M, Flatman S, Beattie C, Ram B. Magnetic resonance imaging screening in acoustic neuroma. Am J Otolaryngol. 2010;31:217–20.
10. Mafee M. Acoustic neuroma and other acoustic nerve disorders: role of MRI and CT: an analysis of 238 cases. Semin Ultrasound CT MRI. 1987;8:256–61.
11. Jackler RK, Shapiro MS, Dillon WP, et al. Gadolinium-DTPA enhanced magnetic resonance imaging in acoustic neuroma diagnosis and management. Otolaryngol Head Neck Surg. 1990;102:670–7.
12. Sweeney AD, Carlson ML, Shepard NT, McCracken DJ, Vivas EX, Neff BA, Olson JJ. Congress of neurological surgeons systematic review and evidence-based guidelines on otologic and audiologic screening for patients with vestibular schwannomas. Neurosurgery. 2018;82:E29–31.
13. Kulkarni M. Constructive interference in steady-state/FIESTA-C clinical applications in neuroimaging. J Med Imaging Radiat Oncol. 2011;55:183–90.
14. Ozgen B, Oguz B, Dolgun A. Diagnostic accuracy of the constructive interference in steady state sequence alone for follow-up imaging of vestibular schwannomas. AJR Am J Roentgenol. 2009;30:985–91.
15. Hingwala D, Chatterjee S, Kesavadas C, Thomas B, Kapilamoorthy TR. Applications of 3D CISS sequence for problem solving in neuroimaging. Indian J Radiol Imaging. 2011;21:90–7.
16. Crowson MG, Rocke DJ, Hoang JK, Weissman JL, Kaylie DM. Cost-effectiveness analysis of a non-contrast screening MRI protocol for vestibular schwannoma in patients with asymmetric sensorineural hearing loss. Neuroradiology. 2017;59:727–36.
17. Hentschel MA, Kunst HPM, Rovers MM, Steens SCA. Diagnostic accuracy of high-resolution T2-weighted MRI vs contrast-enhanced T1-weighted MRI to screen for cerebellopontine angle lesions in symptomatic patients. Clin Otolaryngol. 2017; https://doi.org/10.1111/coa.13051. [Epub ahead of print].
18. Allen RW, Harnsberger HR, Shelton C, et al. Low-cost high-resolution fast spin-echo MR of acoustic schwannoma: an alternative to enhanced conventional spin-echo MR? AJNR Am J Neuroradiol. 1996;17:1205–10.
19. Daniels RL, Swallow C, Shelton C, et al. Causes of unilateral sensorineural hearing loss screened by high-resolution fast spin echo magnetic resonance imaging: review of 1,070 consecutive cases. Am J Otol. 2000;21:173–80.
20. Schmalbrock P, Chakeres DW, Monroe JW, et al. Assessment of internal auditory canal tumors: a comparison of contrast-enhanced T1-weighted and steady-state T2-weighted gradient-echo MR imaging. AJNR Am J Neuroradiol. 1999;20:1207–13.
21. Hermans R, Van der Goten A, De Foer B, Baert AL. MRI screening for acoustic neuroma without gadolinium: value of 3DFT-CISS sequence. Neuroradiology. 1997;39:593–8.
22. Stuckey SL, Harris AJ, Mannolini SM. Detection of acoustic schwannoma: use of constructive interference in the steady state three-dimensional MR. AJNR Am J Neuroradiol. 1996;17:1219–25.
23. Goebell E, Ries T, Kucinski T, et al. Screening for cerebellopontine angle tumors: is a CISS sufficient? Eur Radiol. 2005;15:286–91.
24. Curnes JT. MR imaging of peripheral intracranial neoplasms: extraaxial vs intraaxial masses. J Comput Assist Tomogr. 1987;11:932–7.
25. Brackmann DE, Bartels LJ. Rare tumors of the cerebellopontine angle. Otolaryngol Head Neck Surg. 1980;88:555–9.
26. Hasso AN, Smith DS. The cerebellopontine angle. Semin Ultrasound CT MR. 1989;10:280–301.
27. Lo W. Cerebellopontine angle tumors, categorical course on neoplasms of the central nervous system. Paper presented at the American Society of Neuroradiology; 1990. p. 72–5.
28. Moffat DA, Saunders JE, McElveen JT Jr, et al. Unusual cerebellopontine angle tumours. J Laryngol Otol. 1993;107:1087–98.
29. Press GA, Hesselink JR. MR imaging of cerebellopontine angle and internal auditory canal lesions at 1.5 T. AJR Am J Roentgenol. 1988;150:1371–81.
30. Mikhael MA, Ciric IS, Wolff AP. Differentiation of cerebellopontine angle neuromas and meningiomas with MR imaging. J Comput Assist Tomogr. 1985;9:852–6.
31. Harnsberger HR. Head and neck imaging. 2nd ed. Chicago: Mosby-Year Book; 1995.
32. Charabi S, Mantoni M, Tos M, Thomsen J. Cystic vestibular schwannomas: neuroimaging and growth rate. J Laryngol Otol. 1994;108:375–9.
33. Rubenstein LJ, Russell DS. Pathology of tumors of the nervous system. 5th ed. Baltimore: Williams and Wilkins; 1989.
34. Naidich T. Imaging evaluation of meningiomas: categorical course on CNS neoplasms. Paper presented at the American Society of Neuroradiology; 1990.
35. Gentry LR, Jacoby CG, Turski PA, et al. Cerebellopontine angle-petromastoid mass lesions: comparative study of diagnosis with MR imaging and CT. Radiology. 1987;162:513–20.
36. Nakamura M, Roser F, Mirzai S, et al. Meningiomas of the internal auditory canal. Neurosurgery. 2004;55:119–27.
37. Asaoka K, Barrs DM, Sampson JH, et al. Intracanalicular meningioma mimicking vestibular schwannoma. AJNR Am J Neuroradiol. 2002;23:1493–6.
38. Lo W. Computed tomography of the petrous bone and posterior fossa. New York: Marcel Dekker; 1987.
39. Valavanis A, Schubiger O, Hayek J, Pouliadis G. CT of meningiomas on the posterior surface of the petrous bone. Neuroradiology. 1981;22:111–21.
40. Bourekas EC, Wildenhain P, Lewin JS, et al. The dural tail sign revisited. AJNR Am J Neuroradiol. 1995;16:1514–6.
41. Aoki S, Sasaki Y, Machida T, Tanioka H. Contrast-enhanced MR images in patients with meningioma: importance of enhancement of the dura adjacent to the tumor. AJNR Am J Neuroradiol. 1990;11:935–8.
42. Grey PL, Moffat DA, Hardy DG. Surgical results in unusual cerebellopontine angle tumours. Clin Otolaryngol Allied Sci. 1996;21:237–43.

43. Sriskandan N, Connor SE. The role of radiology in the diagnosis and management of vestibular schwannoma. Clin Radiol. 2011;66:357–65. Epub 2011 Jan 20.
44. Thompson AL, Aviv RI, Chen JM, Nedzelski JM, Yuen HW, Fox AJ, Bharatha A, Bartlett ES, Symons SP. Magnetic resonance imaging of facial nerve schwannoma. Laryngoscope. 2009;119:2428–36.
45. Mundada P, Purohit BS, Kumar TS, Tan TY. Imaging of facial nerve schwannomas: diagnostic pearls and potential pitfalls. Diagn Interv Radiol. 2016;22:40–6.
46. Ishikawa K, Haneda J, Okamoto K. Decreased vestibular signal intensity on 3D-FIESTA in vestibular schwannomas differentiating from meningiomas. Neuroradiology. 2013;55:261–70. Epub 2012 Oct 16.
47. Tampieri D, Melanson D, Ethier R. MR imaging of epidermoid cysts. AJNR Am J Neuroradiol. 1989;10:351–6.
48. Dutt SN, Mirza S, Chavda SV, Irving RM. Radiologic differentiation of intracranial epidermoids from arachnoid cysts. Otol Neurotol. 2002;23:84–92.
49. Tsuchiya K, Mizutani Y, Hachiya J. Preliminary evaluation of fluid-attenuated inversion-recovery MR in the diagnosis of intracranial tumors. AJNR Am J Neuroradiol. 1996;17:1081–6.
50. Tsuruda JS, Chew WM, Moseley ME, Norman D. Diffusion-weighted MR imaging of the brain: value of differentiating between extraaxial cysts and epidermoid tumors. AJNR Am J Neuroradiol. 1990;11:925–31.
51. Aprile I, Iaiza F, Lavaroni A, et al. Analysis of cystic intracranial lesions performed with fluid-attenuated inversion recovery MR imaging. AJNR Am J Neuroradiol. 1999;20:1259–67.
52. Chen S, Ikawa F, Kurisu K, et al. Quantitative MR evaluation of intracranial epidermoid tumors by fast fluid-attenuated inversion recovery imaging and echo-planar diffusion-weighted imaging. AJNR Am J Neuroradiol. 2001;22:1089–96.
53. Liu P, Saida Y, Yoshioka H, Itai Y. MR imaging of epidermoids at the cerebellopontine angle. Magn Reson Med Sci. 2003;2:109–15.
54. Zimmerman RA, Bilaniuk LT, Dolinskas C. Cranial computed tomography of epidermoid and congenital fatty tumors of maldevelopmental origin. J Comput Tomogr. 1979;3:40–50.
55. Dalley RW, Robertson WD, Lapointe JS, Durity FA. Computed tomography of a cerebellopontine angle lipoma. J Comput Assist Tomogr. 1986;10:704–6.
56. Passero S, Rossi S, Giannini F, Nuti D. Brain-stem compression in vertebrobasilar dolichoectasia. A multimodal electrophysiological study. Clin Neurophysiol. 2001;112:1531–9.
57. Smoker WR, Corbett JJ, Gentry LR, et al. High-resolution computed tomography of the basilar artery: 2. Vertebrobasilar dolichoectasia: clinical-pathologic correlation and review. AJNR Am J Neuroradiol. 1986;7:61–72.
58. Akimoto H, Nagaoka T, Nariai T, et al. Preoperative evaluation of neurovascular compression in patients with trigeminal neuralgia by use of three-dimensional reconstruction from two types of high-resolution magnetic resonance imaging. Neurosurgery. 2002;51:956–61.
59. Yoshino N, Akimoto H, Yamada I, et al. Trigeminal neuralgia: evaluation of neuralgic manifestation and site of neurovascular compression with 3D CISS MR imaging and MR angiography. Radiology. 2003;228:539–45.
60. Anderson VC, Berryhill PC, Sandquist MA, et al. High-resolution three-dimensional magnetic resonance angiography and three-dimensional spoiled gradient-recalled imaging in the evaluation of neurovascular compression in patients with trigeminal neuralgia: a double-blind pilot study. Neurosurgery. 2006;58:666–73.
61. Valavanis A. Clinical imaging of the cerebellopontine angle. Berlin: Springer-Verlag; 1986.
62. Olsen WL, Dillon WP, Kelly WM, et al. MR imaging of paragangliomas. AJR Am J Roentgenol. 1987;148:201–4.
63. Lo WW, Solti-Bohman LG, Brackmann DE, Gruskin P. Cholesterol granuloma of the petrous apex: CT diagnosis. Radiology. 1984;153:705–11.
64. Latack JT, Graham MD, Kemink JL, Knake JE. Giant cholesterol cysts of the petrous apex: radiologic features. AJNR Am J Neuroradiol. 1985;6:409–13.
65. Griffin C, DeLaPaz R, Enzmann D. MR and CT correlation of cholesterol cysts of the petrous bone. AJNR Am J Neuroradiol. 1987;8:825–9.
66. Greenberg JJ, Oot RF, Wismer GL, et al. Cholesterol granuloma of the petrous apex: MR and CT evaluation. AJNR Am J Neuroradiol. 1988;9:1205–14.
67. Lee BC, Kneeland JB, Walker RW, et al. MR imaging of brainstem tumors. AJNR Am J Neuroradiol. 1985;6:159–63.
68. Armington WG, Harnsberger HR, Smoker WR, Osborn AG. Normal and diseased acoustic pathway: evaluation with MR imaging. Radiology. 1988;167:509–15.
69. King JT Jr. Epidemiology of aneurysmal subarachnoid hemorrhage. Neuroimaging Clin N Am. 1997;7:659–68.
70. Mayberg MR, Batjer HH, Dacey R, et al. Guidelines for the management of aneurysmal subarachnoid hemorrhage. A statement for healthcare professionals from a special writing group of the Stroke Council, American Heart Association. Stroke. 1994;25:2315–28.
71. Wintermark M, Uske A, Chalaron M, et al. Multislice computerized tomography angiography in the evaluation of intracranial aneurysms: a comparison with intraarterial digital subtraction angiography. J Neurosurg. 2003;98:828–36.
72. Villablanca JP, Jahan R, Hooshi P, et al. Detection and characterization of very small cerebral aneurysms by using 2D and 3D helical CT angiography. AJNR Am J Neuroradiol. 2002;23:1187–98.
73. Jayaraman MV, Mayo-Smith WW, Tung GA, et al. Detection of intracranial aneurysms: multi-detector row CT angiography compared with DSA. Radiology. 2004;230:510–8.
74. Hoh BL, Cheung AC, Rabinov JD, et al. Results of a prospective protocol of computed tomographic angiography in place of catheter angiography as the only diagnostic and pretreatment planning study for cerebral aneurysms by a combined neurovascular team. Neurosurgery. 2004;54:1329–40.
75. Dehdashti AR, Rufenacht DA, Delavelle J, et al. Therapeutic decision and management of aneurysmal subarachnoid haemorrhage based on computed tomographic angiography. Br J Neurosurg. 2003;17:46–53.
76. Hallett JW Jr, Nora JD, Hollier LH, et al. Trends in neurovascular complications of surgical management for carotid body and cervical paragangliomas: a fifty-year experience with 153 tumors. J Vasc Surg. 1988;7:284–91.
77. Tikkakoski T, Luotonen J, Leinonen S, et al. Preoperative embolization in the management of neck paragangliomas. Laryngoscope. 1997;107:821–6.
78. Sanna M, Jain Y, De Donato G, et al. Management of jugular paragangliomas: the Gruppo Otologico experience. Otol Neurotol. 2004;25:797–804.
79. Persky MS, Setton A, Niimi Y, et al. Combined endovascular and surgical treatment of head and neck paragangliomas—a team approach. Head Neck. 2002;24:423–31.
80. Conners J. Interventional neuroradiology: strategies and practical techniques. Philadelphia: W.B. Saunders; 1999.
81. Abud DG, Mounayer C, Benndorf G, et al. Intratumoral injection of cyanoacrylate glue in head and neck paragangliomas. AJNR Am J Neuroradiol. 2004;25:1457–62.
82. Bendszus M, Monoranu CM, Schutz A, et al. Neurologic complications after particle embolization of intracranial meningiomas. AJNR Am J Neuroradiol. 2005;26:1413–9.
83. Rodiek SO, Stolzle A, Lumenta CB. Preoperative embolization of intracranial meningiomas with embosphere microspheres. Minim Invasive Neurosurg. 2004;47:299–305.

84. Dunn IF, Bi WL, Mukundan S, Delman BN, Parish J, Atkins T, Asher AL, Olson JJ. Congress of neurological surgeons systematic review and evidence-based guidelines on the role of imaging in the diagnosis and management of patients with vestibular schwannomas. Neurosurgery. 2018;82:E32–4.
85. Held P, Fellner C, Seitz J, Graf S, Fellner F, Strutz J. The value of T2(*)-weighted MR images for the diagnosis of acoustic neuromas. Eur J Radiol. 1999;30:237–44.
86. Held P, Fellner C, Fellner F, et al. MRI of inner ear and facial nerve pathology using 3D MP-RAGE and 3D CISS sequences. Br J Radiol. 1997;70:558–66.
87. Kim DY, Lee JH, Goh MJ, Sung YS, Choi YJ, Yoon RG, Cho SH, Ahn JH, Park HJ, Baek JH. Clinical significance of an increased cochlear 3D fluid-attenuated inversion recovery signal intensity on an MR imaging examination in patients with acoustic neuroma. AJNR Am J Neuroradiol. 2014;35:1825–9.
88. Rizk AR, Adam A, Gugel I, Schittenhelm J, Tatagiba M, Ebner FH. Implications of vestibular schwannoma consistency: analysis of 140 cases regarding radiologic and clinical features. World Neurosurg. 2017;99:159–63. Epub 2016 Nov 24.
89. Copeland WR, Hoover JM, Morris JM, Driscoll CL, Link MJ. Use of preoperative MRI to predict vestibular schwannoma intraoperative consistency and facial nerve outcome. J Neurol Surg B Skull Base. 2013;74:347–50.
90. Yoshino M, Kin T, Ito A, Saito T, Nakagawa D, Ino K, Kamada K, Mori H, Kunimatsu A, Nakatomi H, Oyama H, Saito N. Combined use of diffusion tensor tractography and multifused contrast-enhanced FIESTA for predicting facial and cochlear nerve positions in relation to vestibular schwannoma. J Neurosurg. 2015;123:1480–8. Epub 2015 May 22.
91. Gerganov VM, Giordano M, Samii M, Samii A. Diffusion tensor imaging-based fiber tracking for prediction of the position of the facial nerve in relation to large vestibular schwannomas. J Neurosurg. 2011;115:1087–93.
92. Song F, Hou Y, Sun G, Chen X, Xu B, Huang JH, Zhang J. In vivo visualization of the facial nerve in patients with acoustic neuroma using diffusion tensor imaging-based fiber tracking. J Neurosurg. 2016;125:787–94. Epub 2016 Jan 1.
93. Jung S, Kim SH, Kim HW, et al. Prediction of facial nerve displacement in extra large vestibular schwannoma. Acta Neurochir (Wien). 1998;140:1143–5.
94. Sartoretti-Schefer S, Kollias S, Valavanis A. Spatial relationship between vestibular schwannoma and facial nerve on three-dimensional T2-weighted fast spin-echo MR images. AJNR Am J Neuroradiol. 2000;21:810–6.
95. Zhang Y, Chen Y, Zou Y, et al. Facial nerve preservation with preoperative identification and intraoperative monitoring in large vestibular schwannoma surgery. Acta Neurochir (Wien). 2013;155:1857–62.
96. Choi KS, Kim MS, Kwon HG, Jang SH, Kim OL. Preoperative identification of facial nerve in vestibular schwannomas surgery using diffusion tensor tractography. J Korean Neurosurg Soc. 2014;56:11–5.
97. Taoka T, Hirabayashi H, Nakagawa H, et al. Displacement of the facial nerve course by vestibular schwannoma: preoperative visualization using diffusion tensor tractography. J Magn Reson Imaging. 2006;24:1005–10.
98. Larson TL, Wong ML. Imaging of the mastoid, middle ear, and internal auditory canal after surgery: what every radiologist should know. Neuroimaging Clin N Am. 2009;19:307–20.
99. Peyre M, Goutagny S, Imbead S, et al. Increased growth rate of vestibular schwannoma after resection of contralateral tumor in neurofibromatosis type 2. Neuro-Oncology. 2011;13:1125–32.
100. Fisher LM, Doherty JK, Lev MH, Slattery WH. Concordance of bilateral vestibular schwannoma growth and hearing changes in neurofibromatosis 2: neurofibromatosis 2 natural history consortium. Otol Neurotol. 2009;30:835–41.
101. Slattery WH 3rd, Fisher LM, Igbal Z, Oppenheimer M. Vestibular schwannoma growth rates in neurofibromatosis type 2 natural history consortium subjects. Otol Neurotol. 2004;25:811–7.
102. Nagano O, Higuchi Y, Serizawa T, et al. Transient expansion of vestibular schwannoma following stereotactic radiosurgery. J Neurosurg. 2008;109:811–6.
103. Nowe V, Michiels JL, Salgado R, et al. High-resolution virtual MR endoscopy of the cerebellopontine angle. AJR Am J Roentgenol. 2004;182:379–84.

Neurology

4

Simone E. Dekker, Chad A. Glenn, Eric M. Bershad, and Jose I. Suarez

Lesions of the cerebellopontine angle (CPA) produce a fascinating array of clinical manifestations. To understand the neurological manifestations produced by pathology in the CPA region, one must have a firm grasp of the corresponding neuroanatomical structures and pathways and of the consequences of their dysfunction. It is important to recognize specific neurological syndromes that may suggest a lesion in the CPA or surrounding anatomical structures, including the brainstem and cerebellum. It is important to realize that the causes underlying neurological dysfunction attributable to this region include not only tumors, but also a myriad of other pathologies such as vascular, infectious, and inflammatory conditions.

Anatomy

Understanding the clinical manifestations produced by CPA lesions requires a firm grasp of the anatomical structures within and surrounding the CPA (Fig. 4.1). The CPA is a wedge-shaped area filled with cerebrospinal fluid (CSF) [1, 2]. The CPA is bordered laterally by the petrous portion of the temporal bone, medially by the middle and lower brainstem (pons and medulla), posteriorly and superiorly by the cerebellum, and inferiorly by cranial nerves (CN) IX, X, and XI with their surrounding arachnoid investments.

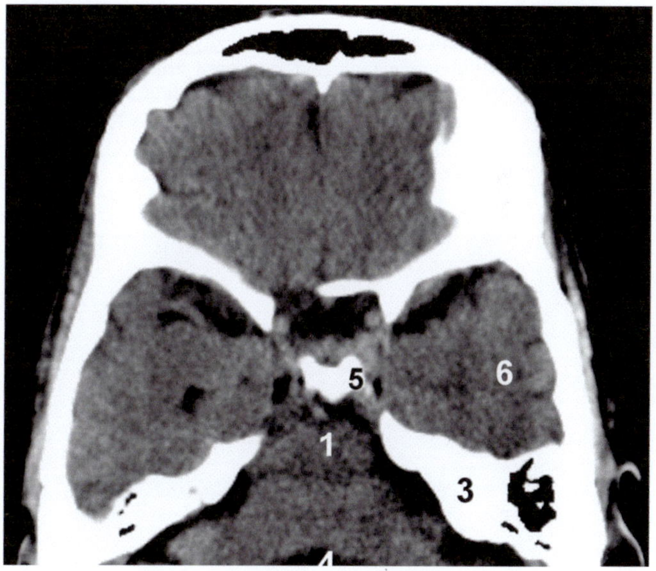

Fig. 4.1 Head CT scan of a patient showing the landmarks of the cerebellopontine angle: (1) pons; (2) cerebellum; (3) petrous temporal bone; (4) fourth ventricle; (5) posterior clinoid process; and (6) temporal lobe

The pons forms part of the medial boundary of the CPA and contains many important neuroanatomical structures and pathways (Fig. 4.2). The dorsal portion of the pons (tegmentum) contains the ascending reticular activating system, which helps maintain alertness. The ventral part of the pons (basis pontis) contains multiple nerve fiber tracts and the corticospinal tract (motor pathway). The caudal pons contains CN VI and VII nuclei in its dorsomedial and ventrolateral portions, respectively (Fig. 4.3). The CN VI nucleus forms the abducens nerve, a pure motor nerve that innervates the ipsilateral lateral rectus and abducts the eye. Dysfunction of the CN VI nucleus or nerve causes paresis of the ipsilateral eye with lateral gaze, whereas the contralateral eye moves

S. E. Dekker (✉)
Department of Neurological Surgery, The Neurological Institute, University Hospitals Cleveland Medical Center, Case Western Reserve University, Cleveland, OH, USA

C. A. Glenn
Comprehensive Brain Tumor Program, Neurosurgery, Stephenson Cancer Center, University of Oklahoma School of Medicine, Oklahoma City, OK, USA

E. M. Bershad
Neurology, Baylor College of Medicine, Houston, TX, USA

Neurosurgery, Baylor College of Medicine, Houston, TX, USA

Space Medicine, Baylor College of Medicine, Houston, TX, USA

J. I. Suarez
Division of Neurosciences Critical Care, Neurology, Johns Hopkins School of Medicine, Baltimore, MD, USA

N. C. Bambakidis et al. (eds.), *Surgery of the Cerebellopontine Angle*, https://doi.org/10.1007/978-3-031-12507-2_4

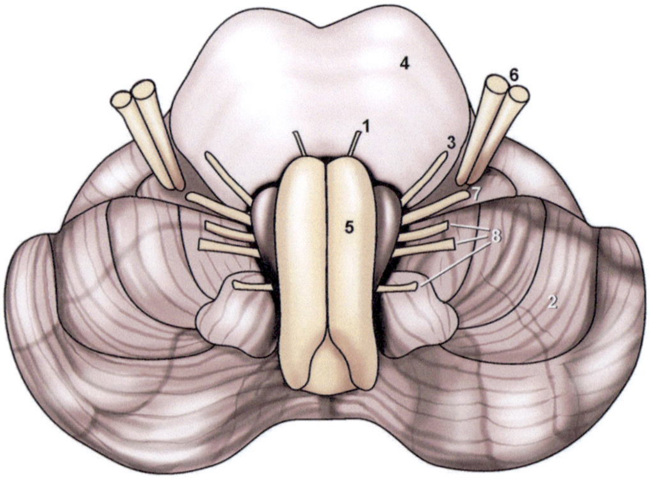

Fig. 4.2 The brainstem and cerebellum viewed from the basal aspect to show the cerebellopontine angle and associated structures: (1) abducens nerve (CN VI); (2) cerebellum; (3) facial nerve (CN VII); (4) pons; (5) pyramid (medulla); (6) vestibulocochlear nerve (CN VIII); (7) glossopharyngeal nerve (CN IX); and (8) roots of vagus (CN X), accessory (CN XI), and hypoglossal (CN XII) nerves

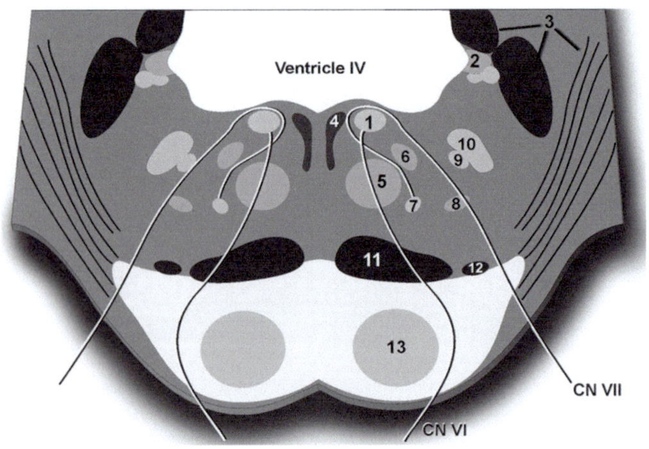

Fig. 4.3 Cross-section of the pons at the level of the cerebellopontine angle: (1) abducens nerve nucleus (CN VI); (2) vestibular nuclei; (3) cerebellar peduncles; (4) medial longitudinal fasciculus; (5) paramedian pontine reticular formation; (6) central tegmental tract; (7) facial nerve nucleus (CN VII); (8) spinothalamic tract; (9) spinal trigeminal nucleus; (10) spinal trigeminal tract; (11) medial lemniscus; (12) lateral lemniscus; and (13) corticospinal tract

normally. The parapontine reticular formation, which is ventromedial to the CN VI nucleus, controls horizontal saccadic eye movements. The motor nucleus of the facial nerve (CN VII) is ventrolateral to the CN VI nuclei. The motor and sensory nuclei of the trigeminal nerve (CN V) and the vestibular and cochlear nuclei are located dorsolaterally. Other tracts within the pons include the medial longitudinal fasciculus, which coordinates conjugate eye movements; the medial lemniscus, which contains sensory fibers for light touch, vibration, and proprioception from the trunk and limbs; and the lateral spinothalamic tract, which contains pain and temperature fibers from the trunk and limbs. The middle cerebellar peduncle connects the ventral pons to the cerebellum.

The contents of the CPA include CN VII and VIII, which cross the CPA before entering the internal auditory canal. The anterior inferior cerebellar artery (AICA) passes through the CPA. Small branches exit the AICA to CN VII and VIII. The labyrinthine artery (internal auditory artery) also exits from AICA. Two venous structures are relevant to the CPA. The petrosal vein drains blood from the cerebellum and lateral brainstem to the greater petrosal sinus, and Labbé's vein drains blood returning from the inferior and lateral surfaces of the temporal lobe.

Etiologies

Understanding the anatomical origins of a CPA lesion can help narrow the differential diagnosis of a lesion and also explain associated neurological manifestations. Likewise, the presenting neurological signs and symptoms can help predict the anatomical location of a lesion. Lesions producing clinical manifestations referable to the CPA may arise from within the CPA itself, or they arise from the internal auditory canal, temporal bone, brainstem, or cerebellum. Table 4.1 summarizes the differential diagnosis of a CPA lesion, stratified by extraaxial, extradural, vascular, and intraaxial origins.

The most common lesions (80–90%) of the CPA are vestibular schwannomas. These tumors arise from the Schwann cell lining of CN VIII within the internal acoustic canal and grow medially into the CPA. Less often, schwannomas arise from CN V or VII, or even from CN IX through CN XII. The second most common lesions (6%) of the CPA region are meningiomas, which may arise from the petrous ridge, tentorium, clivus, or internal acoustic meatus [3, 4].

Primary tumors that arise within the CPA include epidermoids, dermoids, and arachnoid cysts. Rare cysts include neurenteric, neuroepithelial, or neurocysticercosis cysts. Other primary tumors that can originate within the CPA include lipomas or melanocytic tumors. Other primary lesions include abnormal vascular loops, ectasia of the vertebrobasilar artery and branches, and aneurysms. Aneurysms, like tumors, can produce mass effect on CPA structures, thereby causing neurological dysfunction. Metastatic lesions within the CPA can include lung and breast carcinomas, melanomas or other systemic tumors, or carcinomatous meningitis. Infectious lesions within the CPA, which primarily infiltrate the meninges, include tuberculosis and syphilis [5]. Other lesions include granulomatous processes such as sarcoidosis or Wegener's granulomatosis.

Skull-base lesions impinging on the CPA originate mainly from the temporal bone and grow medially into the

Table 4.1 Differential diagnosis

Type of lesion	Lesion
Extraaxial	Vestibular schwannoma
	Trigeminal schwannoma
	Facial nerve schwannoma
	Mixed nerve schwannoma
	Meningioma
	Metastasis
	Melanoma
	Sarcoidosis
	Tuberculosis
	Syphilis
	Epidermoid
	Dermoid
	Arachnoid cyst
	Lipoma
	Erdheim–Chester
Extradural	Paragangliomas
	Cholesterol granulomas
	Cholesteatoma
	Chordoma
	Chondromas
	Chondrosarcoma
	Endolymphatic sac tumor
	Apex petrositis
	Skull-base trauma
Vascular	Vertebrobasilar dolichoectasia
	Vascular loops
	Posterior circulation aneurysms
	Arteriovenous malformation (AVM)
	Cavernous hemangiomas
Intraaxial	Brainstem gliomas
	Metastasis
	Lymphoma
	Medulloblastoma
	Hemangioblastoma
	Choroid plexus papillomas
	Ependymomas
	Dysembryoplastic neuroepithelial tumors
	Multiple sclerosis

CPA. These lesions include cholesterol granulomas, paragangliomas, chondromas, chondrosarcomas, chordomas, and endolymphatic sac tumors. A condition called apex petrositis, which involves an inflammatory lesion of the petrous apex from otitis media, can occur [5]. This entity can manifest with Gradenigo's syndrome, which consists of ear pain, facial numbness, or dysesthesias (CN V), and ipsilateral ocular abduction palsy from CN VI dysfunction [6].

Occasionally, intraaxial lesions can impinge on the CPA. Tumors may include brainstem gliomas, choroid plexus papillomas, lymphomas, hemangioblastomas, ependymomas, medulloblastomas, and dysembryoplastic neuroepithelial tumors. Other intraaxial lesions include vascular lesions such as arteriovenous malformations or cavernous hemangiomas, or demyelinating diseases such as multiple sclerosis.

Clinical Manifestations

The neurological manifestations of CPA lesions depend on multiple factors related to the responsible lesion, including their anatomical origin, size and degree of extension, pathology, and associated mechanism of injury. The timeliness of the clinical presentation may provide clues to the diagnosis. Protracted courses are often present for extraaxial lesions of the CPA (e.g., vestibular schwannomas and meningiomas). Signs of cranial nerve dysfunction develop over the course of years, with hearing loss being most common. A protracted course is also more common with other benign pathologies intrinsic to the brainstem. Rapidly progressive symptom development or sign of dysfunction at multiple levels of the brainstem portends an aggressive pathology. Rapid development of symptoms followed by stability raises concern for a vascular injury.

The anatomical origin of the CPA lesion may help determine the initial presenting neurological symptoms. For example, a vestibular schwannoma usually becomes symptomatic with hearing dysfunction because of the proximity of the cochlear nerve, whereas an intraaxial lesion usually manifests with signs of brainstem dysfunction. The size of the lesion and degree of extension also affect neurological dysfunction. Matthies and Samii determined that certain neurological symptoms in patients with vestibular schwannomas depended on the degree of tumor extension [7]. For example, patients with the largest tumors and extension had a significantly higher incidence of preoperative impaired function of the trigeminal nerve, facial nerve, and deafness.

Differences in the clinical manifestation of CPA lesions can also reflect the pathology involved [3, 4]. The two most common CPA lesions, vestibular schwannomas and meningiomas, demonstrate distinct clinical differences. For example, hearing loss is the most common symptom associated with both vestibular schwannomas and meningiomas (95% vs 60–75%, respectively). However, dysequilibrium seems to be more common with the latter, occurring in as many as 50% of patients, compared with the former. Furthermore, trigeminal nerve symptoms are reported to be prominent in patients with nonacoustic lesions.

Mechanisms of injury by CPA lesions responsible for neurological dysfunction can include direct compression of neurovascular structures (nerves, arteries, and veins); compression of the brainstem; or obstruction of CSF flow. Compression of arteries can result in infarction of the brainstem, cranial nerves, or cochlea. Compression of veins can result in venous infarction and life-threatening cerebral edema. Obstruction of CSF flow can cause hydrocephalus associated with dangerous elevations of intracranial pressure (ICP).

Symptoms of increased ICP include headache, nausea, vomiting, visual blurring, diplopia, lethargy, and confusion.

Signs of elevated ICP include decreased level of consciousness, papilledema (blurring of the optic disk or absence of venous pulsations), unilateral or bilateral CN VI dysfunction, and impairment of upgaze. In the setting of elevated ICP, CN VI dysfunction is considered a nonlocalizing sign and does not necessarily imply pontine dysfunction or direct compression of CN VI. The finding of impaired upgaze suggests hydrocephalus, which causes pressure on the dorsal midbrain where the centers responsible for initiating and maintaining upward gaze are located. It should be noted that the signs and symptoms of hydrocephalus are highly variable with the presence of both slowly and rapidly progressive presentations.

Because vestibular schwannomas are the most common CPA lesion, most literatures on the neurological manifestations of CPA masses refer to these lesions. Matthies and Samii reported the neurological manifestations associated with vestibular schwannomas in an impressive series of 1000 patients [7]. Hearing loss was overwhelmingly the most prevalent symptom and sign (95% and 93%, respectively). Vestibular dysfunction was the second most common symptom and sign (61% and 45–59%, respectively). Symptoms of vestibular dysfunction included vertigo, dizziness, and unsteadiness. Tinnitus occurred in 63% of patients. Headaches, primarily located occipitally, occurred in about 12% of the patients. Less frequent symptoms included impaired facial sensation (CN V, 8%); facial weakness (CN VII, 5%); and lower cranial nerve dysfunction (CN IX–XII) including dysphagia, dysarthria, dysphonia, and shoulder shrug weakness. Other symptoms included nausea, vomiting, and visual disturbances (1–3%). Interestingly, objective dysfunction of the trigeminal nerve, primarily of the maxillary division (V2), occurred in 19% of patients, but was reported subjectively by only 8%. Likewise, facial muscle paresis occurred in 17% objectively, but was reported subjectively by only 5% of the patients.

Neurological Examination of the CPA

The neurological examination of patients with symptoms that may be referable to the CPA must focus on the anatomical structures typically affected by lesions in this region. The standard elements tested in the neurological examination include mental status, cranial nerves, motor function, sensory function, reflexes, coordination, and gait. In patients suspected of having a CPA lesion, the neurological examination must include a detailed evaluation of cranial nerve function and coordination. In general, signs and symptoms of brainstem or upper motor neuron disease present in a delayed fashion in the case of extraaxial pathologies. Early presentation of multiple cranial nerve dysfunction or long tract signs, including hyperreflexia, spasticity, or the presence of abnormal reflexes, should prompt consideration for an intrinsic pathology.

The mental status examination consists of evaluating level of consciousness, orientation, language, memory, and cognition. Determining if there are signs of decreased level of consciousness or cognitive dysfunction is especially important. Large CPA lesions may obstruct the fourth ventricle or foramen of Luschka, causing obstructive hydrocephalus. The impairment in level of consciousness can range from drowsiness to coma.

The motor examination should assess the strength and tone of all extremities. Motor strength is assessed by testing individual muscles and grading them on a standard 5-point scale: 0, no movement; 1, trace movement; 2, movement present but not against gravity; 3, antigravity only; 4, some resistance to examiner; or 5, full strength. The examiner should check muscle strength in at least the major muscle groups, including the deltoids, biceps, triceps, hand grip, hip flexors, knee extensors and flexors, ankle dorsiflexion, and plantar flexion. Asymmetric muscle weakness may indicate damage to the corticospinal tract from brainstem compression or an intraaxial lesion. Increased tone on the same side of the weakness indicates an upper motor neuron corticospinal tract injury as would be expected if a lesion in the CPA damages these pathways. However, signs of brainstem compression usually occur later in the clinical presentation, following signs of cranial nerve dysfunction in the case of extraaxial lesions.

The reflexes should be tested in the biceps, triceps, patellae, and ankles. The examiner should note asymmetrical or abnormally brisk reflexes that would indicate upper motor neuron damage. The patient should be checked for the abnormal reflex, Babinski's sign. To elicit this sign, the examiner strokes the lateral aspect of the sole of the foot posteriorly to anteriorly. Babinski's sign is present when the great toe moves upward (dorsiflexes). This response usually indicates previous damage to the corticospinal tract.

Examination of sensory modalities should focus on trigeminal nerve function, which is discussed in terms of evaluating the cranial nerves. Examination of general sensory function in patients with symptoms suggestive of CPA dysfunction should include assessment of light touch, pinprick, temperature, and vibration in all extremities. Asymmetry of temperature and pinprick sensation usually indicates dysfunction of the lateral spinothalamic tract, whereas decreased vibration indicates medial lemniscus dysfunction.

Coordination and gait are examined to assess cerebellar function. The finger-to-nose maneuver, rapid finger tapping, heel-to-shin, and foot tapping tests may be used in assessing function of the corresponding ipsilateral cerebellar hemisphere. Midline cerebellar function is tested by having the patient walk heel-to-toe in tandem. A useful screening test for ataxia is Romberg's sign, which involves having the patient close his or her eyes with feet together and assessing stability. Romberg's sign is abnormal when the patient sways excessively or falls to one side. The side toward which the patient falls usually indicates the side of cerebellar dysfunction.

The cranial nerve portion of the neurological examination should receive the most attention in patients suspected of having a CPA lesion (Table 4.2). The examiner should develop a specific routine for checking the cranial nerves to ensure efficiency and accuracy of the evaluation. First, the visual fields (CN II) and pupillary light reflex, which contains an afferent limb (CN II) and an efferent limb (CN III), can be checked. Next, the patient should be checked for eyelid ptosis and pupillary miosis (Horner syndrome). If present, this combination may indicate damage to the sympathetic tract, which passes through the lateral pons and medulla.

Ocular motility involves the function of CN III (oculomotor), CN IV (trochlear nerve), and CN VI (abducens nerve). CN III originates in the midbrain and innervates the medial rectus (eye adduction), inferior rectus (depresses eye in abducted position), inferior oblique (elevates eye in adducted position), and superior rectus (elevates eye in abducted position) muscles. CN IV innervates the superior oblique muscle, which depresses the eye in the adducted position.

CN V (trigeminal) function is tested by assessing both sensory and motor components. The sensory fibers of the trigeminal nerve are separated into the ophthalmic (V1), maxillary (V2), and mandibular (V3) divisions. V1 supplies the forehead and portion of the scalp, upper eyelid, and skin of the nose. V2 supplies the skin of the lower eyelid, upper lip, and cheek. V3 supplies the skin of the lower lip, lower jaw, and chin. Each division should be tested individually using a sharp disposable pin and compared with the normal contralateral side.

Table 4.2 Function of cranial nerve

Cranial nerve	Origin	Function
Optic (II)	Retina	Vision, afferent limb pupillary light reflex
Oculomotor (III)	Midbrain	Ocular motility: medial rectus, superior rectus, inferior oblique muscles
		Lid elevation, efferent limb pupillary light reflex
Trochlear (IV)	Caudal midbrain	Ocular motility: superior oblique muscle
Trigeminal (V)	Pons	Facial sensation, jaw movement, and proprioception
Abducens (VI)	Pons	Ocular motility: lateral rectus muscle
Facial (VII)	Pons	Facial movement, taste sensory, efferent limb corneal reflex, parasympathetic function: tearing and salivation
Vestibulocochlear (VIII)	Pontomedullary	Vestibular function and hearing
Glossopharyngeal (IX)	Medulla, lateral	Gag reflex, swallowing, taste, salivation, phonation
Vagus (X)	Medulla, lateral	Gag reflex, swallowing, phonation
Spinal accessory (XI)	Medulla/spinal cord	Head turning, shoulder shrug
Hypoglossal (XII)	Medulla, medial	Tongue movements

CN VII (facial nerve) function is most easily tested by observing the muscles of facial expression. Asymmetry of the patient's face at rest should be noted. The crease at the angle of the nose and upper lip, the nasolabial fold, should be examined bilaterally for subtle signs of flattening. The patient should be asked to raise his or her eyebrows. The examiner then applies downward pressure and should not be able to resist the upward force easily. Similarly, the patient should close his or her eyes tightly, and the examiner should try to open them. In a patient with normal orbicularis oculi strength (CN VII), the examiner should be unable to force the eyes open. Other tests of facial nerve strength include puffing the cheeks (buccinator muscle) and retracting the chin (platysma muscle). CN VII supplies taste sensation to the anterior two-thirds of the tongue, which may manifest as an asymmetric ability to detect fundamental tastes.

The corneal reflex, which is depressed on the side of a lower motor neuron CN VII lesion, should be tested. The corneal reflex involves an afferent limb (CN V) and an efferent limb (CN VII, orbicularis oculi muscle). To test this reflex, the examiner gently stimulates each cornea with a sterile wisp of cotton and observes the briskness of blinking in both ipsilateral and contralateral eyes. An abnormality of CN V (afferent limb) manifests as a reduced blink in both the tested and contralateral side, with a normal blink response in both eyes when only the contralateral side is tested. An abnormality of CN VII (efferent limb) manifests as a reduced blink response on the side ipsilateral to the lesion, a normal contralateral blink response, and a reduced blink response on the contralateral side when only the normal eye is tested. With a combined lesion of CN V and VII, neither eye blinks in response to stimulation of the ipsilateral cornea. When only the cornea on the normal contralateral side is stimulated, the blink is normal only on that side.

CN VIII (vestibulocochlear nerve) contains both vestibular and auditory divisions. In patients with vestibular schwannomas, the cochlear division typically manifests dysfunction because the vestibular system effectively equilibrates to gradual damage to the vestibular nerve.

The cochlear division of CN VIII should be tested audiometrically for pure tone perception and speech discrimination. Patients with a CPA lesion exhibit a retrocochlear pattern of hearing loss in which speech discrimination is impaired disproportionately to pure tone perception. Some bedside screening tests for hearing dysfunction may be helpful as an initial screen of auditory function. The examiner can perform finger rubbing and observe the maximum distance at which the patient can detect the stimulus.

The examiner can also perform the Weber's and Rinne tests to help differentiate between conductive and sensorineuronal hearing loss. The Weber's test involves placing a vibrating tuning fork over the midline of the forehead. In a patient with normal hearing, the vibration is heard equally in both ears because bone conduction is equal bilaterally. In a patient with a unilateral conduction deficit, the vibration is heard louder in the affected ear because the conduction pathways are bypassed and there is a concomitant lack of interfering background noise on that side. In sensorineuronal hearing loss, the vibration is heard louder in the normal ear. The Rinne test, which is performed by placing the stem of a vibrating tuning fork on the mastoid bone, compares air conduction with bone conduction in the abnormal ear. When the patient can no longer hear the vibration, the tines of the vibrating tuning fork are placed 1–2 in. outside the external acoustic meatus. A patient with normal conductive hearing continues to detect the vibration for about twice as long as it was heard on the mastoid bone. In contrast, a patient with abnormal conduction is unable to hear the vibration when the tuning fork is vibrated outside the external acoustic meatus.

Evaluation of the vestibular portion of the CN VIII requires assessment of eye movements to look for evidence of nystagmus, gait examination, and station. As described, Romberg's sign may be abnormal in that the patient sways or falls to the side of the hypofunctioning vestibular nerve. Another test of vestibular function, the Unterberger test, requires the patient to step in place for 1 min. If the patient has a unilateral hypofunctioning vestibular nerve, he or she gradually turns in that direction. In one study of patients with acoustic neuromas, the Unterberger test was more sensitive than Romberg's sign for detecting vestibular abnormalities (71% vs 39%, respectively) [8].

CN IX and CN X (glossopharyngeal and vagus nerves, respectively) are tested simultaneously by checking the gag reflex, elevation of the soft palate, and uvula. The gag reflex and palatal elevation are depressed on the ipsilateral side of a patient with a lesion affecting the nucleus or nerve fascicles of CN IX or CN X. The uvula deviates contralateral to the side of cranial nerve dysfunction because unopposed action of the intact palatal muscles pulls the uvula toward that side.

CN XI (accessory nerve) innervates the sternocleidomastoid and trapezius muscles. Its function can be tested by having the patient turn his or her head against resistance on each side and shrugging the shoulders.

CN XII (hypoglossal nerve) function is evaluated by observing tongue movements and strength. The ventral aspect of the tongue is inspected for signs of atrophy or fasciculation seen ipsilateral to the side of a lower motor neuron hypoglossal lesion.

Additional Testing

When a lesion of the CPA is suspected based on the clinical presentation and physical examination findings, additional testing may aid in narrowing the differential diagnosis as well as guide further treatment. For example, pure tone audiometry can be used to objectively measure bone and air conduction for the frequencies 125, 250, 500, 1000, 2000, 4000, and 8000 Hz. The degree of hearing dysfunction may guide treatment recommendations in the setting of vestibular schwannomas. In addition, caloric stimulation can be performed to measure damage to the superior vestibular nerve through the lateral semi-circular canal. However, this test is not commonly performed in the alert patient and is more commonly used to assess brainstem function in the comatose patient.

As vestibular schwannomas are perhaps the most well-studied pathology of the CPA, further discussion regarding the clinical workup is warranted. Additional tools to evaluate vestibular schwannomas include auditory brainstem response testing and magnetic resonance imaging (MRI). The Congress of Neurological Surgeons Systematic Review and Evidence-Based Guidelines on Otologic and Audiologic Screening for Patients with Vestibular Schwannomas recommends that MRI screening be performed in patients with ≥10 dB of interaural difference at two or more contiguous frequencies or ≥15 dB at one frequency [8]. In addition, MRI can also be used to evaluate patients with sudden sensorineural hearing or asymmetric tinnitus. However, this practice is low yield in terms of vestibular schwannoma diagnosis (<3% and <1%, respectively) [8]. A detailed review of imaging of the CPA is available elsewhere in this text (see Chap. 3).

Brainstem Syndromes

A CPA lesion that extends to the brainstem extraaxially or one that originates intraaxially may become symptomatic with a constellation of neurological findings referable to the brainstem. In this section, some of the classic brainstem syndromes referable to the pons and medulla are reviewed (Table 4.3).

The lateral pontine syndrome (Marie–Foix syndrome) consists of ipsilateral cerebellar ataxia (middle cerebellar peduncle), contralateral hemiparesis (corticospinal tract), and contralateral hemihypesthesia for pain and temperature (spinothalamic tract) [9, 10].

The lateral medullary syndrome (Wallenberg syndrome), which is most often associated with occlusion of the ipsilateral intracranial vertebral artery or the posterior inferior cerebellar artery, may also be associated with neoplasms, demyelinating disease, hematomas, or abscesses. The characteristic findings include ipsilateral facial hypalgesia (spinal trigeminal tract); hypalgesia of the contralateral trunk

Table 4.3 Brainstem syndromes

Syndrome	Location	Findings
Wallenberg syndrome	Lateral medullary	Ipsilateral facial hypalgesia (spinal trigeminal tract) Contralateral trunk and extremity hypalgesia (lateral spinothalamic tract) Ipsilateral palatal, pharyngeal and vocal cord dysfunction with dysarthria and dysphagia (nucleus ambiguus, CN IX, X motor) Ipsilateral Horner syndrome (descending sympathetic fibers) Vertigo, nausea, and vomiting (vestibular nuclei) Ipsilateral cerebellar signs (inferior cerebellar peduncle and cerebellum)
Lateral pontomedullary syndrome	Lateral pontomedullary	Lateral medullary syndrome Ipsilateral facial weakness (CN VII) Ipsilateral tinnitus and/or hearing disturbances (CN VIII)
Marie–Foix syndrome	Lateral pontine	Ipsilateral cerebellar ataxia (middle cerebellar peduncle) Contralateral hemiparesis (corticospinal tract) Contralateral pain and temperature loss (lateral spinothalamic tract)
Foville's syndrome	Dorsal pontine, caudally	Contralateral hemiplegia with facial sparing (corticospinal tract) Ipsilateral peripheral facial palsy (facial nucleus and/or fascicle CN VII) Contralateral forced gaze (parapontine reticular formation ± abducens)
Raymond–Cestan–Chenais syndrome	Dorsal pontine, rostrally	Ataxia and coarse tremor (cerebellar pathways) Contralateral sensory deficit, all modalities (medial lemniscus and spinothalamic tract)
Millard–Gubler syndrome	Ventral pontine, caudally	Contralateral hemiplegia (sparing the face) (corticospinal tract) Ipsilateral abduction impairment (CN VI) Ipsilateral peripheral facial palsy (CN VII)

CN cranial nerve

and extremities (lateral spinothalamic tract); ipsilateral palatal, pharyngeal, and vocal cord dysfunction associated with dysarthria and dysphagia (nucleus ambiguus, CN IX, CN X motor); ipsilateral Horner syndrome (descending sympathetic fibers) of ptosis, miosis, and hypohidrosis; vertigo, nausea, and vomiting (vestibular nuclei); and ipsilateral cerebellar signs (inferior cerebellar peduncle and cerebellum). The presence of all of these findings is unusual. However, the presence of a majority of these findings strongly implicates the lateral medulla as the site of dysfunction [11, 12].

A similar brainstem syndrome, the lateral pontomedullary syndrome, includes the same elements as the lateral medullary syndrome. It also may include ipsilateral facial weakness (CN VII), ipsilateral tinnitus, and/or hearing disturbances (CN VIII) [13, 14].

The dorsal pontine syndrome, Foville's syndrome, occurs when a lesion involves the dorsal pontine tegmentum in the caudal portion of the pons. This syndrome consists of contralateral hemiplegia with facial sparing (corticospinal tract); ipsilateral peripheral facial palsy (facial nucleus and/or fascicle CN VII); and contralateral forced gaze owing to impairment of the ipsilateral parapontine reticular formation, abducens nucleus, or both [15].

Another dorsal pontine syndrome, the Raymond–Cestan–Chenais syndrome, occurs from a lesion involving the dorsal pons rostrally. The typical findings include cerebellar ataxia with a coarse tremor (cerebellar pathways) and contralateral sensory deficit to all modalities (medial lemniscus and spinothalamic tract). With ventral extension, contralateral hemiparesis (corticospinal tract) and/or an ipsilateral gaze palsy occur (parapontine reticular formation) [10, 15].

References

1. Carpenter MB. Core text of neuroanatomy. Baltimore: Williams & Wilkins; 1991.
2. England MA, Wakely J. Color atlas of the brain & spinal cord: an introduction to normal neuroanatomy. St. Louis: Mosby Year Book; 1991.
3. Voss NF, Vrionis FD, Heilman CB, Robertson JH. Meningiomas of the cerebellopontine angle. Surg Neurol. 2000;53:439–46.
4. Mallucci CL, Ward V, Carney AS, et al. Clinical features and outcomes in patients with non-acoustic cerebellopontine angle tumours. J Neurol Neurosurg Psychiatry. 1999;66:768–71.
5. Bonneville F, Sarrazin JL, Marsot-Dupuch K, et al. Unusual lesions of the cerebellopontine angle: a segmental approach. Radiographics. 2001;21:419–38.
6. Dave AV, Diaz-Marchan PJ, Lee AG. Clinical and magnetic resonance imaging features of Gradenigo syndrome. Am J Ophthalmol. 1997;124:568–70.
7. Matthies C, Samii M. Management of 1000 vestibular schwannomas (acoustic neuromas): clinical presentation. Neurosurgery. 1997;40:1–9.
8. Sweeney AD, Carlson ML, Shepard NT, McCracken DJ, Vivas EX, Neff BA, Olson JJ. Congress of Neurological Surgeons systematic review and evidence-based guidelines on otologic and audiologic screening for patients with vestibular schwannomas. Neurosurgery. 2018;82:E29–31.
9. Moffat DA, Harries ML, Baguley DM, Hardy DG. Unterberger's stepping test in acoustic neuroma. J Laryngol Otol. 1989;103:839–41.
10. Brazis PW, Masdeu JC, Biller J. Localization in clinical neurology. Philadelphia: Lippincott Williams & Wilkins; 2006.
11. Kim JS, Lee JH, Suh DC, Lee MC. Spectrum of lateral medullary syndrome. Correlation between clinical findings and magnetic resonance imaging in 33 subjects. Stroke. 1994;25:1405–10.

12. Sacco RL, Freddo L, Bello JA, et al. Wallenberg's lateral medullary syndrome. Clinical-magnetic resonance imaging correlations. Arch Neurol. 1993;50:609–14.
13. Aleksic S, Budzilovich G. Lateral inferior pontine syndrome. Clinico-pathologic study and review of literature. J Neurol Sci. 1973;18:317–22.
14. Fisher CM. Lacunar strokes and infarcts: a review. Neurology. 1982;32:871–6.
15. Silverman IE, Liu GT, Volpe NJ, Galetta SL. The crossed paralyses. The original brain-stem syndromes of Millard-Gubler, Foville, Weber, and Raymond-Cestan. Arch Neurol. 1995;52:635–8.

Part II

Surgical Approaches

Approaches to the Cerebellopontine Angle

5

Shervin Rahimpour, Ali R. Zomorodi, Patrick J. Codd, Max O. Krucoff, Allan H. Friedman, and L. Fernando Gonzalez

Introduction

The cerebellopontine angle (CPA) is formed by the petrosal cerebellar surface, middle cerebellar peduncle, lateral pons, petrosal surface of the petrous bone, and clival portion of the occipital bone. While only accounting for 10–15% of intracranial tumors, CPA tumors are the most common tumors of the posterior fossa. Vestibular schwannomas (VS) account for 85% of masses in this region, while meningiomas, epidermoids (primary cholesteatomas), and trigeminal, facial, and lower cranial nerve schwannomas constitute the majority of non-VS CPA tumors [1]. The three primary approaches to the CPA are the retrosigmoid, translabyrinthine, and middle fossa approaches. The optimal approach for a given patient depends on the tumor's growth pattern (e.g., the middle fossa approach is suboptimal for tumors with extensive growth in the CPA), the patient's hearing status, the surgeon's expertise in a given approach, and the goals of the operation. Furthermore, the density of crucial structures in this region makes careful preoperative assessment and planning essential in complication avoidance [2]. The retrosigmoid approach allows for hearing preservation and resection of lesions with significant extension into the CPA, though it requires cerebellar retraction and offers limited access to the fundus of the internal auditory canal (IAC). In contrast, the translabyrinthine approach requires very little brain retraction and has no limitation on tumor size or IAC exposure but does require sacrificing hearing. The middle fossa approach, while maintaining hearing preservation, is limited by the extension of the mass lesion into the CPA (~10 mm). In this chapter, we elaborate on these approaches and their variations. We emphasize that these approaches are a continuum of trajectories progressing from an exposure of the face of the petrous bone (retrosigmoid approach) to an anterior view of the brainstem (middle fossa approach; Fig. 5.1). Exposure and comparison of the three main approaches in the context of a VS are summarized in Tables 5.1 and 5.2.

S. Rahimpour (✉)
Department of Neurosurgery, University of Utah, Salt Lake City, UT, USA
e-mail: Shervin.Rahimpour@utah.edu

A. R. Zomorodi
Neurosurgery, Duke Health, Duke University School of Medicine, Durham, NC, USA

P. J. Codd
Duke Cancer Center, Duke University Medical Center, Durham, NC, USA

M. O. Krucoff
Neurosurgery, Neurosurgical Oncology, Medical College of Wisconsin, Milwaukee, WI, USA

Biomedical Engineering, Marquette University and Medical College of Wisconsin, Milwaukee, WI, USA

A. H. Friedman
The Preston Robert Tisch Brain Tumor Center, Duke Health, Durham, NC, USA

L. F. Gonzalez
Neurosurgery, Cerebrovascular and Endovascular Neurosurgery, Duke University, Durham, NC, USA

N. C. Bambakidis et al. (eds.), *Surgery of the Cerebellopontine Angle*, https://doi.org/10.1007/978-3-031-12507-2_5

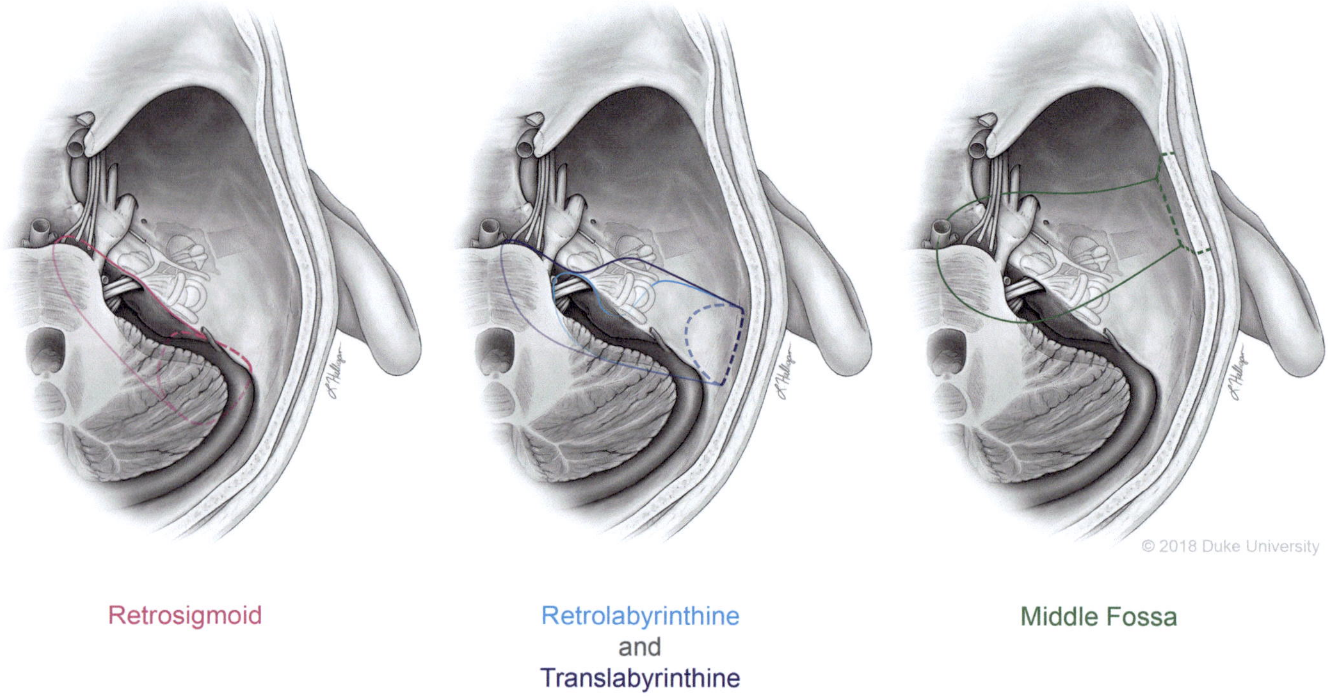

Fig. 5.1 A schematic view of surgical approaches to the cerebellopontine angle (CPA) in the axial plane. CPA exposures gradually progress from a more anterior view of the brainstem (middle fossa approach) to the face of the petrous bone (retrosigmoid approach)

Table 5.1 Summary of surgical approaches to the cerebellopontine angle

Approach	Limits of exposure	Advantages	Disadvantages	Anatomic structures exposed
Middle fossa	Medial—clivus Inferior—lower pons, pontomedullary junction Lateral—IAC Anterior—petrous carotid artery	Extradural petrous apex resection minimizes lobe retraction Preservation of hearing and vestibular apparatus	Risk of hearing loss Temporal lobe retraction	Intrapetrous carotid artery; IAC; pons; basilar artery; AICA; CNs V, VI, VII, and VIII
Retrolabyrinthine	Superior—middle fossa dura/tentorium Inferior—jugular bulb/foramen Posterior—brainstem and cerebellum Anterior—petrous bone Medial—midline/basilar artery	No cerebellar retraction required Anterior view trajectory of brainstem compared to retrosigmoid	Obligatory hearing loss	Labyrinth, sigmoid sinus, CNs VII and VIII
Translabyrinthine	Superior—tentorium Inferior—jugular bulb Anterior—carotid artery Medial—clivus	Minimal brain retraction Anterior viewing trajectory of brainstem	Obligatory hearing loss	Cerebellar hemisphere; pons; upper medulla; CNs V, VI, VII, VIII, IX, X, and XI; cochlea; labyrinth; middle ear; ossicles; petrous internal carotid artery
Retrosigmoid	Superior—tentorium Inferior—foramen magnum Anterior—petrous bone	Preservation of bony labyrinth	May require significant cerebellar retraction, limited view of anterior brainstem	Cerebellar hemisphere; lateral pons; CNs IV, V, VI, VII, VIII, IX, X, and XI; vertebrobasilar complex

AICA anterior inferior cerebellar artery, *CN* cranial nerve, *IAC* internal auditory canal

Table 5.2 Summary of surgical approaches for vestibular schwannomas

Feature	Retrosigmoid	Translabyrinthine	Middle fossa
Size limitation	None	None	Minimal CPA extension
Hearing preservation	Possible	No	Possible
Risk of facial nerve palsy	Dependent on size	Low	Moderate
Risk of CSF leak	Moderate	Moderate	Low
Application	Serviceable hearing, posterior fossa tumor with minimal intracanalicular extension (6 mm)	Nonserviceable hearing, no size limitation	Intracanalicular, less than 10 mm extension into the CPA

CPA cerebellopontine angle, *CSF* cerebrospinal fluid

Retrosigmoid Approach

The retrosigmoid approach is a versatile approach to the CPA and one with which most neurosurgeons are familiar. With various modifications, this approach can provide access to different levels of the CPA, including the tentorial incisura, IAC, posterior part of the petrous bone, jugular foramen, and craniocervical junction (Fig. 5.2). With respect to VS, it allows for the possibility of hearing preservation. Success is dependent on the size of the lesion. Specifically, if the lesion is less than 1 cm in diameter from pons to petrous, the chance of preserving hearing is as high as 83% while this number decreases to 53% for lesions up to 2 cm in size [3]. The major limitation of this approach is the surgeon's ability to follow tumors that have grown across the midline, anteriorly to the brainstem.

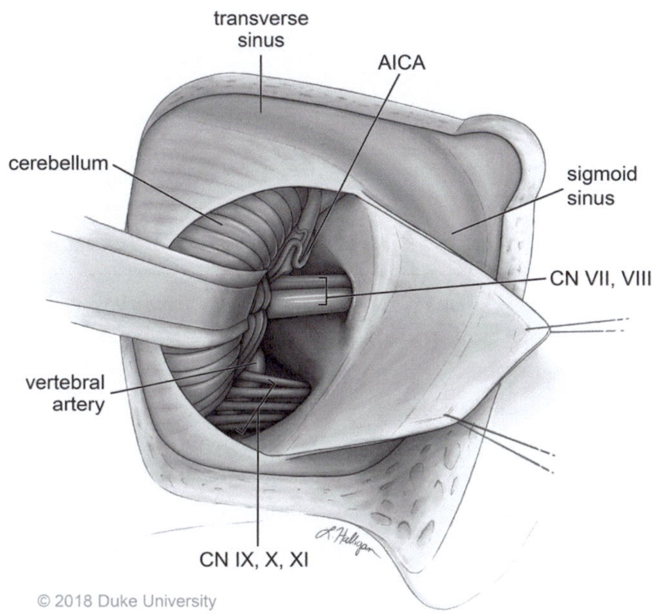

Fig. 5.2 Retrosigmoid exposure of the cerebellopontine angle. Cerebrospinal fluid (CSF) drainage and opening of the lumbar drain minimize the need to retract the cerebellum. In this extended view, lower cranial nerves and vertebral artery are visible

Surgical Technique

Patient positioning can include semi-sitting, prone, three-quarters lateral, lateral oblique, supine oblique, Concorde, or supine with the head turned. The position varies by surgeon comfort and institutional experience. We favor the lateral or park-bench position to avoid risks to the cervical spine and impediment of venous outflow. Adequate padding is used to avoid compression or traction injuries to the peripheral nerves and compression of bony prominences. After induction of anesthesia, we routinely place a lumbar drain to minimize retraction of the cerebellum. The incision for this approach is typically two fingerbreadths behind the pinna. Standard landmarks are used to locate the transverse sinus (imaginary line between the external occipital protuberance and the origin of the zygomatic arch or under the asterion) and the sigmoid (two fingerbreadths behind the ear aimed at the mastoid tip). We start the craniectomy at the transverse sigmoid junction. The junction is exposed and the posterior edge of the sigmoid sinus is skeletonized to permit the surgeon a view along the petrous bone. Venous bleeding is addressed with the use of hemostatic agents, such as Gelfoam®. Unavoidable exposure of the mastoid air cells should be waxed to prevent a cerebrospinal fluid (CSF) leak. Next, the lumbar drain is opened, and ~30 cc of CSF is drained to provide adequate brain relaxation. Dura is opened in a semicircular fashion, with its base facing the sigmoid sinus. The cerebellum surface is covered and protected, after which gentle retraction can be applied. When resecting a VS by this approach, the IAC is opened before the tumor is debulked to avoid bone dust from entering the subarachnoid space. A petrous dural flap and a plate of bone wax can be used to protect the contents of the CPA during drilling. Residue trapping (i.e., with Gelfoam® or bone wax) is an effective means to prevent CSF contamination with products that cause aseptic meningitis and headaches [4]. The drilling of the IAC should not exceed 7 mm as this may violate the vestibule and sacrifice hearing. (The depth in an individual patient can be measured on a preoperative magnetic resonance imaging [MRI] or computed tomography [CT] scan.) Next, the superior and inferior corners of the tumor are removed to interrupt the blood supply. Dissection is started at the upper pole to radically debulk the tumor using ultrasonic aspiration and sharp technique. It is important to not move the tumor mass prior to separating the tumor from the cochlear nerve. Along the brainstem, the origin of the facial nerve will be obscured by the tumor overlying the vestibulocochlear nerve. Proximally, the vestibular portion of the eighth nerve is cut in a "V" shape fashion, which frees the tumor from the inferior and superior vestibular nerves. Gradually, the tumor is thinned and sharply separated from the cochlear nerve. The nerve is kept moist using small pieces of Gelfoam® or cotton patties. Regardless of the approach used, intraoperative monitoring of the vestibulocochlear and facial nerves is used to guide the dissection safely (further discussed below). On closure, all exposed air cells are again covered with bone wax to prevent a CSF leak. The dura is closed in a watertight fashion. The lumbar drain can be left in place postoperatively at the surgeon's discretion to help prevent a leak and aid in healing. An abdominal fat graft can also be used to fill the mastoidectomy. Details of our techniques for complication avoidance have been previously described [2].

Transpetrosal Approaches

The supra/infratentorial exposure was popularized by Naffziger in 1928 [5]. The technique was retrosigmoid and used for decompression of the posterior fossa. Much later, Hitselberger and House used a petrosal approach to the CPA, again targeting only the posterior fossa. Shortly thereafter, King and Morrison combined these approaches (presigmoid–supra/infratentorial exposure), referred to as petrosal approaches of the petroclival region. These techniques have since been advanced with the use of the operating microscope, including the translabyrinthine approach and transcochlear by House and later the transotic approach by Jenkins and Fisch [6, 7]. Approaches from retrosigmoid to transotic provide the surgeon with a progressively flatter trajectory to the clivus. The translabyrinthine approach is useful when greater exposure of the lateral segment of the internal acoustic meatus is needed. The transotic approach can be utilized if further exposure of the temporal bone is needed, which requires skeletonization of the facial nerve and resection of the external acoustic meatus. If exposure of the petrous internal carotid artery is needed, the transcochlear approach can be used, which requires posterior mobilization of the facial nerve and removal of the cochlea (Table 5.3).

Table 5.3 Summary of transpetrosal approaches

Approach	Temporal bone
Retrolabyrinthine	Preserves posterior and superior semicircular canals (preserves hearing); narrow corridor of access.
Transcrusal	Superior and posterior semicircular canals are removed from ampullae to common crus
Translabyrinthine	Vestibule and horizontal canal are opened (hearing sacrificed) and lateral portion of internal acoustic meatus
Transotic	Complete removal of semicircular canals skeletonization of facial nerve
Transcochlear	Transotic, with posterior translation of facial nerve, removal of cochlea and exposure of petrous internal carotid artery

Retrolabyrinthine Approach

First described by Hitselberger and Pulec [8] for trigeminal neurectomy, the retrolabyrinthine approach is a workhorse approach to the CPA. This approach has several advantages, including decreased morbidity and hearing preservation. However, the exposure often does not provide a sufficient working area [9]. Surgically, a C-shaped flap is raised, and the mastoid surface is exposed. The asterion marks the posterior limit of the cortical bone removal. The sigmoid sinus is skeletonized, and the mastoid antrum is opened. The volume of bone inferior to the horizontal semicircular canal localizes the facial nerve. The exposure is defined by uncovering Trautmann's triangle, an area of dura with an inferior vertex (jugular bulb), limited by the sigmoid sinus posteriorly and the otic capsule anteriorly. The origins of the seventh and eighth cranial nerves at the brainstem can be seen in this view. The exposure can be enlarged with a combined retrosigmoid approach, leaving the sinus in the middle of the exposure. The sinus can be sacrificed based on angiographic criteria [10]. The narrow corridor of standard retrolabyrinthine approach as well as potential injury of the endolymphatic sac (running medial to the sigmoid sinus and inferior to the posterior semicircular canal, communicating through the vestibular aqueduct) are its disadvantages. In general, the exposure achieved through the presigmoid approaches is influenced by four specific anatomic characteristics: the level of temporal bone aeration, the size of Trautmann's triangle, the angle of the petrous slope (angle between the anterior sigmoid sinus and the petroclival fissure at the level of the IAC), and the height of the jugular bulb. Aeration can help facilitate intraoperative identification of landmarks (e.g., labyrinth, fallopian canal) opposed to a sclerotic temporal bone, which makes drilling more difficult and time-consuming. The impact of the height of the jugular bulb on the presigmoid approach has been well established. Specifically, a high jugular bulb allows for a smaller working area inferior to the IAC [11]. However, a full assessment of the dural exposure requires determining the distance between the sigmoid sinus to labyrinth and the jugular bulb to petrous ridge. In a study by Tubbs and colleagues, cadaveric specimens were found to have Trautmann's triangle areas ranging from 45 to 210 mm^2 (mean 151 mm^2) [12]. These specimens were categorized into three types, where type 1 (<75 mm^2) had a prohibitively small working area, type 2 (75–149 mm^2) had a potentially workable area, and type 3 (>150 mm^2) had the largest working corridor. In a larger analysis of 177 computed tomography scans, Wong and colleagues established the petrous angle to assess the "openness" of the posterior petrous bone and accessibility of Trautmann's triangle. This analysis revealed that a smaller angle can make a presigmoid approach more difficult. Consideration of these temporal bone characteristics can guide an optimal surgical strategy.

Translabyrinthine Approach

To gain access to the lateral recess of the IAC, hearing must be sacrificed. The translabyrinthine approach is ideal for tumors of all sizes when hearing is severely compromised prior to surgery. Similar to the retrolabyrinthine approach, a C-shaped skin incision is made approximately 1 cm superior to the auricle at the anterior most aspect of the ear behind the sigmoid, extending to the mastoid tip. Drilling follows the retrolabyrinthine approach. The mastoidectomy is completed to the point of exposing the antrum. Next, the incus is identified, which points in the direction of the facial nerve (Fig. 5.3a). The junction between the horizontal and posterior semicircular canals (also known as the vestibule) constitutes the lateral wall of the IAC. It is opened, and the IAC is exposed superiorly, posteriorly, and inferiorly (270° of exposure). Inside the IAC, the vertical crest (Bill's bar) separates the facial nerve and the superior vestibular nerve. The facial nerve is anterior while the superior vestibular nerve is posterior. Early identification of the facial nerve is an advantage of this approach in preserving facial nerve function. Once the dura is opened, the intracanalicular and vertical portions of the facial nerve can be followed through or around the tumor (Fig. 5.3b). In the case of a VS, the superior and inferior vestibular nerves are cut. The tumor is separated from the facial nerve in the IAC. The intracisternal portion of the tumor is stimulated to ensure that the facial nerve has not been displaced posteriorly. The tumor is opened, radically debulked, and separated from cerebellum. Stimulation of the tumor capsule throughout the resection is critical to elucidate the course of the facial nerve around the tumor and preserve function.

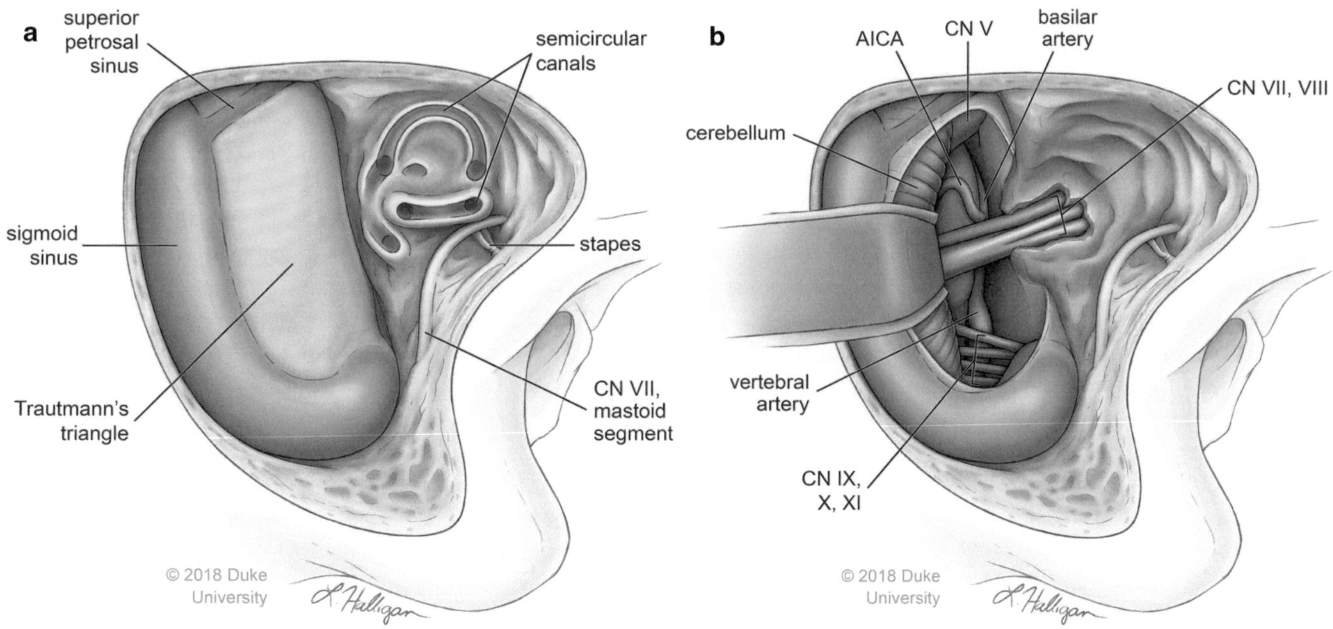

Fig. 5.3 Transpetrosal approaches such as the translabyrinthine approach provide a more anterior view of the brainstem when compared to the retrosigmoid. (**a**) The early stage of the translabyrinthine approach reveals Trautmann's triangle. Note that the tip of the incus points toward the vertical or mastoid portion of the facial nerve. (**b**) The dura is opened and the contents of the posterior fossa are exposed including the anterior inferior cerebellar and basilar arteries as well as lower cranial nerves

Partial labyrinthectomy (also known as the transcrusal approach) has been described by McElveen and Wilkins [13]. To improve exposure, this modified approach sacrifices the superior and inferior canals from ampullae to common crus. Similarly, after identification of the superior and posterior canals, Horgan and colleagues perforate the apex of canals after which the exposed ends are filled with mixtures of bone wax and dust. Drilling is then continued toward the common crus and ampullae [14].

Transcochlear Approach

While not particularly useful for the resection of a VS, the transcochlear approach is a direct approach to the petrous tip, midclival, and prepontine region. This approach maximizes exposure by extending bony removal in the presigmoid and translabyrinthine approaches, which results in a wide corridor to the midclival region and anterior brainstem. The original transcochlear approach as described by House and Hitselberger involves complete skeletonization and mobilization of the facial nerve posteriorly [15]. It requires cutting the greater superficial petrosal nerve (GSPN) as it emerges from the geniculate ganglion. After the nerve is mobilized, the cochlea is entered. A more extensive approach involving facial nerve rerouting and high cervical exposure was introduced by Fisch to treat extensive glomus jugulare tumors [7]. Rerouting or translocation of the facial nerve invariably causes moderate to severe facial nerve deficits. Variations of this approach include the transotic approach in which the facial nerve is not mobilized but the external auditory canal is occluded and resected. Drilling is continued through the petrous apex and inferior petrosal sinus. The petrous internal carotid artery constitutes the lateral aspect of the exposure.

Our group has described a less invasive transjugular approach with fallopian bridge technique in which a thin layer of cortical bone is left to cover the fallopian segment of the facial nerve from genu to the stylomastoid foramen. The mastoid tip is maximally skeletonized and infrajugular drilling is carried down into the occipital condyle until the hypoglossal canal is exposed. Our experience with this less invasive approach has provided adequate tumor resection and improved cranial nerve preservation compared to more extensive approaches [16].

Middle Fossa Approach

First described by Parry in 1904 and later popularized by House, the middle fossa approach is utilized in cases where there is an opportunity for hearing preservation and the lesion is located in the IAC [15, 17]. Importantly, however, intracanalicular lesions on preoperative imaging may be flush against the fundal region (fundal cap VS), which is predictive of poor postoperative hearing outcomes [18]. The presence of CSF in the fundal region on preoperative imaging leads to higher rates of postoperative measurable hearing [18]. This approach provides a direct exposure of the IAC and its contents from a superior trajectory. The subarachnoid/cisternal, intracanalicular, labyrinthine, horizontal, and tympanic segments of the facial nerve can be exposed. Moreover, the facial nerve can be identified early, making it less susceptible to injury during tumor dissection. Drawbacks of this approach include limited exposure of the lower portion of the CPA and the morbidity associated with retraction of the temporal lobe. Additionally, tumors of the inferior vestibular nerve can displace the facial nerve superiorly making it susceptible to injury during tumor dissection. Because the bulk of the tumor will then be located inferior to the tumor in a narrow corridor, the nerve is subjected to greater manipulation, so a higher risk of postoperative facial weakness is present.

Surgical Technique

The patient is placed in the lateral position where the long axis of the head is positioned parallel to the floor, with the ear facing the ceiling and the neck slightly extended. A vertical incision is made anterior to the tragus and perpendicular to the zygomatic arch. Fascia and temporal muscle are exposed and opened with Bovie electrocauterization and then retracted with self-retractors or fishhooks. The superior extent of the exposure is the bone below the squamous suture. The craniotomy, which is square, is planned so that a third is positioned posterior to and the remaining two-thirds are positioned anterior to the external acoustic canal. This strategy will adequately expose the floor of the middle fossa. Particular attention must be paid to ensure the floor is flush to improve visualization and minimize retraction on the temporal lobe. The dura is then elevated in a posterior-to-anterior direction to prevent pulling on the GSPN and damaging the facial nerve. The zygomatic root can be split into thirds, where the anterior third is lateral to the foramen ovale and the mandibular branch of the trigeminal nerve (V3), the middle third is directly lateral to the foramen spinosum and the middle meningeal artery, and the posterior third is lateral to the geniculate ganglion. The petrous bone medial to the GSPN is partially removed using a diamond drill. The IAC is first exposed medially at its meatus. Here there are no important neural or vascular structures between the superior semicircular canal and the gasserian ganglion. The IAC can be exposed for 270°. The surgeon continues the lateral exposure of the IAC, being aware that the cochlea and superior semicircular canal restrict lateral exposure at the fundus. After the

GSPN, arcuate eminence, and petrous ridge are identified, the IAC can be localized using any of the following three techniques:

1. *Garcia–Ibanez technique*: This technique builds off of the relationship between the GSPN and the arcuate eminence. Bisecting this 120° angle provides the site at which drilling the temporal bone exposes the IAC.
2. *Fisch technique*: A similar technique involves drawing a line over the long axis of the arcuate eminence and a subsequent line 60° from the original line. This second line provides the location of the IAC, typically 3–4 mm below the petrous ridge and as much as 7 mm below the floor of the middle fossa.
3. *House technique*: Once the GSPN is identified, the floor of the middle fossa can be drilled to identify the geniculate ganglion and then to follow the labyrinthine portion of the facial nerve medially until the IAC is reached. The function between the geniculate ganglion and the facial nerve is not on the same plane as the IAC; therefore, most of the geniculate ganglion must be uncovered to expose the facial nerve medially. This exposure extends to the posterior limit (superior semicircular canal), anterior limit (petrous ridge), and laterally (cochlea). Once the roof of the IAC has been drilled, the vertical crest (Bill's bar) is identified, which separates the facial nerve from the superior vestibular nerve. Inside the IAC is the meatal portion of the anterior inferior cerebellar artery. This anatomy of the parent vessel can be variable with a percentage of loops (64%) projecting to the meatus or into the IAC [19]. Early identification and preservation of these branches are essential in preservation of hearing.

Extended Middle Fossa Approach

House and Hitselberger first described a region in the middle fossa that could be removed with relative impunity. This technique was modified for the treatment of low-neck basilar tip aneurysms (between the sellar floor and IAC on lateral projection) and resection of petroclival meningiomas. Day and colleagues formalized a geometric construct of compartments in and adjacent to the cavernous sinus. The posteromedial triangle (Kawase's triangle) is limited by the porus trigeminus, cochlea, and the posterior border of the mandibular branch. This region is devoid of vascular or nerve branches. In this approach, the patient is positioned as described for a traditional middle fossa approach. The craniotomy varies depending on the extent of anterior exposure needed to include the posterior portion of the cavernous sinus. The petrous apex is exposed extradurally, and the dura is again elevated in a posterior-to-anterior fashion. Anteriorly,

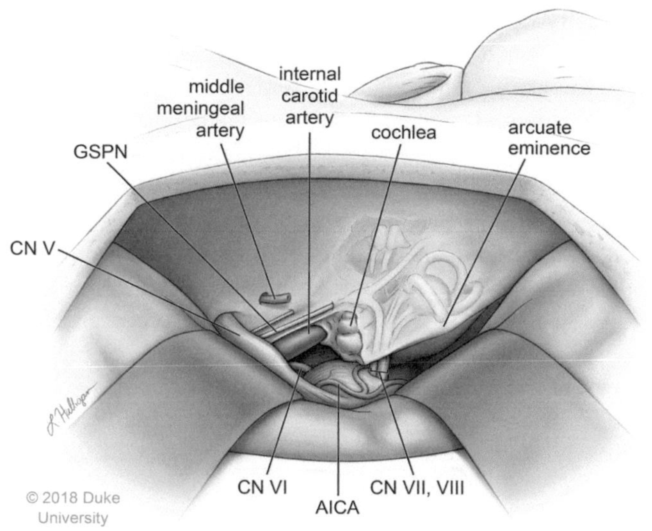

Fig. 5.4 In an extended middle fossa approach, removal of the posteromedial triangle reveals midline structures, including the abducens nerve and basilar artery

the foramen spinosum is identified and the middle meningeal artery coagulated with bipolar cautery.

In this extended exposure, the basilar artery and the emergence of both the anterior inferior cerebellar artery and abducens nerve are visible medially (Fig. 5.4). Posteriorly, the nerves of the IAC are visible. The brainstem is exposed from the medullopontine sulcus and the anterolateral portion of the pons between the trigeminal and facial nerves.

Endoscopic Approach

Endoscopy of the CPA has become an increasingly popular technique, though the inherent complexity and crowdedness of the posterior fossa anatomy has prevented its widespread use. The surgical endoscope was first introduced to CPA surgery in 1917 by Doyen for trigeminal neurectomy. With the advent of the operative microscope, endoscopic techniques took a secondary role. Recently, improved technology targeting lighting, magnification, and angled optics has reinvigorated the use of endoscopy in skull-base surgery. These technical advances over the past 20 years have allowed for combined endoscopic and microsurgical exposures for a variety of different pathologies, including VS, petroclival meningioma, epidermoid tumor, arachnoid cyst, and neurovascular compression syndromes [20–25]. Purely endoscopic approaches have been described for the resection of a VS [26, 27]. When the endoscope is used as a supplementary tool to assist in primarily microscopic procedures, endoscopic assistance helps in expanding the surgical field and improving the visualization around neurovascular corners, thereby increasing the resection volume of CPA lesions.

Especially with angled lenses, trajectories can be visualized distinct from the primary working trajectory. These blind spots are specific to the approach being used. For example, in the retrosigmoid approach, the anterior surface of cranial nerves VII–X, ventral surface of the trigeminal nerve or various foramina, or IAC cannot be visualized. In the middle fossa approach, the inferior and lateral CPA as well as the CPA posterior to the IAC cannot be seen. Takemura and colleagues formally demonstrated superior visualization with endoscopic assistance of the CPA [28]. Specifically, the endoscope improved views of the junction of the trigeminal nerve and the pons, the entrance into the porus of Meckel's cave, and the course of the superior cerebellar artery. Inferiorly, the endoscope improved visualization of the root exit zone of the facial nerve from the brainstem, the medullary junction, and the dural exits of cranial nerves IX–XI. Combined with angled instrumentation, surgical dissections can be performed in these regions that are otherwise obscured by a direct linear viewing trajectory.

One major concern with navigation of an endoscope in the limited corridor of the CPA is injury of the cranial nerves due to trauma or thermal injury. Inadvertent collateral injury to tissues may occur as the result of improper endoscope holding techniques and inappropriate side-to-side motions of the scope. Likewise, insertion of instrumentation blindly behind the viewing space of the endoscope can lead to injury to unseen structures as the instrument is brought to the viewing field. Familiarity with instrumentation and careful handling of both endoscopes and associated instruments are essential for safe endoscopic-assisted surgery.

As previously discussed by Ebner and Abolfotoh [29, 30], adjunctive use of the endoscope emphasizes additional visualization through the same exposure as a microscopic approach compared with the same visualization through a smaller exposure. In general, with any endoscopic approach, particularly with respect to approaches of the CPA, it is imperative that the surgeon be comfortable with the endoscope and CPA anatomy.

Neuromonitoring and Anesthetic Considerations

By virtue of their location, CPA lesions are close to the abducens, facial, vestibulocochlear, glossopharyngeal, and vagus cranial nerves, thus making these nerves susceptible to injury with microsurgical resection. The advent of intraoperative neuromonitoring has led to improvements in structural and functional preservation of the cranial nerves. Several monitoring techniques have been described with particular focus on the facial and vestibulocochlear nerves: electromyography (EMG) for facial nerve monitoring and brainstem auditory evoked potential (BAEP) monitoring for the vestibulocochlear nerve.

Facial Nerve Monitoring

EMG is widely used as a means of monitoring facial nerve function. Monitoring in this modality includes a stimulator probe and sensors for detection of facial muscle contraction. Typically, a two-channel system is used in which a pair of needle electrodes is planted in the orbicularis oris and orbicularis oculi muscles while another is placed in the forehead or shoulder for grounding. Additional channel systems to monitor more facial muscles that may provide increased sensitivity and benefit have been described [31]. Prior to the beginning of the operation, baseline parameters (i.e., motor unit potentials [MUPs], insertion activity) are obtained for comparison. The stimulator probe is then used during the operation, preferably near the brainstem as this area is unaffected by the tumor and resection. The stimulation current can be modulated. When the stimulation current exceeds the action potential threshold of the facial nerve, facial muscles twitch, which triggers a sound alarm, providing immediate feedback for the surgeon. The morphology and frequency of the motor unit potential (MUP) provides insights into facial nerve pathology. A single MUP is a "spike" while a short sequence of MUPs is termed a "burst." When this activity is sustained, it is designated as a "train," and those of particularly high frequency (>30 Hz) are termed "neurotonic." Neurotonic discharges can occur as a result of stimulation, irritation, or damage to the nerve. Specifically, the A-train, which is characterized as a high-frequency train pattern—with the duration lasting milliseconds to seconds, amplitude in the range of 100–200 μV, and short onset and offset—has been associated with postoperative facial nerve deficits. In fact, the duration of the train time has been shown to correlate with worse postoperative facial nerve paresis. EMG is useful for anatomic localization of the facial nerve. In cases where tumor capsule or bone obscures direct visualization of the facial nerve, stimulation at low currents (e.g., 0.2 mA) implies the nerve is exposed whereas higher currents (e.g., 0.5 mA) suggest a sizable tissue barrier. Despite its benefits, EMG does not always translate to true nerve function and runs the added risk of causing electrical injury from overstimulation. Intense or prolonged stimulation can increase the risk of irreparable nerve injury. To that end, low frequency and pulsed stimulation along with judicious use of the stimulator can minimize injury risk.

Vestibulocochlear Nerve Monitoring

Operative damage to the vestibulocochlear nerve can be done by direct or traction injury or ischemic changes (e.g., occlusion, rupture, or vasospasm of the internal auditory artery). BAEP waves are a measure of the bioelectric neural activity associated with stimulation of the vestibulocochlear nerve. In this form of monitoring, scalp and ear electrodes are placed and an auditory click (20–50 Hz) is used as the stimulating apparatus. These responses are typically small in comparison to background brain activity and, as a result, are difficult to detect. Trial averaged signals ideally yield evoked potentials classified as wave I through wave VII, of which waves I through V represent the peripheral cochlear nerve to the inferior colliculus. Waves I, III, and V carry the most clinical significance. Specifically, increased peak latencies, high interaural latency differences, decreased amplitudes, and increased interpeak (waves I–III, III–V, and I–V) latencies are potentially concerning changes intraoperatively. These parameters are warning signs while waves I and V correlate with better postoperative hearing preservation rates. Importantly, the surgeon should keep in mind that, because evoked potentials are average signals from multiple samples (>1000), there may be a time delay (seconds to minutes) in measuring the electrophysiologic effects from the surgery. While BAEP recordings can be altered by trauma, the surgeon should be cognizant of other factors including anesthesia, hypothermia, and irrigation [32]. The utility of BAEP monitoring is largely patient-dependent as some patients may not have detectable BAEPs and others may have abnormal baselines. In these circumstances, electrocorticography (ECoG) and direct cochlear nerve action potential (CNAP) can be more useful as these are "near-field" techniques in which stimulation evokes and records an electrical response close to its origin on the auditory nerve. For ECoG, electrodes are positioned transtympanically on the middle ear promontory or intrameatal electrode. Direct CNAPs measure directly from the acoustic nerve. The recording electrode is placed directly on the acoustic nerve, often proximal to the tumor being resected. Like BAEP and ECoG, a click stimulus is used, and the resulting compound muscle action potential is measured. Technical limitations in the surgical environment may make this method impractical for monitoring. The advantage of these latter techniques is that the acquisition takes less time, leading to a more real-time response. Brainstem auditory evoked responses (BAERs) have predictive value in that a loss of wave V portends a poor hearing outcome, but the inverse is not necessarily the case. One method that has been postulated to account for hearing loss associated with a working vestibulocochlear nerve is loss of the cochlear blood supply via the labyrinthine artery. For example, delayed hearing loss may be a result of vasospasm or swelling, causing occlusion of the artery. There has been some reported utility in topical papaverine or use of postoperative nimodipine in patients with delayed hearing loss [33, 34].

Glossopharyngeal and Vagus Nerve Monitoring

Both the glossopharyngeal and vagus nerves contain sensory, parasympathetic, and motor fibers. It is the motor fibers that are most amenable to neuromonitoring. The motor fibers of the glossopharyngeal nerve originate in the rostral nucleus ambiguus and supply the stylopharyngeus muscle. The motor fibers of the vagus nerve supply the striated musculature of the soft palate, pharynx, and larynx, but not the tensor veli palatini and stylopharyngeus. Monitoring of the glossopharyngeal nerve can be done by placing electrodes in the lateral aspect of the palate to record from the stylopharyngeus muscle. This procedure can be performed with a manually curved needle or adhesive electrodes on a laryngeal mask airway [35]. Monitoring of the vagus nerve can be accomplished by EMG recording from the laryngeal muscles, which can be done by wire electrodes built in the endotracheal tube or laryngoscopic placement of electrodes placed in the laryngeal musculature. Both nerves can be identified by recording the stimulated compound muscle action potential. Stimulation can be performed by using bipolar or monopolar stimulation, with constant current or constant voltage stimulus, each with its own pros and cons [36]. In a study by Topsakal and colleagues, intraoperative monitoring helped identify the course of a nerve and reduced the risk of lower cranial nerve injury [37].

Summary

The CPA can be approached with a variety of different techniques largely based on clinical and imaging factors. Expertise in microneurosurgery and temporal bone anatomy is essential for successful execution. To review, the retrosigmoid approach is the workhorse approach for neurosurgeons and is useful for tumors of all sizes. This approach is limited by the intracanalicular extent of the tumor. For pure intracanalicular tumors, the middle fossa and transpetrosal approaches are reasonable options. If the patient has serviceable hearing, the middle fossa approach is preferable. In the case that hearing is severely compromised, the transpetrosal approaches, such as the translabyrinthine approach, are indicated. Variations of these approaches and combined approaches are indicated for larger tumors, lesions anterior to the pons, clival lesions, and acoustic schwannomas. Endoscopic approaches have become increasingly popular given technical advances, though they remain limited to institutions with experience. Mastering these approaches to the CPA is essential to the armamentarium of a skull-base neurosurgeon.

References

1. Gal TJ, Shinn J, Huang B. Current epidemiology and management trends in acoustic neuroma. Otolaryngol Head Neck Surg. 2010;142:677–81.
2. Rahimpour S, Friedman AH, Fukushima T, Zomorodi AR. Microsurgical resection of vestibular schwannomas: complication avoidance. J Neuro-Oncol. 2016;130:367–75.
3. Post KD, Eisenberg MB, Catalano PJ. Hearing preservation in vestibular schwannoma surgery: what factors influence outcome? J Neurosurg. 1995;83:191–6.
4. Catalano PJ, Jacobowitz O, Post KD. Prevention of headache after retrosigmoid removal of acoustic tumors. Am J Otol. 1996;17:904–8.
5. Naffziger HC. Brain surgery with special reference to exposure of the brain stem and posterior fossa: the principle of intracranial decompression, and relief of impactions in the posterior fossa. Surg Gynecol Obstet. 1928;46:241–8.
6. House WF. Transtemporal bone microsurgical removal of acoustic neuromas. Report of cases. Arch Otolaryngol. 1964;80:617–67.
7. Jenkins HA, Fisch U. The transotic approach to resection of difficult acoustic tumors of the cerebellopontine angle. Am J Otol. 1980;2:70–6.
8. Hitselberger WE, Pulec JL. Trigeminal nerve (posterior root) retrolabyrinthine selective section: operative procedure for intractable pain. Arch Otolaryngol. 1972;96:412–5.
9. Russell SM, Roland JT, Golfinos JG. Retrolabyrinthine craniectomy: the unsung hero of skull base surgery. Skull Base. 2004;14:63–71.
10. Spetzler RF, Daspit CP, Pappas CTE. The combined supra- and infratentorial approach for lesions of the petrous and clival regions; experience with 46 cases. J Neurosurg. 1992;76:588–99.
11. Aslan A, Falcioni M, Russo A, De Donato G, Balyan FR, Taibah A, et al. Anatomical considerations of high jugular bulb in lateral skull base surgery. J Laryngol Otol. 1997;111:333–6.
12. Tubbs RS, Griessenauer C, Loukas M, Ansari SF, Fritsch MH, Gadol AAC. Trautmann's triangle anatomy with application to posterior transpetrosal and other related skull base procedures. Clin Anat. 2014;27:994–8.
13. McElveen JT, Wilkins RH, Erwin AC, Wolford RD. Modifying the translabyrinthine approach to preserve hearing during acoustic tumour surgery. J Laryngol Otol. 1991;105:34–7.
14. Horgan MA, Delashaw JB, Schwartz MS, Kellogg JX, Spektor S, McMenomey SO. Transcrusal approach to the petroclival region with hearing preservation. J Neurosurg. 2001;94:660–6.
15. Monfared A, Mudry A, Jackler R. The history of middle cranial fossa approach to the cerebellopontine angle. Otol Neurotol. 2010;31:691.
16. Nonaka Y, Fukushima T, Watanabe K, Friedman AH, McElveen JT, Cunningham CD, et al. Less invasive transjugular approach with Fallopian bridge technique for facial nerve protection and hearing preservation in surgery of glomus jugulare tumors. Neurosurg Rev. 2013;36:579–86.
17. Parry RH. A case of tinnitus and vertigo treated by division of the auditory nerve. J Laryngol Otol. 1994;19:402–6.
18. Goddard JC, Schwartz MS, Friedman RA. Fundal fluid as a predictor of hearing preservation in the middle cranial fossa approach for vestibular schwannoma. Otol Neurotol. 2010;31:1128–34.
19. Martin RG, Grant JL, Peace D, Theiss C, Rhoton ALJ. Microsurgical relationships of the anterior inferior cerebellar artery and the facial-vestibulocochlear nerve complex. Neurosurgery. 1980;6:483.
20. Schroeder HWS, Oertel J, Gaab MR. Endoscope-assisted microsurgical resection of epidermoid tumors of the cerebellopontine angle. J Neurosurg. 2004;101:227–32.
21. Tatagiba M, Matthies C, Samii M. Microendoscopy of the internal auditory canal in vestibular schwannoma surgery. Neurosurgery. 1996;38:737–40.
22. Tatagiba M, Rigante L, Mesquita Filho P, Ebner FH, Roser F. Endoscopic-assisted posterior intradural petrous apicectomy in petroclival meningiomas: a clinical series and assessment of perioperative morbidity. World Neurosurg. 2015;84:1708–18.
23. Teo C, Nakaji P, Mobbs RJ. Endoscope-assisted microvascular decompression for trigeminal neuralgia: technical case report. Oper Neurosurg. 2006;59:489–90.
24. Charalampaki P, Kafadar AM, Grunert P, Ayyad A, Perneczky A. Vascular decompression of trigeminal and facial nerves in the posterior fossa under endoscope-assisted keyhole conditions. Skull Base. 2007;18:117–28.
25. Kumon Y, Kohno S, Ohue S, Watanabe H, Inoue A, et al. Usefulness of endoscope-assisted microsurgery for removal of vestibular schwannomas. J Neurol Surg B. 2012;73:42–7.
26. Setty P, D'Andrea KP, Stucken EZ, Babu S, LaRouere MJ, Pieper DR. Endoscopic resection of vestibular schwannomas. J Neurol Surg B. 2015;76:230–8.
27. Shahinian HK, Eby JB, Ocon M. Fully endoscopic excision of vestibular schwannomas. Minim Invasive Neurosurg. 2005;47:329–32.
28. Takemura Y, Inoue T, Morishita T, Rhoton AL Jr. Comparison of microscopic and endoscopic approaches to the cerebellopontine angle. World Neurosurg. 2014;82:427–41.
29. Abolfotoh M, Bi WL, Hong C-K, Almefty KK, Boskovitz A, Dunn IF, et al. The combined microscopic-endoscopic technique for radical resection of cerebellopontine angle tumors. J Neurosurg. 2015;123:1301–11.
30. Ebner FH, Koerbel A, Roser F, Hirt B, Tatagiba M. Microsurgical and endoscopic anatomy of the retrosigmoid intradural suprameatal approach to lesions extending from the posterior fossa to the central skull base. Skull Base. 2006;19:319–23.
31. Grayeli AB, Guindi S, Kalamarides M, Garem HE, Smail M, Rey A, et al. Four-channel electromyography of the facial nerve in vestibular schwannoma surgery: sensitivity and prognostic value for short-term facial function outcome. Otol Neurotol. 2005;26:114.
32. Legatt AD. Mechanisms of intraoperative brainstem auditory evoked potential changes. J Clin Neurophysiol. 2002;19:396.
33. Morawski K, et al. Preventing internal auditory artery vasospasm using topical papaverine: an animal study. Otol Neurotol. 2003;24:918–26.
34. Strauss C, et al. Vasoactive treatment for hearing preservation in acoustic neuroma surgery. J Neurosurg. 2001;95:771–7.
35. Singh R, Husain AM. Neurophysiologic intraoperative monitoring of the glossopharyngeal and vagus nerves. J Clin Neurophysiol. 2011;28:582–6.
36. Schlake HP, Goldbrunner RH, Milewski C, Krauss J, Trautner H, Behr R, et al. Intra-operative electromyographic monitoring of the lower cranial motor nerves (LCN IX-XII) in skull base surgery. Clin Neurol Neurosurg. 2001;103:72–82.
37. Topsakal C, Al-Mefty O, Bulsara KR, Williford VS. Intraoperative monitoring of lower cranial nerves in skull base surgery: technical report and review of 123 monitored cases. Neurosurg Rev. 2008;31:45–53.

Combined Surgical Approaches

6

Nicholas C. Bambakidis, Chad A. Glenn, Sam Safavi-Abbasi, and Robert F. Spetzler

The decision regarding which surgical approach to use during exposure of the posterior fossa requires careful analysis by surgeons. The degree of exposure required is critical in determining the optimum route of attack. The need to visualize the lesion and surrounding eloquent structures adequately so that resection can be undertaken safely must be weighed against the potential complications associated with each type of approach. In the axial plane, the skull-base of the posterior fossa can be exposed through multiple directions broadly classified as posterior or lateral approaches (Fig. 6.1a). In the sagittal plane, the options include supratentorial or infratentorial directions (Fig. 6.1b). In both cases, combinations of these approaches may allow the greatest degree of exposure. This strategy maximizes the potential for safe surgical resection of the pathology in question while limiting potential risks to the patient.

Some degree of petrosectomy is usually common to combined approaches to the posterior fossa. Transpetrosal approaches entail some degree of petrous (temporal) bone resection [1]. Such bony removal allows maximal surgical exposure while minimizing brain retraction and typically requires the talents of both a neurosurgeon and a neuro-otologic skull-base surgeon. Combination approaches using an anterior petrosectomy and subtemporal craniotomy (Kawase's approach) allow excellent exposure of the middle

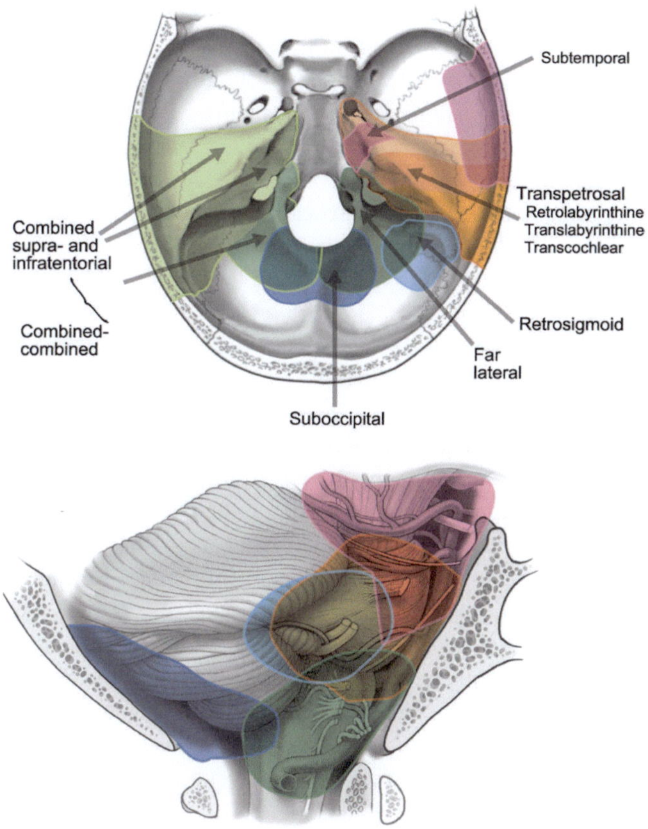

Fig. 6.1 Angles of approach to the posterior fossa in the (**a**) axial and (**b**) sagittal planes can be classified broadly as posterior or lateral and supra- or infratentorial. (Reproduced with permission from Barrow Neurological Institute)

cranial fossa [2]. Likewise, a posterior petrosectomy can be combined with a far-lateral or subtemporal approach or both to provide an unimpeded view of the entire cranial base from the foramen magnum to the clivus to the sphenoid sinus [3–5]. This combined approach allows exposure of cranial nerve (CN) III through CN XII, the anterolateral brainstem, and the posterior fossa vasculature from the vertebral artery to the basilar apex [6].

N. C. Bambakidis (✉)
Neurological Surgery, The Neurological Institute, University Hospitals of Cleveland, Case Western Reserve University School of Medicine, Cleveland, OH, USA
e-mail: Nicholas.Bambakidis2@UHhospitals.org

C. A. Glenn
Comprehensive Brain Tumor Program, Neurosurgery, Stephenson Cancer Center, University of Oklahoma School of Medicine, Oklahoma City, OK, USA

S. Safavi-Abbasi
Flagstaff Neurosurgery, Flagstaff, AZ, USA

R. F. Spetzler
Neurosurgery, Barrow Neurological Institute, Phoenix, AZ, USA

N. C. Bambakidis et al. (eds.), *Surgery of the Cerebellopontine Angle*, https://doi.org/10.1007/978-3-031-12507-2_6

In efforts to minimize brain retraction and cranial nerve manipulation, an endoscopic endonasal approach (EEA) to access the petroclival region has more recently been developed [7–9]. Similar to the team approach utilized for open transpetrosal approaches, the neurosurgeon and a rhinologist trained in endoscopic endonasal skull-base techniques work hand-in-hand. Used alone or in combination with open posterior approaches, an expanded EEA like the endoscopic transclival and the endoscopic transmaxillary transpterygoid has been described for exposure of the clivus and petroclival region. These approaches are most useful when lateral exposure beyond the internal auditory canal (IAC) is unnecessary. Dural exposure along the length of the clivus is obtained from a transclival route. The transpterygoid approach may be combined with an infrasphenoidal transclival exposure to widen the operative field off of the midline. A detailed understanding of endoscopic endonasal anatomy is required as numerous critical neurovascular structures confine the exposure. These critical structures include the cavernous segment of the internal carotid artery (ICA), CN VI as it enters Dorello's canal, the cisternal segment of CN V, the petrous and paraclival segments of the ICA, CNs VII/VIII as they enter the internal auditory canal, and the hypoglossal canal.

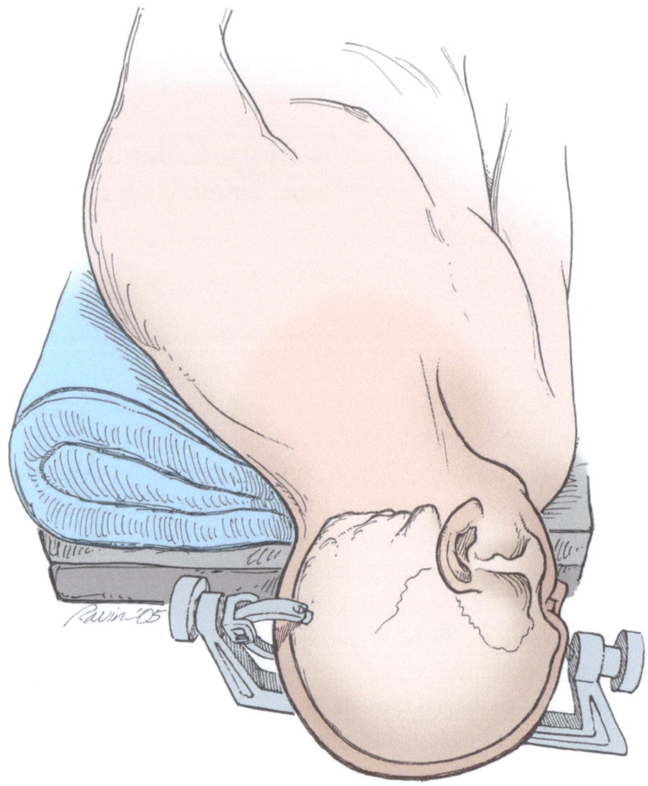

Fig. 6.2 Supine positioning with placement of a log roll under the ipsilateral shoulder. The head is mildly flexed and rotated toward the contralateral shoulder. Elevation of the zygomatic arch allows simultaneous supratentorial and infratemporal exposure. Avoidance of extreme rotation and flexion is important to avoid venous congestion and engorgement. (Reproduced with permission from Barrow Neurological Institute)

General Considerations

For open approaches, we favor placing the patient in a supine position (Fig. 6.2). A shoulder roll allows rotation of the head laterally, accompanied by moderate flexion of the head toward the opposite shoulder. The head is positioned parallel to the floor, and the zygomatic arch is elevated. This simple and straightforward position usually enables excellent visualization of the contents of the posterior fossa. Somatosensory evoked potentials (SSEPs) are monitored while the head is positioned. Changes in the waveforms may indicate compromise of the vascular system or spinal compression. Extreme rotation and flexion, which can cause venous congestion and engorgement, must be avoided.

For large patients in whom contralateral head rotation is precluded due to neck compression or shoulder elevation, a modified park-bench position can be used. In this position, the dependent arm is supported by a sling and the ipsilateral shoulder is taped to minimize its profile. An axillary roll must be used to prevent brachial plexopathy. The park-bench position allows further rotation of the head and elevation of the mastoid process. This position is advantageous for approaching low-lying lesions and provides an operating angle to the anterior brainstem and foramen magnum [10]. In all cases, the patient is taped securely to the operating table to allow maximal flexibility in rotation if required.

Electrophysiological monitoring is used routinely during positioning and throughout surgery. Both brainstem auditory evoked responses and SSEPs of the extremities are measured. Cortical activity can be assessed with electroencephalography. The latter confirms burst suppression during the administration of barbiturates. Facial nerve function is measured through recordings of the orbicularis oris muscle transduced to an audible click. Cerebrospinal fluid (CSF) is drained routinely to increase brain relaxation and to minimize the need for retraction. Postoperative lumbar drainage is associated with a reduction in complications related to CSF leakage [11] and typically continues 3–5 days after surgery.

In general, standard positioning for an EEA requires the patient to be in the supine position with the head elevated and slightly extended to optimize the approach angle. The head is positioned in the midline without rotation. Frameless intraoperative navigation is used to guide the exposure. A lumbar drain may be placed in selected cases. Epinephrine-soaked cottonoids are placed in the nasal cavity prior to beginning the procedure to provide topical decongestion. When necessary, mucosal injections with lidocaine and epinephrine may also be performed. General anesthetic conditions should avoid hypertension intraoperatively as this may lead to excessive venous bleeding.

High-definition straight and angled endoscopes are used throughout the procedure. In general, the straight endoscope is used until the later stages of the procedure. Specialty endoscopic endonasal microinstruments are used as these are typically longer than traditional microinstruments. Endonasal suction monopolar cautery and single-shafted bipolar cautery are used to control bleeding. Venous bleeding is best controlled with hemostatic agents and cellulose packing. Similarly, longer and angled hand pieces for the high-speed drill are critical to these approaches. Diamond burs are preferred over traditional cutting burs in most situations. Most drilling over dural surfaces is continued until the bone has reached an "eggshell" thickness at which time Kerrison rongeurs are used to complete dural exposure.

Three- or four-hand binostril endoscopic endonasal surgery is performed. Resection or lateralization of the ipsilateral middle and inferior turbinates is commonly performed depending on the characteristics of the pathology. To achieve the working room needed in these approaches, a posterior septectomy and a complete ethmoidectomy are often performed. Navigated instruments such as the microdebriders, suction tips, and image-guidance probes greatly aid in identification of anatomic variants as well as in evaluation of extent of resection. An endonasal Doppler ultrasound probe is helpful in identifying the course of the ICA during exposure. Depending on the size and location of the defect, autologous grafts and synthetic materials as well as tissue sealant are used to provide a multilayered closure. Nasoseptal mucosal flaps supported by nasal packing are used in all cases for repair.

Transpetrosal Approaches

Drilling the temporal bone increases exposure of the contents of the posterior and middle fossae. Progressively aggressive bone removal increases the anatomic exposure obtained but likewise is accompanied by increasing rates of complications. Several variations of transpetrosal approaches have been named differently. In general, however, the posterior petrosectomies are divided into the retrolabyrinthine, translabyrinthine, and transcochlear approaches (Table 6.1) and are briefly described [4, 12, 13]. The anterior transpetrosal (Kawase's) approach is not described [2]. In all variations, a mastoidectomy is the initial step of bony exposure. Closure must be meticulous, and dural patch materials and fibrin glue can be used if necessary. The use of abdominal fat grafts and liberal lumbar spinal drainage are critical to prevent postoperative CSF leakage.

The retrolabyrinthine approach involves the least amount of bony resection. The mastoid is drilled posterior to the labyrinth and cochlea, thus preserving hearing. When combined with a far-lateral or retrosigmoid approach, the entire sigmoid sinus is skeletonized. All surrounding dural planes are exposed with a high-powered drill. Care must be taken to avoid injury to the endolymphatic sac, which runs medial to the sigmoid sinus and inferior to the posterior semicircular canal. Damage to this structure can cause hearing loss as a result of leakage of endolymphatic fluid [14].

Once the dura is opened, the contents of the posterior fossa anterior to the sigmoid sinus can be visualized (Fig. 6.3). When the patient's venous anatomy permits [15, 16], additional exposure may be obtained by sacrificing this sinus in combination with a traditional retrosigmoid craniotomy. In our experience, however, the marginal improvement in surgical exposure seldom outweighs the added risk of venous complications and the time required to perform the bony resection. It is ideal for the treatment of vestibular neurectomies (for which the retrolabyrinthine approach was developed), but its applications in other settings are limited.

Additional bone is removed in the translabyrinthine approach (Fig. 6.4a). Bony drilling proceeds much as with the retrolabyrinthine exposure, except that the entire facial nerve is skeletonized completely. The malleus and incus are removed, thus obliterating the middle ear. After a labyrin-

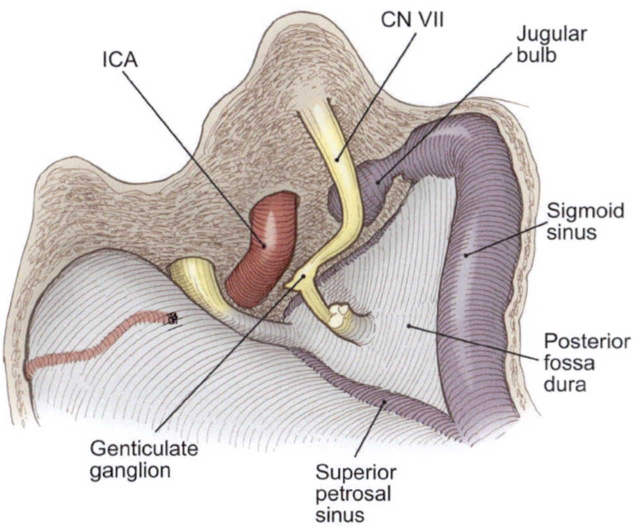

Fig. 6.3 Transcochlear exposure after complete skeletonization of the facial nerve (CN VII). CN VII may be transposed after the superficial petrosal and chorda tympani nerves are sectioned. Alternatively, CN VII may be left in situ after the external auditory canal is occluded. *ICA* internal carotid artery. (Reproduced with permission from Barrow Neurological Institute)

Table 6.1 Features of posterior petrosectomy approaches

Approach	Hearing preservation	Risk to facial nerve	Risk of CSF leak	Extent of exposure
Retrolabyrinthine	Possible	Minimal	Low	Least
Translabyrinthine	No	Minimal	Moderate	Mid
Transcochlear	No	High	Moderate	Most

From Bambakidis NC et al. [60]. Reproduced with permission from *Journal of Neurosurgery*

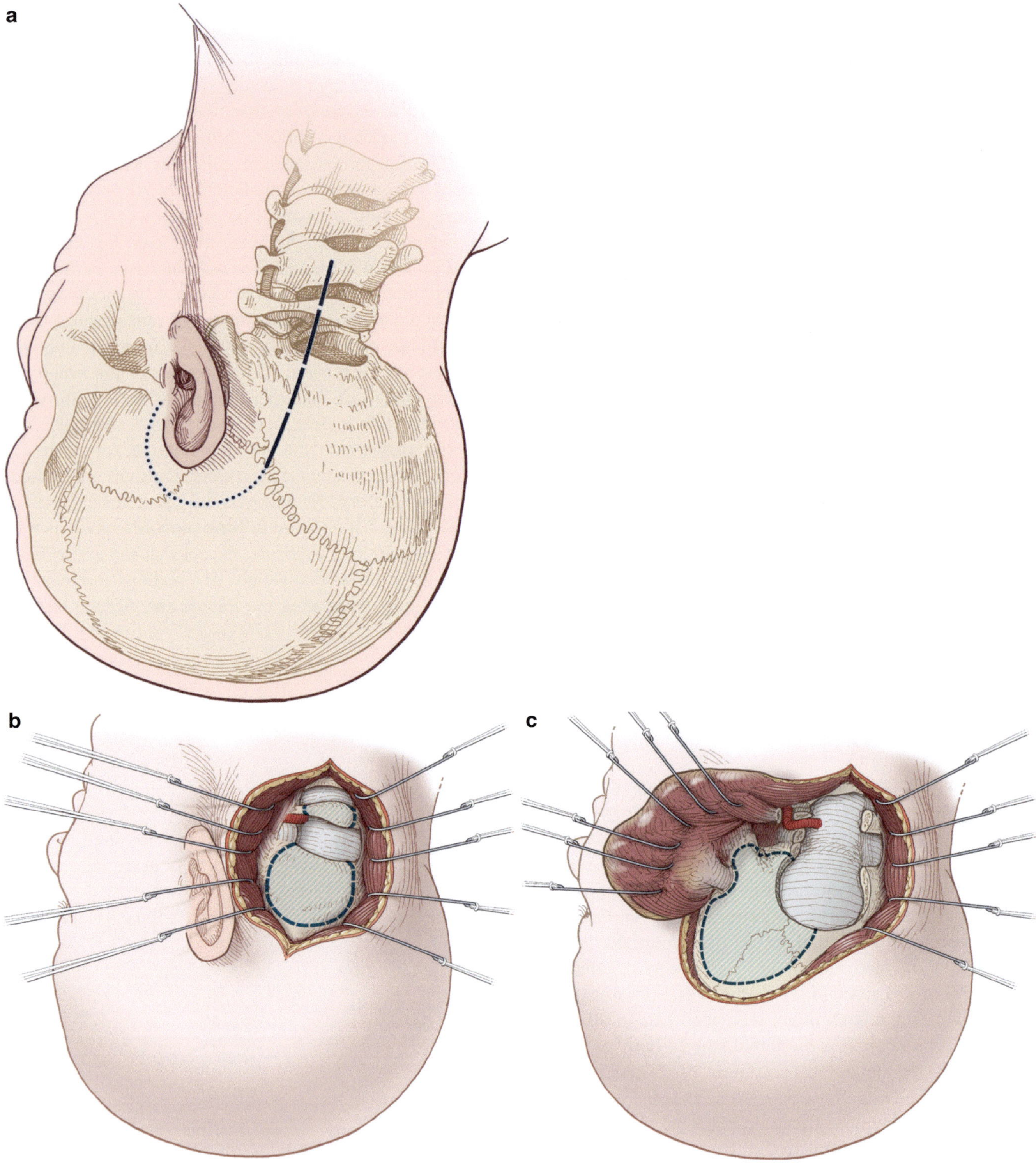

Fig. 6.4 Operative exposure during combined approaches to the posterior fossa. (**a**) The skin incision may extend below the foramen magnum along a paramedian course for the far-lateral exposure (*dashed line*). Extension superiorly in a curvilinear fashion over the pinna to the root of the zygoma allows a subtemporal craniotomy to be incorporated (*dotted line*). (**b**) A paramedian muscle-splitting approach is used to incorporate a far-lateral craniotomy (*dashed line*). Careful dissection of the soft tissue is critical for maintaining the correct surgical orientation and to avoid inadvertent injury to the vertebral artery. (**c**) A subtemporal craniotomy (*dashed line*) can be combined with this approach or can be performed in isolation. Care must be exerted while removing bone over the transverse sinus. (**a**: Modified from Baldwin HZ et al. [3], with permission from *Journal of Neurosurgery*. **b**, **c**: Reproduced with permission from Barrow Neurological Institute)

thectomy is performed (Fig. 6.4b), the dura may be opened to provide a view of the entire subarachnoid, intracanalicular, and vertical portions of the facial nerve. Used in isolation, the translabyrinthine approach is excellent for the resection of acoustic neuromas in patients with preoperative hearing loss. When combined with a far-lateral and Kawase's extended middle fossa approach (transtentorial and anterior transpetrosal approach) [15], excellent visualization of the entire lateral brainstem is obtained.

Expansion of the translabyrinthine approach through removal of the external auditory canal and middle ear and further exposure of the extended facial recess define the transcochlear approach (Fig. 6.3) [13]. Classically described as including transposition of the facial nerve after division of the chorda tympani and greater superficial petrosal nerves, this approach offers the widest approach to the clivus and anterior brainstem. In the transotic variation, the facial nerve is left in situ and the external auditory canal is occluded and resected [17]. This variation may lessen the risk of temporary or even permanent facial paresis associated with translocation.

Combined Open Approaches

The above transpetrosal approaches can be combined with standard craniotomy techniques to obtain unimpeded views of the posterior fossa. The degree of exposure required depends on the location and extent of the lesion. In general, transtemporal approaches are added when lesions are large and extensive, when they involve the anterolateral brainstem or pontomedullary junction, or when they have a supratentorial component. The skin incision is easily incorporated and extended depending on the extent of approach desired (Fig. 6.4a). As noted, the position of the head depends on the rostral–caudal view required. The best view of the region of the foramen magnum and inferior brainstem is afforded by elevating the mastoid so that it is the most prominent point in the surgical field. Conversely, less rotation and greater elevation of the zygoma offer more direct visualization of more rostral structures and of the tentorium.

To incorporate the far-lateral approach, we now use a paramedian incision and muscle-splitting approach (Fig. 6.4b). The incision must be medial enough to allow exposure of the mastoid yet lateral enough to provide midline exposure. When the muscle-splitting approach is used, the soft tissue must be dissected carefully to maintain the correct orientation and to avoid inadvertent injury to the vertebral artery. Constant manual palpation of the mastoid tip and lateral arch of C1 is mandatory. Helpful adjuncts include frameless stereotactic guidance. Subperiosteal dissection exposes the posterior fossa down to the level of the foramen magnum and to the laminae of C1 and C2. The incision and dissection can extend superiorly as desired up to the level of the transverse-sigmoid junction. The skin and muscle edges are reflected bilaterally with the aid of fishhooks.

Once identified, the vertebral artery is dissected from its location above the C1 lamina to its medial entry into the intradural compartment. Most challenging at this point in the procedure is the profuse bleeding, which can be encountered from the venous plexus surrounding the vessel. It is controlled by judicious bipolar coagulation and the generous use of hemostatic agents. A craniotomy may then be performed, as previously described [10]. Careful dissection of the condylar vein away from the foramen magnum allows a generous bone flap to be turned. Ideally, the dissection begins at the foramen magnum laterally and extends to the midline. It continues medially up to the sigmoid sinus and jugular tubercle and courses around to the contralateral side of the foramen magnum. Additional bone may be removed as required. As much as two-thirds of the occipital condyle may be drilled away as needed to increase lateral exposure. Skeletonization of the sigmoid sinus may follow, preceding additional transpetrosal exposure as required to approach the pathology.

A subtemporal craniotomy is easily added by extending the skin incision superiorly and anteriorly in a curvilinear fashion. The myocutaneous flap is dissected down to the level of the zygoma and Henle's spine, and a craniotomy is turned in the usual fashion (Fig. 6.4c). The flap covering the transverse sinus must be turned carefully because the dura is often densely adherent to the bone. Crossing this junction with the drill footplate is seldom advisable. Instead, the sinus is skeletonized carefully with the cutting or diamond bur. Incorporation of both the far-lateral approach and the subtemporal craniotomy with various degrees of petrosectomy allows the entire posterior temporal, retrosigmoid, and lateral suboccipital regions to be included.

After the bone is removed, the dura can be opened in many different ways (Fig. 6.5). The infratentorial opening usually begins in the midline inferiorly and proceeds superiorly and laterally to the junction of the transverse and sigmoid sinuses. A separate linear dural incision along the anterior portion of the sigmoid sinus simultaneously allows visualization of the presigmoid space with minimal cerebellar retraction (Fig. 6.5a). Opening the retrosigmoid dura extending inferiorly below the foramen magnum allows simultaneous visualization of the structures of the inferior posterior fossa and brainstem as in a standard far-lateral approach (Fig. 6.5b). The greatest degree of visualization is obtained by dividing the sigmoid sinus (Fig. 6.5c). However, this maneuver is only possible if the patient's venous anatomy allows drainage of the ipsilateral Labbé's vein into the contralateral transverse and sigmoid sinuses (Fig. 6.6). Subtemporal dural openings begin over the temporal lobe anteriorly and extend posteriorly to the superior petrosal

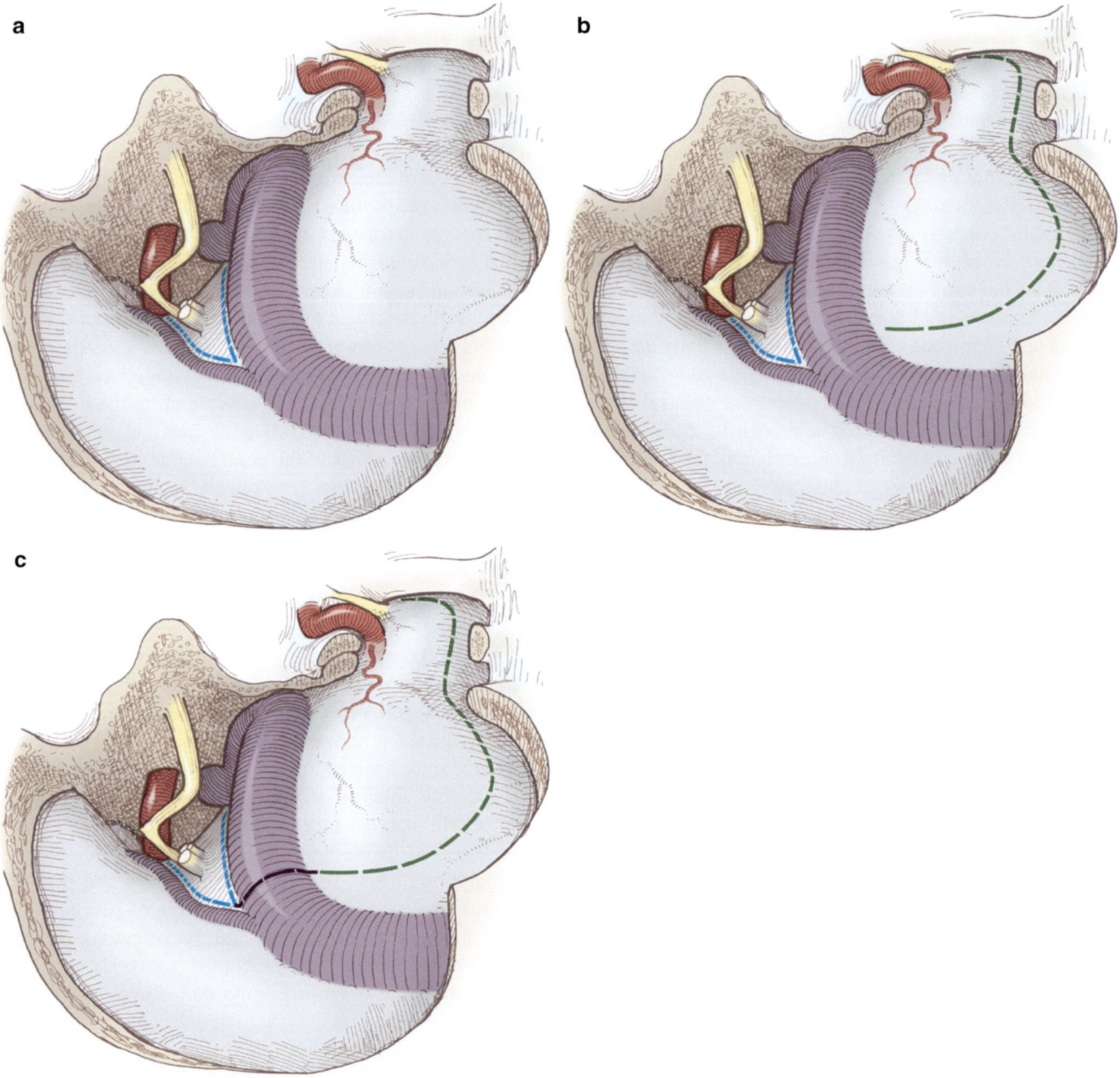

Fig. 6.5 After the transverse and sigmoid sinuses have been skeletonized, the dura may be opened in several ways. (**a**) Opening (*blue dashed line*) along the presigmoid dura allows anatomic visualization with minimal cerebellar retraction. (**b**) Simultaneous cuts in the retrosigmoid dura (*green dashed lined*) may be extended inferiorly to below the foramen magnum. (**c**) Alternatively, the sigmoid sinus may be divided (*purple dashed line*). (Modified from Baldwin HZ et al. [3], with permission from *Journal of Neurosurgery*)

sinuses. Care must be taken to avoid injury to Labbé's vein or to associated veins attached to the temporal dura or tentorium. An additional opening is made anterior to the sigmoid sinus up to the sinodural angle (Citelli's sinodural angle).

The superior petrosal sinus is then divided, and the opening is extended along the tentorium (Fig. 6.7). Care must be taken to avoid damage to the fourth cranial nerve as it courses along the tentorial edge, medial and inferior to the temporal lobe, before its insertion at the medial tentorial edge. If necessary and if the venous anatomy is favorable, the sigmoid sinus can be sacrificed by extending the dural incision across it. Such a maneuver allows an unimpeded view of the contents of the posterior and inferior middle fossae from the inferior brainstem to the upper clivus. The anterosuperior brainstem, cavernous sinus, and Meckel's cave are visualized clearly.

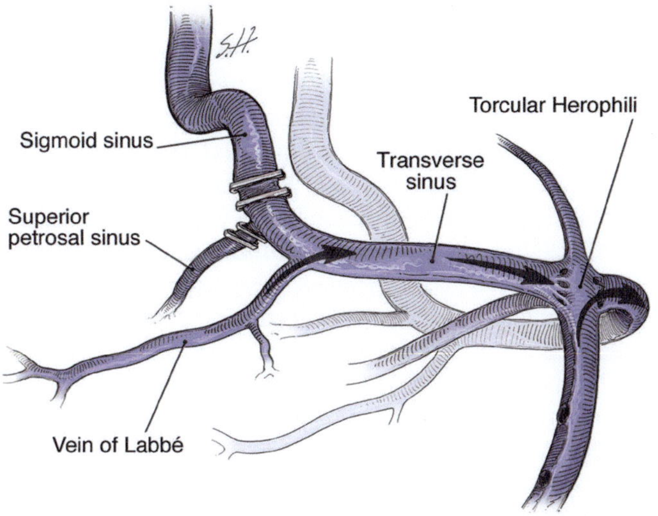

Fig. 6.6 Surgical view of the venous sinuses of the posterior fossa. Before the sigmoid sinus is ligated, patency of the contralateral jugular venous system must be confirmed. After the superior petrosal sinus and sigmoid sinus have been divided, blood is diverted through the torcula down the transverse-sigmoid sinus to the opposite jugular vein. (Reproduced with permission from Barrow Neurological Institute)

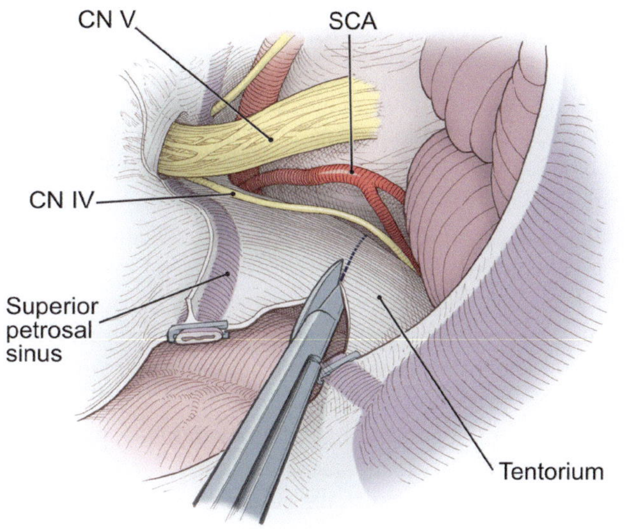

Fig. 6.7 Extent of exposure afforded by a combined transcochlear far-lateral and subtemporal exposure. The superior petrosal sinus has been divided, and further exposure is afforded by division of the tentorium. During this maneuver, care must be taken to avoid damage to the trochlear nerve (CN IV), which courses along the tentorial border. CN V = trigeminal nerve; SCA = superior cerebellar artery. (Reproduced with permission from Barrow Neurological Institute)

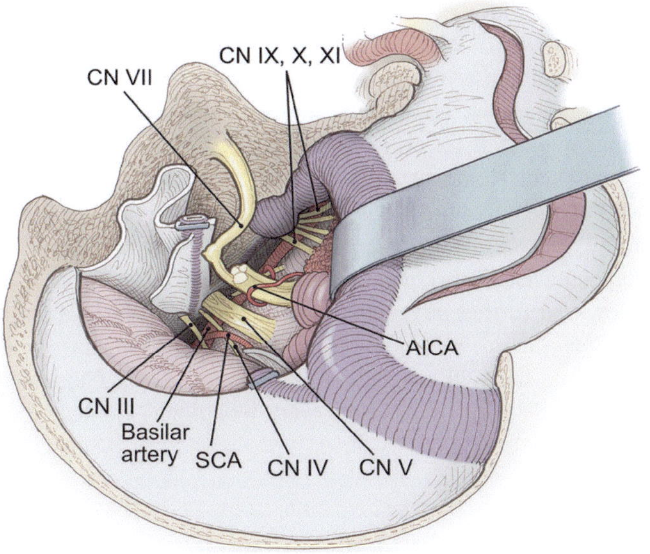

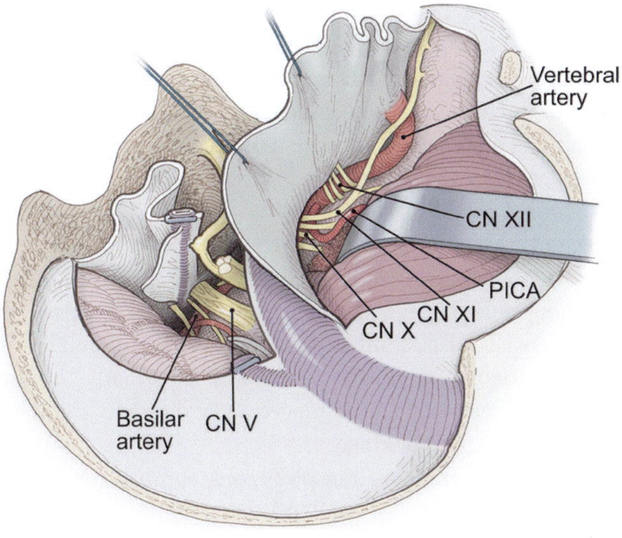

Fig. 6.8 Exposure of the contents of the posterior fossa after combined approaches. Sequential movement of the operating microscope and judicious retraction of the sigmoid sinus (**a**) posteriorly or (**b**) anteriorly affords a view almost as complete as that afforded by its division. This strategy minimizes the risk of venous injury or infarction. AICA = anterior inferior cerebellar artery; CN III = oculomotor nerve; CN IV = trochlear nerve; CN V = trigeminal nerve; CN VII = facial nerve; CN IX = glossopharyngeal nerve; CN X = vagus nerve; CN XI = spinal accessory nerve; CN XII = hypoglossal nerve; PICA = posterior inferior cerebellar artery; SCA = superior cerebellar artery. (Reproduced with permission from Barrow Neurological Institute)

Nevertheless, the venous structures can often be left intact. Sequential movement of the operating microscope and judicious use of the retractor allow adequate visualization while minimizing the risk of venous injury or infarction (Fig. 6.8). The exact approach and degree of exposure must be tailored to the pathology and needs of each individual patient to obtain adequate surgical treatment associated with an acceptable rate of morbidity.

Endoscopic Endonasal Approach to the Petroclival Region

A complete description of the techniques required to perform endoscopic endonasal approaches to the clivus and petroclival region is beyond the scope of this chapter. Numerous resources that provide a comprehensive description of these techniques as well as their variants are available [7–9, 18–22]. Here we will provide a brief overview of the transclival and transpterygoid approaches. Note that for petrous apex lesions projecting medially into the sphenoid sinus, a transsphenoidal approach may be utilized in cases requiring simple biopsy or for drainage procedures.

Access to the sphenoid sinus is common to most endoscopic skull-base techniques, including the transclival approach. In this approach, the anterior wall of the sphenoid sinus is identified and opened widely. Mucosal lining is peeled away from the bony surface of the sinus. Sphenoid sinus septations are drilled until standard anatomic landmarks, such as the optic nerves and ICA prominences, are readily identifiable. The transclival approach begins when the mucosal lining overlying the clivus is reflected exposing the bony surface. High-speed drilling of the clival bone using a diamond bur is performed. Small rongeurs may facilitate dural exposure after drilling is nearing completion. Dural exposure from the sellar floor to the foramen magnum is obtained along the midline. The lateral limitations of exposure are determined by Dorello's canal, the paraclival segment of the ICA, and the occipital condyles bilaterally. Dural opening is made difficult by venous plexus bleeding in some patients. However, aggressive use of bipolar cautery should be avoided as the basilar artery and/or CN VI are in close proximity intradurally. Packing of hemostatic agents achieves hemostasis in most cases. Once intradural, angled endoscopes assist in lateral visualization. Dural repair typically consists of abdominal fat graft with additional overlying autologous or synthetic materials. Finally, a large nasoseptal mucosal flap is placed over the defect and supported with nasal packing.

The transmaxillary transpterygoid approach begins by exposing the posterior wall of the maxillary sinus. This exposure may be performed with a wide antrostomy or by a modified medial maxillectomy. After middle turbinate resection, the sphenopalatine foramen at the crista ethmoidalis is identified and widened with Kerrison rongeurs. The opening is continued to remove the posterior wall of the maxillary sinus, exposing the pterygopalatine fossa (PPF) contents. The PPF is divided into anterior and posterior compartments. The anterior compartment consists of arteries and fat while the posterior compartment consists of neural structures. Gentle fat dissection exposes the vasculature. Depending on the exposure required, the sphenopalatine artery may be cauterized and divided or simply retracted to assist with mobilization of the anterior compartment structures. This exposes the neural structures of the posterior compartment. Exposure is widened medially after drilling the inferior aspect of the medial pterygoid plate. The pterygopalatine ganglion is located in the inferior aspect of the posterior compartment of the PPF just anterior to the Vidian canal and posterior to sphenopalatine arterial branches [8]. The extradural segment of the maxillary nerve (V2) is identified superior and lateral to the pterygopalatine ganglion typically at the level of the sphenopalatine foramen. Further dissection allows V2 to be followed posteriorly identifying the foramen rotundum. The Vidian artery and nerve is located superior to the pterygopalatine ganglion along its path, perpendicular to the sphenopalatine artery. Wide opening of the anterior wall of the sphenoid sinus is performed to identify the lateral extent of the sinus floor. At the junction of the base of the sphenoid sinus floor and the medial pterygoid plate is the pterygoid wedge. The medial aspect of the pterygoid wedge marks the typical location of the Vidian (pterygoid) canal [8, 21]. Elevation of the mucosal lining over the infrasphenoidal clivus completely exposes the canal and allows additional working room. Once the Vidian canal is identified, drilling commences along the inferomedial aspect of the Vidian canal until the depth of the petrous segment of the ICA is determined. As the Vidian artery commonly inserts along the inferior aspect of the ICA at the junction of the horizontal and vertical segments, initial opening of the Vidian canal inferiorly minimizes the risk of inadvertent ICA injury [21]. The remaining superior portion of the Vidian canal may then be removed once the depth of the ICA is established. Removal of the lateral aspect of the posterior wall of the sphenoid sinus exposes the cavernous sinus and allows for slightly greater mobilization of the ICA [22]. Exposure and subsequent mobilization of the petrous ICA allows for further infrapetrous drilling into the petrous apex. Further lateral extension into Meckel's cave has been described but will not be discussed here [8, 9]. Closure is completed using a multilayered technique as described above.

Endoscopic Endonasal Approach Considerations

In recent years, EEAs have been proposed by some as a feasible alternative to more traditional open transpetrosal approaches [7, 18–25]. While each open approach has its own strengths and weaknesses, commonly encountered hurdles to open lateral approaches remain. Lateral approaches to more medially located tumors frequently require the surgeon to work in windows defined by the transverse and sigmoid sinuses as well as the middle and lower CNs. As resection progresses, repetitive maneuvers across the CNs may result in unintended distraction injuries. In addition, tumors in this region may engulf or become adherent to vascular structures requiring meticulous dissection to access the deeper aspects of the tumor. These factors have led to an interest in extending the applications of an EEA into the posterior fossa for tumors near the petroclival region as the operative trajectory provides direct access to the deepest aspect of the tumor at onset.

Despite improvements in surgical technique and approach selection, morbidity following open transpetrosal approaches remains a concern for patients and surgeons alike. Aggressive resection of tumors in this region is associated with significant morbidity as there is frequent involvement of critical neurovascular structures that come into play when the limits of resection are reached [7, 26–29]. This is especially true for petroclival meningiomas where cranial nerve dysfunction remains a common complication of surgery [28–30]. In response, many surgeons advocate for less aggressive resection in an effort to minimize postoperative morbidity [7, 26, 27, 29]. Furthermore, as residual petroclival meningioma is commonly responsive to adjuvant radiosurgery with excellent control rates and minimal morbidity, the argument to pursue gross total resection in all cases is further weakened [7, 30]. In a series of 168 patients with petroclival meningiomas treated with stereotactic radiosurgery, the 10-year progression-free survival rate was 86% with a symptom control rate of 94% over the same period [31]. However, not all pathologies in this region are responsive to adjuvant therapies, which prompts an assessment of the limitations of the multiple surgical approaches to this region.

Expanded EEAs like the endoscopic transclival and endoscopic transpterygoid approaches have been described for the surgical treatment of skull-base malignancies involving the clivus and petroclival region [7–9, 18, 32]. Early reports detailing outcomes after an expanded EEA for the treatment of petrous apex pathologies consisted predominately of inflammatory or cystic lesions as well as encephaloceles [8, 9]. Comparisons between EEAs and more traditional lateral approaches have commonly been made in cadaveric studies [22, 26, 33, 34]. Primary candidates for an expanded EEA harbor lesions along the clivus or petroclival junction without lateral extension beyond the internal auditory canal (IAC) (Fig. 6.9) [7, 18, 33]. These lesions are also more likely to be located in the inferior aspect of the petroclival junction as this region is more easily accessed than the superior portion [22]. While it is true that larger lesions may provide a direct plane for continued lateral resection, open lateral approaches are generally required to access the lateral aspect of the IAC [26]. In addition, lateral tumor extension involving the paraclival, petrous, and/or cavernous segments of the internal carotid artery (ICA) also imposes relative limitations to EEAs. Even in the most experienced hands, endoscopic mobilization of these segments of the ICA is technically demanding [7, 18, 26]. In fact, a notable difference between the EEA and open lateral approach is that the ICA must be dealt with upfront in an EEA. Exposure of the ICA places it at a greater risk for injury. Tumor invasion into the cavernous sinus also poses unique challenges for the surgeon. While larger tumors may occupy the cavernous sinus creating sufficient visualization, smaller tumors invading the cavernous sinus pose a challenge as complete visualization requires enlargement of the opening into the cavernous sinus resulting in further manipulation of the ICA [18]. Should a vascular injury arise during an EEA, the small working angle and difficult visualization make achieving hemostasis difficult.

Limited anatomic studies and small case series have described further extension of EEAs to include extradural petrosectomy as well as medial condylectomy, allowing exposure of the length of the anterolateral brainstem [7–9, 21, 22, 33]. However, application of such expanded approaches has yet to reach common practice. Endoscopic removal of the clivus and exposure of the posterior fossa dura behind the petroclival junction expose CN VI as it courses into Dorello's canal at the medial aspect of the petrous ridge (Fig. 6.10) [7]. CN VI is at risk for injury at dural opening as it courses extradurally into the cavernous sinus. In addition, petroclival meningiomas may displace this nerve medially, interposing it directly between the surgeon and the tumor [7, 26]. In a series of 17 patients with petroclival meningiomas treated via an EEA, CN VI dysfunction was present in 47% postoperatively [7]. An additional challenge to endoscopic resection of tumors involving the lower clivus involves preservation of CN XII should a condylectomy be necessary [18]. Hypoglossal dysfunction and the potential for occipitocervical instability are necessary considerations.

While a less aggressive approach may be feasible for tumors responsive to adjuvant therapies, primary malignancies in this region often require aggressive resection. In a recent series of 42 patients diagnosed with clival chordomas or chondrosarcomas, gross total resection via an expanded EEA was obtained in only 66.7% with a postoperative CSF leak occurring in 16.7% of patients, requiring an additional surgery for reconstructive repair [18]. In this series, patients with tumors invading the cavernous sinus developed worse outcomes postoperatively than those with more medially located tumors, likely due to the morbidity associated with cavernous sinus entry. The authors found paramedian extension of the tumor to be a significant predictor of incomplete resection. For pathologies in which the goal is gross total resection, careful consideration must be offered when deciding the correct surgical approach. While an expanded EEA may be utilized alone or in a staged fashion, the surgeon's understanding of the lateral limitations of these approaches is important in optimizing surgical outcomes. In cases of

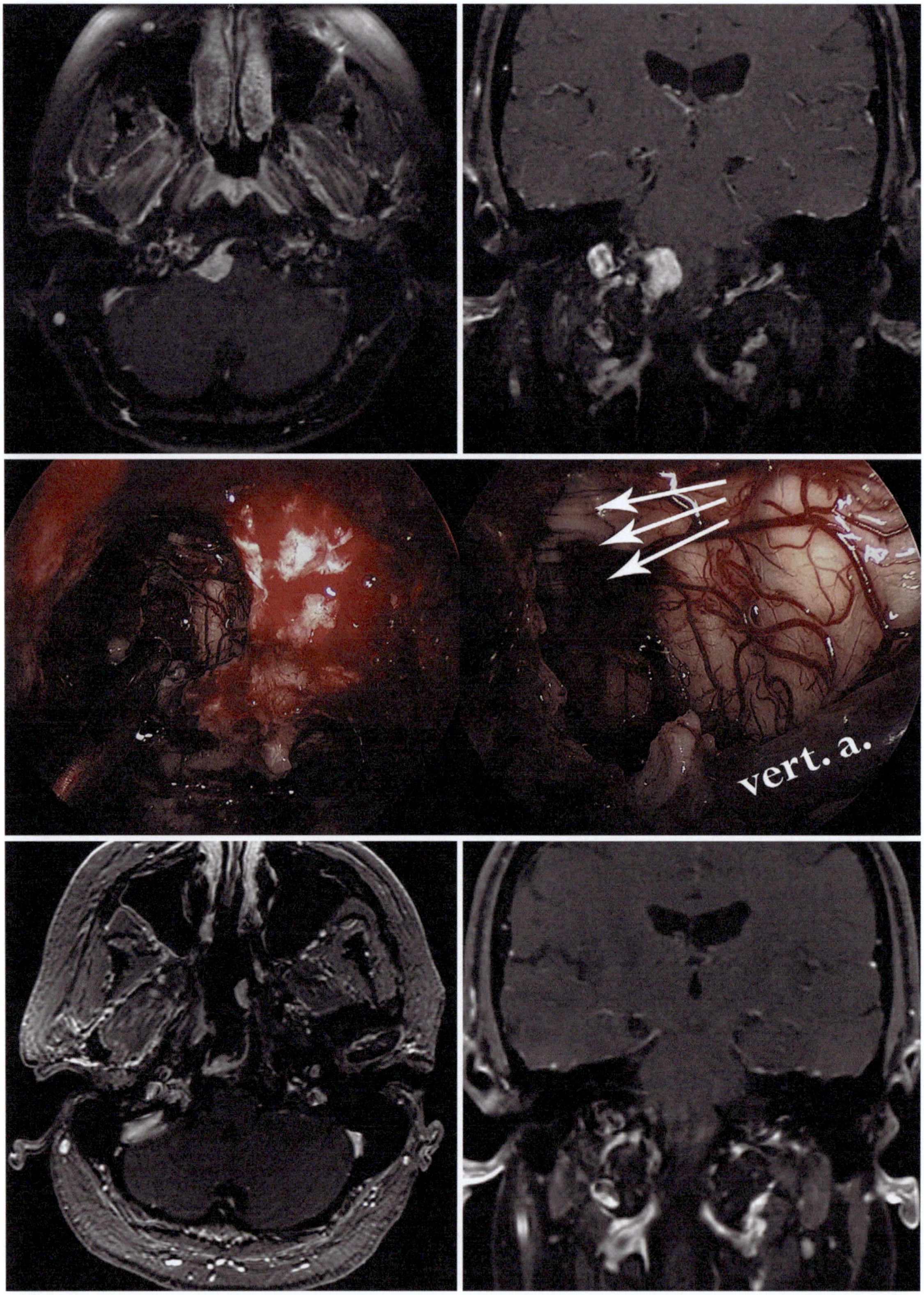

Fig. 6.9 Endoscopic endonasal approach for resection of a petroclival meningioma. (*Top*) Preoperative axial and coronal T1-weighted contrast-enhanced magnetic resonance imaging (MRI) demonstrating an enhancing lesion in the right petroclival region. (*Middle*) Intraoperative endoscopic view following resection of the lesion. Note the vertebral artery and lower cranial nerves are visualized (arrows). (*Bottom*) Postoperative axial and coronal T1-weighted contrast-enhanced MRI demonstrating gross total resection of the lesion [7]. (Reprinted from World Neurosurgery, 99, Koutourousiou M, Fernandez-Miranda JC, Vaz-Guimaraes Filho F, et al., Outcomes of Endonasal and Lateral Approaches to Petroclival Meningiomas, 500–517, 2017, with permission from Elsevier)

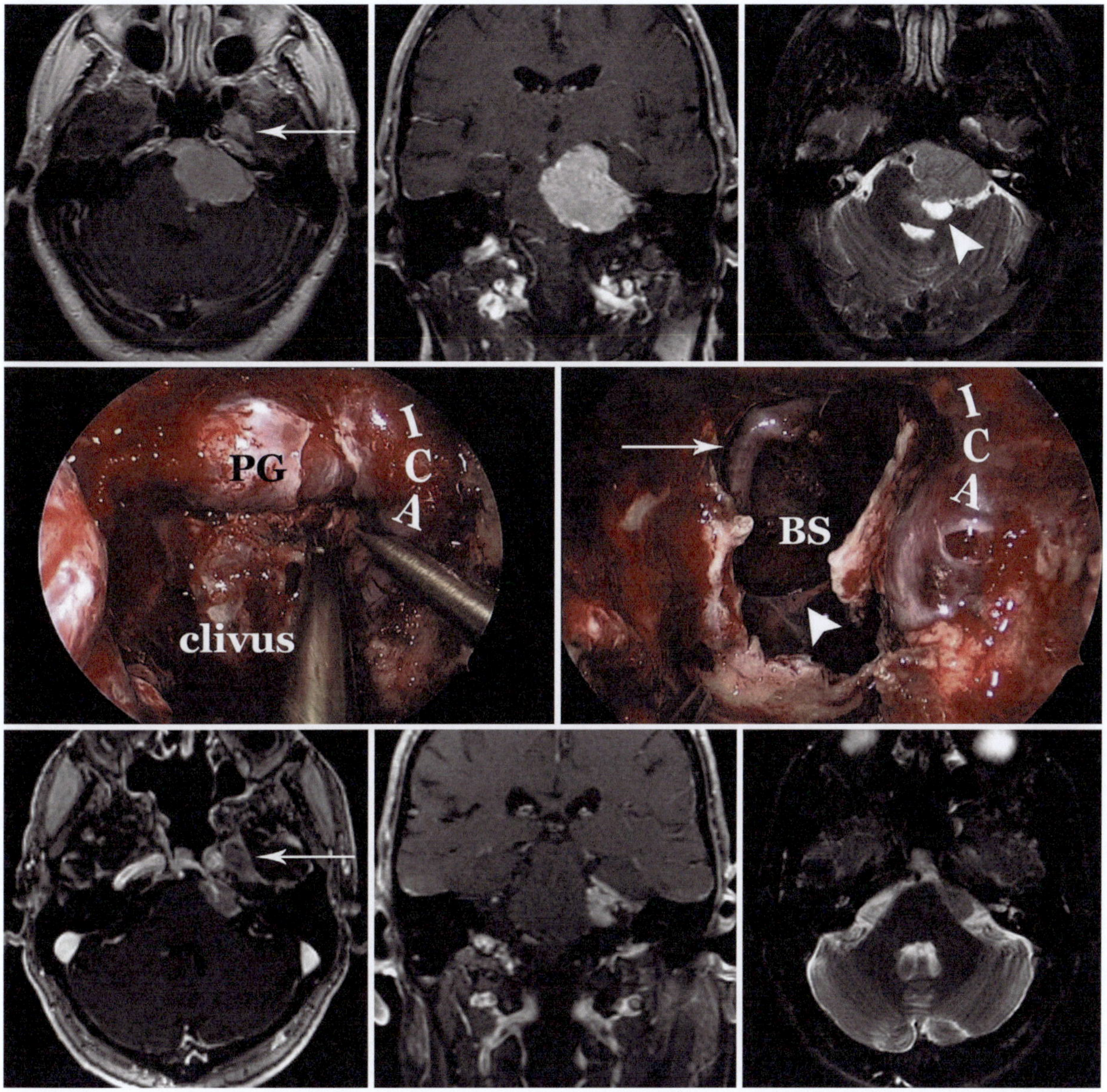

Fig. 6.10 Endoscopic endonasal approach for partial resection of a petroclival meningioma. (*Top*) Preoperative axial and coronal T1-weighted contrast-enhanced and T2-weighted MRI demonstrating an enhancing lesion in the left petroclival region extending into Meckel's cave (*arrow*). A posterior cystic component of the lesion is noted with mass effect on the brainstem (*arrowhead*). (*Middle*) Intraoperative endoscopic view. (*Left*) The clivus, dura overlying the pituitary gland (PG), left internal carotid artery (ICA), and petroclival junction (probe) are exposed. (*Right*) Following resection, the basilar artery (*arrow*), brainstem (BS), left abducens nerve (*arrowhead*), and the skeletonized left ICA are visualized. (*Bottom*) Postoperative axial and coronal T1-weighted contrast-enhanced and T2-weighted MRI demonstrating partial resection of the lesion [7]. (Reprinted from World Neurosurgery, 99, Koutourousiou M, Fernandez-Miranda JC, Vaz-Guimaraes Filho F, et al., Outcomes of Endonasal and Lateral Approaches to Petroclival Meningiomas, 500–517, 2017, with permission from Elsevier)

tumor location at or beyond the IAC, open posterior approaches provide the most direct access.

As with open approaches, appropriate repair of the acquired skull-base defect is critical to success. Reconstruction of skull-base defects following an expanded EEA remains a challenge even with the use of inlays, onlays, and vascularized pedicle flaps [7, 26]. The risk of CSF leak following an expanded EEA for intradural tumors in the petroclival region is higher than that reported for open approaches with rates of 22–41% in the modern era [7, 35]. EEAs for resection of primarily extradural clival malignancies still resulted in CSF leak in 16.7% in another report [18]. In contrast, a large series of 500 open posterior fossa cases reported a postoperative CSF leak rate of 13% for all pathologies [28]. Others have reported a CSF leak rate of just 4% following open resection of petroclival meningiomas [36]. Despite technical advances, the higher risk of CSF leak following expanded EEAs remains an important consideration in approach selection.

In summary, surgical resection of posterior fossa tumors near the petroclival region and anterolateral brainstem is an emerging application of expanded EEAs. Similar to the unique surgical skillset required for transpetrosal approaches, an EEA in this region requires a specialized team with advanced anatomical knowledge and experience as the intraoperative views and techniques are less familiar to most surgeons. Although the literature is still limited, the potential for lessened postoperative morbidity in the form of CN VII/VIII dysfunction is an appealing aspect of the EEA [7]. However, this appeal must be weighed against the maneuverability of a smaller surgical exposure, potential for significant vascular injury with limited means of achieving hemostasis, and, at present, higher rates of postoperative CSF leak for intradural pathologies.

Surgical Decision-Making

Tailoring the exact approach to an individual patient requires detailed anatomical consideration of the individual pathology. A frank assessment of the degree of surgical resection that is reasonable and expected is necessary. Often, the surgical team's experience with a particular approach dictates its use to the exclusion of otherwise viable alternatives. Numerous studies have described the different types of open approaches available for accessing the skull base [2, 5, 37–45]. These reports usually include a wide variety of opinions about the precise and best indication for each approach, depending on the authors' unique experiences and biases.

Erkmen and colleagues discussed the treatment of 97 patients with petroclival tumors treated with open approaches [46]. Their recommended approach depends on the location of the tumor along the clivus and in relation to the IAC. They recommend the orbitozygomatic approach for tumors located medial to the IAC without extensive posterior fossa involvement. The presence of tumors lateral to the IAC requires the use of a posterior transtentorial petrosal approach. The latter approach can be expanded to the middle fossa and combined with an anterior petrosectomy when tumors extend into the middle cranial fossa and cavernous sinus. This variation is particularly preferable in patients with serviceable hearing. They reserved the transcochlear approach for patients with preoperative hearing loss.

While the literature for open approaches to the petroclival region is robust, there is a growing body of literature supporting the role of the expanded EEA in accessing the clival and petroclival regions [7, 8, 18, 26, 32, 33]. Despite these advancements, it is important to understand the anatomic boundaries for exposure when using an expanded EEA. In general, tumor extension laterally beyond the IAC signifies the extreme boundary for an EEA to middle clivus tumors. Koutourousiou and colleagues discussed the surgical treatment of 32 patients with petroclival meningiomas treated with lateral open approaches, expanded endoscopic endonasal approaches, or a combination of the two [7]. Importantly, this series did not include tumors lateral to the upper clivus for which a pterional or frontotemporal orbitozygomatic approach is generally required. The lateral approaches consisted of the retrosigmoid or the far-lateral transcondylar. The retrosigmoid approach was used for tumors primarily along the petrous ridge with or without involvement of the IAC, while the far-lateral approach was used when the tumor extended inferiorly and laterally beyond the jugular foramen or hypoglossal canal. For midline tumors (i.e., those without lateral extension beyond the IAC, jugular foramen, or hypoglossal canal), an anterior EEA was utilized. For tumors requiring multiple approaches, an EEA was used in combination with either a retrosigmoid or far-lateral approach.

When reporting their results, many authors have emphasized the importance of preserving facial nerve and hearing function. Shen and colleagues described their experience with 71 meningiomas [47]. Of these, 94% were removed completely. Combined surgical approaches were used in 47% of the cases, but this proportion diminished substantially over the course of the study. This decrease coincided with an increasing priority to preserve hearing. Kaylie and colleagues preserved hearing in eight of ten patients who underwent a transcrusal approach to the petroclival region [48]. The addition of a partial labyrinthectomy to a standard presigmoid petrosal approach has also been advocated, with the rate of hearing preservation reported to be higher than 80% [49]. While hearing preservation techniques have improved outcomes, the fact remains that exposure of CNs VII–VIII places these nerves at risk. Preservation of facial nerve function is a primary goal when approaching tumors in this region. Tumors that are more laterally positioned may involve the IAC and, as such, a posterior open approach is necessary. However, many tumors in this region are located more medially and do not involve the IAC. One major difference between the EEA and traditional open lateral approaches to the petroclival region involves exposure of CNs VII–VIII. Lateral approaches require dissection of the VII–VIII complex in the majority of cases even when these nerves are not involved in the tumor. In a recent series of 26 patients with petroclival meningiomas treated with a retrosigmoid supracerebellar transtentorial approach, early facial nerve palsy and hearing loss developed in 12% and 15%, respectively [29]. Long-term, persistent CN VII and VIII dysfunction were present in 4% and 12%, respectively. Furthermore, extensive drilling as in transpetrosal approaches to more inferomedial lesions requires the surgeon to repetitively work past these nerves, risking inadvertent injury. Another recent series reporting immediate postoperative outcomes in 60 patients with petroclival meningiomas treated with a combined transpetrosal approach demonstrated facial nerve palsy and hearing loss in 45% and 32%, respectively [30]. Long-term outcomes were not reported. On the contrary, an EEA to more medially located lesions does not require exposure of CNs VII–VIII. A recent study reported outcomes on 17 patients with petroclival meningiomas resected via an expanded EEA [7]. In this group, there were no instances of postoperative facial nerve palsy or hearing loss, which is in sharp contrast to the open approach studies described above. Owing to the effectiveness of adjuvant radiosurgery, the authors state that their primary goal in these cases was to achieve brainstem decompression and minimize cranial nerve dysfunction. Their stated goals were evident as gross total resection was achieved in 3 (17.6%) of the 17 cases. However, owing to limited published series, the long-term recurrence rate following this treatment approach is not yet available [7, 26]. Lastly, with regard to hearing preservation in an expanded EEA, inadvertent obstruction of the Eustachian tube may result in mechanical hearing loss [9, 22].

The retrosigmoid approach has been described as an alternative to combined approaches for the treatment of skull-base tumors [29, 41, 50–54]. Anatomical studies in cadavers have compared the working area provided with the petroclival surface between the retrosigmoid and combined petrosal approaches [55]. Siwanuwatn and colleagues found no significant difference in either working area or angle of attack to the petroclival surface without the inclusion of a complete transcochlear exposure [55]. The axis of approach via the retrosigmoid approach is from a dorsal aspect along the plane of the petrous bone. Therefore, they suggested that the increase in bony removal afforded by the combined approaches, in the absence of a complete petrosectomy, is not extensive enough to increase the working area significantly. However, because some tumors grow posteriorly and compress the brainstem and neurovascular structures laterally, they create a "natural retraction" and an opening toward the upper portions of the clivus. This capacity for increased visualization may allow excellent surgical access via the simple retrosigmoid approach, obviating the need for additional bony removal.

Opening the tentorium in a traditional retrosigmoid approach allows for additional superior and anterior visualization. In a recent series authors reported that the retrosigmoid supracerebellar transtentorial approach provided adequate exposure for resection of petroclival meningiomas without a large middle fossa component [29]. The removal of the suprameatal tubercle has also been purported to increase exposure of the petroclival region, namely the middle fossa [56]. Authors have reported that by drilling the suprameatal tubercle and the petrous bone superior and anterior to the IAC, exposure of the trigeminal nerve in Meckel's cave was obtained [54]. As alluded to above, the choice of approach is often determined by the surgeon's experience as it is clear from the literature that there is often more than one way to access this location.

A major factor in the degree of resection that can be achieved safely is the consistency of the lesion and its involvement with major neurovascular structures. Bricolo and colleagues emphasized this point in their use of the retrosigmoid approach alone to treat 65% of 110 skull-base tumors [51]. Of 84 cases treated by Goel and Muzumdar over 11 years, 28 were treated with the retrosigmoid approach [52]. Their rate of gross total resection was 75% for moderately sized (mean diameter, 4 cm) tumors, most of which extended laterally beyond the IAC. Five patients (18%) developed new facial nerve deficits. Regardless of the surgical approach used, it cannot be overemphasized that the major determinants of the ability to achieve excellent resection associated with low morbidity are the presence of an arachnoid plane around the tumor, the consistency of the tumor, and the degree of its involvement with critical neurovascular structures. In a review of 137 patients, Little and colleagues demonstrated that independent factors associated with postoperative neurological morbidity included a history of prior resection and the presence of tumors described as being adherent or fibrous [44]. The authors describe the evolution of their treatment in pursuing near total resection in these patients rather than gross total resection in an effort to decrease the rates of neurological deficits. This treatment philosophy is further strengthened when the pathology being treated is responsive to adjuvant therapies as in the majority of skull-base meningiomas. Importantly, therapies like stereotactic radiosurgery are excellent treatments for many patients, but they do not treat symptomatic mass effect. Careful consideration of the pitfalls of each approach and responsiveness of the pathology being treated must be taken into account to maximize the benefit of surgery while minimizing morbidity.

The potential for a lower incidence of facial nerve palsy and hearing loss in selected patients is the greatest strength of expanded EEAs for treating tumors in the petroclival region. Midline tumors may be amenable to resection via an EEA especially when they are soft and suckable, but lateral tumor location or extension will likely necessitate an open lateral approach. With the limited operative exposure common to EEAs, gross total resection is made difficult for large or firm tumors. This point was described in a cadaveric study comparing the volume of petrosectomy achieved from an open anterior approach to that from an expanded EEA [22]. The authors found that the volume of bone removed during an open approach was slightly more than double that from an expanded EEA. While this study did not include posterior approaches, it is enlightening that the expanded EEA allowed access to only the inferior aspect of the petrous apex as the C3 segment of the ICA limited superior exposure. For primary malignancies or tumors in this region not responsive to

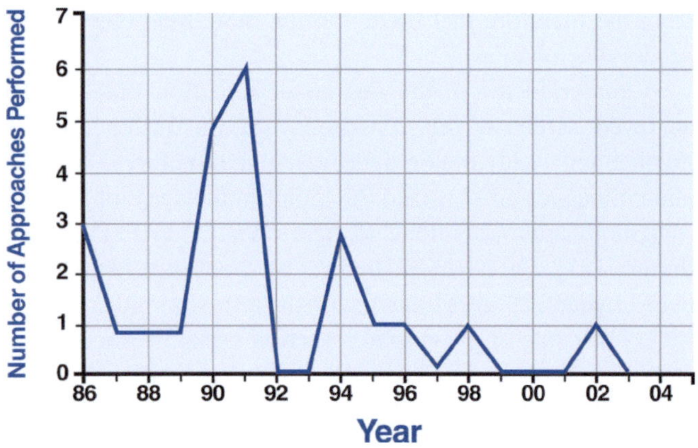

Fig. 6.11 Number of combined petrosal and transcochlear approaches performed in the treatment of petroclival meningiomas at Barrow Neurological Institute as a function of time. Most procedures were performed before 1996 [57]. (Reproduced with permission from Lippincott-Williams & Wilkins)

radiation therapies, the ability to achieve a maximal resection becomes a greater consideration. The higher risk of CSF leak following an EEA must also be considered when selecting this approach.

Although initially very aggressive in using combined approaches to treat a variety of skull-base tumors and vascular lesions [5], our management strategy has changed significantly over the course of time. In a recent retrospective analysis of 64 patients with petroclival tumors treated at our institution over the past 20 years [57], the use of combined petrosal approaches led to greater rates of gross total resection at the cost of an increase in complication rates. At the limits of our brief follow-up, progression-free survival remains excellent in all groups that we followed, regardless of the approach used. The addition of stereotactic radiosurgical treatment for the use of tumor control has significantly affected our treatment algorithm, and the number of combined cases performed in the treatment of petroclival meningiomas has declined significantly (Fig. 6.11).

Nevertheless, the combined approaches continue to be valuable tools in the management of complex skull-base lesions. They are regularly used to treat patients with complex vascular lesions of the posterior fossa [58–60].

Acknowledgments The authors thank Mark Schornak, Spencer Phippen, Deborah Ravin, and Stephen Harrison for their anatomical drawings.

References

1. Horgan MA, Anderson GJ, Kellogg JX, et al. Classification and quantification of the petrosal approach to the petroclival region. J Neurosurg. 2000;93:108–12.
2. Kawase T, Shiobara R, Toya S. Anterior transpetrosal transtentorial approach for sphenopetroclival meningiomas: surgical method and results in 10 patients. Neurosurgery. 1991;28:869–75.
3. Baldwin HZ, Miller CG, van Loveren HR, et al. The far lateral/combined supra and infratentorial approach. A human cadaveric prosection model for routes of access to the petroclival region and ventral brain stem. J Neurosurg. 1994;81:60–8.
4. Hitselberger WE, House WF. A combined approach to the cerebellopontine angle. A suboccipital-petrosal approach. Arch Otolaryngol. 1966;84:267–85.
5. Spetzler RF, Daspit CP, Pappas CT. The combined supra and infratentorial approach for lesions of the petrous and clival regions: experience with 46 cases. J Neurosurg. 1992;76:588–99.
6. Baldwin HZ, Spetzler RF, Daspit CP. Extended transpetrosal approaches to the craniovertebral junction. In: Dickman CA, Spetzler RF, Sonntag VKH, editors. Surgery of the craniovertebral junction. New York: Thieme; 1998. p. 491–506.
7. Koutourousiou M, Fernandez-Miranda JC, Vaz-Guimaraes Filho F, et al. Outcomes of endonasal and lateral approaches to petroclival meningiomas. World Neurosurg. 2017;99:500–17.
8. Hofstetter CP, Singh A, Anand VK, Kacker A, Schwartz TH. The endoscopic, endonasal, transmaxillary transpterygoid approach to the pterygopalatine fossa, infratemporal fossa, petrous apex, and the Meckel cave. J Neurosurg. 2010;113:967–74.
9. Zanation AM, Snyderman CH, Carrau RL, Gardner PA, Prevedello DM, Kassam AB. Endoscopic endonasal surgery for petrous apex lesions. Laryngoscope. 2009;119:19–25.
10. Thompson BG, Spetzler RF. Far-lateral suboccipital approach to the craniovertebral junction. In: Dickman CA, Spetzler RF, Sonntag VKH, editors. Surgery of the craniovertebral junction. New York: Thieme; 1998. p. 467–81.
11. Laing RJ, Smielewski P, Czosnyka M. A study of perioperative lumbar cerebrospinal fluid pressure in patient undergoing acoustic neuroma surgery. Skull Base Surg. 2000;10:179–85.
12. House WF. Translabyrinthine approach. In: House WF, Luetje CM, editors. Acoustic tumors. Baltimore: University Park Press; 1979. p. 43–87.
13. House WF, Hitselberger WE. The transcochlear approach to the skull base. Arch Otolaryngol. 1976;102:334–42.
14. Ammirati M, Spallone A, Feghali J, et al. The endolymphatic sac: microsurgical topographic anatomy. Neurosurgery. 1995;36:416–9.
15. Kawase T, Toya S, Shiobara R, Mine T. Transpetrosal approach for aneurysms of the lower basilar artery. J Neurosurg. 1985;63:857–61.
16. Maceri DR, Giannotta SL. The combined retrolabyrinthine/retrosigmoid approach. Oper Tech Neurosurg. 1999;2:48–51.
17. Fisch U. Infratemporal fossa approach to tumours of the temporal bone and base of the skull. J Laryngol Otol. 1978;92:949–67.
18. Kim YH, Jeon C, Se YB, et al. Clinical outcomes of an endoscopic transclival and transpetrosal approach for primary skull base malignancies involving the clivus. J Neurosurg. 2018;128(5):1454–62.
19. Kassam A, Snyderman CH, Mintz A, Gardner P, Carrau RL. Expanded endonasal approach: the rostrocaudal axis. Part I. Crista galli to the sella turcica. Neurosurg Focus. 2005;19(1):E3.
20. Kassam A, Snyderman CH, Mintz A, Gardner P, Carrau RL. Expanded endonasal approach: the rostrocaudal axis. Part II. Posterior clinoids to the foramen magnum. Neurosurg Focus. 2005;19(1):E4.
21. Kassam AB, Vescan AD, Carrau RL, et al. Expanded endonasal approach: vidian canal as a landmark to the petrous internal carotid artery. J Neurosurg. 2008;108(1):177–83.
22. Van Gompel JJ, Alikhani P, Tabor MH, et al. Anterior inferior petrosectomy: defining the role of endonasal endoscopic techniques for petrous apex approaches. J Neurosurg. 2014;120:1321–5.
23. Kassam AB, Prevedello DM, Carrau RL, et al. The front door to Meckel's cave: an anteromedial corridor via expanded endoscopic endonasal approach—technical considerations and clinical series. Neurosurgery. 2009;64(3 Suppl):ons71–82.
24. Kassam AB, Prevedello DM, Carrau RL, Snyderman CH, Gardner P, Rhoton AL Jr. An anteromedial corridor to Meckel's cave via expanded endoscopic endonasal approach: technical considerations and clinical series. Neurosurgery. 2009;64:ons171–83.

25. Kassam AB, Snyderman C, Gardner P, Carrau R, Spiro R. The expanded endonasal approach: a fully endoscopic transnasal approach and resection of the odontoid process: technical case report. Neurosurgery. 2005;57(ONS Suppl 1):ONS213–4.
26. Mason E, Rompaey JV, Solares CA, Figueroa R, Prevedello D. Subtemporal retrolabyrinthine (posterior petrosal) versus endoscopic endonasal approach to the petroclival region: an anatomical and computed tomography study. J Neurol Surg B Skull Base. 2016;77:231–7.
27. Janjua MB, Caruso JP, Greenfield JP, Souweidane MM, Schwartz TH. The combined transpetrosal approach: anatomic study and literature review. J Clin Neurosci. 2017;41:36–40.
28. Dubey A, Sung WS, Shaya M, et al. Complications of posterior cranial fossa surgery—an institutional experience of 500 patients. Surg Neurol. 2009;72:369–75.
29. Watanabe T, Katayama Y, Fukushima T, Kawamata T. Lateral supracerebellar transtentorial approach for petroclival meningiomas: operative technique and outcome. J Neurosurg. 2011;115:49–54.
30. Morisako H, Goto T, Ohata K. Petroclival meningiomas resected via a combined transpetrosal approach: surgical outcomes in 60 cases and a new scoring system for clinical evaluation. J Neurosurg. 2015;122:373–80.
31. Flannery TJ, Kano H, Lunsford LD, Sirin S, Tormenti M, Niranjan A, et al. Long-term control of petroclival meningiomas through radiosurgery. J Neurosurg. 2010;112:957–64.
32. Jean WC, Felbaum DR, Anaizi A, DeKlotz TR. Endoscopic endonasal approach for transclival resection of a petroclival meningioma: a technical note. Cureus. 2016;8:e641.
33. d'Avella E, Angileri F, de Notaris M, et al. Extended endoscopic endonasal transclival approach to the ventrolateral brainstem and related cisternal spaces: anatomical study. Neurosurg Rev. 2014;37:253–60; discussion 260.
34. Oyama K, Prevedello DM, Ditzel Filho LF, et al. Anatomic comparison of the endonasal and transpetrosal approaches for interpeduncular fossa access. Neurosurg Focus. 2014;37:E12.
35. Pinheiro-Neto CD, Paluzzi A, Fernandez-Miranda JC, Scopel TF, Wang EW, Gardner PA, et al. Extended dissection of the septal flap pedicle for ipsilateral endoscopic transpterygoid approaches. Laryngoscope. 2014;124:391–6.
36. Nanda A, Javalkar V, Banerjee AD. Petroclival meningiomas: study on outcomes, complications and recurrence rates. J Neurosurg. 2011;114:1268–77.
37. Mayberg MR, Symon L. Meningiomas of the clivus and apical petrous bone. Report of 35 cases. J Neurosurg. 1986;65:160–7.
38. Couldwell WT, Fukushima T, Giannotta SL, Weiss MH. Petroclival meningiomas: surgical experience in 109 cases. J Neurosurg. 1996;84:20–8.
39. Al Mefty O, Fox JL, Smith RR. Petrosal approach for petroclival meningiomas. Neurosurgery. 1988;22:510–7.
40. Sekhar LN, Swamy NK, Jaiswal V, et al. Surgical excision of meningiomas involving the clivus: preoperative and intraoperative features as predictors of postoperative functional deterioration. J Neurosurg. 1994;81:860–8.
41. Samii M, Ammirati M, Mahran A, et al. Surgery of petroclival meningiomas: report of 24 cases. Neurosurgery. 1989;24:12–7.
42. Hakuba A, Nishimura S, Tanaka K, et al. Clivus meningioma: six cases of total removal. Neurol Med Chir (Tokyo). 1977;17:63–77.
43. Sekhar LN, Jannetta PJ, Burkhart LE, Janosky JE. Meningiomas involving the clivus: a six-year experience with 41 patients. Neurosurgery. 1990;27:764–81.
44. Little KM, Friedman AH, Sampson JH, et al. Surgical management of petroclival meningiomas: defining resection goals based on risk of neurological morbidity and tumor recurrence rates in 137 patients. Neurosurgery. 2005;56:546–59.
45. Seifert V, Raabe A, Zimmermann M. Conservative (labyrinth-preserving) transpetrosal approach to the clivus and petroclival region–indications, complications, results and lessons learned. Acta Neurochir (Wien). 2003;145:631–42.
46. Erkmen K, Pravdenkova S, Al MO. Surgical management of petroclival meningiomas: factors determining the choice of approach. Neurosurg Focus. 2005;19:E7.
47. Shen T, Friedman RA, Brackmann DE, et al. The evolution of surgical approaches for posterior fossa meningiomas. Otol Neurotol. 2004;25:394–7.
48. Kaylie DM, Horgan MA, Delashaw JB, McMenomey SO. Hearing preservation with the transcrusal approach to the petroclival region. Otol Neurotol. 2004;25:594–8.
49. Sekhar LN, Schessel DA, Bucur SD, et al. Partial labyrinthectomy petrous apicectomy approach to neoplastic and vascular lesions of the petroclival area. Neurosurgery. 1999;44:537–50.
50. Samii M, Tatagiba M. Experience with 36 surgical cases of petroclival meningiomas. Acta Neurochir (Wien). 1992;118:27–32.
51. Bricolo AP, Turazzi S, Talacchi A, Cristofori L. Microsurgical removal of petroclival meningiomas: a report of 33 patients. Neurosurgery. 1992;31:813–28.
52. Goel A, Muzumdar D. Conventional posterior fossa approach for surgery on petroclival meningiomas: a report on an experience with 28 cases. Surg Neurol. 2004;62:332–8.
53. Spallone A, Makhmudov UB, Mukhamedjanov DJ, Tcherekajev VA. Petroclival meningioma. An attempt to define the role of skull base approaches in their surgical management. Surg Neurol. 1999;51:412–9.
54. Samii M, Tatagiba M, Carvalho GA. Retrosigmoid intradural suprameatal approach to Meckel's cave and the middle fossa: surgical technique and outcome. J Neurosurg. 2000;92:235–41.
55. Siwanuwatn R, Deshmukh P, Figueiredo EG, et al. Quantitative analysis of the working area and angle of attack for the retrosigmoid, combined petrosal, and transcochlear approaches to the petroclival region. J Neurosurg. 2006;104:137–42.
56. Seoane E, Rhoton AL Jr. Suprameatal extension of the retrosigmoid approach: microsurgical anatomy. Neurosurgery. 1999;44:553–60.
57. Bambakidis NC, Kumar UK, Kim LJ, et al. The evolution of surgical approaches in the treatment of petroclival meningiomas: a single-center retrospective review. Neurosurgery. 2007;61(5 suppl):202–11.
58. Gonzalez LF, Amin-Hanjani S, Bambakidis NC, Spetzler RF. Skull base approaches to the basilar artery. Neurosurg Focus. 2005;19:E3.
59. Porter RW, Detwiler PW, Spetzler RF, et al. Cavernous malformations of the brainstem: experience with 100 patients. J Neurosurg. 1999;90:50–8.
60. Bambakidis NC, Gonzalez LF, Amin-Hanjani S, et al. Combined skull base approaches to the posterior fossa. Technical note. Neurosurg Focus. 2005;19:E8.

Functional Surgery of the Cerebellopontine Angle

7

P. Ashley Wackym, Shekar N. Kurpad, Wesley A. King, and Anil Nanda

Although most surgery of the cerebellopontine angle (CPA) deals with neoplastic diseases, it is important for contemporary skull-base surgeons to remain proficient in the surgical management of diseases that disrupt cranial nerve function. In addition to the use of the operating microscope, over the past quarter century, we have found that the adjunctive use of endoscopy greatly facilitates optimal outcomes. Endoscopes have the ability to provide high magnification and illumination of the operative field. However, in contrast to the operative microscope, the endoscopic view is not limited to the linear line of sight. Thus, with flexible and angled endoscopes the surgeon can look "around corners," beyond obstructing tissue and structures. Initial reports of endoscope-assisted otologic and neurotologic surgery have been published, and the limits of these techniques continue to be explored [1–8]. This chapter describes the combined use of microsurgery and endoscopy during neurectomy for the treatment of chronic peripheral vestibular dysfunction, geniculate neuralgia, glossopharyngeal neuralgia, cranial nerve microvascular decompression procedures, and placement of auditory brainstem implants (ABI).

P. A. Wackym (✉)
Department of Otolaryngology—Head and Neck Surgery, Rutgers Robert Wood Johnson Medical School, New Brunswick, NJ, USA
e-mail: wackym@neurotology.org

S. N. Kurpad
Department of Neurosurgery, Froedtert & Medical College of Wisconsin, Milwaukee, WI, USA

W. A. King
Center for Minimally Invasive Brain Pituitary and Skull Base Surgery, Department of Neurosurgery, Cedars Sinai Medical Center, Los Angeles, CA, USA

Orofacial Pain Program, School of Dentistry at UCLA, Los Angeles, CA, USA

A. Nanda
Department of Neurosurgery, Rutgers—New Jersey Medical School, New Brunswick, NJ, USA

Neurosurgical Services, Robert Wood Johnson Barnabas Health, New Brunswick, NJ, USA

Vestibular Neurectomy

The rationale for unilateral deafferentation of a dysfunctional vestibular labyrinth is that the central nervous system (CNS) is better able to compensate for a complete loss of vestibular function than for a fluctuating partial loss. The single most common peripheral vestibular disorder requiring vestibular neurectomy is Menière disease, although most patients with this disease are managed successfully with medical therapy [9, 10]. Rarely, recurrent vestibular neuronitis or traumatic labyrinthitis requires unilateral ablation of vestibular function to achieve compensation. When patients have a useful cochlear function, vestibular neurectomy has the advantage of preserving hearing. A survey of the American Otological Society and the American Neurotology Society performed in the early 1990s showed that almost 3000 vestibular neurectomies had been performed in the United States since the introduction of the operating microscope [11]. More recently, it has been advocated that cochlear implantation is performed at the same time as translabyrinthine vestibular neurectomy for Menière disease [12].

Contraindications to vestibular neurectomy include bilateral peripheral vestibular disease, vertigo from an only hearing ear, and indications of CNS pathology such as multiple sclerosis, physiologic old age, and poor medical condition. Elderly patients have more difficulty in compensating than younger patients. Therefore, treatment options should be considered carefully before proceeding to ablative surgical procedures. However, destructive vestibular procedures remain an important treatment option for elderly patients disabled by vertigo of peripheral origin. The distinct advantages associated with each surgical approach are briefly reviewed in the context of the application of endoscopic techniques to this procedure.

Jean-Martin Charcot, who was a contemporary of Prosper Menière and director of the famous Salpêtrière Hospital neurological clinic in Paris, has been credited with first suggesting intracranial division of the auditory nerve to eliminate the symptoms of Menière disease in 1874. Walter Dandy

N. C. Bambakidis et al. (eds.), *Surgery of the Cerebellopontine Angle*, https://doi.org/10.1007/978-3-031-12507-2_7

most consistently attributed this suggestion to Charcot. However, after translating the original French manuscript, Jackler suggested that this attribution is inaccurate [13].

It was not until October 6, 1908, in Philadelphia, that Frazier completed this procedure in a patient with persistent aural vertigo [14]. A passage from Frazier's report [14] summarizes an issue that remains critical in the surgical management of patients with Menière disease: "Before this operation is undertaken in the future, one should determine by every means of precision whether the case falls in the category for which this form of treatment is especially applicable."

Walter Dandy first recognized that selective neurectomy of the vestibular nerve was possible: "In one of the patients … the vestibular and cochlear branches of the auditory nerve were separate and distinct. Such an anatomic variation would lend itself to division of the vestibular nerve without injuring the cochlear nerve and the hearing" [15]. In July 1932, Kenneth McKenzie of Montreal first selectively sectioned the vestibular nerve while preserving hearing [16]. In February 1933, Hugh Cairns of London performed a similar operation, and Dandy performed this selective neurectomy in March 1933 [17, 18]. Dandy, however, popularized the procedure, performing 607 neurectomies in 587 patients with Menière disease from 1924 to 1946 [18]. The use of the middle cranial fossa approach to section the vestibular nerve was first reported in 1904 [19].

Since the introduction of selective neurectomy, there have been numerous advances in surgical deafferentation of the peripheral vestibular system. For a broader perspective, readers are referred to a recent review of this topic [20]. Our initial 14 cases of endoscope-assisted vestibular neurectomy, reported by Wackym and colleagues [3, 21], are reviewed below with the addition of another case.

Clinical Material and Methods

Fifteen patients with intractable unilateral Menière disease underwent a retrosigmoid craniotomy for neurectomy of the vestibular nerve (Table 7.1). During each endoscopic procedure, a Hopkins telescope was used to study anatomical relationships in the posterior fossa and to assist the neurectomy. All patients undergoing vestibular neurectomy underwent preoperative and postoperative audiometric evaluation. Electronystagmography (ENG) was performed in fourteen patients before surgery and in nine patients after surgery. The 1995 American Academy of Otolaryngology Head and Neck Surgery Committee on Hearing and Equilibrium guidelines for the diagnosis and evaluation of therapy in Menière disease were used [22].

Table 7.1 Fifteen patients with Menière disease undergoing vestibular neurectomy (AAO-HNS, 1995 reporting criteria [22])

				Electronystagmography (canal paresis)[b]	
Subject	Age/sex	Stage[a]	Side	Preop (%)	Postop (%)
1	49/F	4	AD	44	100
2	56/F	1	AS	82	100
3	62/F	2	AS	73	100
4	43/F	1	AS	26	100
5	34/F	1	AS	29	100
6	16/F	2	AD	28	100
7	62/F	3	AD	78	100
8	60/F	3	AS	84	100
9	34/F	3	AD	29	na
10	55/F	4	AS	0	na
11	34/F	3	AD	0	na
12	60/F	1	AS	90	na
13	36/F	3	AD	38	na
14	45/M	3	AS	na	na
15	41/F	2	AS	88	100

AD auris dexter, *AS* auris sinister, *na* not available

[a] Staging is based on the four-tone average (pure-tone thresholds) at 0.5, 1, 2, and 3 kHz. Stage 1 (≤25 dB), Stage 2 (26–40 dB), Stage 3 (41–70 dB), Stage 4 (>70 dB)

[b] Canal paresis of affected ear based on caloric irrigation

Operative Technique for Vestibular Neurectomy

Each patient was positioned supine with the head turned in the opposite direction of the affected ear. After 1 g/kg mannitol and 10 mg decadron were administered intravenously, the patient was hyperventilated to achieve maximum cerebellar relaxation. A 4–6-cm linear skin incision was made 10–15 mm posteromedial from the estimated position of the sigmoid sinus. The incision began just above the level of the transverse sinus and extended caudally for 6 cm (Fig. 7.1a). After the nuchal muscles were incised and the periosteum was elevated, a single Adson cerebellar or articulated Weitlaner retractor was placed into the wound.

A retrosigmoid (suboccipital) approach was performed in all patients. The craniotomy measured 18–25 mm in diameter (Fig. 7.1b). After the craniotomy or craniectomy was performed, the dura was opened using a Y-shaped incision and secured to the adjacent soft tissue. The cerebellum was elevated gently to expose the lateral medullary cistern so that cerebrospinal fluid (CSF) could be released when the cistern was opened. Moist cottonoids were placed on the lateral surface of the cerebellum before it was retracted medially to expose the CPA and vestibulocochlear nerve/facial nerve complex (Fig. 7.1b). The cerebellum was maintained in this position by gravity or by a small Greenberg, Leyla, or De Martel retractor blade.

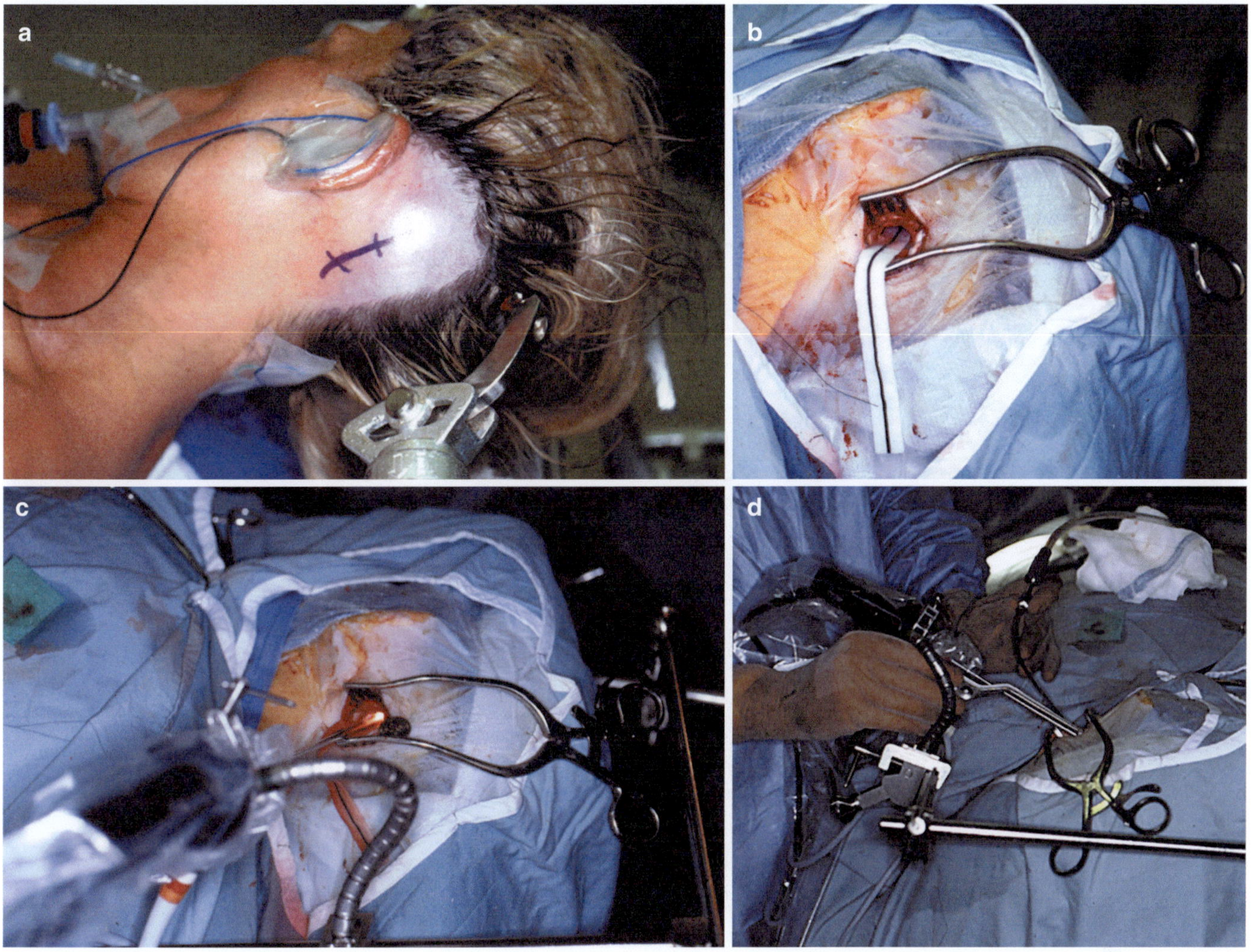

Fig. 7.1 Endoscopic vestibular neurectomy for Menière disease. (**a**) A 4-cm linear incision extends caudally from the transverse sinus. The Mayfield head holder is used to attach the endoscope holder. During the vestibular neurectomy, the auditory brainstem evoked response and facial nerve electromyography are monitored. (**b**) The craniectomy is shown with a cottonoid, measuring 0.5 × 3 in., in place over the cerebellum. (**c**) Endoscope is shown entering the posterior fossa via the craniectomy and is maintained in position using an endoscope holder. Sterilized dime shows scale. (**d**) With the use of an articulated endoscope holder, the operating surgeon is free to use both hands in performing the neurectomy. (Published with permission, copyright © 2007 P. A. Wackym, MD)

In patients with useful preoperative hearing, the auditory brainstem response (ABR) was monitored intraoperatively. All subjects underwent unilateral needle electromyography (EMG) of the orbicularis oris and oculi muscles. A team composed of a neurotologist and a neurosurgeon performed each procedure. If the vestibulocochlear nerve and facial nerve complex could be visualized adequately, the remainder of the vestibular neurectomy was performed while one surgeon held the endoscope and another surgeon identified the vestibular nerve and completed the neurectomy. Alternatively, an articulated endoscope holder (Codman, Randolph, MA) was used while the neurectomy was performed (Fig. 7.1c, d).

Initially, all patients underwent an examination performed with the rigid Hopkins rod endoscopes (4 mm, 0°; 4 mm or 2.7 mm, 30°; Karl Storz, Culver City, CA or Gyrus Medical, Inc., Memphis, TN). Specific attention was paid to cranial nerves V through XI, the internal auditory canal (IAC), and the vascular anatomy (Fig. 7.2a). The surgeon attempted to identify the cleavage plane between the cochlear and vestibular nerves. When this division was not evident, 30°, 45°, or 70° endoscopes were used to identify this plane within the IAC. In no case was a transmeatal approach (i.e., opening the IAC) required.

The vestibular nerve was identified visually. The location of the facial nerve was confirmed by stimulating the nerve

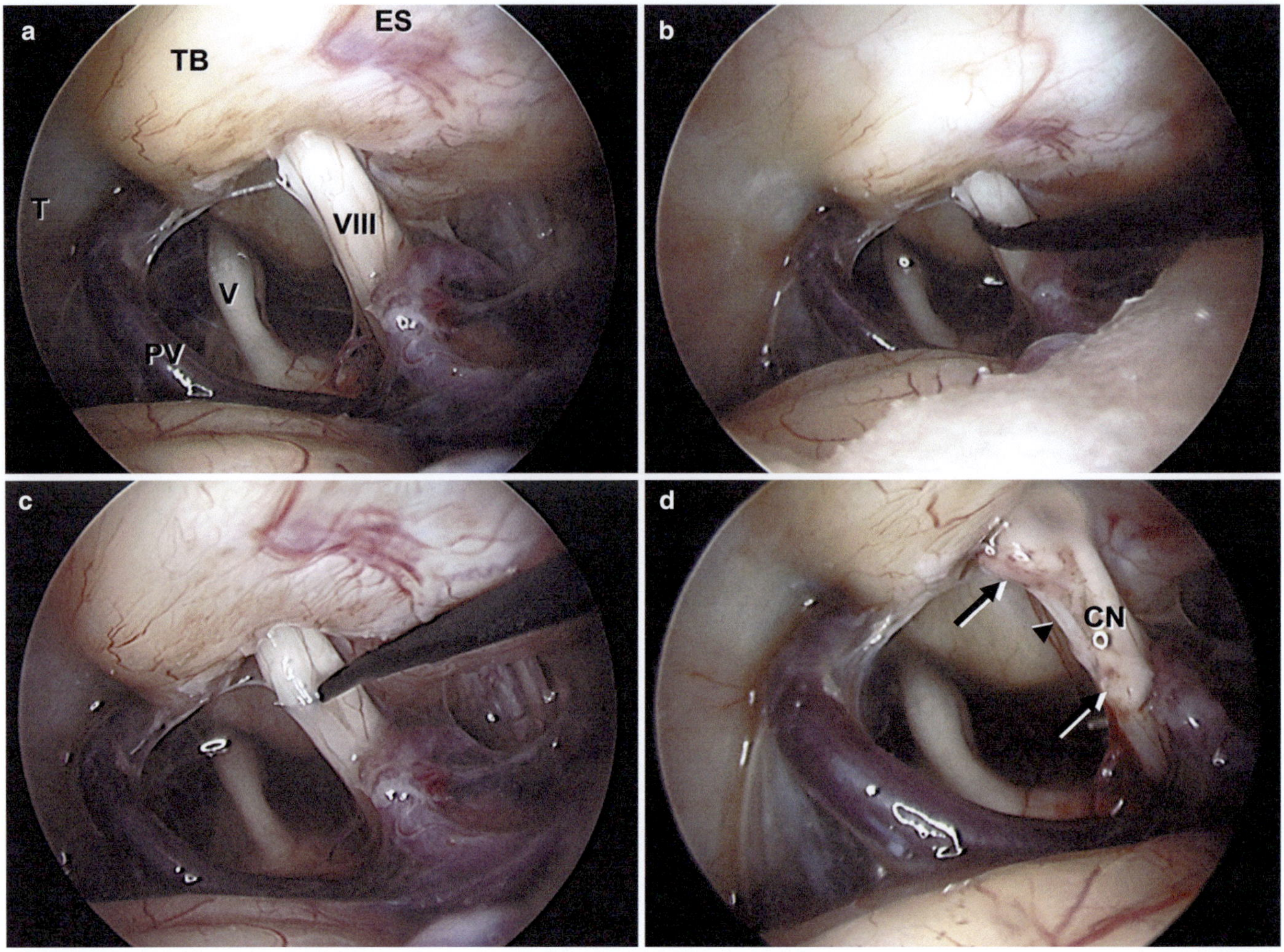

Fig. 7.2 Endoscopic vestibular neurectomy for Ménière disease on the right side. (**a**) An initial survey is performed with a 0° endoscope to gain orientation within the posterior fossa. ES = endolymphatic sac; PV = petrosal vein forming the superior petrosal sinus; T = tentorium; TB = posterior face of the temporal bone; V = trigeminal nerve; VIII = eighth cranial nerve complex. (**b**) The facial nerve is confirmed using a stimulus dissection instrument to deliver a 0.05 mA square wave current with a frequency of 4 times/s, each 100 μs in duration. Simultaneously, the EMG is recorded from the orbicularis oculi and oris muscles. (**c**) After the cleavage plane between the vestibular and cochlear nerves is identified, a stimulus dissection instrument is used to isolate the vestibular nerve from the cochlear and facial nerves. The neurectomy is completed, and a segment of the vestibular nerve is resected to avoid the possibility of regeneration. (**d**) The cut ends of the right vestibular nerve (arrows) are seen via a 0° endoscope. Arrowhead = facial nerve; CN = cochlear nerve. (Published with permission, copyright © 2007 P. A. Wackym, MD)

with 0.05 mA current and recording the EMG activity of the orbicularis oculi and oris muscles (Fig. 7.2b). The vestibular nerve was then sharply sectioned (Fig. 7.2c). While the vestibular nerve was retracted using microsuction in a lateral-to-medial direction, the vestibular nerve was sectioned again to complete the neurectomy (Fig. 7.2d). A 3-chip camera was attached to the lens of the endoscope, and the image was displayed on a 21-in. flat-panel video monitor and recorded on a digital capture system. After the dura was closed, a cranioplasty was performed using hydroxyapatite cement (Norian SRS, Synthes Inc., West Chester, PA) supported by a titanium mesh framework (Synthes Maxillofacial, Paoli, PA), and the wound was closed in layers.

Outcomes of Vestibular Neurectomy

Complete neurectomy was achieved in all 15 patients. Without the need for significant retraction of the cerebellum or brainstem, endoscopy improved the identification of the nervus intermedius; the facial, cochlear, and vestibular nerves; and adjacent neurovascular relationships (Fig. 7.3). Furthermore, the cleavage plane between the cochlear and vestibular nerves medial to or within the IAC could not be identified through the microscope in three cases. However, the plane was identified endoscopically (using a 30°, 45°, or 70° endoscope) in all cases (Fig. 7.3a). After the cleavage plane between the cochlear and vestibular nerves within

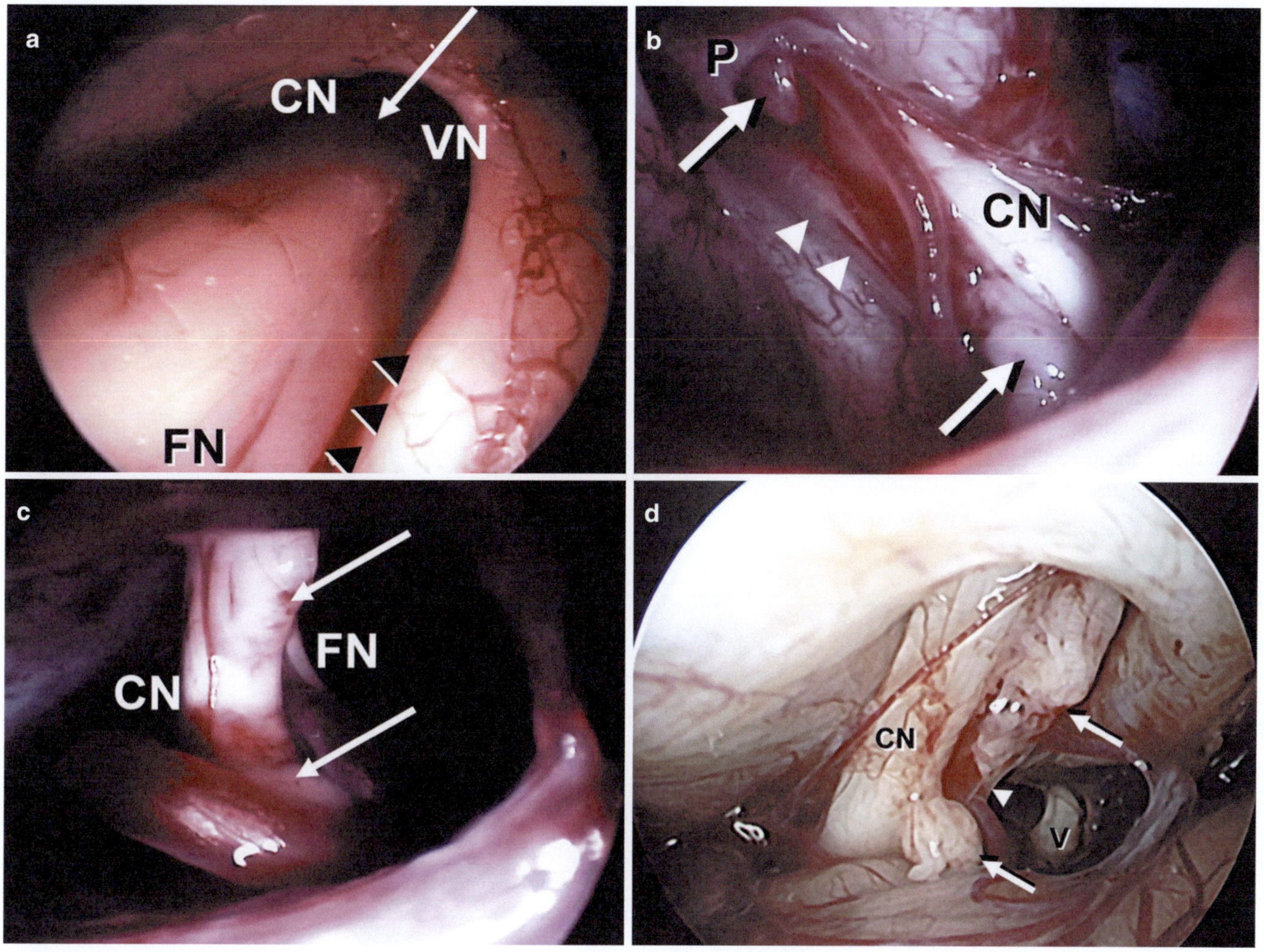

Fig. 7.3 (**a**) Variation, endoscopic vestibular neurectomy for left Menière disease. When a cleavage plane cannot be identified medial to the internal auditory canal (IAC), a 30°, 45°, or 70° endoscope can be used to identify the cleavage plane (arrow) between the cochlear nerve (CN) and the vestibular nerve (VN) within the IAC. Arrowheads = nervus intermedius; FN = facial nerve. (**b**) Variation, endoscopic vestibular neurectomy for right Menière disease. The cut ends of the vestibular nerve (arrows) are visualized through a 30° endoscope, beneath a large branch of the anterior inferior cerebellar artery (AICA) looping through the porus acusticus (P) into the IAC. Arrowheads = facial nerve; CN = cochlear nerve. (**c**) Variation, endoscopic vestibular neurectomy for left Menière disease. A 0° endoscopic view after vestibular neurectomy shows the cut ends of the vestibular nerve (arrows) and the cochlear nerve (CN). Multiple looping branches from the AICA, one of which separates the CN and vestibular nerve from the facial nerve (FN), are visible. (**d**) Complication of endoscopic vestibular neurectomy for left Menière disease. One patient from our series suffered irreversible profound hearing loss during retractor placement. After neurectomy, an intact cochlear nerve (CN) and facial nerve (arrowhead) are seen adjacent to the cut ends of the vestibular nerve (arrows). V = trigeminal nerve. (Published with permission, copyright © 2007 P. A. Wackym, MD)

the IAC was identified, it was developed medially before the neurectomy was performed. Vascular loops and branches of the anterior inferior cerebellar artery (AICA) passing into the IAC were also better appreciated (Fig. 7.3b–d).

In the group of Menière disease patients treated with vestibular neurectomy (Table 7.1), every subject had either recurrent vertigo or otolithic crises of Tumarkin (three patients suffered from both types of vertigo). Although all patients had relief of symptoms from their ipsilateral ear postoperatively, two patients later developed Menière disease in the contralateral ear.

Complete vestibular deafferentation was confirmed in the nine patients who underwent postoperative ENG. None of the patients experienced postoperative CSF leakage, headache, or facial paresis or paralysis. One patient suffered complete hearing loss during placement of the retractor, likely caused by vascular insufficiency of the cochlea. Despite removal of the retractor when changes were observed in the patient's ABR and placement of papaverine on the arteries feeding the vestibulocochlear complex, no measurable hearing returned. Complete vestibular deafferentation was achieved with anatomic preservation of the facial and cochlear nerves (Fig. 7.3d).

Advantages and Disadvantages of Different Approaches for Vestibular Neurectomy

The advantages and limitations of the various approaches to vestibular neurectomy have been reviewed [23]. These approaches include the middle cranial fossa and the posterior fossa approaches, of which there are a number of variations: the retrolabyrinthine approach, the retrosigmoid-IAC approach, and the combined retrolabyrinthine-retrosigmoid approach [11, 24].

The middle cranial fossa approach provides the only exposure that allows the primary afferent vestibular ganglia to be resected. This resection accomplishes two goals: (1) complete deafferentation of the vestibular periphery while preserving auditory function and (2) elimination of the possibility of vestibular nerve regeneration.

Posterior fossa approaches have two significant advantages over the middle cranial fossa approach for vestibular neurectomy: the risks of both facial nerve injury and hearing loss are decreased. However, a posterior fossa vestibular neurectomy has two primary disadvantages. First, the vestibular nerve fibers commingle with cochlear nerve fibers proximal to Scarpa ganglia. Consequently, both incomplete vestibular deafferentation and partial hearing loss are possible (Fig. 7.4) [25, 26]. Second, when the vestibular nerve is sectioned, the potential for regeneration exists. In contrast with a middle cranial fossa vestibular neurectomy, resection of the primary afferent somata within Scarpa ganglia eliminates the possibility of regeneration [27, 28].

We resect a segment of the vestibular nerve (Fig. 7.3) to avoid the possibility of regeneration. In contrast to the 98% rate of elimination of vertigo reported to be associated with

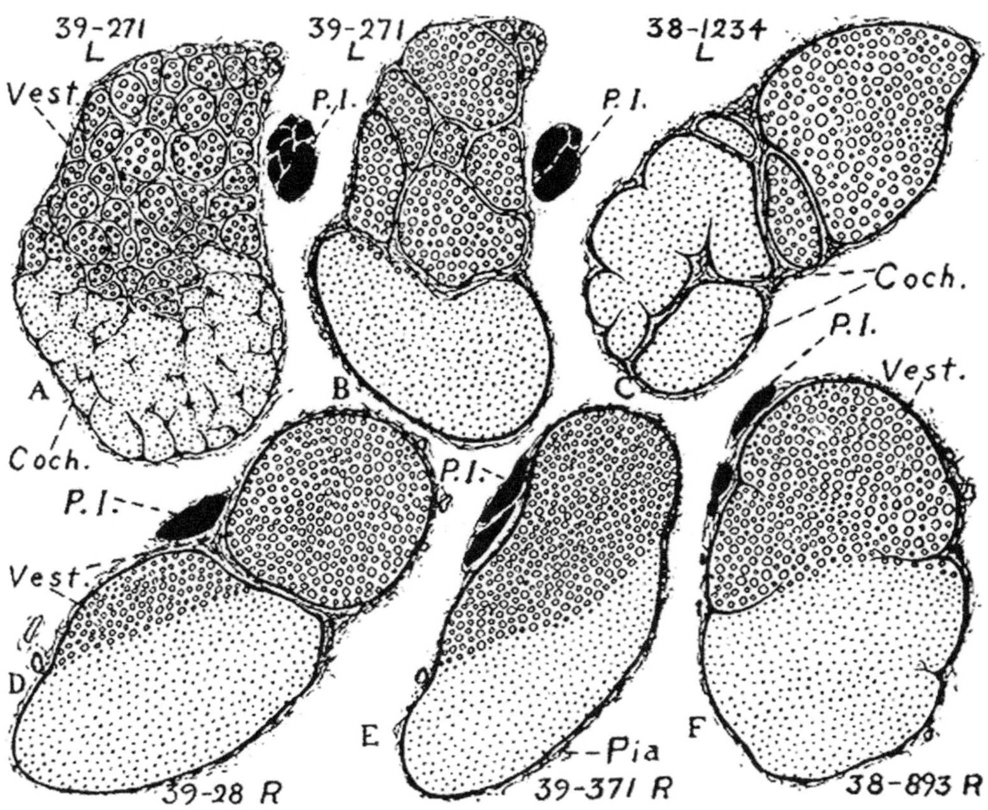

Fig. 7.4 Tracings of a pathological image showing the cable-like patterns of the eighth cranial nerve, in cross sections, from human adults. The cochlear (Coch.) and vestibular (Vest.) regions are distinguished from each other by different types of stippling. The solid white areas (P.I.) represent the pars intermedia (nervus intermedius or Wrisberg nerve) of the seventh cranial nerve. (**a**) Cross section slightly central to the vestibular ganglia. Both cochlear and vestibular portions consist of many small bundles and the cochlear nerve beginning to fuse. (**b**) A section of the same nerve as shown in (**a**), 2 mm further centrally, shows not only complete fusion of the cochlear nerve but several vestibular fasciculi. The vestibular bundles ultimately fuse with each other and with the cochlear component until a single trunk is formed, similar to (**e**). (**c**) A case in which neither the cochlear nor vestibular nerves are fused completely through most of their course in the internal auditory meatus and subarachnoid space. (**d**) Example showing the eighth cranial nerve represented by two distinct trunks, one of which was apparently purely vestibular. The other was mostly cochlear but with a prominent vestibular region amounting to about one-fifth of the cross-sectional area of the cochlear trunk. (**e**) Example of a common condition in which there is a single trunk, little more than half of which (upon microscopic examination) is found to be vestibular and the rest cochlear. (**f**) A case where incomplete glial septa approximately indicate the division between the cochlear and vestibular trunks. There are usually at least a few vestibular fibers on the cochlear side of such septa. (Adapted from Rasmussen [25])

middle cranial fossa vestibular neurectomy [29], 90–92% of patients undergoing posterior fossa vestibular neurectomy are relieved of vertigo [11, 24]. This difference may reflect imperfect patient selection or incomplete transection of the vestibular nerve.

The incidence of early CSF leakage associated with vestibular neurectomy is reported to be about 10% [11]. The retrosigmoid-IAC approach has been associated with postoperative headache, described as severe, in 75% of patients [11, 30]. The cause of the headache is unclear, although bone dust has been suspected. Both of these complications are related to opening the IAC. With the procedure described herein, this transmeatal approach is unnecessary [31]. However, the size of our series is modest. In some cases, if the cleavage plane between the cochlear and vestibular nerves cannot be seen within the IAC using a 30°, 45°, or 70° endoscope, the IAC may need to be opened. One of our patients suffered profound hearing loss during retractor placement. In the literature on microvascular decompression, the incidence of ipsilateral hearing loss attributed to cerebellar retraction ranges from 2% to 8% of patients [32, 33].

Neurectomy of the Nervus Intermedius

Endoscope-assisted surgery can be used to perform rhizotomy of other cranial nerves. An example of another application, neurectomy of the nervus intermedius for intractable geniculate neuralgia, is presented below.

Case Report

A 47-year-old woman who had experienced unilateral right otalgia for 4 months was initially treated for presumed otitis externa with ototopical agents and prednisone, without relief. She was then referred for further evaluation. An audiogram demonstrated normal thresholds, discrimination, and tympanometric results. Her otologic, neurotologic, and complete head and neck examination were within normal limits. Computed tomography (CT) of the temporal bones and magnetic resonance imaging (MRI) with gadolinium enhancement of the temporal bones, IACs, and skull base were unremarkable. An evaluation by an oral surgeon failed to reveal temporomandibular joint arthropathy. A 12-month trial of carbamazepine (Tegretol) followed by baclofen (Lioresal) and gabapentin (Neurontin) was completed with no change in her otalgia. Her erythrocyte sedimentation rate, titer for Lyme disease, and values from a full laboratory evaluation were normal. The patient underwent a retrosigmoid posterior fossa craniotomy with endoscope-assisted section of the nervus intermedius for presumed geniculate neuralgia (Fig. 7.5). Fifteen years after surgical intervention, the patient reports that her otalgia had resolved and had not recurred. Sensation was decreased but not absent in the right posterior concha. She had no other neurologic deficits.

Diagnosis of Geniculate Neuralgia

Geniculate neuralgia as the cause of primary otalgia is rare. However, anatomic and clinical studies have shown a clear sensory component to the seventh cranial nerve that can be implicated in geniculate neuralgia (Fig. 7.6) [34]. Sensory innervation to the cutaneous areas of the internal and external ear is complex: the ear is the locus for cranial nerves V, IX, X, the nervus intermedius (i.e., Wrisberg nerve) [35], and the upper cervical dorsal roots. Cases refractory to conservative therapy can be managed surgically. As cited by Hunt [34], the index case of primary otalgia treated by section of the nervus intermedius, which was reported by Clark and Taylor, served to establish geniculate neuralgia as a definite clinical entity.

Before a patient is diagnosed with geniculate neuralgia, an extensive differential diagnosis should be entertained. Otitis; temporomandibular joint disease; Eagle syndrome; carcinoma of the nasopharynx, temporal bone, external auditory canal, or pinna; vascular lesions; and referred pain from the CPA, larynx, and pharynx must be eliminated clinically and diagnostically. Complete neurologic, otologic, and dental evaluations are paramount.

Functional Anatomy

Attempts at sensory ablation have focused on section of the nervus intermedius with or without section of other cranial nerves, section of the greater superficial petrosal nerve, and resection of the geniculate ganglion [36]. Others have found vascular loops associated with these cranial nerves and advocate their decompression or section of the nervus intermedius combined with microvascular decompression of other cranial nerves [36]. In major series, success rates associated with sectioning of the nervus intermedius range from 72% to 90% [36, 37].

The facial nerve has two major components: a larger motor component supplies the facial musculature, and a smaller component, the nervus intermedius, contains sensory and parasympathetic nerve fibers. The nervus intermedius has distinct features and can be considered a separate cranial nerve. Its sensory portion is responsible for taste sensation on the anterior two-thirds of the tongue as well as for sensation of the external auditory canal and concha. The parasympathetic portion of the nerve supplies secretomotor fibers to the lacrimal, submandibular, sublingual, nasal, and palatine glands.

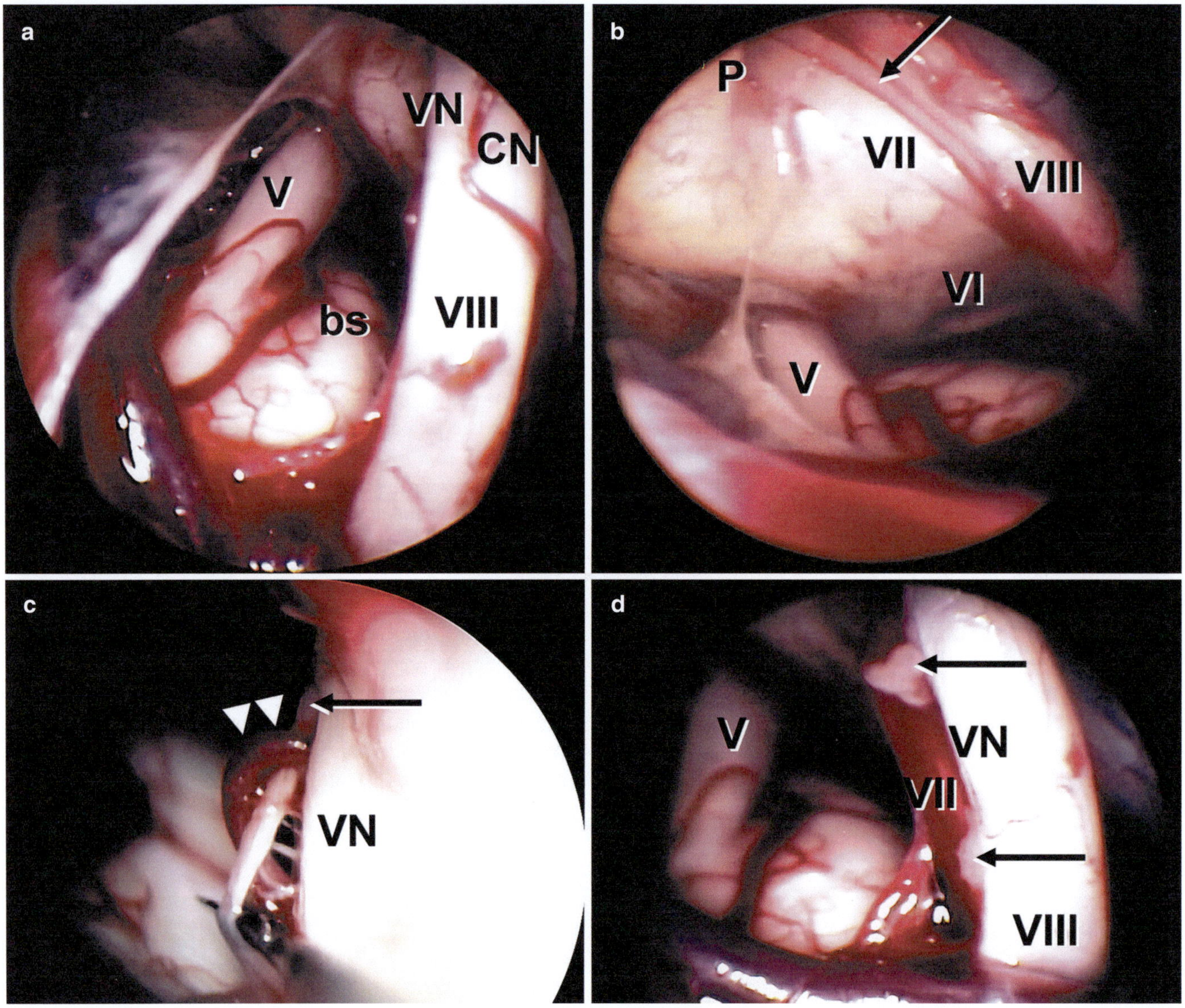

Fig. 7.5 Endoscopic view of the right nervus intermedius within the posterior fossa, in relationship to the trigeminal (V), abducens (VI), facial (VII), and cochleovestibular (VIII) nerves. (**a**) Initial view into the posterior fossa and cerebellopontine angle. The cleavage plane between the vestibular nerve (VN) and cochlear nerve (CN) can be seen distal to the vestibulocochlear nerve (VIII). *bs* brainstem. (**b**) Intermediate segment of the nervus intermedius (arrow) seen entering the porus acusticus (P). (**c**) In this patient, the nervus intermedius (arrow) is separated from the vestibular nerve (VN) by a looping branch of the anterior inferior cerebellar artery (arrowheads) before neurectomy. (**d**) Cut ends of the nervus intermedius (long arrows) are seen between cranial nerves VII and VIII. The anterior inferior cerebellar artery is visible in the foreground at the root entry zone of the vestibulocochlear nerve. The trigeminal nerve (V) is seen in the background. (Published with permission, copyright © 2007 P. A. Wackym, MD)

As described by Rhoton and colleagues [38], the nervus intermedius can be divided into three principle segments. The proximal portion is adherent to the eighth cranial nerve just anterior to the superior vestibular nerve at the brainstem. The intermediate segment lies free between the seventh and eighth cranial nerves (Fig. 7.5). The distal segment becomes incorporated into the seventh cranial nerve, usually within the porus acusticus (Fig. 7.3a).

In cadaveric studies, Rhoton and colleagues found that in most instances the nervus intermedius existed as a single nerve trunk. In the remainder, it was composed of as many as four rootlets. In about 20% of the cases, the nervus intermedius was adherent to the eighth cranial nerve throughout the area between the brainstem and porus acusticus. If the use of a 30°, 45° or 70° endoscope fails to identify this plane in these cases, the posterior lip of the internal auditory canal must be unroofed to allow access. Arteries coursing to supply the brainstem dorsal to the eighth cranial nerve may be found passing between the seventh and eighth cranial nerves as far laterally as the internal auditory meatus. In 5 of their

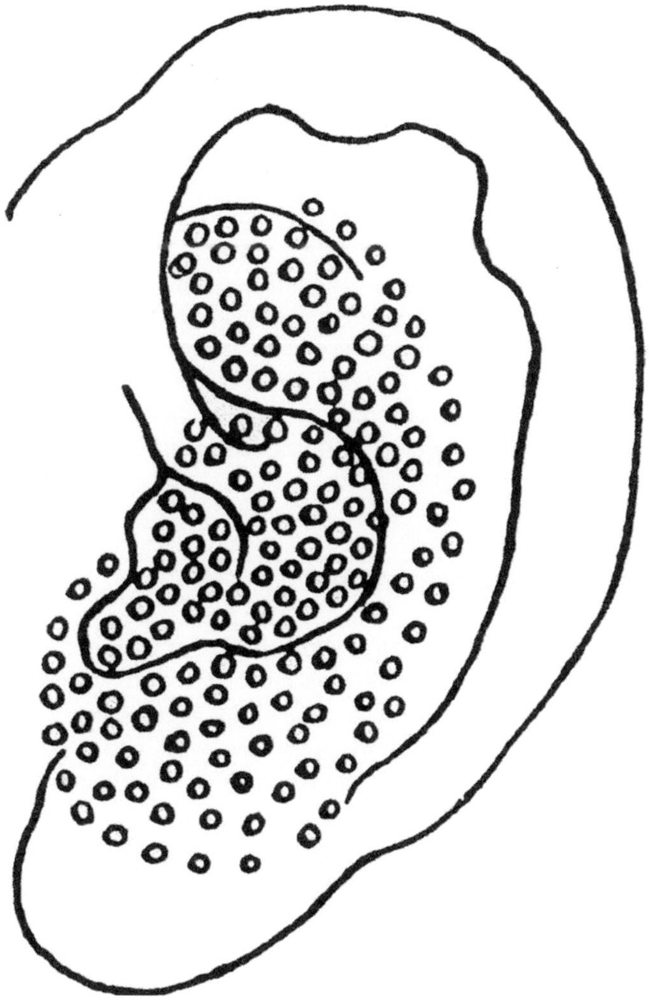

Fig. 7.6 J. Ramsay Hunt described the distribution of the sensory component of the seventh cranial nerve in his clinical studies of patients with Herpes zoster oticus. This figure from his 1937 paper illustrates the sensory distribution of the nervus intermedius in the auricle [34]

37 cases, a branch of the AICA was seen to enter the internal acoustic meatus with the seventh and eighth cranial nerves, giving rise to the labyrinthine artery, which looped back to supply the brainstem.

Neurectomy of the Glossopharyngeal Nerve

Natural History and Clinical Manifestations of Glossopharyngeal Neuralgia

The definitive origin of glossopharyngeal (vagoglossopharyngeal) neuralgia is unknown. Its peak age of onset is between 40 and 60 years. Glossopharyngeal neuralgia affects men as frequently as women. It is almost always unilateral, and it is most common on the left side (about a 3:2 ratio). It is 70–100 times less common than trigeminal neuralgia.

Glossopharyngeal neuralgia is characterized by paroxysms of pain in the sensory distribution of the ninth cranial nerve. On the basis of the distribution of the ninth cranial nerve, pain may be experienced primarily in the ear (otalgia) or in the throat (pharyngeal) or, rarely, in both locations. In 10–15% of individuals, painful paroxysms may be associated with bradycardia or asystole.

Except for the location of the pain and sensory stimuli that induce it, the attacks are identical to those of trigeminal neuralgia. Attacks are typified by a series of lancinating, electric-like jabs of pain in the region of the tonsil or posterior third of the tongue. Painful paroxysms may occur spontaneously or be triggered by a non-noxious sensory stimulus or event such as swallowing.

Initially, long pain-free intervals occur, but the episodes of neuralgia usually become more frequent with time. Paroxysms also often occur in clusters, which may recur through days, weeks, or months.

Radiation to the external auditory meatus or angle of the mandible may make it difficult to differentiate glossopharyngeal neuralgia from trigeminal neuralgia involving the third division of the trigeminal nerve or from pain arising from the nervus intermedius. Occasionally, glossopharyngeal neuralgia and trigeminal neuralgia of the third division may coexist and require surgical manipulation of both fifth and ninth cranial nerves [39].

Like trigeminal neuralgia, glossopharyngeal neuralgia may occur as a result of a structural lesion involving the glossopharyngeal nerve (secondary neuralgia) or as an idiopathic event (primary glossopharyngeal neuralgia). Neoplasms account for most cases of secondary glossopharyngeal neuralgia and are usually extracranial and malignant.

Functional Anatomy

The glossopharyngeal nerve leaves the lateral surface of the medulla, dorsal to the inferior olivary nucleus, and courses through the cephalad portion of the jugular foramen. It is separated from the fibers of the tenth and eleventh cranial nerves by a distinct dural septum. The ganglia of the glossopharyngeal nerve lie within the jugular foramen.

The glossopharyngeal nerve is a mixed nerve. The general somatic afferent fibers supply sensation to the back of the ear. Their cell bodies are in the superior ganglion, and the central connections terminate in the spinal nucleus of the trigeminal nerve. The general visceral afferent fibers supply sensation to the carotid sinus, carotid body, eustachian tube, pharynx, and tongue. The cell bodies are in the inferior (petrosal) ganglion, and the central connections terminate in the solitary tract. The special visceral afferent fibers from the taste receptors of the posterior third of the tongue, in like manner, have cell bodies in the inferior (petrosal) ganglion and terminate in the solitary tract. The general visceral efferent fibers, which supply the parasympathetic innervation to the parotid gland, arise in the inferior salivatory nucleus and terminate in the otic ganglion. The special visceral efferent fibers, which innervate the stylopharyngeus muscle of the pharynx, originate in the nucleus ambiguus.

Differential Diagnosis

Glossopharyngeal neuralgia can sometimes be confused with geniculate neuralgia or mandibular trigeminal neuralgia [40]. When dilemmas arise about the nerves that are the origin of the neuralgia, differential temporary blocks using 10% cocaine may be used to enable neurological localization. A cocaine block of the pharynx relieves the pain associated with the ninth cranial nerve, whereas a cocaine block of the pyriform fossa relieves neuralgia associated with the superior laryngeal branch of the vagus nerve. Blocking the foramen ovale with bupivacaine determines whether a component of the pain is caused by the third division of the trigeminal nerve. A tetracaine block of the jugular foramen blocks all afferent impulses via the ninth and tenth cranial nerves and helps diagnosis in the rare patient suffering from pain mediated by the nervus intermedius component of the seventh cranial nerve [40]. Some have also advocated combining glossopharyngeal neurectomy with partial vagus nerve rhizotomy. Ma and colleagues reviewed their series of 103 patients undergoing glossopharyngeal neurectomy [41]. They found that the long-term complication rate was far lower in glossopharyngeal neurectomy alone compared to their patients who underwent glossopharyngeal neurectomy plus partial vagus rhizotomy (3.8% versus 35.8%, respectively).

Treatment Options

General treatment options for glossopharyngeal neuralgia include medical management with carbamazepine [39], phenytoin [39], or baclofen [42]. If medical treatment fails, surgical options include a block of the ninth cranial nerve at the jugular foramen, microvascular decompression, and neurectomy of the glossopharyngeal nerve [40]. Repetitive alcohol or radiofrequency blocks are effective for the treatment of trigeminal neuralgia. However, significant vagal deficits render this option untenable for the treatment of glossopharyngeal neuralgia.

Various authors advocate microvascular decompression, but the results are mixed. Microvascular decompression risks intraoperative cardiac abnormalities and may be associated with a postoperative recurrence of pain. Hypertensive crises and intra- and extracerebellar hemorrhage have been associated with manipulation of the ninth and tenth cranial nerves during microvascular decompression [43]. Both the literature and the experience of the authors suggest that sectioning nerve rootlets in the posterior fossa offers a more precise mechanism to address refractory pain syndromes unresponsive to medical therapy [40], as originally suggested by Dandy in 1927 [44].

Preoperative Preparation

In planning surgical treatment, the surgical team must remain aware of the clinical phenomena associated with hypersensitivity of the dorsal motor nucleus of the vagus nerve. These symptoms include cardiac arrest, syncope, and seizures. These potential adverse events should be discussed thoroughly with the patient.

Prophylactic antibiotic coverage is administered. The patient is prepared with leads placed to monitor intraoperative somatosensory and auditory evoked potentials. As for all posterior fossa procedures, at least two intravenous access sites are recommended. General anesthesia is induced, and an arterial line is placed. A right atrial catheter is placed if the sitting position is to be used. Adequate anesthesia is administered for pin placement. If necessary, additional local anesthesia can be administered.

Patient Positioning

The sitting or lateral decubitus position may be used. In the lateral decubitus position (Fig. 7.7a), the lower axilla is supported by a roll (the authors typically use a 1-L bag of saline wrapped in a blanket). The patient's head is flexed forward and laterally, away from the operative site. The ipsilateral shoulder is retracted toward the feet using cloth tape. Care is taken to avoid excessive retraction, which may be associated with brachial plexus injury. A pillow is placed between the flexed knees. With the use of muscle relaxants, the weight of the arms is sometimes sufficient to cause stretch injuries of the brachial plexus. Several retractor systems are available. The authors prefer to use the Leyla bar. The table attachment is secured before the skin incision is made.

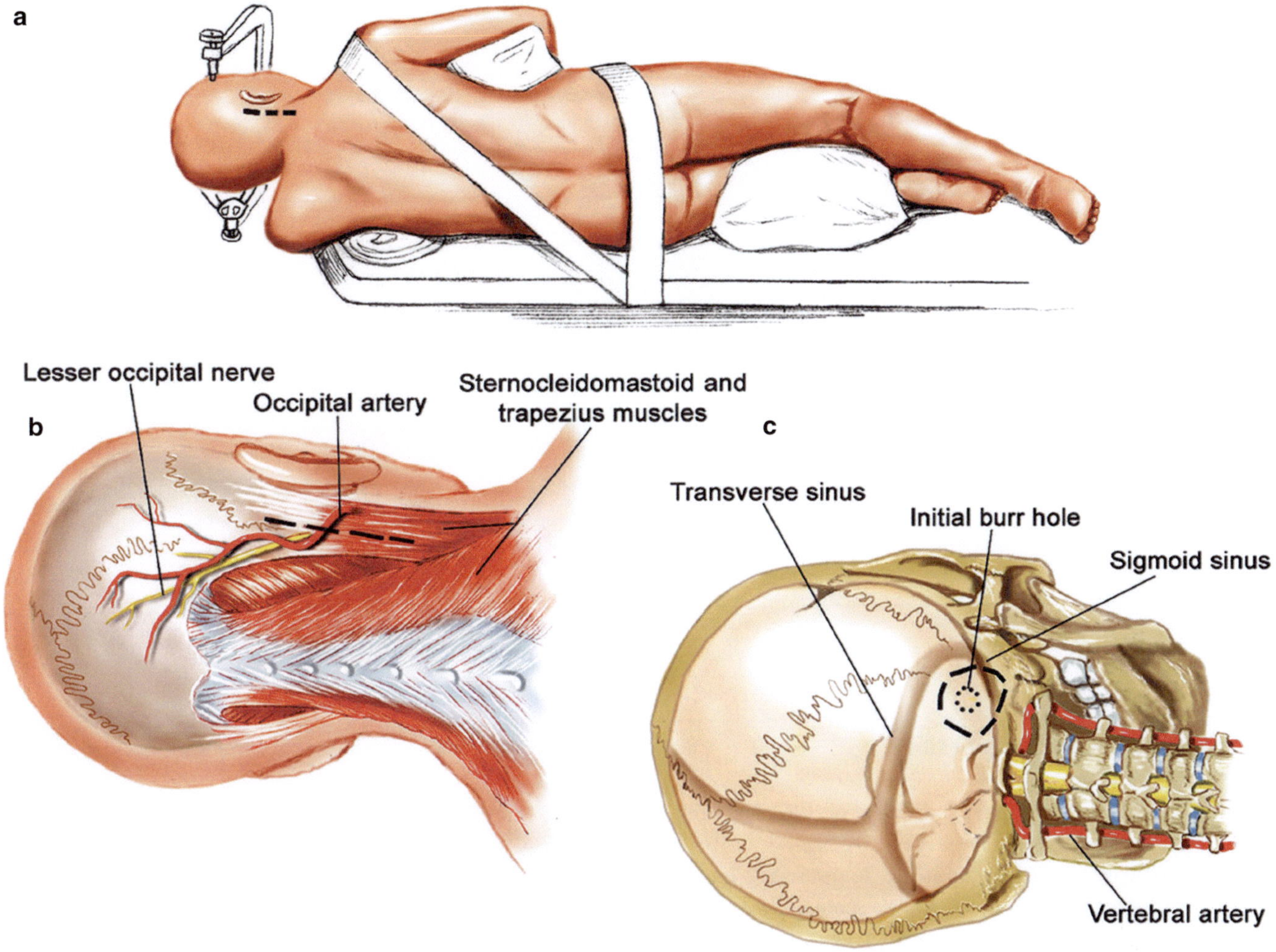

Fig. 7.7 Patient positioning, scalp incision, and craniectomy. (**a**) Lateral decubitus position. (**b**) Skin incision relative to the muscles. (**c**) Craniectomy. Note location of the sigmoid sinus and foramen magnum. (Published with permission, copyright © 2007 S. N. Kurpad, MD)

Care should be exerted to ensure that the crossbar is completely removed from the surgical field.

Operative Technique

A linear or S-shaped incision is made over the occipital bone (Fig. 7.7b). A 3-cm craniectomy is performed using a high-speed drill to incorporate the portion of the occipital bone that lies directly adjacent to the foramen magnum (Fig. 7.7c). The dural margin remains adherent to the edges of the craniectomy. The dura is opened in a cruciate manner and sutured back over the craniectomy margin to the pericranium, occipital fascia, or muscle layer. Epidural oozing is controlled with Surgicel® strips (Johnson & Johnson Medical Device Companies, New Brunswick, NJ, USA).

The operating microscope is brought in under high magnification. Using a medium-sized malleable retractor blade, the cerebellar hemisphere is elevated to expose the arachnoid of the cisterna magna, which is opened. The resulting drainage of CSF maximizes atraumatic cerebellar relaxation. The ninth cranial nerve in the jugular foramen is almost always separated by a dural septum from the tenth and eleventh cranial nerves and jugular vein (Fig. 7.8). The ninth cranial nerve and upper sixth to eighth of the filaments of the tenth cranial nerve are sectioned with the aid of a spatula or with a blunt hook and bipolar coagulation. The dural opening is closed primarily or by using pericranium, fascia lata, or homologous dura as a graft.

Postoperatively, sensation over the pharynx and taste over the posterior third of the tongue are usually diminished. The gag reflex is abolished on the side of the divided nerve. Swallowing may sometimes be disturbed transiently. In our experience, only one of five patients has experienced prolonged swallowing difficulties.

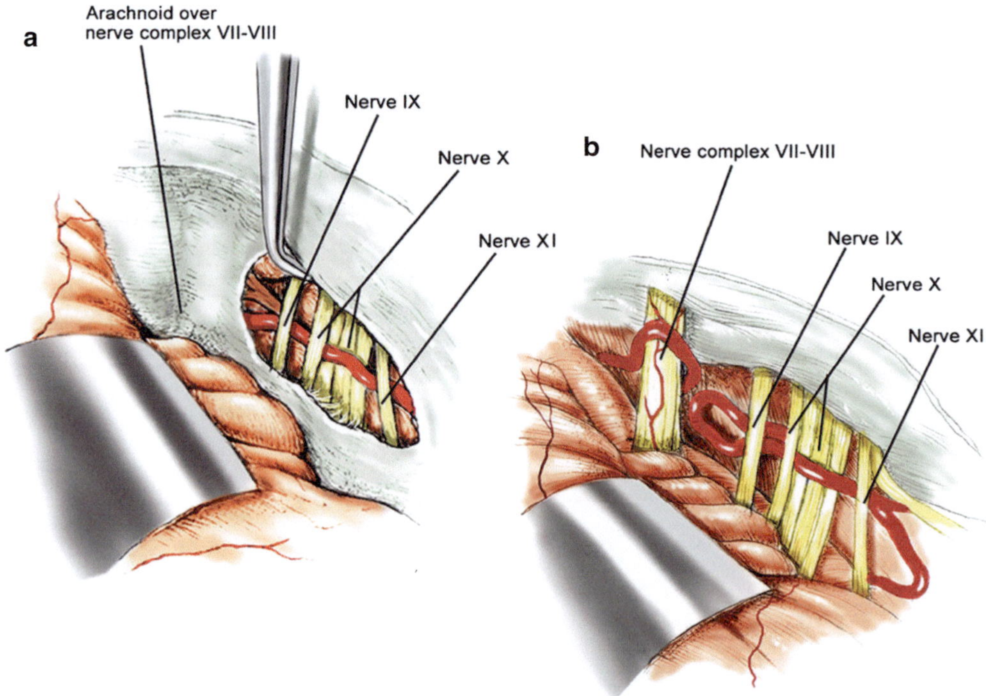

Fig. 7.8 Artist's illustration showing the intraoperative microscopic view of the cerebellopontine angle. (**a**) Cranial nerves IX and X are separated by dural septum. (**b**) Relationships of the lower cranial nerves to the posterior inferior cerebellar artery. (Published with permission, copyright © 2007 S. N. Kurpad, MD)

Microvascular Decompression

Microvascular compression syndromes of the trigeminal, facial, cochlear, and vestibular nerves have been described as the origin of trigeminal neuralgia (tic douloureux), hemifacial spasm, subjective tinnitus, and vestibular dysfunction, respectively [45]. We have performed endoscope-assisted microvascular decompression for the treatment of all of these entities, except vascular loop-induced vestibulopathy (Figs. 7.9, 7.10, and 7.11). In all cases, symptoms resolved or improved. However, it should be noted that van den Berge and colleagues completed a systematic review and meta-analysis of 35 studies (572 patients) undergoing microvascular decompression for tinnitus or vertigo [46]. They concluded, due to the low success rates, that microvascular decompression cannot be considered a standard treatment method for tinnitus or vertigo.

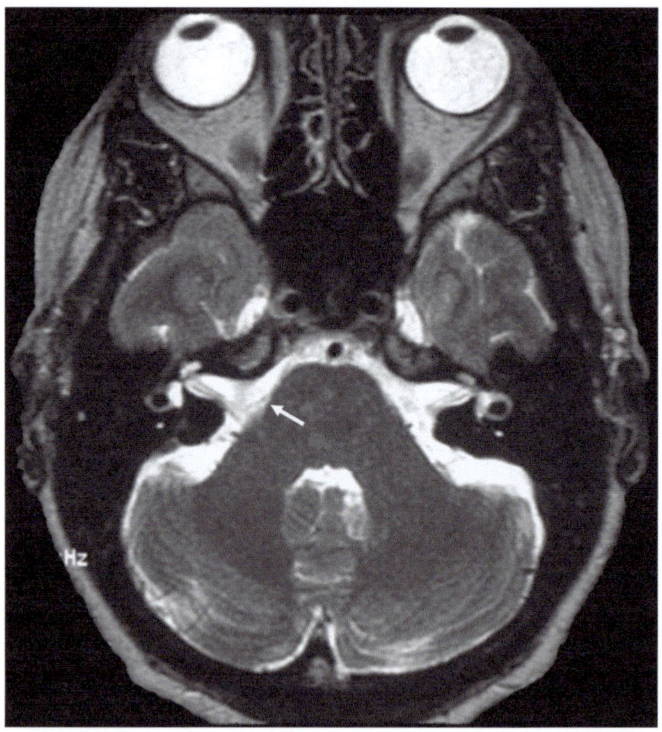

Fig. 7.9 T2-weighted axial MRI shows vessel crossing the right root entry zone of the eighth cranial nerve complex (arrow). Normal cochlea, vestibular apparatus, and cochlear and inferior vestibular nerves are shown. (Published with permission, copyright © 2007 P. A. Wackym, MD)

Case Report: Microvascular Decompression for Tinnitus

A 54-year-old woman presented with intractable right unilateral tinnitus after several years of unsuccessful medical management. Based on MRI studies, she did not have a vestibular schwannoma. However, MRI showed a large vessel crossing the root entry zone of the vestibulocochlear complex (Fig. 7.9). She elected to undergo microvascular decompression using endoscopic techniques. Intraoperatively, the ABR and facial nerve were monitored. A small incision and craniotomy, as described in the earlier section on vestibular neurectomy, were completed (Fig. 7.10a). Upon inspection of the CPA, a vein was found to be compressing the root entry

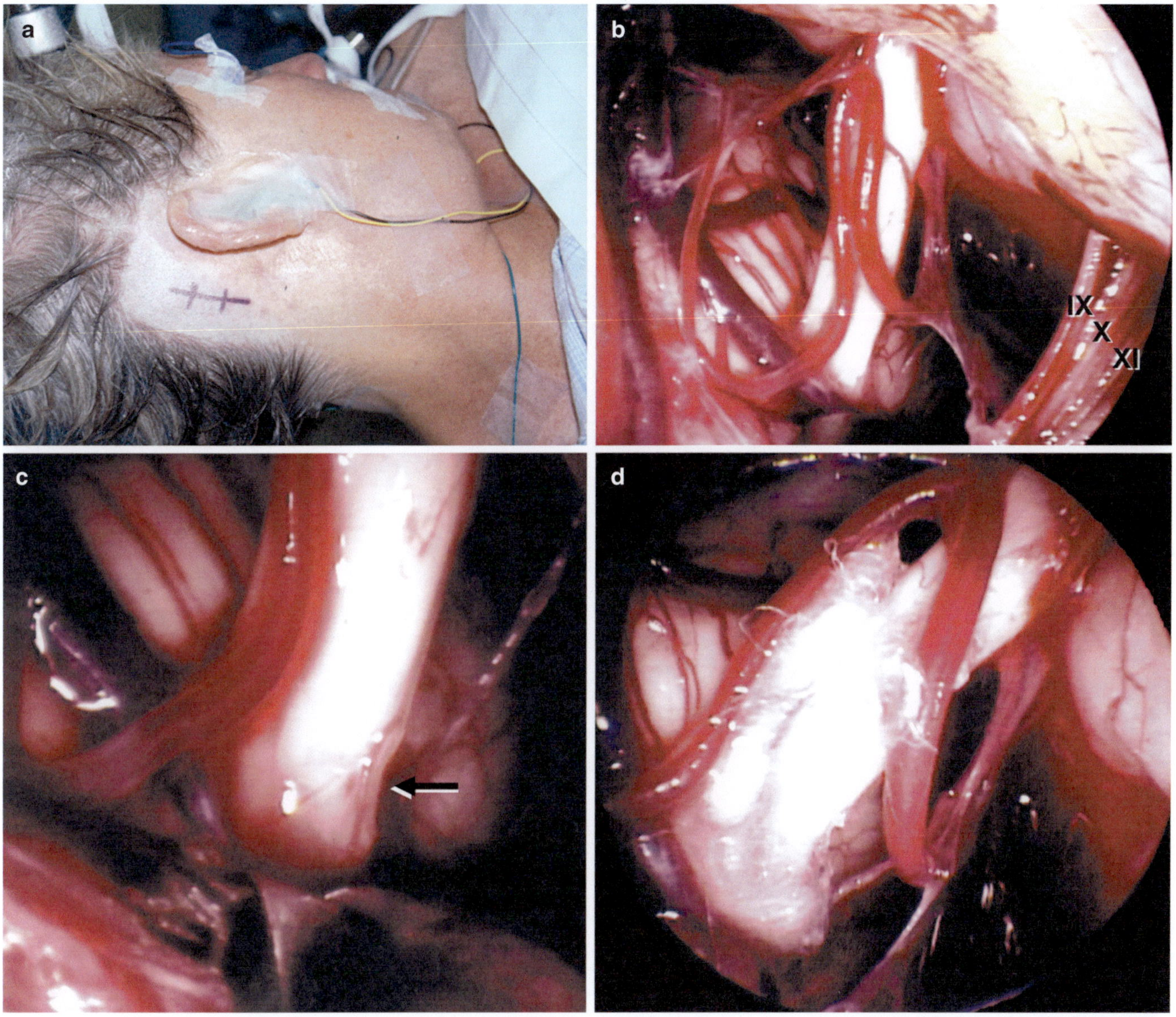

Fig. 7.10 Endoscopic microvascular decompression for intractable tinnitus in the right ear. (**a**) A 3–4-cm linear incision is designed to extend caudally from the transverse sinus. The Mayfield head holder is used to attach the endoscope holder. The intraoperative auditory brainstem evoked response is monitored, and facial nerve electromyography is performed during the microvascular decompression procedure. (**b**) Initial endoscopic view of the eighth cranial nerve complex (center of field) and cranial nerves IX, X, and XI entering the jugular foramen (right of field). Numerous arterial branches from the anterior inferior cerebellar artery (AICA) are seen over the vestibulocochlear nerve. A single vein crosses the root entry zone of the cochlear nerve. (**c**) After the vein crossing the root entry zone is mobilized, indentation and demyelination of the cochlear nerve are apparent (arrow). (**d**) Polytetrafluoroethylene (Teflon) felt is placed between the vestibular and cochlear nerves and the branches from the AICA and the vein crossing the root entry zone of the vestibulocochlear nerve. (Published with permission, copyright © 2007 P. A. Wackym, MD)

zone of the cochlear nerve and numerous branches of the AICA surrounded the vestibulocochlear nerve (Fig. 7.10b). After the vein was mobilized and elevated, the cochlear nerve was seen to be demyelinated and indented at the compression site (Fig. 7.10c). Teflon (polytetrafluoroethylene) felt was placed between the mobilized vessels and the vestibulocochlear nerve complex (Fig. 7.10d).

Postoperatively, the patient experienced subjective improvement of her tinnitus. The character of her tinnitus changed to a higher frequency that was much less intense and only occurred intermittently. Approximately 1 year after surgery, she experienced a 20–25 dB decrease in her pure tone average in the affected ear. Eighteen years after surgery, she had experienced no further changes.

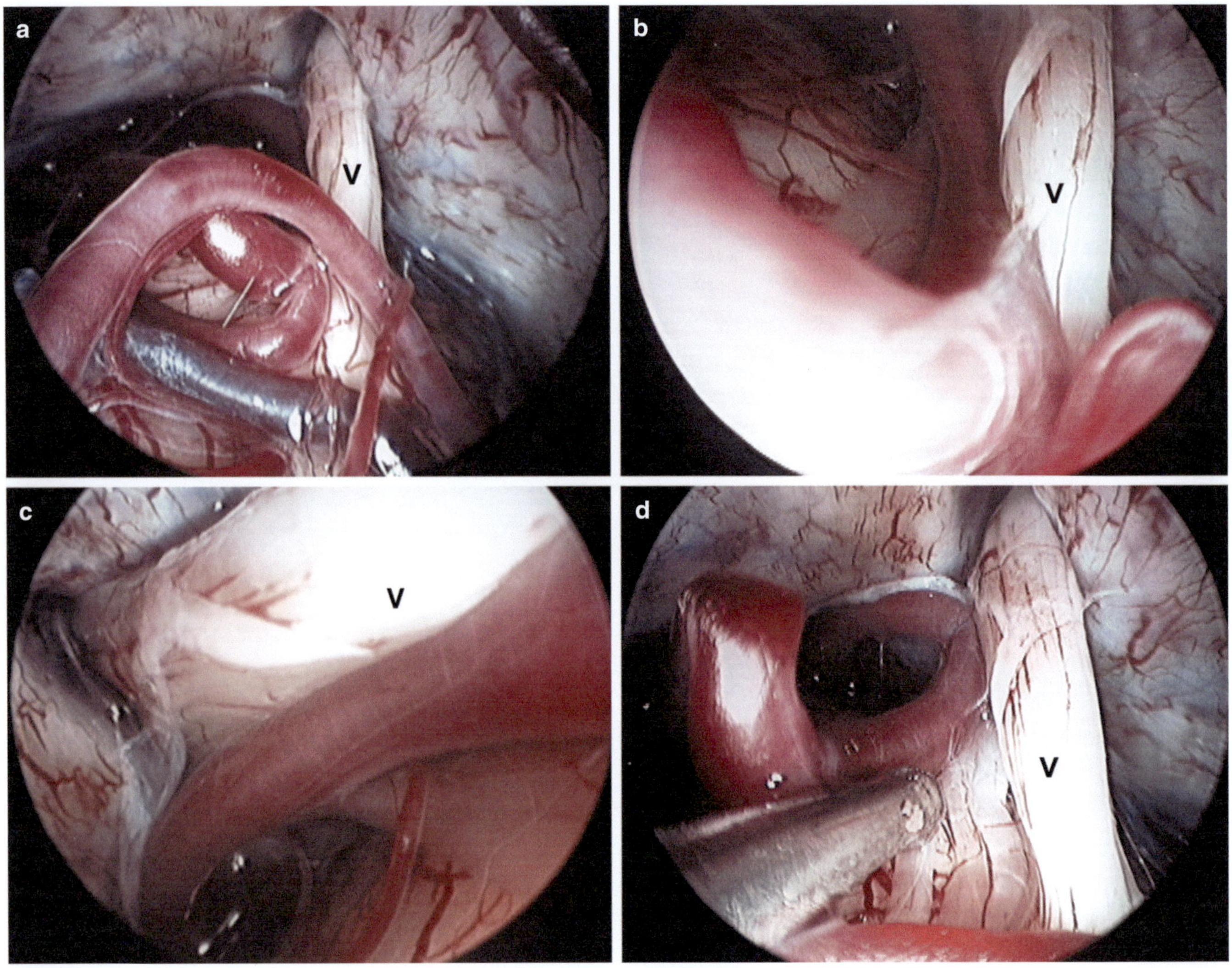

Fig. 7.11 Microvascular decompression for right trigeminal neuralgia. (**a**) Initial endoscopic view on exposure of the right cerebellopontine angle, using a 4 mm 0° endoscope. Multiple arteries and veins are in contact with the trigeminal nerve (V) at the entry zone to the brainstem. (**b**) Panoramic examination of the trigeminal nerve (V) using the 30° endoscope demonstrates compression by a large superior cerebellar artery. (**c**) After the large superior cerebellar artery compressing the trigeminal nerve (V) is elevated, the view through a 30° endoscope demonstrates the displacement of the artery from the nerve. (**d**) Panoramic examination of the nerve using the 0° endoscope after decompression of the trigeminal nerve (V). (Published with permission, copyright © 2007 P. A. Wackym, MD)

Authors' Experience: Microvascular Decompression for Trigeminal Neuralgia or Hemifacial Spasm

Although the authors have a much greater depth of experience, for this chapter we will summarize 30 patients with trigeminal neuralgia and seven patients with hemifacial spasm who had failed medical management and underwent endoscope-assisted microvascular decompression. Anatomic compression of the nerve entry or exit zone was confirmed in all 37 patients. In each case, an arterial loop was considered responsible for the patient's clinical symptoms. The superior cerebellar artery was the offending vessel in patients with trigeminal neuralgia, and the AICA was the offending vessel in patients with hemifacial spasm. In several cases, multiple vessels—both arteries and veins—were identified adjacent to the dysfunctional cranial nerve at its junction with the brainstem (Fig. 7.11). When using the microscope alone, it was difficult to identify the compressive vessel. However, in all cases, endoscopy clarified the exact site of the clinically significant compression.

Endoscopy as a Surgical Adjunct During Microvascular Decompression

Trigeminal neuralgia, hemifacial spasm, glossopharyngeal neuralgia, tinnitus, and disabling positional vertigo have all been associated with vascular compression [43]. Microvascular decompression involves separating the compressive vessel from its point of contact with the cranial nerve root entry or exit zone and interposition of a prosthesis (usually Teflon felt) to prevent further nerve compression.

Extensive experience has shown that 62–64% of patients with trigeminal neuralgia have a compressive artery, 12–24% have a compressive vein, 13–14% have both a compressive artery and a vein, and 8% have either a tumor or vascular malformation compressing the trigeminal nerve [47]. The initial failure rate for microvascular decompression for trigeminal neuralgia is 2–7%. The incidence of recurrence is 3.5% per year [48–50]. In 1996 Barker and colleagues reported 1185 patients who underwent microvascular decompression for trigeminal neuralgia with a mean follow-up of 6.2 years. Thirty percent of their patients experienced a major recurrence, and 11% required a second microvascular decompression [51]. Lu and colleagues completed a systematic review and meta-analysis of 683 patients (13 studies) treated by stereotactic radiosurgery who were compared with 670 patients treated by microvascular decompression for medically refractive trigeminal neuralgia [52]. They found that both stereotactic radiosurgery and microvascular decompression alleviate pain in medically refractive trigeminal neuralgia patients; however, microvascular decompression results in superior rates of short- and long-term pain relief, facial numbness, and dysesthesia control and less recurrence among those in whom pain freedom was achieved, at the cost of greater postoperative complications compared with SRS.

The absence of a clear site of arterial compression has been associated with high recurrence rates [51, 53]. Patients found to have only venous compression and no arterial compression are most likely to suffer a recurrence [51]. Kureshi and Wilkins reported their surgical experience with 31 posterior fossa reexplorations for recurrent or persistent trigeminal neuralgia and hemifacial spasm [54]. In three (10%) cases, they discovered new or previously unrealized arterial compression of neural structures. Similarly, of 116 who underwent reoperation after their first microvascular decompression failed, a previously unseen arterial compression was identified in 65.5% [55]. Liao and colleagues discovered persistent vascular compression in three of five patients undergoing repeat microvascular decompression [56].

Some have doubted that microvascular compression of a cranial nerve can be the cause of trigeminal neuralgia and other cranial nerve dysfunction syndromes. However, during decompression procedures, identification of an arterial vessel compressing the trigeminal nerve in patients with trigeminal neuralgia or the facial nerve in patients with hemifacial spasm increases cure rates and decreases recurrence rates compared with cases in which a specific artery is not identified. We believe that some microvascular decompressive procedures fail because the offending vessel is not identified during the primary operation.

Some of these failures occur because the microscope provides incomplete information about the anatomic relationship between the nerves and vessels. The 0° endoscope provides a panoramic view of the CPA, and an angled endoscope enables the surgeon to "look around corners." Magnan and colleagues used an endoscope to treat 60 patients with hemifacial spasm. The operating microscope was able to visualize the offending vessel in 28% of cases, whereas the endoscope was effective in 93% of the same cases [57]. We believe that the adjunctive use of the endoscope in microvascular decompressive procedures improves surgical outcomes.

Auditory Brainstem Implantation

During recent decades, the restoration of hearing in individuals with clinically significant hearing loss from a wide range of causes has advanced dramatically. At present, surgical intervention in the form of cochlear implants can provide useful auditory perception in individuals deriving little or no benefit from hearing aids; however, these auditory prostheses require an intact cochlear nerve to conduct the electrical signals to the brainstem. The restoration of auditory perception in individuals deafened by loss of the vestibulocochlear nerve is currently being provided by ABIs.

The ABI is a device consisting of several electrodes placed on the surface of the brainstem so that the cochlear nuclei can be stimulated directly [58, 59]. Externally, the ABI is coupled with a digital sound processor similar to that of a cochlear implant. Such stimulation can provide useful perception of environmental sounds and even open-set speech comprehension [58, 59]. However, there is also evidence that patients receiving an ABI who do not have neurofibromatosis type II (NF2), such as patients with a temporal bone fracture and no functional cochlear nerve, perform at a much higher level as measured by open-set speech discrimination testing than those who do not have an ABI [60].

Only one ABI is available commercially in the United States. Cochlear Americas' (Englewood, CO) ABI is approved in the United States by the Federal Drug Administration (FDA) for use in individuals 17 years or older with NF2 undergoing resection of a vestibular schwannoma (acoustic neuroma) or in patients undergoing resection of an acoustic neuroma in an only-hearing ear [61]. When both cochlear nerves must be sacrificed during resection of bilateral tumors, patients with NF2 are left with complete sensorineural deafness [62].

Cochlear Americas' array is a 21-electrode device with the electrodes embedded in a silastic paddle backed with Dacron mesh. This device is also used intraoperatively as a stimulating electrode for the electrically evoked auditory brainstem response (EABR) to help identify the optimal position for the electrode paddle [58]. The recommended protocol with this device is to use a translabyrinthine approach to the tumor and subsequent implantation of the ABI [58]. An FDA clinical trial of a new electrode array with a penetrating electrode was completed, and several patients have now received this device.

Optimal placement of the electrode onto the cochlear nucleus is difficult because this complex cannot be directly visualized through the operating microscope via the surgical approaches used to resect these tumors. However, the use of the endoscope during the placement of an ABI electrode array has been explored to accomplish this goal [63, 64]. Our team has taken a multidisciplinary approach in ABI electrode placement using endoscopic guidance and electrophysiologic mapping to optimize electrode placement. This strategy has increased the number of active electrodes, reduced the number of electrodes producing side effects, and reduced the number of nonactive electrodes.

Translabyrinthine Approach

The translabyrinthine dissection should be performed in standard fashion with an operating microscope and basic otologic instruments. In brief, a complete mastoidectomy is performed, and the facial nerve and semicircular canals are identified. The vestibular labyrinth is removed, and the dura of the posterior and middle fossae is exposed. Working from the ampulla of the superior semicircular canal, the surgeon skeletonizes the IAC. The jugular bulb is identified and should be decompressed thoroughly to provide direct visualization of the rostral fibers of the glossopharyngeal nerve. Doing so allows the identification of an important landmark and provides access for the endoscope during implantation. The posterior fossa dura is then incised and reflected to expose the cerebellum and flocculus.

At this point, the tumor would be removed. Additional intraoperative challenges are typically encountered as a result of the distortion of landmarks produced by compression or extirpation of the tumor. In such case, the use of the landmarks described is even more critical because a stepwise approach may allow identification of the implant site in a grossly distorted CPA.

A 0° endoscope is advanced into the operative field and used to identify the flocculus and the vestibulocochlear and glossopharyngeal nerves (Fig. 7.12). In some individuals, the choroid plexus may be visible over or just inferior to the flocculus. The vestibulocochlear and glossopharyngeal nerves appear to converge behind the flocculus at an imaginary point near the dorsal cochlear nucleus. A 30° or 45° endoscope can now be passed over (i.e., lateral) the flocculus to visualize the choroid plexus. The choroid plexus can be traced medially to the rhomboid lip and foramen of Luschka. Use of the angled endoscope allows this task to be accomplished with minimal retraction on the flocculus, thereby helping to preserve the taenia chordae. Under endoscopic visualization, the McCabe flap knife (V. Mueller, CareFusion, San Diego, CA, USA) is used to gently retract the choroid and to expose the surface of the brainstem and lateral recess of the fourth ventricle. The surface of the brainstem within the recess glistens characteristically due to the overlying ependyma.

The endoscope should be stabilized at the periphery of the operative field to allow the electrode and instruments to be introduced and manipulated. It can be positioned superiorly against the tegmen or inferiorly against the bony ridge remaining over the tympanic and mastoid facial nerve. Decompression of the jugular bulb creates adequate space for the distal aspect of the endoscope to be maneuvered. The

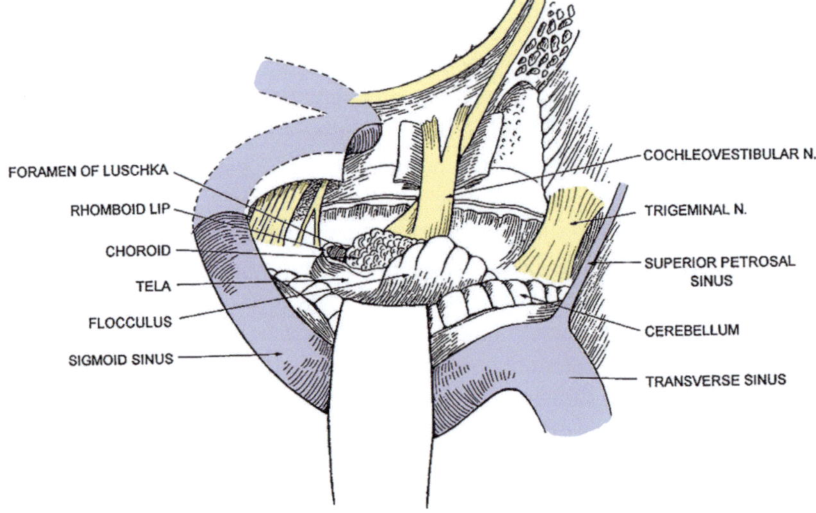

Fig. 7.12 Illustration detailing the landmarks visible near the cochlear nucleus via the translabyrinthine approach. *N* nerve. (Published with permission, copyright © 2007 P. A. Wackym, MD)

position of the endoscope is determined by the side of the patient being operated on and by the dominant hand of the surgeon. There is a tendency for the temperature of the distal endoscope to increase, which can cause neural stimulation and potentially neural damage. Therefore, the endoscope must be positioned near the facial nerve with care, and evoked potentials should be monitored closely.

The implant is introduced into the site with a Rosen needle or a No. 11 Rhoton dissector (V. Mueller). The paddle is directed into the foramen of Luschka. The angled endoscope allows the entire length of the electrode array to be visualized to ensure full contact with the brainstem. The position of the implant can be recorded with digital image capture and digital video to help correlate anatomy with the results of electrophysiologic testing.

The distal portion of the electrode extends through the surgical defect to the receiver/stimulator. This maneuver is similar to that performed with a cochlear implant, and the electrode is implanted in the same manner. The defect is closed in standard translabyrinthine fashion, and routine postoperative management is followed.

Retrosigmoid Approach

The retrosigmoid or suboccipital approach is performed in the standard manner. The opening should be large enough to extirpate the tumor safely. When an ABI is placed for non-NF2 applications, the opening can be smaller. The use of the endoscope actually permits a smaller craniotomy to be used than would be needed with the operating microscope. However, the optical modality used for tumor removal should take precedence and determine the surgical approach. The dura is incised and reflected to expose the cerebellum. A cerebellar retractor is placed to provide access to the CPA. In this description, it is assumed that the lateral medullary cistern is opened and the bone over the IAC is drilled to expose a tumor.

The principal criticism of the retrosigmoid approach for placement of an ABI is the perceived need for extensive cerebellar retraction to expose the implant site. However, endoscopic visualization of the lateral recess of the fourth ventricle usually requires less retraction than a translabyrinthine approach. A 30° or 45° endoscope can be passed along the cerebellar retractor to "look" medially into the implant site even if the site is not visible directly through the craniotomy.

In the retrosigmoid approach, the landmarks for the dorsal cochlear nucleus are identical to those used in the translabyrinthine approach. However, the perspective is shifted in a slightly caudal direction, and visualization of the surface of the brainstem within the recess is less oblique. Consequently, it is easier to identify the ABI electrode contact site (Fig. 7.13). As in the translabyrinthine approach, the operating microscope is introduced first to identify the flocculus and vestibulocochlear and glossopharyngeal nerves. The root entry zone of the eighth cranial nerve is hidden behind the flocculus, but the entry of the glossopharyngeal rootlets may be apparent.

Once the surgeon is oriented to the gross anatomy, the 30° or 45° endoscope can be introduced to look "around" the flocculus. The root entry zones and the choroid plexus emerging from the foramen of Luschka should be clearly visible. The flocculus can now be retracted with the McCabe flap knife to expose the rhomboid lip, lateral recess, and glistening brainstem surface overlying the dorsal cochlear nucleus. Visualization of a small amount of taenia chordae further helps define the cochlear nuclear complex.

At either the superior or inferior aspect of the field, the endoscope should be stabilized against the cerebellar

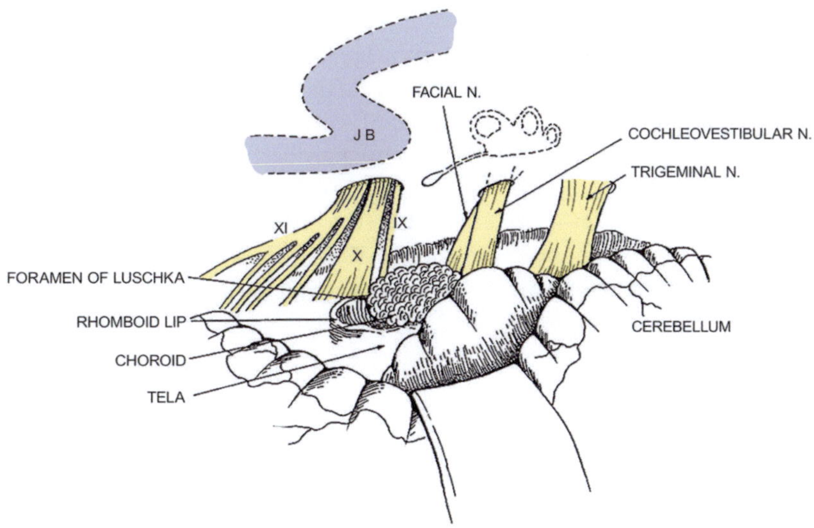

Fig. 7.13 Illustration detailing the landmarks visible near the cochlear nucleus via the retrosigmoid approach. IX = glossopharyngeal nerve fibers; X = vagal nerve fibers; XI = spinal accessory nerve fibers; JB = jugular bulb (*ghosted in position*); N = nerve. (Published with permission, copyright © 2007 P. A. Wackym, MD)

retractor. The side of the operation and the dominant hand of the surgeon determine which aspect is used. The ABI is advanced to the implant site with a Rosen needle or a No. 11 Rhoton dissector and maneuvered into the foramen of Luschka. We have found that using this instrument, combined with the less oblique approach to the brainstem, makes the placement of the implant relatively easy. The position of the implant can be confirmed with the endoscope.

Once the ABI is initially placed under endoscopic guidance, the EABR is tested. Repositioning the electrode array under endoscopic control and retesting the EABR optimize the placement of the electrode. This process typically requires 30–60 min. However, in one of our cases, this process required 3 h.

Authors' Clinical Experience

To date, our team has placed seven ABIs in six patients, five with NF2 and one with a nonfunctional cochlear nerve caused by a temporal bone fracture (Fig. 7.14). The same multidisciplinary approach to placement of the ABI electrode was used in all patients. As described elsewhere, the electrode paddle was placed endoscopically by the same surgeon (Wackym) [63, 64]. Intraoperative EABR was performed using the paradigm suggested by Cochlear Americas, with the exception that mapping was repeated until placement of the electrode was optimal, as defined by the maximum number of active auditory electrodes using EABR.

Localization of the brainstem surface overlying the dorsal cochlear nucleus can be challenging. Brackmann and colleagues noted that in lower mammals the dorsal nucleus forms a characteristic "bulge" on the brainstem surface, which they have not observed in humans [65]. We have intermittently seen this surface bulge in both cadaveric specimens and in our patients undergoing endoscopic placement of an ABI; consequently, this landmark may be inconsistent at best [63, 64]. Further complicating localization of the dorsal cochlear nucleus is its position within the lateral recess of the fourth ventricle, an area reported *not* to be directly visible within the surgical field of the standard translabyrinthine approach [66]. The site of implantation also may be obscured in a translabyrinthine dissection [65]. Because this region is difficult to localize in a clinical setting, the importance of surgical landmarks to guide the surgeon has been stressed [63, 64]. We have found that the retrosigmoid approach provides the best view of the cochlear nucleus complex via the operating microscope. Rhoton's group agreed with our conclusion that adjunctive endoscope use is helpful in auditory brainstem implant placement and that either the translabyrinthine or retrosigmoid approach can be effectively used [67].

Although others have also used EABR to optimize the placement of the electrode array, we have typically spent 30–60 min in mapping this ideal location. However, we have also taken 3 h to accomplish this task. As measured by the number of active electrodes and by the number of electrodes that are nonresponsive or that produce side effects, this multidisciplinary approach has produced excellent outcomes. As this series expands, it may be possible to generalize these principles.

Highlights of Auditory Brainstem Implantation

A systematic approach to locating the dorsal cochlear nucleus is needed to position the ABI appropriately on the brainstem surface. This step is particularly important when tumor or surgical extirpation has altered the normal appearance of the CPA. The 0° and 30° endoscopes provide high-resolution views of these landmarks and allow the CPA to be examined with minimal retraction or manipulation. This strategy enables the preservation of delicate structures, which can further delineate the dorsal cochlear nucleus.

In the translabyrinthine and retrosigmoid approaches, identical landmarks are used and followed to localize the implant site:

- The flocculus and eighth and ninth cranial nerves are identified.
- The region between the root entry zones of these nerves and rostral to the flocculus contains the choroid plexus.
- The choroid plexus can be followed into the foramen of Luschka, and thus to the lateral recess of the fourth ventricle.
- The fold of the tela choroidea forming the rhomboid lip further delineates the foramen of Luschka.
- The root entry zone of the eighth cranial nerve "points" to the region of the cochlear nuclear complex.
- If preserved, the tinea chordae attaches at the junction of the dorsal and inferior ventral cochlear nuclei.
- The brainstem surface in the recess over the cochlear nuclear complex has a glistening ependymal layer.
- The brainstem overlying the dorsal cochlear nucleus may bulge slightly.

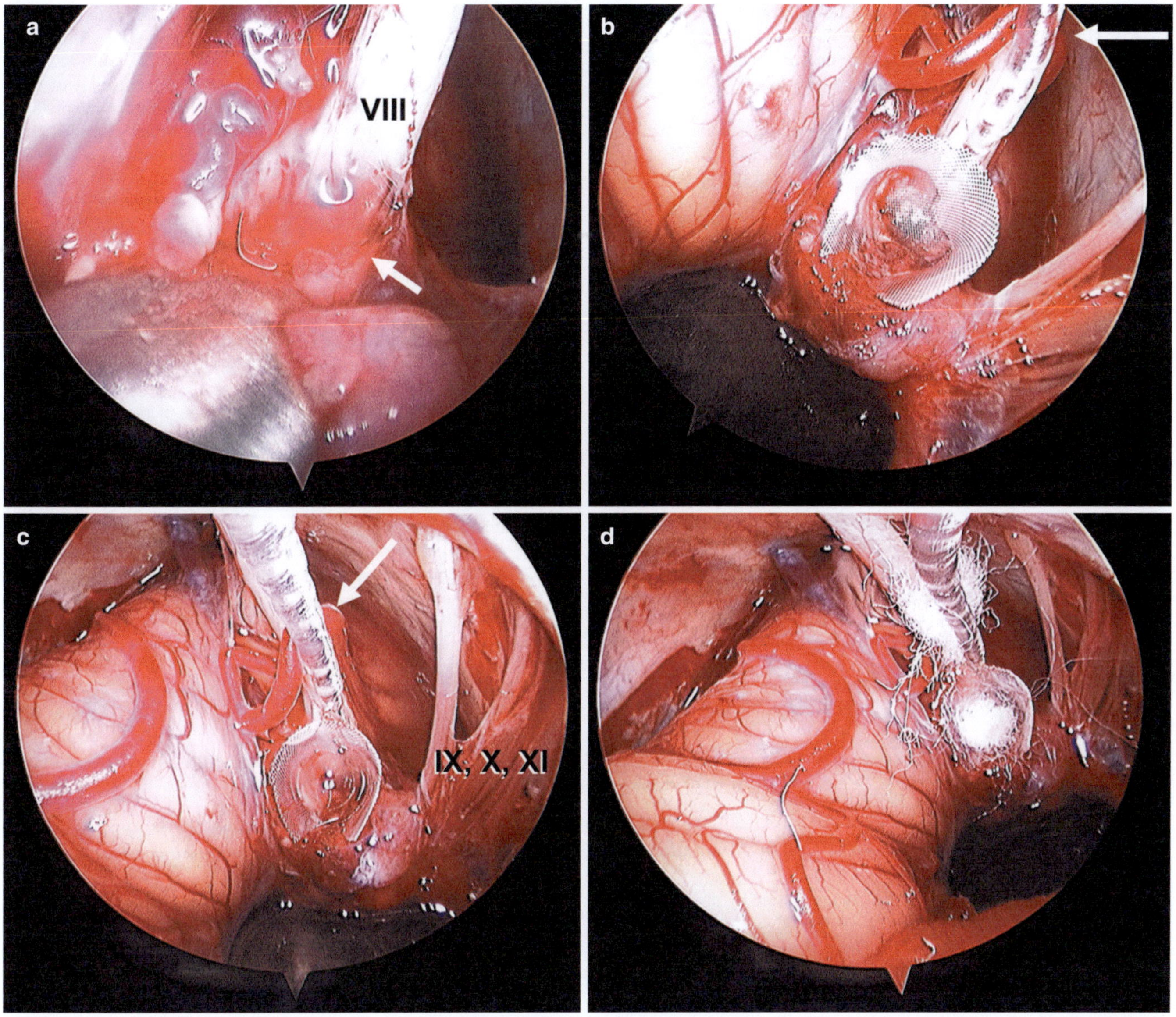

Fig. 7.14 In December 2006, a 52-year-old man with bilateral temporal bone fractures and a nonfunctional right cochlear nerve underwent a right retrosigmoid approach and ABI placement using a 45° endoscope and evoked auditory brainstem response guidance. (**a**) View of cochlear nucleus before placement of the ABI. The rhomboid lip (arrow) is visible in relationship to the lateral recess and vestibulocochlear nerve (VIII). The flocculus is visible in the bottom center of the field. (**b**) ABI in position over the cochlear nucleus. The Dacron mesh wings are bowed around the inside of the rhomboid lip. A loop of the anterior inferior cerebellar artery (AICA) is visible between the electrode array and cranial nerve VIII (arrow). (**c**) CSF wells up through the foramen of Luschka (center of field). Cranial nerves IX, X, and XI are seen in relationship to the ABI electrode paddle. The extent of the AICA loop (arrow) is visible. (**d**) Polytetrafluoroethylene (Teflon) felt placed between the vestibulocochlear nerve and the loop of AICA as well as within the lateral recess. (Published with permission, copyright © 2007 P. A. Wackym, MD)

Summary and Conclusions

Functional surgery of the CPA has the potential to relieve or to partially restore a wide variety of cranial nerve dysfunction involving the trigeminal, facial, cochlear, vestibular, and glossopharyngeal nerves. Adherence to fundamental skull-base microsurgical principles and careful patient selection, coupled with the adjunctive use of endoscopy and electrophysiological monitoring, are essential to achieve optimal patient outcomes.

References

1. King WA, Frazee JG, DeSalles AAF, editors. Endoscopy of the central and peripheral nervous system. New York: Thieme Medical Publishers; 1998. p. 1–259.
2. Wackym PA, Rice DH, Schaefer SD, editors. Minimally invasive surgery of the head, neck, and cranial base. Philadelphia: Lippincott Williams & Wilkins; 2002. p. 1–559.
3. Wackym PA, King WA, Barker FG, Poe DS. Endoscope-assisted vestibular neurectomy. Laryngoscope. 1998;108:1787–93.

4. O'Donoghue GM, O'Flynn P. Endoscopic anatomy of the cerebellopontine angle. Am J Otol. 1993;14:122–5.
5. McKennan KX. Endoscopy of the internal auditory canal during hearing conservation acoustic tumor surgery. Am J Otol. 1993;14:259–62.
6. Mangnan J, Chays A, Lepetre C, et al. Surgical perspectives of endoscopy of the cerebellopontine angle. Am J Otol. 1994;15:366–70.
7. Bottrill ID, Poe DS. Endoscopic-assisted ear surgery. Am J Otol. 1995;16:158–63.
8. Rosenberg SI. Endoscopic otologic surgery. Otolaryngol Clin North Am. 1996;29:291–300.
9. Glasscock ME III, Gulya AJ, Pensak ML, Black JN Jr. Medical and surgical management of Meniere's disease. Am J Otol. 1984;5:536–42.
10. Santos PM, Hall RA, Snyder JM, et al. Diuretic and diet effect on Ménière's disease evaluated by the 1985 Committee on Hearing and Equilibrium guidelines. Otolaryngol Head Neck Surg. 1993;109:680–9.
11. Silverstein H, Wanamaker H, Flanzer J, Rosenberg S. Vestibular neurectomy in the United States—1990. Am J Otol. 1992;13:23–30.
12. Canzi P, Manfrin M, Perotti M, Aprile F, et al. Translabyrinthine vestibular neurectomy and simultaneous cochlear implant for Ménière's disease. Acta Neurochir (Wien). 2017;159(1):123–30.
13. Jackler RK. Endoscope-assisted vestibular neurectomy [letter; comment]. Laryngoscope. 1999;109:1010–1.
14. Frazier CH. Intracranial division of the auditory nerve for persistent aural vertigo. Surg Gynecol Obstet. 1912;15:524–9.
15. Dandy WE. Ménière's disease: its diagnosis and a method of treatment. Arch Surg. 1928;16:1127–52.
16. McKenzie KG. Intracranial division of the vestibular portion of the auditory nerve for Ménière's disease. Can Med Assoc J. 1936;34:369–81.
17. Dandy WE. Treatment of Ménière's disease by section of only the vestibular portion of the acoustic nerve. Bull Johns Hopkins Hosp. 1933;53:52–5.
18. Green RE. Surgical treatment of vertigo, with follow-up on Walter Dandy's cases. Neurological aspects. Clin Neurosurg. 1958;6:141–51.
19. Parry RH. A case of tinnitus and vertigo treated by division of the auditory nerve. J Laryngol Otol. 1904;19:402–7.
20. Silverstein H, Rosenberg S, Arruda J, Isaacson JE. Surgical ablation of the vestibular system in the treatment of Ménière's disease. Otolaryngol Clin North Am. 1997;30:1075–95.
21. Wackym PA, King WA, Meyer GA, et al. Endoscope-assisted surgery of the trigeminal, facial, cochlear or vestibular nerve. In: Wackym PA, Rice DH, Schaefer SD, editors. Minimally invasive surgery of the head, neck, and cranial base. Philadelphia: Lippincott Williams & Wilkins; 2002. p. 101–16.
22. Committee on hearing and equilibrium guidelines for the diagnosis and evaluation of therapy in Ménière's disease. Otolaryngol Head Neck Surg. 1995;113:181–5.
23. Wackym PA, Monsell EM. Revision vestibular surgery. In: Carrasco V, Pillsbury III HC, editors. Revision otologic surgery. New York: Thieme Medical Publishers; 1997. p. 109–33.
24. Silverstein H, Norrel H, Rosenberg S. An evolution of approach in vestibular neurectomy. Otolaryngol Head Neck Surg. 1990;102:374–81.
25. Rasmussen GL. Studies of the VIIIth cranial nerve of man. Laryngoscope. 1940;50:67–83.
26. Silverstein H. Cochlear and vestibular gross and histologic anatomy (as seen from the postauricular approach). Otolaryngol Head Neck Surg. 1984;92:207–11.
27. Newman A, Honrubia V. Regeneration of the eighth cranial nerve in the bullfrog, Rana catesbeiana. Exp Neurol. 1992;115:115–20.
28. Monsell EM, Brackmann DE, Linthicum FH. Why do vestibular destructive procedures sometimes fail? Otolaryngol Head Neck Surg. 1988;99:472–9.
29. Kronenberg J, Fisch U, Dillier N. Long-term evaluation of hearing after transtemporal supralabyrinthine vestibular neurectomy. In: Nadol Jr JB, editor. The second international symposium on Ménière's disease. New York: Kugler & Ghedini Publications; 1989. p. 481–8.
30. Silverstein H, Rosenberg SI. Retrolabyrinthine/retrosigmoid vestibular neurectomy. In: Brackmann DE, editor. Otologic surgery. Philadelphia: W.B. Saunders; 1994. p. 490–500.
31. Saim L, McKenna MJ, Nadol JB Jr. Tubal and tympanic openings of the peritubal cells: implications for cerebrospinal fluid otorhinorrhea. Am J Otol. 1996;17:335–9.
32. Bederson J, Wilson C. Evaluation of microvascular decompression and partial sensory rhizotomy in 252 cases of trigeminal neuralgia. J Neurosurg. 1989;71:359–67.
33. Fritz W, Shafer J, Klein H. Hearing loss after microvascular decompression for trigeminal neuralgia. J Neurosurg. 1988;69:367–70.
34. Hunt JR. Geniculate neuralgia (neuralgia of the nervus facialis). Arch Neurol Psychiatry. 1937;37:253–83.
35. Lustig LR, Jackler RK, Mandelcorn R. The history of otology through its eponyms I: anatomy. Am J Otol. 1998;19:371–89.
36. Rupa V, Saunders RL, Weider DJ. Geniculate neuralgia: the surgical management of primary otalgia. J Neurosurg. 1991;75:505–11.
37. Lovely TJ, Janetta PJ. Surgical management of geniculate neuralgia. Am J Otol. 1997;18:512–7.
38. Rhoton AL Jr, Kobayashi S, Hollinshead WH. Nervus intermedius. J Neurosurg. 1968;29:609–18.
39. Rushton JG, Stevens JC, Miller RH. Glossopharyngeal (vagoglossopharyngeal) neuralgia: a study of 217 cases. Arch Neurol. 1981;38:201–5.
40. Onofrio B. Glossopharyngeal neurectomy. In: AANS operative atlas, vol. 1. 3rd ed. Park Ridge, IL: American Association of Neurological Surgeons; 1991. p. 301–4.
41. Ma Y, Li YF, Wang QC, Wang B, Huang HT. Neurosurgical treatment of glossopharyngeal neuralgia: analysis of 103 cases. J Neurosurg. 2016;124(4):1088–92.
42. Gybels JM, Sweet WH. Neurosurgical management of persistent pain. In: Schmidek HH, Sweet WH, editors. Physiological and pathological mechanisms of human pain. Basel: Karger; 1989. p. 88–103.
43. Resnick DK, Jannetta PJ, Bissonnette D, et al. Microvascular decompression for glossopharyngeal neuralgia. Neurosurgery. 1995;36:64–9.
44. Dandy WE. Glossopharyngeal neuralgia (tic douloureux). Its diagnosis and treatment. Arch Surg. 1927;15:198–214.
45. Schwaber MK. Vascular compression syndromes. In: Jackler RK, Brackmann DE, editors. Neurotology. Philadelphia: Mosby; 2005. p. 892–911.
46. van den Berge MJC, van Dijk JMC, Posthumus IA, et al. Microvascular decompression of the cochleovestibular nerve for treatment of tinnitus and vertigo: a systematic review and meta-analysis of individual patient data. J Neurosurg. 2017;127(3):588–601.
47. Rohrer D, Burchiel K. Trigeminal neuralgia and other trigeminal dysfunction syndromes. In: Barrow D, editor. Surgery of the cranial nerves of the posterior fossa. Park Ridge, IL: American Association of Neurological Surgeons; 1993. p. 201–17.
48. Apfelbaum R. Surgery for tic douloureux. Clin Neurosurg. 1984;31:346–50.
49. Burchiel K, Clarke H, Haglund M. Long-term efficacy of microvascular decompression in trigeminal neuralgia. J Neurosurg. 1988;69:35–8.

50. Sweet W. Trigeminal neuralgia: problems as to cause and consequent conclusions regarding treatment. In: Wilkins RH, Rengachary S, editors. Neurosurgery update II. New York: McGraw-Hill; 1991. p. 366–72.
51. Barker FG, Jannetta PJ, Bissonette DJ, et al. The long-term outcome of microvascular decompression for trigeminal neuralgia. N Engl J Med. 1996;334:1077–83.
52. Lu VM, Duvall JB, Phan K, Jonker BP. First treatment and retreatment of medically refractive trigeminal neuralgia by stereotactic radiosurgery versus microvascular decompression: a systematic review and meta-analysis. Br J Neurosurg. 2018;32:355–64.
53. Mendoza N, Illingworth RD. Trigeminal neuralgia treated by microvascular decompression: a long-term follow-up study. Br J Neurosurg. 1995;9:13–9.
54. Kureshi SA, Wilkins RH. Posterior fossa reexploration for persistent or recurrent trigeminal neuralgia or hemifacial spasm: surgical findings and therapeutic implications. Neurosurgery. 1998;43:1111–7.
55. Wilkins RH. Cranial nerve dysfunction syndromes: evidence for microvascular compression. In: Barrow D, editor. Surgery of the cranial nerves of the posterior fossa. Park Ridge, IL: American Association of Neurological Surgeons; 1993. p. 155–63.
56. Liao JJ, Cheng WC, Chang CN, et al. Reoperation for recurrent trigeminal neuralgia after microvascular decompression. Surg Neurol. 1997;47:562–70.
57. Magnan J, Caces F, Locatelli P, Chays A. Hemifacial spasm: endoscopic vascular decompression. Otolaryngol Head Neck Surg. 1997;117:308–14.
58. Otto SR, Shannon RV, Brackmann DE, et al. The multichannel auditory brain stem implant: performance in twenty patients. Otolaryngol Head Neck Surg. 1998;118:291–303.
59. Laszig R, Sollmann WP. Marangos N The restoration of hearing in neurofibromatosis type 2. J Laryngol Otol. 1995;109:385–9.
60. Colletti V, Shannon RV. Open set speech perception with auditory brainstem implant? Laryngoscope. 2005;115:1974–8.
61. Otto SR, Brackmann DE, Staller S, Menapace CM. The multichannel auditory brainstem implant: 6-month coinvestigator results. Adv Otorhinolaryngol. 1997;52:1–7.
62. Miyamoto RT, Campbell RL, Fritsch M, Lochmueller G. Preservation of hearing in neurofibromatosis 2. Otolaryngol Head Neck Surg. 1990;103:619–24.
63. Friedland DR, Wackym PA. Evaluation of surgical approaches to endoscopic auditory brainstem implantation. Laryngoscope. 1999;109:175–80.
64. Wackym PA, Firszt JB, Runge-Samuelson CL. Auditory brainstem implantation. In: Wackym PA, guest editor. Cochlear and brainstem implantation. Oper tech otolaryngol head neck surg, vol 16. 2005. p. 159–63.
65. Brackmann DE, Hitselberger WE, Nelson RA, et al. Auditory brainstem implant: I. Issues in surgical implantation. Otolaryngol Head Neck Surg. 1993;108:624–33.
66. Kuroki A, Moller AR. Microsurgical anatomy around the foramen of Luschka in relation to intraoperative recording of auditory evoked potentials from the cochlear nuclei. J Neurosurg. 1995;82:933–9.
67. Komune N, Yagmurlu K, Matsuo S, Miki K, Abe H, Rhoton AL Jr. Auditory brainstem implantation: anatomy and approaches. Neurosurgery. 2015;11(Suppl 2):306–20; discussion 320–1.

Endoscopy in the Cerebellopontine Angle

8

Steven B. Carr, Charles Teo, Pankaj A. Gore, Steve W. Chang, and Peter Nakaji

Over the past few decades, the integration of endoscopic techniques into many aspects of cranial surgery, including that of the X, has gained widespread acceptance. However, the use of the endoscope in this region is not new. In 1917, Doyen [1] introduced an endoscope to the cerebellopontine angle (CPA) during a suboccipital approach for a trigeminal neurectomy. Although the endoscopes of the premicrosurgical era probably provided the best visualization of the critical neurovascular anatomy that had yet been developed, their safe use was hindered by several factors. Early endoscopes were bulky and rudimentary. The light source was by necessity located at the tip, and the resulting heat posed a significant risk to critical structures. The viewing eyepiece was integrated into the endoscope and, therefore, compromised the sterile field. Despite innovations in design in the 1950s, including the Hopkins rod-lens and fiber optic light sources, endoscopes were not popular with neurosurgeons of that era. In the 1960s, the introduction of the operating microscope to neurosurgery vastly improved illumination and magnification and allowed bimanual manipulation of instruments. The microscope made surgeons realize that what they could do in surgery had been greatly limited by their inability to adequately visualize the anatomy and pathology of interest. The microscope rose in popularity, and the role of endoscopy in neurosurgery was further marginalized.

The resurgence of endoscopy in numerous medical specialties resulted directly from technological improvements. Illumination was improved by the creation of better light sources, particularly those driven by fiber optics. The invention of the charge-coupled device allowed visualization of high-quality endoscopic images on a television screen. As a result, the field of neuroendoscopy has advanced from its initial forays into hydrocephalus management to become a complex discipline with unique advantages and surgical applications that reach the innermost depths of the central nervous system.

The modern place of endoscopic neurosurgical techniques in addressing CPA pathology is simple in concept as it parallels the advantages of the use of endoscopes elsewhere in the central nervous system. The appeal of minimally invasive endoscopic operations is in how they can allow smaller incisions and craniotomies compared with open procedures, decreasing both approach-related impact and morbidity. However, the standard with which endoscopy must compete is high, using a standard 2-cm retrosigmoid craniotomy, a surgeon can accomplish much within the CPA, and the exposure required by an endoscope in this setting is the same or not much less. The real benefits of the endoscope are its panoramic view, high magnification, superb illumination, and ability to "look around corners." Spencer and colleagues [2] reported that the endoscope provides 1.5–2.5 times greater volume of view compared with the operating microscope. These characteristics make the endoscope a useful tool for addressing pathology within the CPA with potentially greater efficacy than use of the operating microscope alone. In many settings, its best use is as an adjunct to the microscope. In other cases, the endoscope can be used as an independent tool.

S. B. Carr
Division of Neurological Surgery, Department of Neurosurgery, University of Missouri School of Medicine, Columbia, MO, USA

C. Teo
Centre for Minimally Invasive Neurosurgery, Prince of Wales Private Hospital, Randwick, NSW, Australia

P. A. Gore
Division of Neurological Surgery, The Oregon Clinic, Providence Brain and Spine Institute, Portland, OR, USA

S. W. Chang
Department of Neurosurgery, Barrow Neurological Institute, St. Joseph's Hospital and Medical Center, Phoenix, AZ, USA

P. Nakaji (✉)
Department of Neurosurgery, University of Arizona College of Medicine—Banner, Phoenix, AZ, USA

Surgery, University of Arizona College of Medicine—Phoenix, Phoenix, AZ, USA

Neurosurgery, Neuroscience Institute, Phoenix, AZ, USA
e-mail: Peter.Nakaji@bannerhealth.com

N. C. Bambakidis et al. (eds.), *Surgery of the Cerebellopontine Angle*, https://doi.org/10.1007/978-3-031-12507-2_8

Equipment

A standard endoscopic system appropriate for use within the CPA contains 0°, 30°, and 70° rigid endoscopes, a fiber optic light source, a high-definition video camera, a digital recorder with video and still image–capture capabilities, and a high-resolution monitor. The light source, recorder, and monitor should all be housed in a mobile cabinet to facilitate transport. We prefer a well-balanced pistol-grip Perneczky-style endoscope because of its high-quality images and favorable ergonomics. Other authors prefer pen-style endoscopes because they can be manipulated like microsurgical instruments and used for dissection [3].

The 0° endoscope provides a high-magnification view of structures along the line of sight. It provides an excellent panoramic view and delivers light close to the target, but it offers only limited improvement over the microscope in its ability to visualize objects outside the direct line of sight. The 30° endoscope adds the ability to look around corners adjacent to the line of sight; however, the surgeon should be aware that different trajectories may be required to manipulate the endoscope and microsurgical instruments simultaneously. With few exceptions, we discourage the routine use of the 70° endoscope within the CPA. This endoscope provides an even wider view perpendicular to the trajectory of the scope, but it provides a poor view directly ahead, placing structures directly in front of or behind the bevel of the tip at risk. The 70° endoscope should be introduced only in the setting of endoscopic-assisted surgery, with an assistant carefully monitoring its trajectory through the microscope. More recent innovations, such as the variable-view endoscope, which has the ability to rotate the tip lens from low to high angulation without changing the shape of the endoscope tip, may help to decrease the risk compared with introducing an endoscope with a view already fixed at a high angulation [4].

Overview of Endoscopic Techniques

Hopf and Perneczky [5] classified the intracranial application of endoscopy based on whether the endoscope is used independently or in conjunction with the microscope and based on the route of instrument manipulation. In modern parlance, *endoscopic-controlled surgery* describes an operation where no microscope is used; the video image provided by the endoscope guides all manipulation. *Endoscopic-assisted surgery* describes the use of the endoscope in conjunction with the microscope via the same operative corridor. In both endoscopic-controlled and endoscopic-assisted surgery, microsurgical instruments are used adjacent to the endoscope. This method allows far more effective dissection, haptic instrument feedback, and control of bleeding compared with the transendoscopic instruments used during endoscopic neurosurgery performed through working channels incorporated into the endoscope (e.g., as used for endoscopic colloid cyst resection). When a pneumatic scope holder is used or an experienced surgical assistant participates, the neurosurgeon can manipulate instruments with both hands. Lastly, the evolution of sophisticated keyhole instruments that may have a single shaft and a variety of angulations has helped to advance our minimally invasive capabilities.

The range of pathologies in the CPA that can be addressed with endoscopic techniques is now quite diverse and includes fenestration of cysts; removal of epidermoid and other CP angle tumors; microvascular decompression (MVD) of the trigeminal, facial, and hypoglossal nerves; inspection during removal of vestibular schwannomas; sealing of bony defects after CPA drilling; and other pathologies.

Operative Technique

For most endoscopic-assisted approaches to the CPA, the operating room setup and technique are determined by the planned microsurgical approach. Monitoring of somatosensory evoked potentials, brainstem auditory evoked potentials, and the facial nerve is standard protocol. The patient is positioned in the supine, lateral decubitus, or park bench position. In the supine position, the head is turned away from the surgical site until the sagittal plane is parallel to the floor, anatomy permitting, with the chin mildly flexed and the neck mildly extended. If possible, the shoulder should be positioned below the plane of the surgical site to avoid obstructing the surgeon's hand. The head is placed in three-point pin fixation and rigidly fixed to the operating table. Optional use of a lumbar drain to divert cerebrospinal fluid (CSF) can facilitate intraoperative brain relaxation and postoperative wound healing in high-risk patients, particularly those with a large habitus and high venous pressures; however, when addressing most pathologies, a lumbar drain is usually unnecessary.

The mobile cabinet containing the endoscope monitor is positioned either contralateral to the side of surgery at about the level of the patient's knees or above the patient's head (Fig. 8.1). Using either of these positions, the surgeon can rapidly change the view between the microscope and monitor without significant head movement. Endoscopic image projection into the microscope eyepiece is available on some microscopes. These systems allow the image to be inserted into part of the microscope view to be inserted into one eyepiece, or to replace the view in both eyepieces. Surgeons vary in their preference of receiving visual input in this way. Many find a separate monitor easier to use.

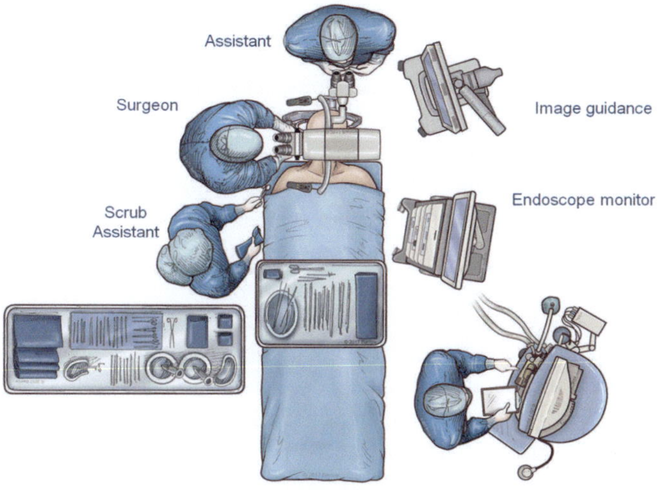

Fig. 8.1 Room setup and placement of the microscope during cerebellopontine angle microscopy with endoscopic assistance. Typically, the microscope is positioned on the same side as the surgeon and the endoscope is placed directly across from the surgeon in clear view. Alternatively, the monitor can be placed on the other side of the microscope, beyond the end of the bed (not shown). (*Used with permission from Barrow Neurological Institute, Phoenix, Arizona*)

Frameless stereotactic image guidance enables precise localization of the transverse-sigmoid junction and is used for most retrosigmoid craniotomies. Typically, a bur hole is placed immediately posteroinferior to the transverse-sigmoid junction, a craniotomy or craniectomy is fashioned slightly removed from the sinuses, and the transverse-sigmoid junction is gradually exposed as its edge is carefully approached. In the case of MVD, no more than 2 cm of bony exposure is required. For tumors, larger craniotomies or transpetrosal approaches may be necessary depending on the individual pathology.

Obtaining cerebellar relaxation before the dura is opened can ease the approach to the CPA and is usually satisfactorily facilitated by lumbar drainage of CSF and head elevation. Administration of mannitol (0.5–1.0 g/kg), maintenance of mild hyperventilation (pCO_2 28–32 mmHg), and administration of low-dose barbiturates or propofol can be useful maneuvers if head elevation and CSF drainage are insufficient.

The use of the endoscope is tailored to the specific pathology being addressed. Typically, we use the microscope as the primary mode of visualization and rely on the endoscope to visualize structures at the margin of or beyond the microscopic field of view. Tasks such as arachnoid dissection and tumor resection are most safely accomplished with bimanual control under the microscope. Several authors have successfully used endoscopic-controlled microsurgery for MVD [6–8] and even tumor resection [9] without using the microscope at all. However, in our experience, endoscopic-controlled surgery within the field of view that could have been afforded by the microscope often adds unnecessary risk to delicate structures without offering a substantial operative advantage because using the endoscope alone for visualization shows only structures at or beyond the tip of the endoscope, compared to the full corridor of visualization up to the site of interest seen through the microscope. Additionally, for a surgeon who does not utilize an endoscope holder, the intradural dissection must be performed with one hand, which is inherently disadvantageous. In fact, even if an endoscope holder is used to allow bimanual dissection, the shaft of the endoscope can become an additional physical obstacle. When the holder is placed at the top of a triangle with the working instruments at the two angles of the base of the triangle, it is less of an obstacle. Nevertheless, the endoscope can limit the working space available. Thus, in our experience the ideal application of the endoscope is as an adjunct tool to see structures outside the microscopic field of view.

Refraction at the air-fluid interface can significantly impair visualization. Thus, ideally the endoscope should be used in air or, less preferably, completely submerged in clear CSF or lactated Ringer's solution. A completely bloodless field is a prerequisite for submerged use of the endoscope, as any blood will generally substantially degrade the view. In the CPA, it is usually possible to drain enough cisternal CSF to allow work to be performed solely in an air medium.

Avoiding Complications with the Endoscope

Initially, the learning curve for using an endoscope is best ascended within the laboratory setting. Practice in the laboratory allows the surgeon to become familiar with the endoscopic equipment and to rapidly troubleshoot equipment problems that may arise within the operating room. Appropriate technique is essential to avoid complications. Before the endoscope is introduced, the orientation of the camera to the video image must be verified. This step is easily accomplished by examining any object with writing on it. It is essential that the operator learn to maintain the orientation of the camera regardless of the position of the endoscope. Disorientation is the greatest single risk associated with endoscopy.

Within the CPA, lateral or sweeping movements of the endoscope present substantial risks to adjacent cranial nerves and vascular structures and should be avoided categorically. Rather, redirecting should be performed by moving the endoscope in and out as opposed to side-to-side. Structures visible through the endoscope are not at significant risk. Once the tip of the endoscope passes a structure, it is no longer in the field of view and is therefore in potential danger. When the endoscope is superior to the acousticofacial complex, the petrotentorial angle can be used as a relatively safe zone to which the endoscope may drift. This maneuver is safer if the petrosal vein is sacrificed prophylactically. Typically, if an endoscope needs to be redirected or the camera rotated, it should be withdrawn to a safe extent from the CPA, adjusted, its orientation reconfirmed, and then reinserted.

When a microsurgical instrument is introduced in conjunction with the endoscope, the surgeon must recall that the shafts of both the endoscope and the instrument pose a potential risk of collision with neurovascular structures. The endoscope and instrument should be introduced side by side in a near-parallel trajectory. The endoscope should trail the instrument slightly, keeping the instrument in view at all times. If a less acute angle between the endoscope and the instrument is used, the surgeon or assistant should monitor the shafts via the microscope. A long focal length is used with the microscope to allow sufficient space to manipulate the endoscope.

The presence of a skilled assistant who can hold and maneuver the endoscope restores bimanual instrument control to the surgeon. Although several groups routinely use endoscopic holders [7, 10, 11], we find that these devices do not provide sufficient free mobility and fine control for routine use in this application compared with a human assistant.

Specific Applications of the Endoscope in the CPA: Cranial Nerve Decompression

Trigeminal Neuralgia

Of the various interventions used in the treatment of trigeminal neuralgia, MVD is associated with the highest long-term success rates and the lowest incidence of facial dysesthesias [12]. Jannetta, the key pioneer in MVD and senior author on the largest reported experience with MVD, has written that the surgeon performing this operation must keep two principles in mind [13]. The first is that "there must be a vessel and it is my job to find it" [13]. The second is that the length of the dorsal root entry zone can vary and may extend from the brainstem to a more distal position of the nerve. Reported immediate success rates with this operation range from 82% to 94% [14, 15]. The reported incidence of negative or equivocal microsurgical retrosigmoid explorations ranges from 6% to 18% [16–19]. We hypothesize that the unsatisfactory results associated with MVD are related to incomplete identification of neurovascular conflicts or to incomplete decompression of an identified conflict [20, 21].

A growing body of literature suggests that endoscopy improves the identification of neurovascular conflicts and the outcomes of MVD. Kabil and colleagues [6] reported 255 endoscopic-controlled MVD procedures; at 3 months, symptoms had resolved completely in 95% of the patients. In their series of 21 patients with trigeminal neuralgia who underwent endoscopic-assisted MVD, Jarrahy and colleagues [22] found 51 neurovascular conflicts, 27% of which could be identified only with the endoscope. In this series, decompression was performed under the microscope and then examined with the endoscope. In 24% of the patients, endoscopy demonstrated that further maneuvers were required to obtain adequate decompression. Given that 85% of the patients had complete or partial relief after surgery, the authors concluded that "despite a surgically better perspective and objectively improved detection of pathology, overall surgical results are unchanged by the addition of endoscopy" [22]. El-Garem and colleagues [23] reported similar findings in their series of 42 patients who underwent endoscopic-assisted MVD. Neurovascular conflicts were identified in all patients, 84% of whom experienced complete or partial relief. Another group reported vascular conflicts were not apparent with the microscope but were discovered using the endoscope in 15% of patients [24].

Teo and colleagues [21] implicated only arterial compression in the pathogenesis of trigeminal neuralgia in 114 patients treated with endoscopic-assisted MVD. Veins were spared even when they deformed the trigeminal nerve. In 25% of their patients, endoscopy only poorly improved visualization of arterial compression compared with the view through the microscope. In 8% of their patients, no vessel was identified with the microscope. In all patients of this latter group, the endoscope demonstrated a vessel located proximally in the groove between the dorsal root entry zone of the trigeminal nerve and cerebellum. Once viewed under the endoscope, 15% of the decompressions considered adequate under the microscope were found to be insufficient. At a mean follow-up of 29 months, 99.1% of patients had achieved complete or partial relief of their neuralgia symptoms. In comparing microscopic to fully endoscopic MVD for trigeminal neuralgia, Lee and colleagues [25] found similar pain outcomes; however, in addition, patients in whom fully endoscopic MVD was performed experienced a lower rate of postoperative headache.

For the treatment of trigeminal neuralgia, a high retrosigmoid craniotomy is fashioned to permit a lateral supracerebellar infratentorial approach. For several reasons, the trigeminal nerve is best approached microsurgically from the tentorial surface rather than from the petrous surface. First, there is less chance of placing traction on the facial nerve when the cerebellum is retracted rostrocaudally rather than mediolaterally. Second, the superior cerebellar artery, the most common compressive vessel, often impinges the trigeminal nerve from the medial side [26] and is best visualized from the tentorial surface [27]. Compression from the anterior inferior cerebellar artery occurs at the caudolateral aspect of the trigeminal nerve but is still well visualized from the tentorial surface [27].

Once arachnoid dissection is completed under the microscope, the endoscope is introduced (Fig. 8.2a). The 30° endoscope allows visualization of the entire cisternal segment of the trigeminal nerve, from the pons to the Meckel cave, and allows visualization of regions of the nerve that are poorly seen with the microscope [7, 20]. It is first introduced with the bevel pointed inferiorly and is used to inspect the trigeminal nerve from above. The endoscope is then rotated so that the bevel faces medially and is used to inspect the most dorsal aspect of the root entry zone. Through the microscope, the overlying cerebellum often hides this area of compression by the superior cerebellar artery. The endoscope is then directed laterally and used to examine the entry of the nerve into the Meckel cave. The veins in this region are preserved unless they greatly deform the nerve, split the nerve, or obstruct visualization of the entire nerve. With the bevel of the endoscope facing superiorly, the trigeminal nerve is inspected from below. This maneuver can put the seventh and eighth cranial nerves at risk. Consequently, an assistant should monitor the shaft of the endoscope through the microscope.

Once a compressive vessel or vessels are identified, further decompression is usually performed under microscopic visualization. A Teflon or Ivalon sponge is interposed between the nerve and offending vessel. The endoscope is again brought into the surgical field to evaluate the decompression. Closure proceeds in standard fashion.

Hemifacial Spasm

The incidence of hemifacial spasm, estimated at 0.8 cases per 100,000 persons per year [28], is much less than that of trigeminal neuralgia. Nevertheless, several moderately sized series of endoscopic-assisted MVD of the facial nerve have been published [29, 30]. In a series of 60 patients, Magnan and colleagues [29] gained an additional 72% accuracy in the identification of neurovascular conflicts involving the facial nerve when using the endoscope compared with using the microscope. Samii and colleagues [31] have reported a 23% incidence of multiple compressive neurovascular conflicts in patients with hemifacial spasm. However, asymptomatic vessel loops impinging on the facial nerve are estimated to be present in 38% of patients [32]. These authors' work supports the claim that the endoscope provides higher magnification, superior illumination, and the

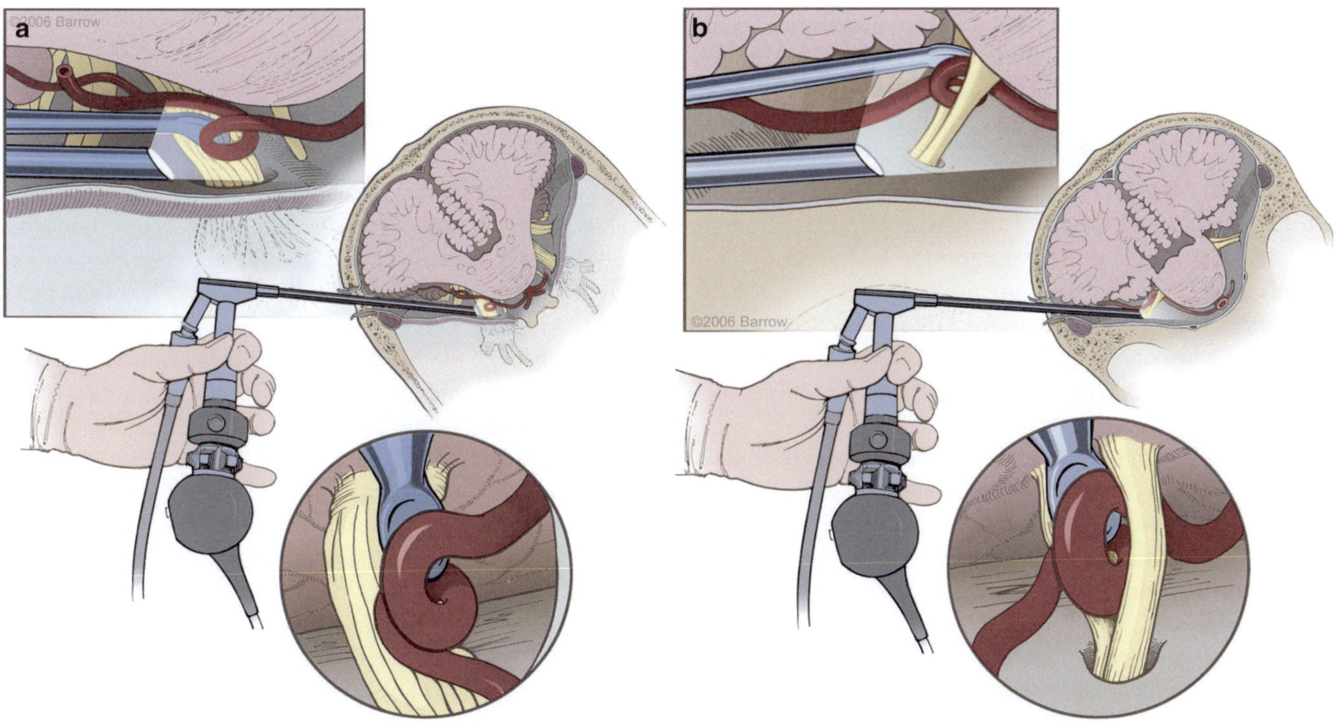

Fig. 8.2 (**a**) In endoscope-assisted or endoscope-controlled surgery, the endoscope is held in one hand, while a second instrument is maneuvered with another. An endoscope-assisted retrosigmoid craniotomy for microvascular decompression for trigeminal neuralgia is shown (*middle*). A 30° endoscope is held with the view angled back toward the root entry zone (*top*, illustrated view through microscope), while a No. 4 Penfield dissector is used to lift the vessel off the trigeminal nerve (*bottom*, illustrated view through endoscope). (**b**) A similar technique is used to decompress the facial nerve to treat hemifacial spasm (*middle*). In this case, the vessel courses between the nerves (*top*, illustrated view through microscope; *bottom*, illustrated view through endoscope). The 30° view helps in safely mobilizing the loop touching the brainstem, which is usually anterior to the nerve and out of the view of the microscope. (*Used with permission from Barrow Neurological Institute, Phoenix, Arizona*)

ability to view the facial nerve from angles unavailable to the microscope. Compression is often from the medial side, where microscopic exposure is challenging. Identification of gross changes in the appearance of the facial nerve suggestive of pathologic rather than incidental impingement is facilitated with the endoscope [29]. Use of the endoscope during inspection also minimizes retraction and manipulation of the acousticofacial complex [11, 29, 33].

Badr-El-Dine and colleagues [30] reported 80 patients with hemifacial spasm who underwent endoscope-assisted MVD. The authors stated that "the capacity of the endoscope to detect a neurovascular conflict is [100% and] superior to the best results obtained by the operative microscope" [30]. In the above two studies, 88–96% of patients had complete or substantial relief 1 year or longer after the procedure. This finding is similar to the range of 91–95% good outcomes reported in the largest microsurgical series [31, 34–36]. Endoscope-controlled MVD for hemifacial spasm has been reported by a few groups. In Cheng and colleagues' series [24], all ten patients treated under pure endoscopic visualization had a good outcome. An earlier case series [37] reported symptom recovery in all three patients treated with endoscope-controlled MVD, without long-term complications.

The microsurgical and endoscopic techniques used to treat hemifacial spasm are similar to those used for trigeminal neuralgia. The craniotomy to treat a hemifacial spasm is made about 1 cm lower than that used for trigeminal neuralgia because the dorsal root entry zone of the facial nerve should be approached inferior to the origin of the eighth cranial nerve and flocculus. Typically, the compressive vessel is on the anterocaudal aspect of the dorsal root entry zone of the facial nerve [34] directly against the brainstem. Even if vessels are found laterally, superiorly, or medially, a close inspection of the medial face of the root entry zone is mandatory. The endoscope helps visualize precisely this portion of the nerve, which is difficult to see through the microscope (Fig. 8.2b).

The initial arachnoid dissection proceeds under the microscope. Again, the 30° endoscope is the most useful choice. Initially, it is inserted with the bevel directed laterally to identify the rare neurovascular conflict on the distal aspect of the nerve. The endoscope is then directed medially to visualize the dorsal root entry zone and most common site of compression. Because the offending vessel occupies a medial location, it is sometimes easier to decompress the nerve and place the sponge under endoscopic visualization.

Glossopharyngeal Neuralgia

Although the reported experience with glossopharyngeal neuralgia is small, the endoscope can readily be used during MVD of the glossopharyngeal nerve. The vascular compression is often medial to the ninth cranial nerve, and decompression is most easily performed under endoscopic visualization. Jarrahy and colleagues [33] have reported good outcomes after endoscope-controlled MVD of the glossopharyngeal nerve. Broggi and colleagues [38] reported their series of MVD for neurovascular conflicts, in which one patient was being treated for glossopharyngeal neuralgia and in whom an offending vessel not visible with the microscope was identified by endoscopy.

Specific Applications of the Endoscope in the CPA: CPA Masses

The high magnification, illumination, and angled view offered by the endoscope can prove useful when addressing tumors of the CPA. Tumors located at the most medial aspect of the CPA or with components behind eloquent neurovascular structures can be beyond the line of sight of the microscope and only visualized with the endoscope (Fig. 8.3). In a series with Al-Mefty as the senior author, residual tumor was discovered using the endoscope intraoperatively after what was felt to be a gross total resection using the microscope in 69% of patients harboring CPA tumors of various types [39].

Vestibular Schwannoma

During retrosigmoid or retrolabyrinthine approaches to vestibular schwannomas, the endoscope has been shown to safely improve visualization of the facial nerve [40], lateral internal auditory canal (IAC), and open air cells of the mastoid [3, 11]. The lateral IAC can be especially difficult to visualize through the microscope with these approaches. The endoscope has been reported to be useful in retrieving intracanalicular tumor from within the IAC without sacrificing hearing or facial nerve function [41]. Use of the 30° endoscope can limit the amount of bony drilling required to sufficiently expose and view the lateral IAC [11, 42]. More recently, both a flexible surgeon-controlled tip [43] and variable-view rotating lens rigid endoscope [4] have been reported to improve visualization within the IAC.

Although we do not recommend widespread adoption of endoscope-controlled vestibular schwannoma resection, some authors have reported good results resecting vestibular schwannomas even under pure endoscopic control [3, 42, 44]. Regardless of the extent to which the endoscope was used during dissection or resection, we recommend using the endoscope to inspect the bone where drilling has been performed to ensure any open mastoid air cells are waxed adequately before closure (Fig. 8.4).

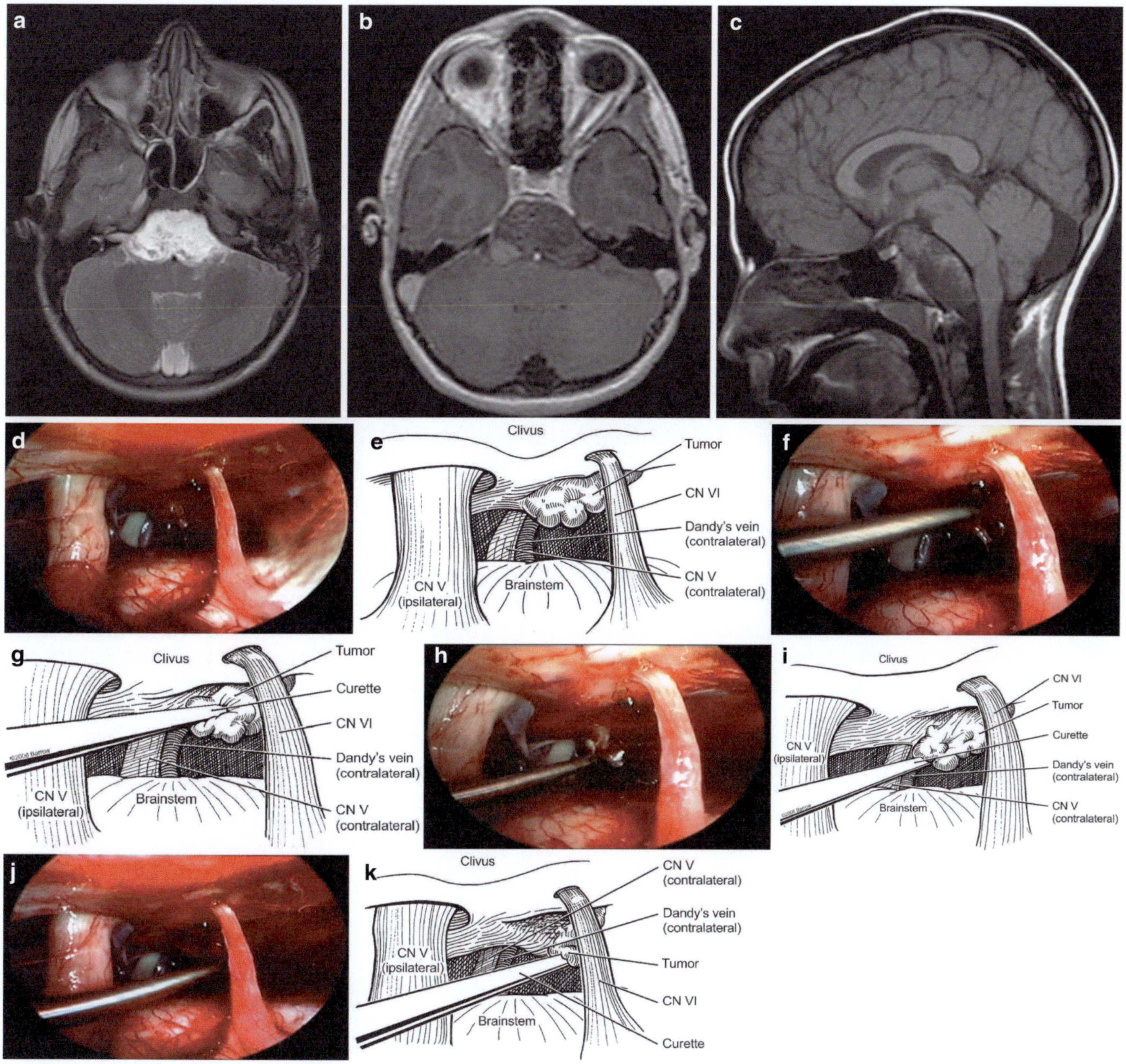

Fig. 8.3 Endoscope-assisted debulking of a large intradural chordoma. (**a**) Axial T2-weighted and (**b**) T1-weighted magnetic resonance images (MRIs) with contrast show minimal enhancement at right ambient cistern. (**c**) Sagittal T1-weighted MRI without contrast shows a mass effect on the pons and medulla. (**d**) Endoscopic view and (**e**) corresponding illustration after second-stage microscopic debulking via a right retrosigmoid craniotomy. The 30° angled endoscope allows visualization of cranial extensions of tumor and contralateral recesses. Most of the tumor has been debulked, but the remnants along the cranial-caudal extensions of the retroclival cisterns were not visible under microscopic visualization. The remnants were removed with a microcurette with direct visualization of all neurovascular structures, including the contralateral trigeminal nerve (CN V), Dandy's vein, and abducens nerve (CN VI). (**f**, **h**, **j**) Sequential endoscopic images and (**g**, **i**, **k**) corresponding illustrations of tumor remnant being removed from the upper clivus. (*Used with permission from Barrow Neurological Institute, Phoenix, Arizona*)

Meningioma

Meningiomas can arise in the posterior fossa and are one of the most common tumors encountered in the CPA. Schroeder and colleagues [45] published their experience with treating skull-base meningiomas with endoscopic assistance, of which 23 were located in the CPA. With the endoscope, they found tumor that was not visible with the microscope in 56% of those cases. Al-Mefty's group reported its support for endoscope assistance in meningioma resection, in which

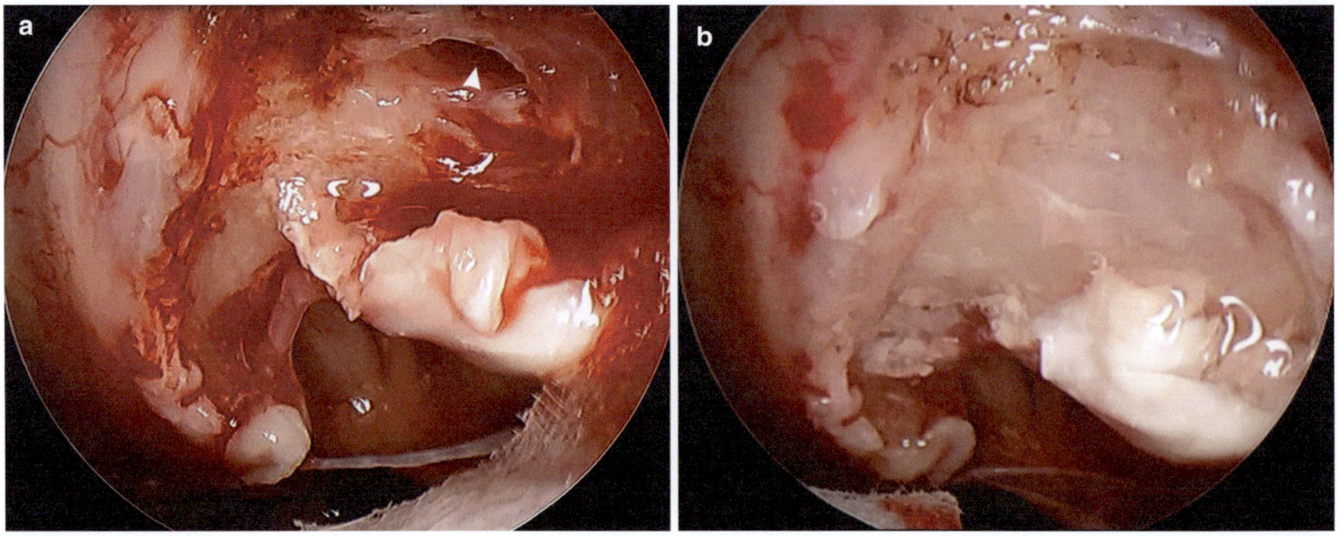

Fig. 8.4 The endoscope can be used to visualize the IAC after drilling to identify unwaxed air cells. (**a**) A view of the IAC through the 30° endoscope reveals an open-air cell (arrowhead). (**b**) The same view after covering the IAC wall with wax under endoscopic visualization. (*Used with permission from Barrow Neurological Institute, Phoenix, Arizona*)

78% of presumed microscopic gross total resections were found to have residual tumor upon endoscopic inspection [39]. They recommended introducing the endoscope as late as possible in the dissection because of the bloody character of CPA meningioma resection and to avoid difficulties with bone dust from drilling, both of which can necessitate frequent lens cleaning. While meningiomas may not be ideal tumors to resect fully endoscopically in the current era, the procedure has been reported [46].

Epidermoid

Epidermoid tumors are most commonly found in the posterior fossa and specifically tend to arise within the CPA. Due to their soft flaky consistency, avascular character, and tendency to insinuate themselves in tight skull-base locations such as the CPA, epidermoids are well suited for application of endoscopic surgical techniques. Epidermoids are generally considered insensitive to nonsurgical treatment and have a high rate of recurrence when gross total resection is unable to be achieved [47].

As a result, surgeons have been striving to maximize safe resection by using tools such as the endoscope. In fact, one group reported that residual tumor was discovered using endoscopic visualization after what was felt to be gross total resection using the microscope in 85% of CPA epidermoid resections [48]. In a separate series, Schroeder and colleagues [10] found that they were able to achieve more complete resections without recurrence or complication in 100% of their patients with CPA epidermoids in whom they performed endoscope-assisted resection. While endoscope-controlled resection of CPA epidermoids has been reported and can be successful [9], the risks and benefits of endoscopy currently favor an endoscope-assisted approach to CPA epidermoid resection.

Epidermoid tumors can often extend into the contralateral CPA or into the supratentorial compartment. The angled endoscopes help in the identification and resection of epidermoid desquamate extending into other cranial compartments and can reduce the need for more than one surgical approach [10, 49].

Arachnoid Cysts

CPA cysts can be amenable to fenestration by all of the endoscopic treatment modalities [5, 50–53], including transendoscopic. By performing CPA arachnoid cyst fenestration transendoscopically, only a bur hole exposure is required. However, the transendoscopic instruments used with this modality can prove unwieldy for addressing a thick cyst wall. Endoscope-assisted and endoscope-controlled techniques allow the use of standard microsurgical instruments and permit improved hemostatic control, and, while they require a relatively larger bony exposure and dural opening, wider fenestrations are easier to achieve with microsurgical instruments [50]. Gangemi and colleagues [52] have advocated fenestrating CPA cysts into the prepontine cistern between the trigeminal nerve and acousticofacial nerve complex. Alternatively, the cisterna magna provides a safe reservoir for fenestration. Frameless image guidance can be invaluable in targeting the bur hole, trajectory, and site of fenestration. When a catheter is placed therapeutically in the CPA, the endoscope also can be used for visual guidance [52].

Conclusion

Almost any neurosurgical procedure involving the CPA can be supplemented with endoscopy. It remains for the surgeon to decide whether the benefits of improved magnification, illumination, and ability to "look around corners" justify the potential risks for an individual case. It is imperative that novice neuroendoscopists become thoroughly comfortable with the endoscopic equipment and its operation in the laboratory setting before attempting its use in their clinical setting. To the novice, the endoscope can prove unwieldy, fatiguing, and disorienting, and the potential loss of bimanual control can present a further stumbling block. We strongly believe that these obstacles can be readily overcome with appropriate preparation and experience and we believe that the benefits of incorporating the endoscope in CPA surgery can improve the safety and efficacy of our interventions.

References

1. Doyen E. Surgical therapeutics and operative technique. London: Bailliere, Tindall and Cox; 1917.
2. Spencer WR, Das K, Nwagu C, et al. Approaches to the sellar and parasellar region: anatomic comparison of the microscope versus endoscope. Laryngoscope. 1999;109(5):791–4.
3. King WA, Frazee JG, Teo C, Wackym PA. Endoscopic treatment of cranial base lesions. New York: Thieme; 1998.
4. Ebner FH, Roser F, Roder C, Tatagiba M, Schuhmann MU. Rigid, variable-view endoscope in neurosurgery: first intraoperative experience. Surg Innov. 2015;22(4):390–3.
5. Hopf NJ, Perneczky A. Endoscopic neurosurgery and endoscope-assisted microneurosurgery for the treatment of intracranial cysts. Neurosurgery. 1998;43(6):1330–6; discussion 1336–7.
6. Kabil MS, Eby JB, Shahinian HK. Endoscopic vascular decompression versus microvascular decompression of the trigeminal nerve. Minim Invasive Neurosurg. 2005;48(4):207–12.
7. Jarrahy R, Eby JB, Cha ST, Shahinian HK. Fully endoscopic vascular decompression of the trigeminal nerve. Minim Invasive Neurosurg. 2002;45(1):32–5.
8. Piazza M, Lee JY. Endoscopic and microscopic microvascular decompression. Neurosurg Clin N Am. 2016;27(3):305–13.
9. Peng Y, Yu L, Li Y, Fan J, Qiu M, Qi S. Pure endoscopic removal of epidermoid tumors of the cerebellopontine angle. Childs Nerv Syst. 2014;30(7):1261–7.
10. Schroeder HW, Oertel J, Gaab MR. Endoscope-assisted microsurgical resection of epidermoid tumors of the cerebellopontine angle. J Neurosurg. 2004;101(2):227–32.
11. Goksu N, Bayazit Y, Kemaloglu Y. Endoscopy of the posterior fossa and dissection of acoustic neuroma. J Neurosurg. 1999;91(5):776–80.
12. Jannetta PJ, Levy EI. Trigeminal neuralgia: microvascular decompression of the trigeminal nerve for tic douloureux. Philadelphia: W.B. Saunders; 2004.
13. McLaughlin MR, Jannetta PJ, Clyde BL, Subach BR, Comey CH, Resnick DK. Microvascular decompression of cranial nerves: lessons learned after 4400 operations. J Neurosurg. 1999;90(1):1–8.
14. Barker FG 2nd, Jannetta PJ, Bissonette DJ, Larkins MV, Jho HD. The long-term outcome of microvascular decompression for trigeminal neuralgia. N Engl J Med. 1996;334(17):1077–83.
15. Klun B. Microvascular decompression and partial sensory rhizotomy in the treatment of trigeminal neuralgia: personal experience with 220 patients. Neurosurgery. 1992;30(1):49–52.
16. Jannetta PJ. Microvascular decompression. In: Rovit RL, Murali R, Jannetta PJ, editors. Trigeminal neuralgia. Baltimore: Williams & Wilkins; 1990. p. 201–2.
17. van Loveren H, Tew JM Jr, Keller JT, Nurre MA. A 10-year experience in the treatment of trigeminal neuralgia. Comparison of percutaneous stereotaxic rhizotomy and posterior fossa exploration. J Neurosurg. 1982;57(6):757–64.
18. Kolluri S, Heros RC. Microvascular decompression for trigeminal neuralgia. A five-year follow-up study. Surg Neurol. 1984;22(3):235–40.
19. Richards P, Shawdon H, Illingworth R. Operative findings on microsurgical exploration of the cerebello-pontine angle in trigeminal neuralgia. J Neurol Neurosurg Psychiatry. 1983;46(12):1098–101.
20. Nakaji P, Teo C. Endoscopic-assisted microvascular decompression of the cranial nerves: operative technique. Oper Tech Neurosurg. 2005;8:186–92.
21. Teo C, Nakaji P, Mobbs RJ. Endoscope-assisted microvascular decompression for trigeminal neuralgia: technical case report. Neurosurgery. 2006;59(4 Suppl 2):ONSE489–90; discussion ONSE490.
22. Jarrahy R, Berci G, Shahinian HK. Endoscope-assisted microvascular decompression of the trigeminal nerve. Otolaryngol Head Neck Surg. 2000;123(3):218–23.
23. El-Garem HF, Badr-El-Dine M, Talaat AM, Magnan J. Endoscopy as a tool in minimally invasive trigeminal neuralgia surgery. Otol Neurotol. 2002;23(2):132–5.
24. Cheng WY, Chao SC, Shen CC. Endoscopic microvascular decompression of the hemifacial spasm. Surg Neurol. 2008;70(Suppl 1):40–6.
25. Lee JYK, Pierce JT, Sandhu SK, Petrov D, Yang AI. Endoscopic versus microscopic microvascular decompression for trigeminal neuralgia: equivalent pain outcomes with possibly decreased postoperative headache after endoscopic surgery. J Neurosurg. 2017;126(5):1676–84.
26. Matsushima T, Fukui M, Suzuki S, Rhoton AL Jr. The microsurgical anatomy of the infratentorial lateral supracerebellar approach to the trigeminal nerve for tic douloureux. Neurosurgery. 1989;24(6):890–5.
27. Hitotsumatsu T, Matsushima T, Inoue T. Microvascular decompression for treatment of trigeminal neuralgia, hemifacial spasm, and glossopharyngeal neuralgia: three surgical approach variations: technical note. Neurosurgery. 2003;53(6):1436–41; discussion 1442–3.
28. Auger RG, Whisnant JP. Hemifacial spasm in Rochester and Olmsted County, Minnesota, 1960 to 1984. Arch Neurol. 1990;47(11):1233–4.
29. Magnan J, Caces F, Locatelli P, Chays A. Hemifacial spasm: endoscopic vascular decompression. Otolaryngol Head Neck Surg. 1997;117(4):308–14.
30. Badr-El-Dine M, El-Garem HF, Talaat AM, Magnan J. Endoscopically assisted minimally invasive microvascular decompression of hemifacial spasm. Otol Neurotol. 2002;23(2):122–8.
31. Samii M, Gunther T, Iaconetta G, Muehling M, Vorkapic P, Samii A. Microvascular decompression to treat hemifacial spasm: long-term results for a consecutive series of 143 patients. Neurosurgery. 2002;50(4):712–8; discussion 718–9.

32. Magnan J, Bremond G, Chays A, Gignac D, Florence A. Vestibular neurotomy by retrosigmoid approach: technique, indications, and results. Am J Otol. 1991;12(2):101–4.
33. Jarrahy R, Cha ST, Eby JB, Berci G, Shahinian HK. Fully endoscopic vascular decompression of the glossopharyngeal nerve. J Craniofac Surg. 2002;13(1):90–5.
34. Huang CI, Chen IH, Lee LS. Microvascular decompression for hemifacial spasm: analyses of operative findings and results in 310 patients. Neurosurgery. 1992;30(1):53–6; discussion 56–7.
35. Chung SS, Chang JH, Choi JY, Chang JW, Park YG. Microvascular decompression for hemifacial spasm: a long-term follow-up of 1,169 consecutive cases. Stereotact Funct Neurosurg. 2001;77(1–4):190–3.
36. Barker FG 2nd, Jannetta PJ, Bissonette DJ, Shields PT, Larkins MV, Jho HD. Microvascular decompression for hemifacial spasm. J Neurosurg. 1995;82(2):201–10.
37. Eby JB, Cha ST, Shahinian HK. Fully endoscopic vascular decompression of the facial nerve for hemifacial spasm. Skull Base. 2001;11(3):189–97.
38. Broggi M, Acerbi F, Ferroli P, Tringali G, Schiariti M, Broggi G. Microvascular decompression for neurovascular conflicts in the cerebellopontine angle: which role for endoscopy? Acta Neurochir (Wien). 2013;155(9):1709–16.
39. Abolfotoh M, Bi WL, Hong CK, et al. The combined microscopic-endoscopic technique for radical resection of cerebellopontine angle tumors. J Neurosurg. 2015;123(5):1301–11.
40. Gerganov VM, Giordano M, Herold C, Samii A, Samii M. An electrophysiological study on the safety of the endoscope-assisted microsurgical removal of vestibular schwannomas. Eur J Surg Oncol. 2010;36(4):422–7.
41. Kumon Y, Kohno S, Ohue S, et al. Usefulness of endoscope-assisted microsurgery for removal of vestibular schwannomas. J Neurol Surg B Skull Base. 2012;73(1):42–7.
42. Rosenberg SI, Silverstein H, Willcox TO, Gordon MA. Endoscopy in otology and neurotology. Am J Otol. 1994;15(2):168–72.
43. Corrivetti F, Cacciotti G, Giacobbo Scavo C, Roperto R, Mastronardi L. Flexible endoscopic-assisted microsurgical radical resection of intracanalicular vestibular schwannomas by a retrosigmoid approach: operative technique. World Neurosurg. 2018;115:229–33.
44. Shahinian HK, Ra Y. 527 fully endoscopic resections of vestibular schwannomas. Minim Invasive Neurosurg. 2011;54(2):61–7.
45. Schroeder HW, Hickmann AK, Baldauf J. Endoscope-assisted microsurgical resection of skull base meningiomas. Neurosurg Rev. 2011;34(4):441–5.
46. Vaz-Guimaraes F, Gardner PA, Fernandez-Miranda JC. Fully endoscopic retrosigmoid approach for posterior petrous meningioma and trigeminal microvascular decompression. Acta Neurochir (Wien). 2015;157(4):611–5; discussion 615.
47. Gopalakrishnan CV, Ansari KA, Nair S, Menon G. Long term outcome in surgically treated posterior fossa epidermoids. Clin Neurol Neurosurg. 2014;117:93–9.
48. Tuchman A, Platt A, Winer J, Pham M, Giannotta S, Zada G. Endoscopic-assisted resection of intracranial epidermoid tumors. World Neurosurg. 2014;82(3-4):450–4.
49. Darrouzet V, Franco-Vidal V, Hilton M, et al. Surgery of cerebellopontine angle epidermoid cysts: role of the widened retrolabyrinthine approach combined with endoscopy. Otolaryngol Head Neck Surg. 2004;131(1):120–5.
50. Godano U, Mascari C, Consales A, Calbucci F. Endoscope-controlled microneurosurgery for the treatment of intracranial fluid cysts. Childs Nerv Syst. 2004;20(11-12):839–41.
51. Gaab MR, Schroeder HWS. Arachnoid cysts. In: King WA, Frazee JG, De Salles AAF, editors. Endoscopy of the central and peripheral nervous system. New York: Thieme; 1998. p. 136–46.
52. Gangemi M, Maiuri F, Colella G, Sardo L. Endoscopic surgery for large posterior fossa arachnoid cysts. Minim Invasive Neurosurg. 2001;44(1):21–4.
53. Ottaviani F, Neglia CB, Scotti A, Capaccio P. Arachnoid cyst of the cranial posterior fossa causing sensorineural hearing loss and tinnitus: a case report. Eur Arch Otorhinolaryngol. 2002;259(6):306–8.

Part III

Vestibular Schwannomas

9 Biology and Genetics of Vestibular Schwannomas in Tumors of the Cerebellopontine Angle

Dunia Abdul-Aziz, Nicholas A. Dewyer, and D. Bradley Welling

Advances in molecular biology have improved our understanding of the origin of vestibular schwannomas. The identification of mutations in the neurofibromatosis type 2 gene (*NF2*) as the underlying genetic cause of vestibular schwannomas has driven research into the molecular events leading to tumor formation. (Note: The italicized "*NF2*" represents the human neurofibromatosis type 2 gene specifically, while "NF2" is used to indicate the human disease of neurofibromatosis type 2, and "*Nf2*" indicates the homolog expressed in rodents). The clinical characteristics of both sporadic vestibular schwannomas and neurofibromatosis type 2 syndrome have been related to alterations in *NF2*. This gene encodes the protein "merlin," a tumor suppressor that is involved in cell signaling pathways regulating growth and proliferation. These molecular studies have identified potential therapeutic targets, and here we review these recent advances in the context of vestibular schwannoma biology.

Background

Histologically, vestibular schwannomas are tumors of the neural sheath that originate on the superior or inferior vestibular branches of cranial nerve (CN) VIII. These tumors arise within the internal auditory canal and can extend into the cerebellopontine angle. They have been called both "acoustic neuromas" and "vestibular schwannomas," but the latter term is preferred because these tumors are not neuromas and only rarely arise from the acoustic (cochlear) nerve (nomenclature adopted at the National Institutes of Health [NIH] Consensus Development Conference) [1]. Vestibular schwannomas can occur as sporadic unilateral tumors or as bilateral tumors. The development of bilateral vestibular schwannomas is pathognomonic for the hereditary disorder NF2. Various types of vestibular schwannomas can be loosely grouped as unilateral sporadic vestibular schwannomas or as bilateral or *NF2*-associated schwannomas. Vestibular schwannomas with true cysts (cystic schwannomas) typically have a more aggressive phenotype, which may be distinguished from more benign unilateral sporadic schwannomas. Mutations in the *NF2* gene are characteristic of all three tumor types, while differences between the tumor types are only beginning to be identified at the molecular level [2, 3].

Schwannomas typically occur as solitary tumors, which make up the majority of cases (>90%). The detected incidence of unilateral vestibular schwannomas has increased to approximately 20 persons per million per year [4, 5]. Sporadic tumors usually occur in the fourth and fifth decades with a mean age of 50 years at presentation. Symptomatically, they manifest most commonly with hearing loss, tinnitus, and vertigo due to compression of the cochlear and invasion of the vestibular branches of CN VIII. While CN VII is often stretched and splayed by the tumor, facial paralysis is uncommon. Compression of other adjacent nerves at the brainstem, namely CN V, can result in facial paresthesia. Although histologically benign, large tumors can compress the brainstem and result in hydrocephalus, herniation, and death in rare cases (Fig. 9.1).

Clinically, NF2 is a highly penetrant autosomal dominant disease (Online Mendelian Inheritance in Man [OMIM] #101000) affecting 1 in 33,000 people [6, 7]. Patients who inherit a pathologic mutation in the *NF2* tumor-suppressor gene located on chromosome 22q12 have a 95% chance of developing bilateral vestibular schwannomas. However, about one-half of the patients with NF2 are caused by *de*

D. Abdul-Aziz (✉) · D. B. Welling
Massachusetts Eye and Ear, Boston, MA, USA

Otolaryngology—Head and Neck Surgery, Harvard Medical School, Boston, MA, USA
e-mail: Dunia_Abdul-Aziz@MEEI.HARVARD.EDU

N. A. Dewyer
Department of Otolaryngology—Head and Neck Surgery, Department of Otology, Neurotology, and Skull Base Surgery, Department of Audiology, University of Arizona College of Medicine, Tucson, AZ, USA

N. C. Bambakidis et al. (eds.), *Surgery of the Cerebellopontine Angle*, https://doi.org/10.1007/978-3-031-12507-2_9

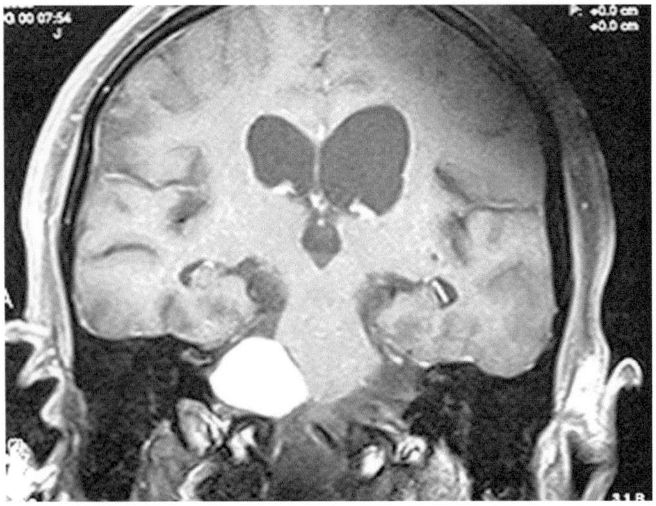

Fig. 9.1 Coronal T1-weighted MRI with gadolinium contrast shows a solid unilateral vestibular schwannoma associated with slight shift of the brainstem

novo mutations and lack a family history of NF2. NF2 follows the Knudson two-hit hypothesis with the first "hit" involving the inherited or *de novo* mutation and an additional second "hit" developing as a somatic mutation resulting in loss of heterozygosity [7–9]. Other disease features of NF2 include intracranial meningiomas, ependymomas, spinal schwannomas, and presenile lens opacities (Fig. 9.2) [10–12]. The onset of symptoms usually presents between the ages of 11 and 30 years, but some patients may present in their fifth or sixth decade. NF2 is not to be confused with neurofibromatosis type 1 (NF1) or von Recklinghausen disease (OMIM #162200), which is associated with multiple peripheral neurofibromas and is caused by a mutation in the *NF1* tumor-suppressor gene on chromosome 17.

Occasionally, segmental or mosaic categories of NF2 are included to describe another category of NF2 [13]. The cause of segmental NF2 may be due to somatic mosaicism, where a mutation occurs later in embryogenesis rather than in the

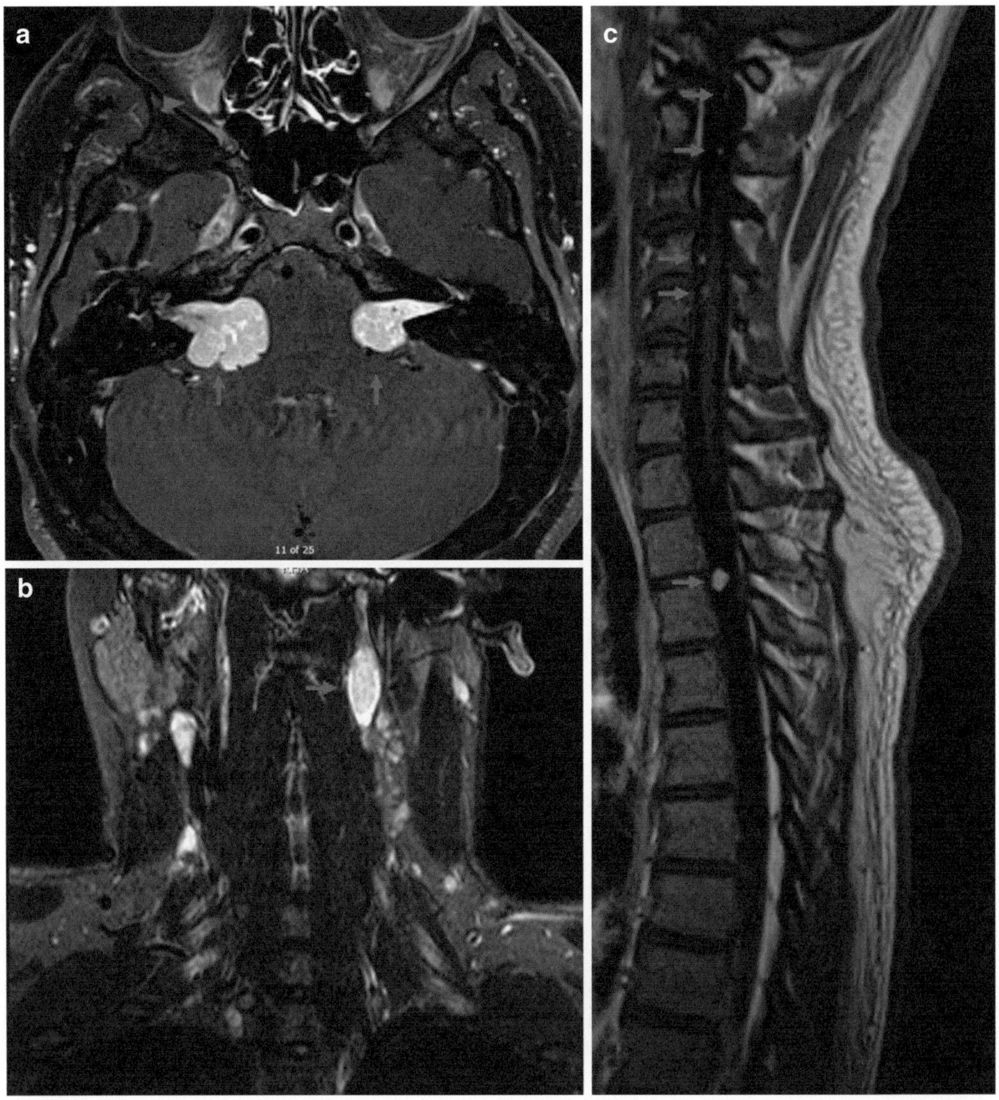

Fig. 9.2 Contrast-enhanced T1-weighted MRIs of a patient with NF2 demonstrate (**a**) bilateral vestibular schwannomas (arrows) and optic nerve tumor (arrowhead), (**b**) vagal nerve schwannoma (arrow) in the left carotid space of the neck, and (**c**) multiple enhancing lesions in the spinal cord representing likely ependymomas and schwannomas (arrows)

germline DNA, in which case only a portion of a patient's cells carries the mutation, and the disease is manifest in limited areas of the body [14, 15]. In contrast, patients with familial NF2 inherit one mutation from a parent at conception and all cells carry one mutant allele. Kluwe and colleagues estimated that mosaicism may account for 25% of NF2 cases of any subtype among patients whose parents did not display the disease [14].

Patients with somatic mosaicism can display bilateral vestibular schwannomas if the postzygotic mutation occurred early in embryogenesis. However, they may also display an atypical presentation, or *segmental* NF2, in which the patient has a unilateral vestibular schwannoma and an additional ipsilateral intracranial tumor, such as a meningioma. In such cases, the postzygotic mutation occurred later in development [16]. Unlike the traditional forms of NF2, the risk of passing NF2 caused by mosaicism to future offspring is low.

Schwannomatosis (OMIM #162091) was first described in 1973 and is characterized by multiple schwannomas and (to a lesser extent) meningiomas, but vestibular schwannomas are distinctly absent [17]. Patients with schwannomatosis often become symptomatic with intractable pain rather than with cranial nerve deficits. They do not develop other intracranial tumors or malignancies. MacCollin and colleagues noted that about one-third of patients with schwannomatosis had tumors in an anatomically limited distribution, such as a single limb, several contiguous segments of the spine, or half of the body [18]. Sporadic cases of schwannomatosis are as common as NF2. In contrast to NF1 and NF2, which are autosomal dominant and highly penetrant, few cases of familial schwannomatosis have been identified. The molecular origins of schwannomatosis point to mutations in the SMARCB1 gene also found on chromosome 22, and these mutations can occur concurrently with biallelic somatic inactivation of the *NF2* gene [17].

Although current surgical and radiation treatments for vestibular schwannomas are generally effective at controlling compressive symptoms, treatment-related morbidity such as hearing loss and facial paralysis continues to be problematic. Recent discoveries and advances in the molecular biology of vestibular schwannomas, with focus on the *NF2* gene, are reviewed below with the goal of identifying specific medical options for treatment of this disease.

The *NF2* Gene

Vestibular schwannomas harbor mutations in the tumor suppressor gene, *NF2*, resulting in abnormal production of merlin protein, which underlies the pathogenesis of the disease both in inherited and sporadic cases [19, 20]. In 1993, two independent groups, Rouleau and colleagues and Trofatter and colleagues used linkage analysis and positional cloning to localize the *NF2* gene to chromosome 22 band q12 in patients with NF2 [21, 22]. Since then, mutations in the *NF2* gene have also been found in sporadic unilateral schwannomas and cystic schwannomas [20, 23–27]. Furthermore, mutations within the *NF2* gene have often been identified in meningiomas and occasionally in other cancers, including melanoma, mesothelioma, and breast cancer [7, 28–31].

Structure and Function of the NF2 Protein, Merlin

The *NF2* gene contains 17 exons and the protein product called merlin (an acronym for moesin-ezrin-radixin-like) or schwannomin, a name derived from schwannoma [21, 22]. The *NF2* gene is transcribed into multiple RNA species by alternative splicing. Multiple isoforms have been identified, with two common isoforms described that differ by the absence (type I merlin) or presence (type II merlin) of exon 16. Isoform I is the predominant and longest isoform, with 595 amino acids. Isoform II contains all 17 exons, with 590 amino acids and with inclusion of exon 16 into the mRNA resulting in a new stop codon [32–35].

Merlin shares a high degree of homology to the erythrocyte protein 4.1-related superfamily, which acts to link the actin cytoskeleton to the plasma membrane [21, 22]. In particular, relative conservation of the N-terminal domain known as the FERM domain (F for 4.1 protein, E for ezrin, R for radixin, and M for moesin) characterizes the gene family [35, 36]. In merlin, the FERM domain is followed by a coil–coil domain and a charged carboxyl-terminus (C-terminus) domain (Fig. 9.3) [36–38]. The key functions of merlin may be mediated by the highly conserved FERM domain and the unique C-terminus of the protein, which distinguishes it from other ERM proteins. Unlike other ERM proteins that have an actin-binding site in the C-terminus, merlin has a unique actin-binding site in the N-terminus.

Merlin's growth regulatory function is related to its conformation and protein–protein interactions. Like other ERM proteins, merlin forms intramolecular and intermolecular associations that mediate its activities. Merlin's conformational states and protein–protein interactions are regulated by phosphorylation of specific amino acid residues in the protein, including Serine 10, Threonine 280, Serine 315, and Serine 518 [3]. Phosphorylation of Ser518 has been the most studied [39, 40]. In a simplified model (Fig. 9.3), phosphorylated Ser518 renders merlin in an open state where it serves as a cell membrane scaffold interacting with other receptors to mediate signaling events promoting proliferation. Phosphorylation also inactivates merlin by targeting merlin for polyubiquitination and proteasomal degradation [41, 42]. In turn, dephosphorylated merlin enables self-association of the N- and C-terminal domains and a more "closed" active

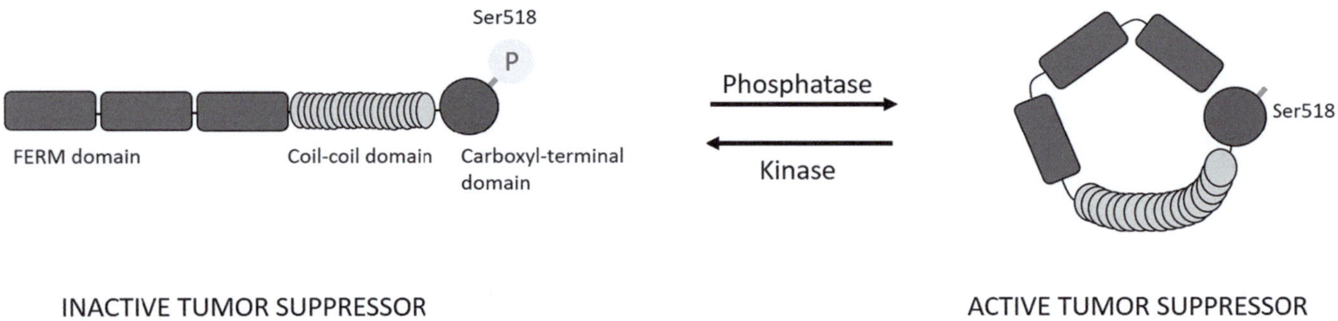

Fig. 9.3 Schematic diagram illustrates merlin's structural domains and regulation by phosphorylation at Serine 518 (Ser518). Phosphorylation of merlin at Ser518 results in an open configuration that renders merlin inactive as a tumor suppressor. Dephosphorylation of Ser518 allows the association between merlin's N-terminal and C-terminal domains, resulting in a "closed" configuration that is an active tumor suppressor

form, which mediates tumor suppressor function (Fig. 9.3) [41, 43].

Phosphorylation of merlin thus represents a posttranslational mechanism through which merlin's growth inhibitory activity is regulated [41, 44]. During growth, merlin exists in an inactive, phosphorylated state; when dephosphorylated and active, merlin signals growth arrest. Ser518 dephosphorylation and phosphorylation are respectively mediated by myosin phosphatase MYPT1-PP1δ and by protein kinases, including P21-activated kinases (PAKs) and protein kinase A (PKA) (Fig. 9.3) [40]. Thus, pathologic loss of merlin function can occur through various mechanisms involving merlin itself or its regulators.

NF2 Mutations and Their Clinical Correlation

Given the varied clinical manifestations of NF2 and sporadic VS, genotype–phenotype correlations have been explored [14, 23, 25, 26, 40, 44–46]. The frequency, type, and distribution of *NF2* mutations differ between sporadic and familial NF2 tumors. The effect of these mutations on the resultant protein product, merlin, shows some degree of correlation with clinical severity [47]. Namely, deletion mutations that cause truncation of merlin produce a more severe phenotype in NF2 pedigrees, whereas missense mutations, mosaic mutations, or small in-frame insertions in the *NF2*-coding region may be associated with a milder phenotype [14, 23, 24, 40, 44, 47]. The location of the mutation within the gene may also be important because missense mutations within merlin's α-helical domain appear to associate with a less severe phenotype than those within the conserved FERM domain (Fig. 9.3) [37]. The genotype–phenotype correlations are complex. Clinical studies indicate that phenotypic expression is more similar within families than between them, but even within families, significant variability exists [48]. The age at onset of NF2, the age at onset of hearing loss, and the number of intracranial meningiomas all have a significant intrafamilial correlation [37]. Whether the variability observed between families occurs by chance, epigenetic phenomena, environmental factors, or genetic differences at other loci is unknown [49]. More information regarding the impact of the underlying genetic aberrations in VS and their interplay with other pathways can help guide individualized counseling regarding prognosis and management.

Merlin Acts as a Tumor Suppressor

Merlin has a multifunctional role in translating and regulating extracellular cues into intracellular signals that control cell fate, morphology, and proliferation. Contact inhibition of cell proliferation—a phenomenon whereby the growth of cells is arrested with increasing density of cell-to-cell interactions—is an important mechanism of regulation of tissue growth, differentiation, and development [50]. Loss of this regulatory mechanism contributes to tumorogenesis and is a hallmark of cancer [51, 52]. As a linker between transmembrane proteins and the actin-cytoskeleton, merlin is naturally positioned to regulate cell proliferation in response to outside signals (Fig. 9.4).

Merlin overexpression causes growth suppression. Vestibular schwannoma cells with *NF2* inactivation have dramatic aberrations in cell spreading [53]. To date, merlin has been shown to interact with several pathways, including hyaluronic acid-CD44, Ras-related C3 botulinum toxin substrate 1 (Rac1), receptor tyrosine kinase (RTK), phosphatidylinositol 3-kinase (PI3K)/Akt serine/threonine kinase (Akt), mammalian target of rapamycin (mTOR), erbin (erbB2-interacting protein), and hippo pathways [40, 50, 52, 54–62]. How these interactions relate to the tumor-suppressor activity of merlin is an area of active research. Some of the key pathways involving merlin are summarized below to illustrate merlin's multifaceted role in controlling proliferative cell signaling.

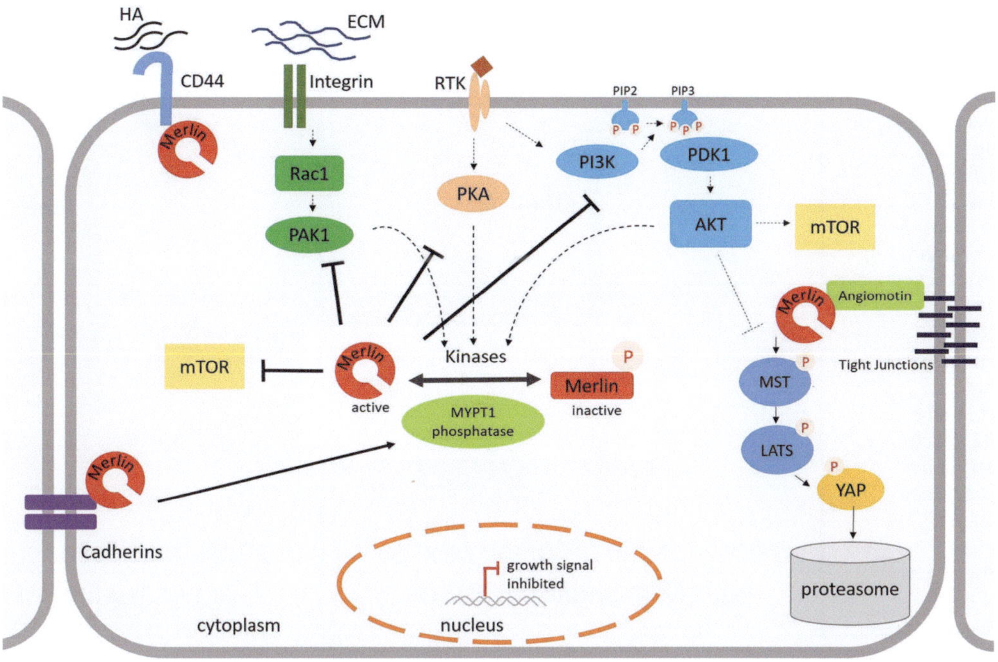

Fig. 9.4 Model shows merlin's tumor suppressor function and interactions with several pathways. Several extracellular signals mediated through interaction with the extracellular matrix (ECM) and its components, such as hyaluronic acid (HA) as well as with adjacent cells via cadherins and tight junctions, are integrated in the cell to signal growth arrest. Merlin stabilizes cadherins at the cell membrane, which in turn is inhibited from phosphorylation by cadherin binding. HA-mediated signaling via CD44 further promotes active merlin tumor suppressor function. Dephosphorylated merlin has an inhibitory function on Rac1/Pak1, protein kinase A (PKA) and PI3K/PDK1/Akt and mTOR pathways. In a promitogenic state, these kinase pathways are active (dashed lines), which phosphorylate and inactivate merlin. Tight junctions activate Hippo pathway, which interacts with active merlin to mediate YAP phosphorylation, leading to its sequestration in the cytoplasm and degradation

Molecular Roles of the Merlin Tumor Suppressor and Consequence of Its Loss in Vestibular Schwannomas

Merlin and CD44-Mediated Contact Inhibition of Cellular Proliferation

Merlin's growth inhibitory effects are activated in conditions of increased cell density. This function is dependent in part on its protein interaction with CD44, a transmembrane hyaluronate receptor [50, 63–65]. Hyaluronan (HA) is a mucopolysaccharide that is abundant in the extracellular matrix surrounding cells, and CD44 is a major cell membrane receptor that binds HA [65]. It is important for directing intercellular and cell–matrix signaling and is commonly upregulated in cancer cells, including cancer stem cells, where it portends poor prognosis both in terms of tumor progression and metastasis [50]. Under low cell density, pro-proliferative conditions, CD44 forms a complex with ERM proteins and phosphorylated, inactive merlin. With increased cell density, HA binds to CD44 to induce merlin dephosphorylation, which activates merlin's tumor suppressive activities inside the cell to signal growth arrest. In turn, merlin exerts its tumor suppressor function in part by negative regulation of CD44 [50]. Overexpression of merlin in Tr6BC1 schwannoma cells inhibits HA binding to CD44 and CD44-mediated growth, while overexpression of a mutant form of merlin unable to bind CD44 is unable to inhibit schwannoma growth [16, 65]. These findings describe a model in which cellular environment and density signal a codependent merlin-CD44 molecular switch from growth to arrest (Fig. 9.5). Aberrancies in this pathway, such as through loss of merlin protein or abnormal phosphorylation, result in a pro-proliferative signal that may contribute to tumorigenesis.

Merlin-Rac1 Mediated Cytoskeletal Interactions

Merlin and CD44 are involved in a complex interplay with other cytoskeletal signals, including integrins and cadherins, and these pathways represent another route for cell cycle control under the direction of the extracellular microenvironment [40, 50, 66]. In conditions of low cell density, pro-growth signals are initiated by integrins and receptor tyrosine kinases; they are transduced by Rho family small GTPases—Cdc42 and Rac1—two essential regulators of cell migration

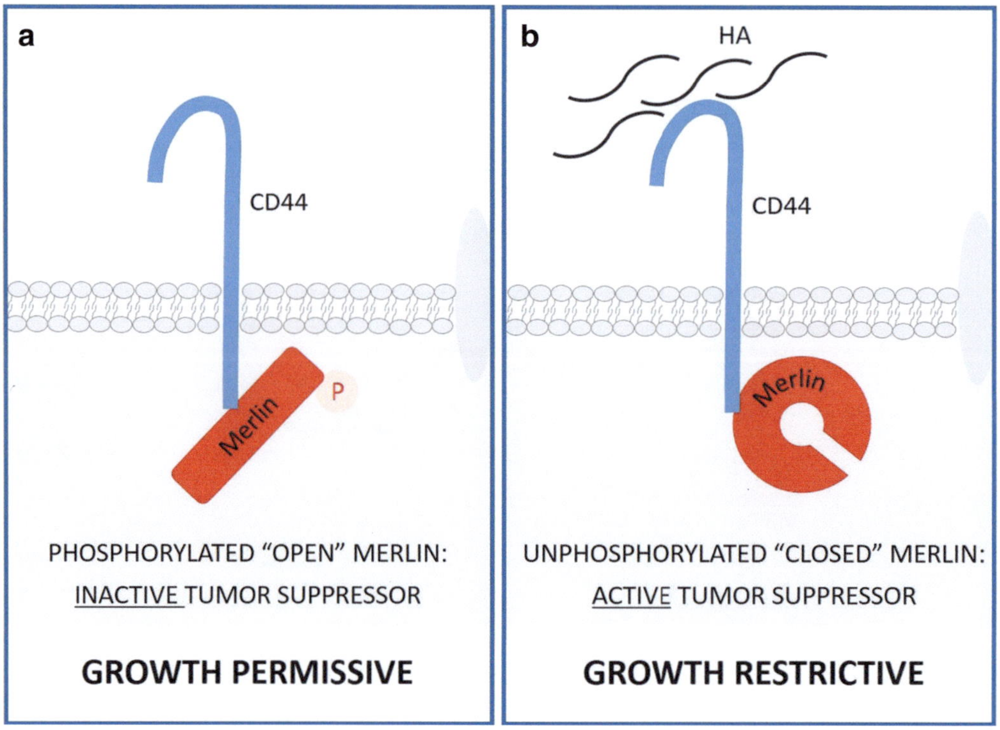

Fig. 9.5 Model illustrates the interaction between merlin and CD44. (**a**) In a growth-permissive state, merlin is phosphorylated by a cascade of kinases, including Rac1. Phosphorylated merlin associates with CD44's cytoplasmic tail and exists in an inactive "open" form to promote cell growth and survival. (**b**) In a growth-restrictive state, CD44 mediates signaling from the outside environment (e.g., hyaluronic acid [HA] in the extracellular matrix), which results in dephosphorylation of merlin. Unphosphorylated merlin assumes a "closed" and active confirmation through the association of the N- and C-termini of the protein, which mediates growth arrest

as well as in cell invasion in cancer. Rac1 activates Pak1, which phosphorylates merlin Ser518, resulting in an open inactive configuration. A negative feedback loop exists whereby active merlin suppresses Pak1 activation (Fig. 9.4). Pak1 inhibition is mediated by binding of merlin's FERM domain to the Pak1-Cdc42/Rac1 binding domain [67, 68]. Thus, inactivation or loss of merlin facilitates aberrant Rac1/Pak1 signaling, which is mitogenic and triggers cytoskeletal remodeling [69]. Indeed, cultured schwannoma and meningioma cells have abundant cytoskeletal actin projection and membrane ruffles, which are characteristic of fibroblasts expressing the excess amount of Rac [69–71].

Merlin Activates the Mammalian Hippo Pathway to Induce Growth Arrest

The Hippo signaling pathway is a major mechanism of organ-size control that regulates cell growth and apoptosis [72, 73]. Merlin has been found to be a key upstream regulator of this pathway, providing another important mechanism through which merlin transduces extracellular signals to regulate cell growth [57]. The Hippo pathway is a kinase cascade composed of two core kinases (MST1/2 and LATS1/2) [72]. MST1/2 phosphorylate LATS1/2 which in turn phosphorylate and inactivate the oncoproteins Yes-associated protein (YAP) and transcriptional activator with PDZ binding motif (TAZ) [72]. Phosphorylated-YAP/TAZ are sequestered in the cytoplasm and unable to enter into the nucleus to activate the TEAD transcription factor to signal growth (Fig. 9.6) [73]. Phosphorylation also primes YAP/TAZ for proteasomal degradation [74]. Increased YAP expression is prevalent in certain tumors, and loss of hippo kinases (MST1/2) or overexpression of YAP in a mouse liver model results in a massive expansion of liver size and cancer [74]. Merlin directly activates the mammalian Hippo kinases, MST1/2, and also recruits LATS1/2 to the cell membrane (where it binds to merlin's FERM domain) to be phosphorylated by MST1/2, which renders YAP/TAZ inactive [57]. Using transgenic mice models to study the role of merlin in tumorigenesis in the liver, genetic deletion of merlin in hepatocytes resulted in liver hyperplasia and hepatocellular carcinoma [75]. The overgrowth of merlin mutant livers was greatly suppressed by loss of YAP, indicating a critical role for merlin in antagonizing YAP activity as well as demonstrating YAP as a major effector of merlin in controlling growth [75]. Within the Hippo cascade, merlin has several interacting protein partners, including angiomotin—a cell membrane protein located in tight junctions of cells [57, 71]. Angiomotin binds to and activates merlin to promote its binding to LATS1/2 to activate the Hippo cascade. In turn, phosphorylation of Ser518 prevents angiomotin binding to merlin, which in turn is unable to activate the Hippo pathway, leaving YAP/TAZ free to mediate mitogenic signaling in the nucleus [57]. Indeed, angiomotin provides yet another mechanism through which adherens and tight junctions can

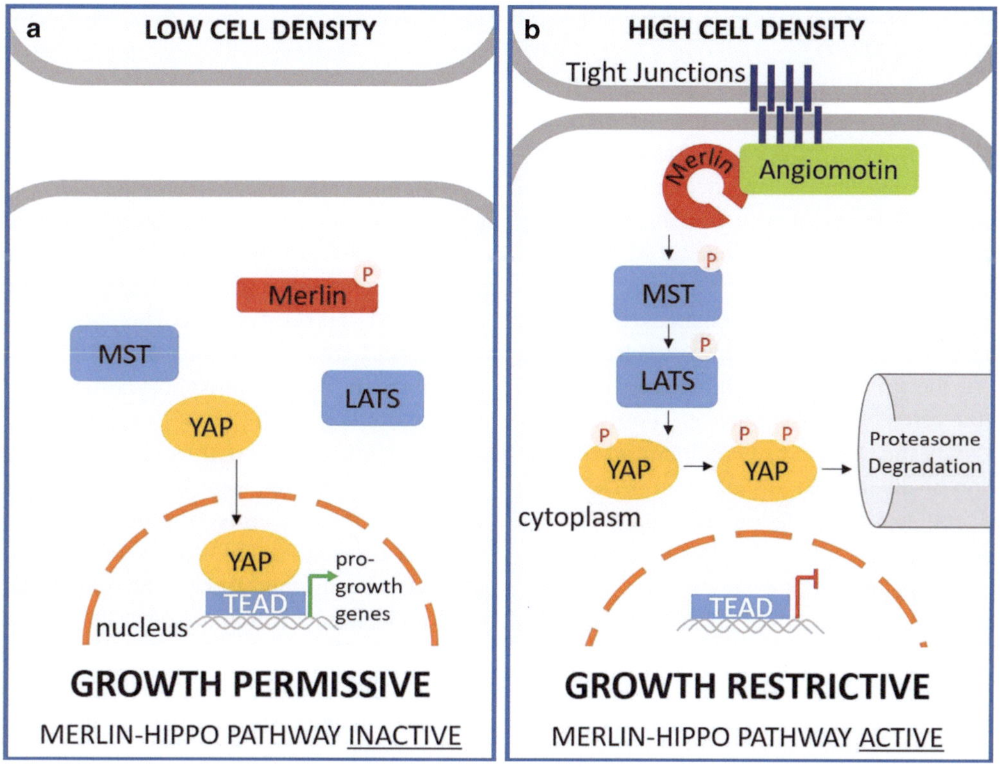

Fig. 9.6 Model illustrates merlin and Hippo pathway. The Hippo pathway consists of a cascade of kinases (MST, LATS) that result in phosphorylation of the transcriptional coactivators YAP/TAZ, which renders them inactive, sequestered in the cytoplasm and targeted for proteasomal degradation. (**a**) In growth-permissive conditions, merlin is phosphorylated and inactive. YAP is active in the nucleus where it interacts with transcription factors to promote promitogenic signaling. (**b**) In growth-restrictive conditions, such as high cell density, tight junctions between cells activate angiomotin. Dephosphorylated/active merlin interacts with angiomotin to mediate Hippo pathway activation, with phosphorylation of MST and LATS kinase cascade, which phosphorylate YAP (and TAZ, not depicted). Phosphorylated YAP is unable to enter the nucleus to mediate growth signaling and is targeted to degradation

signal through the merlin/Hippo pathways to antagonize the YAP/TAZ proliferative signal.

Merlin Inhibits the Mammalian Target of Rapamycin Pathway

Merlin's tumor-suppressive function is also mediated in part through inhibition of the mammalian target of rapamycin (mTOR), a critical pathway for cell growth and proliferation [56, 71, 76]. Constitutive mTOR complex 1 (mTORC1) activation has been demonstrated in NF2-schwannomas and meningiomas [3]. The loss of merlin activates PI3K, which starts a signaling cascade resulting in activation of mTOR and cell proliferation (Fig. 9.4) [56]. In experimental merlin deficient cells, reexpression of merlin attenuates mTORC1 activity [56]. The mTORC1 inhibitor, rapamycin, inhibits the proliferation of meningioma cells from NF2 patients [56]. Merlin mediates its tumor suppressor effects through the mTOR pathway—a fundamental mediator of cellular growth and proliferation—and this trait has motivated clinical trials testing known mTOR drugs in treatment of VS [61, 77, 78].

Additional Merlin-Mediated Pathways

While the majority of merlin's actions are mediated at the cellular membrane where it integrates extracellular responses, merlin's tumor suppressor function extends to other pathways, discussion of which is beyond the scope of this chapter. The reader is referred to the most current research articles for an in-depth study of these pathways [40]. What is clear is that merlin loss of function, whether through genetic mutation or phosphorylation-mediated inactivation, results in aberrant growth-permissive signals that promote tumor formation. Understanding of these molecular pathways is important as they lay the foundations for the identification of possible therapeutic targets.

Epigenetic Alterations in Vestibular Schwannomas

DNA mutations in the *NF2* gene are the hallmark of both sporadic and bilateral vestibular schwannomas [20, 79]. In two recently reported whole exome sequencing of sporadic vestibular schwannomas, *NF2* mutations were found in 67%

to 77% of all tumors [20, 79]. In addition, other mutations were identified involving *ARID1A*, *ARID1B*, *TSC1*, *TSC2*, *CDC27*, and *USP8*, highlighting the heterogeneous nature of the disease and the involvement of several other pathways [20, 79]. Interestingly, a subset of these tumors with genetically normal NF2 gene had significantly decreased levels of NF2 transcription (mRNA) and merlin protein, suggesting epigenetic changes may play a role in silencing NF2 or other genes [20, 79, 80].

Epigenetic regulation refers to the changes that occur "on" the DNA that influences the gene expression by altering the accessibility of the gene to transcriptional machinery—without altering the primary DNA sequence. These changes include methylation of the DNA at CpG regions and acetylation or methylation of the histone proteins that package the DNA. Disrupted epigenetic regulation has emerged as a prominent mechanism of tumorigenesis as well as the pathogenesis of other disease states [81].

Aberrant DNA methylation—both global DNA hypomethylation and/or promoter hypermethylation—was the first described epigenetic mark associated with cancer. While early studies looking at aberrant DNA hypermethylation of NF2 gene in VS suggested that it may also play a role in NF2 silencing, this role has not been demonstrated in more recent studies by us and others of both VS and meningioma specimens [82]. Nevertheless, abnormal DNA hypomethylation was shown to affect other genes including HOX homeobox genes, microRNA-21, and Met proto-oncogene [80]. A recent study investigating mutation and methylation changes of NF2 and Hippo pathway genes LATS1/2 and YAP in 82 sporadic schwannomas found both genetic and methylation abnormalities to describe the majority of these tumors, specifically *NF2* mutations (55% of tumors), *LATS1* mutations (2%), *LATS2* mutations (1%), and abnormal promoter methylation of *LATS1* (17%) and *LATS2* (30%) [83]. This finding points to the importance of the hippo pathway described above as well as to the complex genetic and epigenetic changes underlying VS development.

Histone Modifications and the Role of Histone Deacetylase Inhibitors

In addition to reversible changes to the methylation status of DNA, alterations to the acetylation and methylation of specific histone proteins around the DNA significantly influence gene expression, and together these modifications represent the "epigenetic" signature of a gene [81]. As cancer cells can be associated with global epigenetic changes (generally toward a more stem cell-like chromatin signature), specific drugs have been designed to target these pathways. However, histone deacetylases (HDACs) and other histone-modifying enzymes can have broader effects beyond altering histone/DNA regions, including modifying proteins outside the nucleus. For example, HDAC inhibitors mediate effects beyond histone acetylation: they target protein pathways in the cell, including transcription factors in the nucleus and structural proteins in the cytoplasm [84]. We have studied a specific HDAC inhibitor, AR42 (formerly OSU-HDAC42; Arno Therapeutics, Parsippany, NJ), and found that it inhibits the PI3-kinase/Akt pathway, resulting in Akt dephosphorylation and suppression of schwannoma growth [84–86]. Indeed, loss of merlin results in activation of this pathway, which is reversed with an HDAC or PDK1 inhibitor [84]. VS xenografts treated with AR-42 showed the arrest of proliferation in cell culture and reduction in size in a mouse model [84, 86]. HDAC inhibitors have been found to have broad cellular effects outside of direct histone modifications. This impact was recently shown in cell cultures of merlin-deficient human Schwann cells, where HDAC inhibitors showed a dramatic increase in kinase activity and selectively induced mTOR-centered kinase subnetworks [61]. These findings support a broad effect of HDAC on pathways relevant to VS tumorogenesis, and a clinical trial studying the effect of AR42 is ongoing [61, 85].

Vascular Endothelial Growth Factor in VS

Beyond the cellular level, tumor cells must maintain a nutrient supply to sustain continued growth and proliferation. Tumors growing larger than 2 mm within the central nervous system require a structured blood supply for the delivery of nutrients and oxygen. Vascular endothelial growth factor (VEGF) is a key mediator of angiogenesis and vascular permeability [87, 88]. In VS, VEGF signaling has been found to be abnormally upregulated, suggesting this to be a fundamental and potentially targetable mechanism for promoting vascular ingrowth [88–90]. Plotkins and colleagues demonstrated the efficacy of bevacizumab—the first monoclonal antibody against VEGF approved by the Food and Drug Administration—in not only arresting but also shrinking tumor size in 55% NF2 patients with a growing VS [91]. Several studies have since supported these findings [92–94]. Long term duration and dose of bevacizumab remain controversial and is limited by adverse side effects [92, 95]. However, the efficacy of bevacizumab, even in the short term, is promising and provides impetus for continued investigation for single or combinatorial molecular-based therapy for NF2.

Bench to Bedside: Molecular Targets of VS Therapy

While significant insight has been gained into the molecular biology of NF2 and the role of merlin in driving tumorogenesis, there remain no effective targeted drug therapies specific to vestibular schwannomas. Conventional therapies entail surgical resection or stereotactic radiation and, while effective in non-NF2 patients, carry significant morbidity in NF2 patients who have bilateral VS and other tumors throughout the body. A targeted approach tailored to the underlying pathophysiology of these tumors represents an important goal. To date, such efforts have found limited success clinically. Several clinical investigations have been undertaken and target pathways involved in NF2 tumorigenesis (Table 9.1) [3, 61]. Tumor-specific therapies targeting NF2-deficient tumors have proved challenging in part because these tumors are slow-growing, complicating the ability to identify therapies that have selective toxicity against merlin-deficient tumors while sparing normal cells. To begin to address these challenges, the Synodos for NF2 Consortium (www.synapse.org/SynodosNF2) was recently created [61]. In an effort to streamline *in vitro* and *in vivo* studies of drug targets, the consortium created a validated set of cell lines containing matched pairs of meningioma and schwannoma cells with and without merlin expression as well as two *in vivo* murine models of meningioma and schwannoma. The consortium tested 19 drugs that are currently in clinical trial for NF2 patients and represent key merlin-related pathways, including HDAC, mTOR, MAPK/ERK kinase (MEK), and PI3K (Table 9.1). While there was no selective toxicity based on merlin status induced by these drugs *in vitro*, three drugs (CUDC-907 [dual PI3K/HDAC inhibitor], panobinostat [HDAC inhibitor], and GSK2126458 [dual PI3K/mTOR inhibitor]) showed promising antiproliferation properties *in vitro*. However, while GSK2126458 and panobinostat seemed to have an effect on growth in the *in vivo* meningioma model, none of the three agents showed an effect in the *in vivo* schwannoma model. These results suggest that the underlying cells of origin (arachnoid vs Schwann cells) influence tumor biology and response as well as attest to the role of a tumor 3D microenvironment, which is not fully recapitulated in a 2D cell culture system, and the limitations of the murine models in planning therapeutic trials. Indeed, additional efforts to investigate other potential targets and combination therapies are ongoing.

Table 9.1 Summary of FDA approved drugs and their targets selected [61]

Compound	Target(s)
LY2157299	TGF-beta/SMAD [96]
Ganetespib (STA-9090)	HSP [97]
Panobinostat (LBH589)	HDAC [84, 86]
Vorinostat (SAHA)	Autophagy, HDAC [84, 86]
AR-42	HDAC [84, 86]
Lapatinib ditosylate	HER2, EGFR [98, 99]
Axitinib	VEGFR, PDGFR, c-Kit [91, 92, 100, 101]
AZD2014	mTOR [56, 77, 78, 102, 103]
OSU-03012 (AR-12)	PDK-1 [59, 100]
Perifosine (KRX-0401)	AKT [59, 104–106]
Erevolimus	mTOR [56, 77, 78, 102, 103]
GSK2126458 (GSK458)	P13K, mTOR [56, 59]
GDC-0980 (RG7422)	P13K, mTOR [56, 59]
CUDC-907	P13K, HDAC [3, 59, 63, 85]
GDC-0941	P13K [59, 63]
Selumetinib (AZD6244)	MEK [98]
Trametinib (GSK 1120212)	MEK [98]
Visodegib (GDC-0449)	Sonic hedgehog [106–108]
Bortezomib	Proteasome [109]

Modified with permission from The Synodos for NF2 Consortium et al. (2018) Traditional and Systems Biology Based Drug Discovery for the Rare Tumor Syndrome Neurofibromatosis Type 2. *PLOS*: 1–26. https://doi.org/10.1371/journal.pone.0197350.t002

Summary

Vestibular schwannomas are tumors that arise in sporadic and familiar forms with varied clinical manifestations. Loss of function of the NF2 tumor suppressor, merlin, is the fundamental driver of VS tumorogenesis. The characterization of merlin's function and its interactions with other proteins and signaling pathways have opened the door to a molecular understanding of the pathogenesis of VS, revealing a complex network of pathways involving the integration of extracellular signals and cell–cell interactions with intracellular growth and proliferative gene expression changes, the details of which are still being clarified. These findings are the foundation for clinical translation into possible therapeutic targets. Thus far—aside from anti-VEGF therapy, which targets tumor angiogenesis and is used in NF2 patients, surgery, and stereotactic radiation—there is no medical treatment for VS. Many clinical trials are ongoing. Given the realization of merlin's involvement in multiple signaling pathways, successful treatment strategies may require combinatorial therapy. The hope is that, as we increase our understanding of the biology of these tumors, we can identify specific targets to treat patients with NF2 as well as sporadic VS.

Acknowledgments The work performed in this chapter by the authors was supported by the National Institute of Deafness and Communicative Disorders and the Department of Defense Neurofibromatosis Research Program.

References

1. National Institutes of Health. Acoustic neuroma. NIH Consens Statement. 1991;9:1–24.
2. Evans DGR. Neurofibromatosis type 2 (NF2): a clinical and molecular review. Orphanet J Rare Dis. 2009;4:16.
3. Petrilli AM, Fernández-Valle C. Role of Merlin/NF2 inactivation in tumor biology. Oncogene. 2015;35:537–48.
4. Howitz MF, Johansen TCM, Charabi S, Olsen JH. Incidence of vestibular schwannoma in Denmark, 1977-1995. Am J Otol. 2000;21:690–4.
5. Stangerup SE, Tos M, Thomsen J, Cayé-Thomasen P. True incidence of vestibular schwannoma? Neurosurgery. 2010;67:1335–40.
6. Evans DG, Huson SM, Donnai D, Neary W, Blair V, Teare D, Newton V, Strachan T, Ramsden R, Harris R. A genetic study of type 2 neurofibromatosis in the United Kingdom. I. Prevalence, mutation rate, fitness, and confirmation of maternal transmission effect on severity. J Med Genet. 1992;29:841–6.
7. Schroeder RD, Angelo LS, Kurzrock R. NF2/merlin in hereditary neurofibromatosis 2 versus cancer: biologic mechanisms and clinical associations. Oncotarget. 2014;5:67–77.
8. Berger AH, Knudson AG, Pandolfi PP. A continuum model for tumour suppression. Nature. 2011;476:163–9.
9. Knudson AG. Mutation and cancer: statistical study of retinoblastoma. Proc Natl Acad Sci U S A. 1971;68:820–3.
10. Fontaine B, Rouleau GA, Seizinger BR, et al. Molecular genetics of neurofibromatosis 2 and related tumors (acoustic neuroma and meningioma). Ann NY Acad Sci. 1991;615:338–43.
11. Kaiser-Kupfer MI, Freidlin V, Datiles MB, et al. The association of posterior capsular lens opacities with bilateral acoustic neuromas in patients with neurofibromatosis type 2. Arch Ophthalmol. 1989;107:541–4.
12. Martuza RL, Eldridge R. Neurofibromatosis 2 (bilateral acoustic neurofibromatosis). N Engl J Med. 1988;318:684–8.
13. Evans DG, Wallace AJ, Wu CL, et al. Somatic mosaicism: a common cause of classic disease in tumor-prone syndromes? Lessons from type 2 neurofibromatosis. Am J Hum Genet. 1998;63:727–36.
14. Kluwe L, Mautner V, Heinrich B, et al. Molecular study of frequency of mosaicism in neurofibromatosis 2 patients with bilateral vestibular schwannomas. J Med Genet. 2003;40:109–14.
15. Ruggieri M, Praticò AD, Serra A, et al. Childhood neurofibromatosis type 2 (NF2) and related disorders: from bench to bedside and biologically targeted therapies. Acta Otorhinolaryngol Ital. 2016;36:345–67.
16. Moyhuddin A, Baser ME, Watson C, et al. Somatic mosaicism in neurofibromatosis 2: prevalence and risk of disease transmission to offspring. J Med Genet. 2003;40:459–63.
17. Evans DG, Bowers NL, Tobi S, et al. Schwannomatosis: a genetic and epidemiological study. J Neurol Neurosurg Psychiatry. 2018;89:1215–9.
18. MacCollin M, Willett C, Heinrich B, et al. Familial schwannomatosis: exclusion of the NF2 locus as the germline event. Neurology. 2003;60:1968–74.
19. Lee JD, Kwon TJ, Kim UK, Lee WS. Genetic and epigenetic alterations of the NF2 gene in sporadic vestibular schwannomas. PLoS One. 2012;7:e30418.
20. Håvik HL, Bruland O, Myrseth E, et al. Genetic landscape of sporadic vestibular schwannoma. J Neurosurg. 2018;128:911–22.
21. Rouleau GA, Merel P, Lutchman M, et al. Alteration in a new gene encoding a putative membrane-organizing protein causes neurofibromatosis type 2. Nature. 1993;363:515–21.
22. Trofatter JA, MacCollin MM, Rutter JL, et al. A novel moesin-, ezrin-, radixin-like gene is a candidate for the neurofibromatosis 2 tumor suppressor. Cell. 1993;72:791–800.
23. Welling DB, Guida M, Goll F, et al. Mutational spectrum in the neurofibromatosis type 2 gene in sporadic and familial schwannomas. Hum Genet. 1996;98:189–93.
24. Welling DB. Clinical manifestations of mutations in the neurofibromatosis type 2 gene in vestibular schwannomas (acoustic neuromas). Laryngoscope. 1998;108:178–89.
25. Irving RM, Harada T, Moffat DA, et al. Somatic neurofibromatosis type 2 gene mutations and growth characteristics in vestibular schwannoma. Am J Otol. 1997;18:754–60.
26. Jacoby LB, MacCollin M, Barone R, Ramesh V, Gusella JF. Frequency and distribution of NF2 mutations in schwannomas. Genes Chromosomes Cancer. 1996;17:45–55.
27. Lasota J, Fetsch JF, Wozniak A, et al. The neurofibromatosis type 2 gene is mutated in perineurial cell tumors: a molecular genetic study of eight cases. Am J Pathol. 2001;158:1223–9.
28. Bianchi AB, Hara T, Ramesh V, et al. Mutations in transcript isoforms of the neurofibromatosis 2 gene in multiple human tumour types. Nat Genet. 1994;6:185–92.
29. Ruttledge MH, Sarrazin J, Rangaratnam S, et al. Evidence for the complete inactivation of the NF2 gene in the majority of sporadic meningiomas. Nat Genet. 1994;6:180–4.
30. Sekido Y, Pass HI, Bader S, et al. Neurofibromatosis type 2 (NF2) gene is somatically mutated in mesothelioma but not in lung cancer. Cancer Res. 1995;55:1227–31.
31. Sanson M, Marineau C, Desmaze C, et al. Germline deletion in a neurofibromatosis type 2 kindred inactivates the NF2 gene and a candidate meningioma locus. Hum Mol Genet. 1993;2:1215–20.
32. Hara T, Bianchi AB, Seizinger BR, Kley N. Molecular cloning and characterization of alternatively spliced transcripts of the mouse neurofibromatosis 2 gene. Cancer Res. 1994;54:330–5.
33. Jacoby LB, MacCollin M, Louis DN, et al. Exon scanning for mutation of the NF2 gene in schwannomas. Hum Mol Genet. 1994;3:413–9.
34. Pykett MJ, Murphy M, Harnish PR, George DL. The neurofibromatosis 2 (NF2) tumor suppressor gene encodes multiple alternatively spliced transcripts. Hum Mol Genet. 1994;3:559–64.
35. Golovnina K, Blinov A, Akhmametyeva EM, Omelyanchuk LV, Chang LS. Evolution and origin of merlin, the product of the neurofibromatosis type 2 (NF2) tumor-suppressor gene. BMC Evol Biol. 2005;5:69.
36. Chishti AH, Kim AC, Marfatia SM, et al. The FERM domain: a unique module involved in the linkage of cytoplasmic proteins to the membrane. Trends Biochem Sci. 1998;23:281–2.
37. Bruder CE, Hirvelä C, Tapia-Paez I, et al. High-resolution deletion analysis of constitutional DNA from neurofibromatosis type 2 (NF2) patients using microarray-CGH. Hum Mol Genet. 2001;10:271–82.
38. Shimizu T, Seto A, Maita N, et al. Structural basis for neurofibromatosis type 2. J Biol Chem. 2002;277:10332–6.
39. Jin H, Sperka T, Herrlich P, Morrison H. Tumorigenic transformation by CPI-17 through inhibition of a merlin phosphatase. Nature. 2006;442:576–9.

40. de Vries M, van der Mey AGL, Hogendoorn PCW. Tumor biology of vestibular schwannoma: a review of experimental data on the determinants of tumor genesis and growth characteristics. Otol Neurotol. 2015;36:1128–36.
41. Ye K. Phosphorylation of merlin regulates its stability and tumor suppressive activity. Cell Adhes Migr. 2007;1:196–8.
42. Laulajainen M, Muranen T, Nyman TA, Carpén O, Grönholm M. Multistep phosphorylation by oncogenic kinases enhances the degradation of the NF2 tumor suppressor merlin. Neoplasia. 2011;13:643–52.
43. Bretscher A, Reczek D, Berryman M. Ezrin: a protein requiring conformational activation to link microfilaments to the plasma membrane in the assembly of cell surface structures. J Cell Sci. 1997;110:3011–8.
44. Gutmann DH, Haipek CA, Hoang LK. Neurofibromatosis 2 tumor suppressor protein, merlin, forms two functionally important intramolecular associations. J Neurosci Res. 1999;58:706–16.
45. Bianchi AB, Mitsunaga SI, Cheng JQ, et al. High frequency of inactivating mutations in the neurofibromatosis type 2 gene (NF2) in primary malignant mesotheliomas. Proc Natl Acad Sci U S A. 1995;92:10854–8.
46. Bourn D, Evans G, Mason S, et al. Eleven novel mutations in the NF2 tumour suppressor gene. Hum Genet. 1995;95:572–4.
47. Halliday D, Emmanouil B, Pretorius P, et al. Genetic Severity Score predicts clinical phenotype in NF2. J Med Genet. 2017;54:657–64.
48. Zhao Y, et al. Intrafamilial correlation of clinical manifestations in neurofibromatosis 2 (NF2). Genet Epidemiol. 2002;23:245–59.
49. Zucman-Rossi J, et al. NF2 gene in neurofibromatosis type 2 patients. Hum Mol Genet. 1998;7:2095–101.
50. Stamenkovic I, Yu Q. Merlin, a "magic" linker between extracellular cues and intracellular signaling pathways that regulate cell motility, proliferation, and survival. Curr Protein Pept Sci. 2010;11:471–84.
51. Puliafito A, et al. Collective and single cell behavior in epithelial contact inhibition. Proc Natl Acad Sci. 2012;109:739–44.
52. Morrison H, et al. The NF2 tumor suppressor gene product, merlin, mediates contact inhibition of growth through interactions with CD44. Genes Dev. 2001;15:968–80.
53. Pelton PD, et al. Ruffling membrane, stress fiber, cell spreading and proliferation abnormalities in human Schwannoma cells. Oncogene. 1998;17:2195–209.
54. Sherman L, et al. Interdomain binding mediates tumor growth suppression by the NF2 gene product. Oncogene. 1997;15:2505–9.
55. Tikoo A, Varga M, Ramesh V, Gusella J, Maruta H. An anti-Ras function of neurofibromatosis type 2 gene product (NF2/Merlin). J Biol Chem. 1994;269:23387–90.
56. James MF, et al. NF2/Merlin is a novel negative regulator of mTOR complex 1, and activation of mTORC1 is associated with meningioma and schwannoma growth. Mol Cell Biol. 2009;29:4250–61.
57. Li Y, et al. Angiomotin binding-induced activation of Merlin/NF2 in the Hippo pathway. Cell Res. 2015;25:801–17.
58. Rong R, Tang X, Gutmann DH, Ye K. Neurofibromatosis 2 (NF2) tumor suppressor merlin inhibits phosphatidylinositol 3-kinase through binding to PIKE-L. Proc Natl Acad Sci U S A. 2004;101:18200–5.
59. Jacob A, et al. Phosphatidylinositol 3-kinase/AKT pathway activation in human vestibular schwannoma. Otol Neurotol. 2008;29:58–68.
60. Welling DB, Packer MD, Chang LS. Molecular studies of vestibular schwannomas: a review. Curr Opin Otol Head Neck Surg. 2007;15:341–6.
61. The Synodos for NF2 Consortium, Allaway R, Angus SP, Beauchamp RL, Blakeley JO, Bott M, et al. Traditional and systems biology based drug discovery for the rare tumor syndrome neurofibromatosis type 2. PLoS ONE 2018;13(6):e0197350.
62. Rangwala R, Banine F, Borg JP, Sherman LS. Erbin regulates mitogen-activated protein (MAP) kinase activation and MAP kinase-dependent interactions between merlin and adherens junction protein complexes in Schwann cells. J Biol Chem. 2005;280:11790–7.
63. Morrison H, et al. Merlin/neurofibromatosis type 2 suppresses growth by inhibiting the activation of Ras and Rac. Cancer Res. 2007;67:520–7.
64. Sainio M, et al. Neurofibromatosis 2 tumor suppressor protein colocalizes with ezrin and CD44 and associates with actin-containing cytoskeleton. J Cell Sci. 1997;110:2249–60.
65. Bai Y, Liu YJ, et al. Inhibition of the hyaluronan-CD44 interaction by merlin contributes to the tumor-suppressor activity of merlin. Oncogene. 2006;26:836–50.
66. Shaw RJ, et al. The Nf2 tumor suppressor, merlin, functions in Rac-dependent signaling. Dev Cell. 2001;1:63–72.
67. Xiao GH, Chernoff J, Testa JR. NF2: the wizardry of merlin. Genes Chromosomes Cancer. 2003;38:389–99.
68. Xiao GH, Beeser A, Chernoff J, Testa JR. p21-activated kinase links Rac/Cdc42 signaling to merlin. J Biol Chem. 2002;277:883–6.
69. Kaempchen K. Upregulation of the Rac1/JNK signaling pathway in primary human schwannoma cells. Hum Mol Genet. 2003;12:1211–21.
70. Sixt M. Cell migration: fibroblasts find a new way to get ahead: figure 1. J Cell Biol. 2012;197:347–9.
71. Li W, Cooper J, Karajannis MA, Giancotti FG. Merlin: a tumour suppressor with functions at the cell cortex and in the nucleus. EMBO Rep. 2012;13:204–15.
72. Yu FX, Zhao B, Guan KL. Hippo pathway in organ size control, tissue homeostasis, and cancer. Cell. 2015;163:811–28.
73. Piccolo S, Dupont S, Cordenonsi M. The biology of YAP/TAZ: hippo signaling and beyond. Physiol Rev. 2014;94:1287–312.
74. Song H, et al. Mammalian Mst1 and Mst2 kinases play essential roles in organ size control and tumor suppression. Proc Natl Acad Sci. 2010;107:1431–6.
75. Zhang N, et al. The Merlin/NF2 tumor suppressor functions through the YAP oncoprotein to regulate tissue homeostasis in mammals. Dev Cell. 2010;19:27–38.
76. Saxton RA, Sabatini DM. mTOR signaling in growth, metabolism, and disease. Cell. 2017;168:960–76.
77. Goutagny S. A 4-year phase II study of everolimus in NF2 patients with growing vestibular schwannomas. J Neuro Oncol. 2017;133:443–5.
78. Karajannis MA, et al. Phase II study of everolimus in children and adults with neurofibromatosis type 2 and progressive vestibular schwannomas. Neuro Oncol. 2013;16:292–7.
79. Agnihotri S, et al. The genomic landscape of schwannoma. Nat Genet. 2016;48:1339–48.
80. Torres-Martín M, et al. Genome-wide methylation analysis in vestibular schwannomas shows putative mechanisms of gene expression modulation and global hypomethylation at the HOX gene cluster. Genes Chromosomes Cancer. 2014;54:197–209.
81. Mohammad HP, Baylin SB. Linking cell signaling and the epigenetic machinery. Nat Biotechnol. 2010;28:1033–8.
82. Hansson CM, et al. Comprehensive genetic and epigenetic analysis of sporadic meningioma for macro-mutations on 22q and micro-mutations within the NF2 locus. BMC Genomics. 2007;8:16.
83. Oh JE, et al. Alterations in the NF2/LATS1/LATS2/YAP pathway in schwannomas. J Neuropathol Exp Neurol. 2015;74:952–9.
84. Bush ML, et al. AR42, a novel histone deacetylase inhibitor, as a potential therapy for vestibular schwannomas and meningiomas. Neuro Oncol. 2011;13:983–99.
85. Jacob A, et al. Preclinical validation of AR42, a novel histone deacetylase inhibitor, as treatment for vestibular schwannomas. Laryngoscope. 2011;122:174–89.

86. Burns SS, et al. Histone deacetylase inhibitor AR-42 differentially affects cell-cycle transit in meningeal and meningioma cells, potently inhibiting NF2-deficient meningioma growth. Cancer Res. 2013;73:792–803.
87. Folkman J. Seminars in medicine of the Beth Israel Hospital, Boston. Clinical applications of research on angiogenesis. N Engl J Med. 1995;333:1757–63.
88. Ferrara N, Gerber HP, LeCouter J. The biology of VEGF and its receptors. Nat Med. 2003;9:669–76.
89. Dilwali S, Roberts D, Stankovic KM. Interplay between VEGF-A and cMET signaling in human vestibular schwannomas and schwann cells. Cancer Biol Ther. 2014;16:170–5.
90. Cayé-Thomasen P, et al. VEGF and VEGF receptor-1 concentration in vestibular schwannoma homogenates correlates to tumor growth rate. Otol Neurotol. 2005;26:98–101.
91. Plotkin SR, et al. Hearing improvement after bevacizumab in patients with neurofibromatosis type 2. N Engl J Med. 2009;361:358–67.
92. Blakeley JO, et al. Efficacy and biomarker study of bevacizumab for hearing loss resulting from neurofibromatosis type 2–associated vestibular schwannomas. J Clin Oncol. 2016;34:1669–75.
93. Morris KA, et al. Bevacizumab in neurofibromatosis type 2 (NF2) related vestibular schwannomas: a nationally coordinated approach to delivery and prospective evaluation. NOPRAC. 2016;3:281–9.
94. Liu P, et al. Low-dose bevacizumab induces radiographic regression of vestibular schwannomas in neurofibromatosis type 2: a case report and literature review. Oncol Lett. 2016;11:2981–6.
95. Plotkin SR, et al. Bevacizumab for progressive vestibular schwannoma in neurofibromatosis type 2: a retrospective review of 31 patients. Otol Neurotol. 2012;33:1046–52.
96. Fujii M, et al. Convergent signaling in the regulation of connective tissue growth factor in malignant mesothelioma: TGFβ signaling and defects in the Hippo signaling cascade. Cell Cycle. 2014;11:3373–9.
97. Tanaka K, et al. Therapeutic potential of HSP90 inhibition for neurofibromatosis type 2. Clin Cancer Res. 2013;19:3856–70.
98. Ammoun S, Ristic NM, Matthies C, Hilton DA, Hanemann CO. Neurobiology of disease. Neurobiol Dis. 2010;37:141–6.
99. Karajannis MA, et al. Phase II trial of lapatinib in adult and pediatric patients with neurofibromatosis type 2 and progressive vestibular schwannomas. Neuro Oncol. 2012;14:1163–70.
100. Ammoun S, Flaiz C, Ristic N, Schuldt J, Hanemann CO. Dissecting and targeting the growth factor-dependent and growth factor-independent sxtracellular signal-regulated kinase pathway in human schwannoma. Cancer Res. 2008;68:5236–45.
101. Wong HK, et al. Anti-vascular endothelial growth factor therapies as a novel therapeutic approach to treating neurofibromatosis-related tumors. Cancer Res. 2010;70:3483–93.
102. Beauchamp RL, et al. A high-throughput kinome screen reveals serum/glucocorticoid-regulated kinase 1 as a therapeutic target for NF2-deficient meningiomas. Oncotarget. 2015;6:16981–97.
103. James MF, Stivison E, Beauchamp R, et al. Regulation of mTOR complex 2 signaling in neurofibromatosis 2-deficient target cell types. Mol Cancer Res. 2012;10:649–59.
104. Petrilli AM, et al. A chemical biology approach identified PI3K as a potential therapeutic target for neurofibromatosis type 2. Am J Transl Res. 2014;6:471–93.
105. Ammoun S, et al. The role of insulin-like growth factors signaling in merlin-deficient human schwannomas. Glia. 2012;60:1721–33.
106. Brastianos PK, et al. Genomic sequencing of meningiomas identifies oncogenic SMO and AKT1 mutations. Nat Genet. 2013;45:285–9.
107. Morrow KA, et al. Loss of tumor suppressor merlin results in aberrant activation of Wnt/β-catenin signaling in cancer. Oncotarget. 2016;7:17991–8005.
108. Clark VE, et al. Genomic analysis of non-NF2 meningiomas reveals mutations in TRAF7, KLF4, AKT1, and SMO. Science. 2013;339:1077–80.
109. Koschny R, Boehm C, Sprick MR, et al. Bortezomib sensitizes primary meningioma cells to TRAIL-induced apoptosis by enhancing formation of the death-inducing signaling complex. J Neuropathol Exp Neurol. 2014;73:1034–46.

Treatment Options for Acoustic Neuroma, Including Stereotactic Radiosurgery

10

Panagiotis Kerezoudis, Peter A. Weisskopf, Colin L. W. Driscoll, and Michael J. Link

Introduction

Vestibular schwannoma (VS) represents a challenging intracranial tumor to treat. Almost a century ago, the most prominent neurosurgeons in Europe reported operative mortality rates greater than 70% [1–3]. Harvey Cushing, in the US, advocated for a wide bilateral posterior fossa decompression and intracapsular internal decompression of the tumor to achieve a safe subtotal resection (STR) and reduced the operative mortality to ~20% [4, 5]. Walter Dandy, on the other hand, described a unilateral craniectomy and complete tumor removal with the necessary sacrifice of cranial nerves VII and VIII but obviating the risk of tumor regrowth and need for additional treatment [6–9]. Over the next several decades, the integration of the operating microscope, improvement in neuroanesthetic techniques, and development of intraoperative electromyographic (EMG) monitoring have markedly improved the outcome from microsurgical resection of VS.

P. Kerezoudis (✉)
Department of Neurologic Surgery, Mayo Clinic, Rochester, MN, USA
e-mail: Kerezoudis.Panagiotis@mayo.edu

P. A. Weisskopf
Department of Surgery, Department of Neurosurgery, Department of Otolaryngology, Head and Neck Cancer Center, Mayo Clinic, Phoenix, AZ, USA

C. L. W. Driscoll
Department of Otolaryngology—Head and Neck Surgery, Mayo Clinic, Rochester, MN, USA

M. J. Link
Department of Neurologic Surgery, Mayo Clinic, Rochester, MN, USA

Department of Otorhinolaryngology, Mayo Clinic, Rochester, MN, USA

Lars Leksell from Sweden, internationally recognized as the father of stereotactic radiosurgery, treated his first patient with VS at the Karolinska Hospital in 1969 [10]. He reported 81% tumor control rate at a median follow-up of 3.7 years. The first Gamma Knife center in the United States was established at the University of Pittsburgh, which reported their 4-year data with 134 treated patients in 1993 [11]. The 4-year actuarial tumor control rate was 89.2% using a median marginal radiation dose of 17 Gy.

Currently, no prospective randomized controlled trials exist to directly compare the outcomes following radiosurgical and microneurosurgical options for acoustic neuromas; in the absence of class I evidence, three management strategies are available to this patient population: observation, stereotactic radiotherapy/radiosurgery, and microsurgical resection. This chapter provides an overview of the outcomes of each approach with respect to tumor control and preservation of cranial nerve function; particular emphasis is provided regarding stereotactic radiosurgery and fractionated radiotherapy.

Observation

There is a wealth of data in the medical literature to support the rationale for careful observation. Two systematic reviews based on 21 and 26 studies, respectively, with more than 1300 patients found the average annual growth rate of acoustic neuromas to be 1.2–1.9 mm, with 43–46% of tumors showing some degree of growth and only 18–20% requiring intervention at a mean follow-up of approximately 3 years [12, 13]. Tumor size at diagnosis, presence of disequilibrium, and cerebellopontine angle location rather than pure intracanalicular tumors have been reported to be associated with a higher risk of progression, thereby necessitating intervention [14, 15]. It should also be noted that some studies have reported that 3–11% of tumors will spontaneously regress without any form of intervention [13, 16, 17]. As

N. C. Bambakidis et al. (eds.), *Surgery of the Cerebellopontine Angle*, https://doi.org/10.1007/978-3-031-12507-2_10

such, elderly patients with small tumors represent the ideal population to be observed, especially on the grounds of increasing mean age at the time of diagnosis, that is, from 49 years in 1976 to 58 years in 2008 [18].

Patients who opt for watchful waiting are followed up with serial magnetic resonance imaging (MRI) and audiograms, typically every 6 months for the first year, then annually until year 5, and then biennially indefinitely. While the initial MRI scan should include gadolinium (Gd) to make sure there are not additional intracranial tumors, the follow-up scans can be thin-slice, heavily T2-weighted, steady state images without Gd as some recent reports suggest that Gd may accumulate in the brain—an increasing concern for some patients [19]. Evidence of tumor growth, that is, >2.5 mm/year, regardless of tumor size, is usually an indication for therapeutic intervention. If the patient cannot tolerate MRI, high-resolution computed tomography scanning with and without contrast is an option. Additionally, recently published guidelines suggest that, for intracanalicular or small tumors (<2 cm in the posterior fossa) without tinnitus, observation does not have a negative impact on tumor growth or hearing preservation compared to treatment [20]. However, according to data from the Acoustic Neuroma Association observation is associated with worsening of symptomatic tinnitus, whereas tinnitus severity is reduced with microsurgical resection or radiosurgery [21].

In an important observational study by Stangerup and colleagues, 932 patients were allocated with "wait and scan" with annual imaging and audiological examination over a follow-up period exceeding 10 years [22]. The authors found that the level of hearing preservation during follow-up correlated with speech discrimination (according to the American Academy of Otolaryngology-Head and Neck Surgery classification [AAO-HNS] [23]) at the time of diagnosis: 87% chance of maintaining good hearing (speech discrimination over 70%) for patients with perfect speech discrimination compared to 54% for patients with minor (1–10%) and 33% for those with moderate (21–30%) speech discrimination loss at the time of diagnosis [22, 23].

The same group recently showed that, in 156 patients with intracanalicular VS, tumor growth had occurred in 37% and growth into the cerebellopontine angle in 23% of patients after a mean follow-up of 9.5 years, while the proportion of patients with good hearing decreased from 52% to 22% [24]. Our institutional experience revealed a volumetric increase >20% from baseline AAO-HNS tumor size >2 mm at a median radiographic follow-up of 4.1 years. In addition, almost 70% of patients exhibited some degree of volumetric growth after a median of 1.1 years.

Finally, another important consideration is how tumor progression during the observation period may affect future treatment options. Two studies by Flint and colleagues and Shin and colleagues found that approximately 11–33% of observed patients will lose eligibility for hearing preservation surgery [17, 25]. In addition, Hajioff and colleagues reviewed the 10-year outcome data from 72 patients with unilateral VS that were managed conservatively, 25 of which required surgical intervention during the study period [14]. Interestingly, they demonstrated similar outcomes in patients who failed conservative management and those who underwent primary treatment without a period of observation [14].

In summary, observation is preferred for elderly patients, patients with small tumors and good hearing function, those who are poor surgical candidates, and those who refuse treatment. Based on a review by Telian and colleagues, the following factors should be taken into account when observation is recommended: patient's life expectancy, tumor size and growth rate, neurofibromatosis type 2 status, preoperative hearing in both ears, and risk of complications, particularly hearing loss and facial nerve paralysis as a result of surgery [26].

Stereotactic Radiation and Radiosurgery

Radiation can be delivered to VS using either stereotactic radiosurgery (SRS) (≤5 fractions) or stereotactic radiotherapy (>5 fractions) (Table 10.1). Considerable contention

Table 10.1 Summary of characteristics of each radiosurgery modality employed for acoustic neuromas

	Type of radiation		
Characteristic	Stereotactic radiosurgery (GK, LINAC)	Fractionated radiotherapy	Proton beam
Number of sessions	1–5	30–33 fractions (daily treatment for 5–6 weeks)	Variable
Total dosage	12–13 Gy	40–57.6 Gy	54–60 cobalt Gy equivalents
Head frame used	Invasive or "face masks"	Noninvasive relocatable head frame	Noninvasive
Margin for uncertainty	Not needed	1–2 mm for planning target volume	Not needed
Tumor size amenable to treatment	Up to 3 cm in diameter	Can treat tumors larger than 3 cm	Variable
Tumor control rates	>90%	94–100%	84–100%
Hearing preservation[a]	23–74%	61–98%	31–42%
Facial nerve preservation	92–100%	~94%	91–100%
Trigeminal preservation	92–100%	~95%	89–100%

GK Gamma Knife, *LINAC* linear-based accelerator system
[a] Depending on length of follow-up

exists in the literature regarding the comparative effectiveness of the two modalities for the management of patients with small to medium-sized tumors. Shared decision making should be based on patient preference between a minimally invasive 1-day procedure and up to 5–6 weeks of daily treatment, technology availability, and tumor size [27].

Stereotactic Radiosurgery

Stereotactic radiosurgery can be performed using either Leksell Gamma Knife® (Elekta Instruments, Norcross, GA, USA) or Linear Accelerator (LINAC) systems, such as X-knife (Radionics Inc., Burlington, MA, USA), Novalis® (BrainLAB, Heimstetten, Germany), Versa HD™ (Elekta Instruments, Norcross, GA, USA) and Cyberknife® (Accuray Inc., Sunnyvale, CA, USA). Gamma Knife uses a fixed number of cobalt radiation sources to deliver very focused radiation with steep fall-off beyond the target volume (Fig. 10.1). A stereotactic headframe is placed under local anesthesia that serves as both reference fiducials for stereotactic imaging and fixation in the device during treatment [28]. More recently, thanks to advances in computer software and machine hardware, "face masks" have been used to immobilize the patient thereby eliminating the need for a rigid frame (frameless stereotactic radiosurgery) while achieving a similar degree of precision. LINAC systems also make use of a stereotactic head frame; however, instead of relying on multiple fixed radiation sources, the arc radiation delivery system moves (Figs. 10.2 and 10.3). In newer systems, the patient's bed moves along with the arcs in order to shape target volume and improve dose conformality. With respect to ionized particles emitted, these can either be photons, protons, or carbon ions.

A landmark paper by the Pittsburgh group in 1998 demonstrated the excellent long-term (5–10 years) tumor control

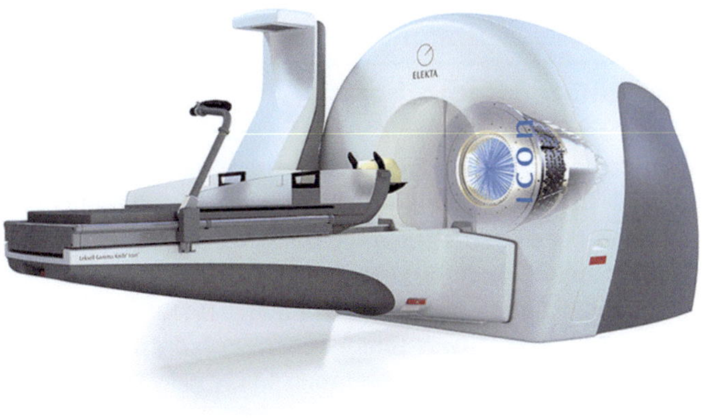

Fig. 10.1 The Leksell Gamma Knife® model Icon™ (Elekta Inc., Atlanta, GA) unit. (Reproduction of photograph courtesy of Elekta, Inc.)

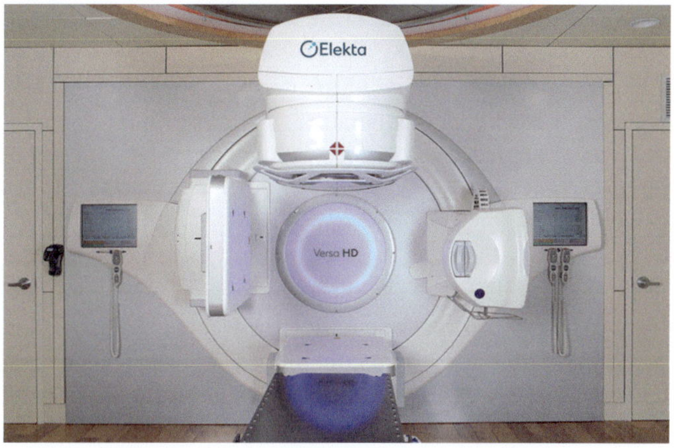

Fig. 10.2 The Versa HD™ (Elekta Inc., Atlanta, GA) is a linear accelerator with a multi-leaf collimating system, which allows for precision shaping of the beam to the treatment area. (Reproduction of photograph courtesy of Elekta, Inc.)

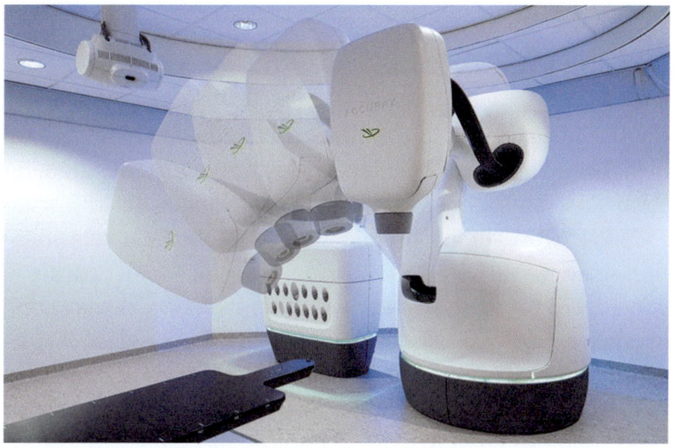

Fig. 10.3 The Cyberknife® (Accuray Inc., Sunnyvale, CA, USA) is a linear accelerator mounted on a six-axis robot that delivers radiation at the target from different positions. The system allows for the detection of patient movement and correction of dose delivery in real time. (Image courtesy of Accuray Incorporated—©2018 Accuray Incorporated. All Rights Reserved)

rates (i.e., 95%) that can be achieved with stereotactic radiosurgery [29]. In addition, function was noted to be preserved in 84% and 85% of patients with intact trigeminal and facial nerves at presentation, respectively, with 63% actuarial recovery rate of facial nerve deficit at 8 years. Subsequently, stereotactic radiosurgery and radiotherapy have become a very viable alternative to microsurgical removal of small to medium-sized VS.

Tumor Control Rates

Although there is an established body of literature on the effectiveness of radiosurgery for VS, the optimal parameters, including appropriate time of treatment, treatment modality (Gamma Knife vs. LINAC vs. proton beam) as well as dose and dosing scheme are still a matter of contention. A comprehensive review of the literature, including both retrospective and prospective studies, shows similar favorable radiosurgical failure rates ranging from 1.4% to 10.8% [30–39].

Following stereotactic radiosurgery, patients should be followed up with MRI scans and audiograms every 6 months for the first year, then annually for the next 2 years, then every other year for 4 years, then every 3 years for 6 years, and continuing in a similar pattern for the next few decades. Patients should also be informed that a transient increase in tumor volume after radiosurgery is an expected phenomenon (mean interval 13.4 months); therefore, additional treatments should not be hastily recommended [20, 40]. Median time to salvage microsurgery has been reported at 30–37 months (range 3–153 months) [31, 41, 42].

Hearing Preservation

Published hearing results following stereotactic radiosurgery have been highly variable among institutional series ranging from 23% to 74%, depending on the length of follow-up [30–39]. Most studies use the Gardner-Robertson classification scale (I–V, from good hearing to deaf), where hearing is considered preserved when it is class I (0–30 dB pure tone average and 70–100% speech discrimination) or class II (31–50 dB pure tone average and 50–69% speech discrimination). The American Academy of Otolaryngology-Head and Neck Surgery (AAO-HNS) scale uses the same criteria for defining useful hearing [23].

A pooled analysis by Coughlin and colleagues with almost 2200 patients showed a 58% crude hearing preservation rate after an average follow-up of 46.6 months [43]. Regarding longer-term outcomes, according to our experience, only 23% of patients maintained useful hearing (AAO-HNS Class A/B) at 10 years [39]. Similarly, Hasegawa and colleagues observed that hearing function remain unchanged in 68% of patients, while the useful hearing was preserved in 37% of cases [44].

Excellent pretreatment hearing remains the most predictive factor of preserved serviceable hearing irrespective of the cochlear dose. Proposed strategies suggest reducing the radiation dose to the cochlea with the rationale of improving hearing outcomes; however, this strategy may require that we reduce the marginal dose, thereby intentionally undertreating the lateral portion of the tumor and compromising long-term tumor control [45]. Several studies have identified a cochlear dose between 3.0 and 5.3 Gy as the optimal threshold, beyond which risk of losing serviceable hearing increases significantly [36, 37, 46, 47].

Cranial Nerve Function

Besides the vestibulocochlear nerves, the cranial nerves mostly at risk following stereotactic radiosurgery are the trigeminal and the facial nerves. Several reviews have identified tumor size and the delivered marginal dose to be important prognostic factors for subsequent risk of cranial neuropathy [31, 48–50]. Evidence has consistently shown that a marginal tumor dose of 12–13 Gy is associated with excellent trigeminal and facial nerve preservation rates, which range from 92% to 100% [30, 31, 48, 51–58]. These rates are lower, though, in patients who have undergone microsurgical resection prior to radiosurgery [50].

Linskey and colleagues hypothesized that it is the CN length, rather than tumor volume and dose that determines the risk of cranial neuropathy following SRS [59]. Specifically, they found the pons-petrous distance and the mid-porous transverse tumor diameter to independently correlate with the risk of neuropathy. Consequently, the maximal diameter allowable for radiosurgery is generally accepted as 3 cm; however, some centers may still treat larger lesions by administering a dose lower than 12 Gy or employing fractionation. Data regarding the function of the vestibular nerve are more limited. A detailed examination of vestibular function by Fukuoka and colleagues showed that almost 90% of patients had some degree of vestibular dysfunction before radiosurgery and that treatment did not significantly affect vestibular function [52]. In addition, persistent dizziness was observed in 2% of patients. Similarly, Combs and colleagues reported that patients presenting with dizziness noticed no improvement following treatment [60]. In a series of 117 patients by Murphy and colleagues, 4% of patients reported new vertigo and 18% had new gait imbalance [61]. Finally, Badakhshi and colleagues conducted a retrospective analysis of 190 patients treated with a LINAC-based, image-guided system and found that 14% of patients had worse symptoms compared to baseline, while 29% had symptom relief.

Fractionated Radiotherapy

Fractionated radiotherapy refers to radiation delivered in multiple fractions. When it is delivered in a small number of fractions (i.e., 2–5) it is referred to as hypofractionated. Wallner and colleagues were the first to report the use of fractionated radiotherapy as an adjunct treatment to STR and biopsy [62]. Local tumor recurrence decreased from 46% to 6% when doses greater than 45 Gy were delivered to the postoperative bed, with an actuarial 15-year tumor control rate equal to 94% [62]. Accordingly, the first report with 20-year data noted a tumor control rate of 88% at 5 years and 85% at 15 years; the mean radiation dosage was 51 Gy with an average of 1.8 Gy per fraction and a 1–2 mm margin on the contrast-enhanced tumor image on MRI [27, 63–67].

With the popularization of stereotactic techniques, advanced radiotherapy technologies have allowed for more conformal dose distributions. Stereotactic radiotherapy emerged as an attractive option after reports of high rates of cranial neuropathy following initially high single-fraction doses (i.e., 16 Gy) [30]. Tumors with a pons-petrous distance >1 cm and mid-porous transverse diameter >2 cm were the first ones to be treated [59, 68]. Several stereotactic radiotherapy schemes have been reported in the literature for the treatment of VS [28, 41, 60, 64, 69–71]. Current dosing schemes typically range from 1.8 to 2.0 Gy per fraction for a total maximum dose of 40.0–57.6 Gy.

Reported local tumor control rates are estimated at 94–100% [41, 61]. Similarly, trigeminal and facial nerve preservation rates range from 84–100% and 96–100%, respectively [72]. Fractionating the total radiation dosage into a series of smaller doses aims to minimize injury to adjacent cranial nerves, particularly the cochlear nerve. Though inconsistently measured, hearing preservation rates are estimated at 61–98%, based on a systematic review by Jian and colleagues of modern series (843 patients with a median follow-up ranging from 1.6 to 9 years) [72].

It is worth mentioning that in the largest contemporary series by Aoyama and colleagues and by Litre and colleagues, with a total 356 patients who underwent fractionated stereotactic radiotherapy (median total dose of 50 Gy in sessions of 1.8–2 Gy), tumor growth necessitating new intervention was noted in 4.8% at a median follow-up of 60–72 months [73, 74]. Hearing deterioration (Gardner-Robertson class I–II to III–V) was observed in 45%, facial nerve deterioration in 2.5–2.7%, and trigeminal nerve deterioration in 2–3.6% of patients.

Data on hypofractionated radiotherapy (five sessions) is more limited. According to a systematic review by Nguyen and colleagues of 228 patients treated with LINAC-based systems (total dose of 20–25 Gy), estimated pooled tumor control rates average 95%, while hearing, facial nerve, and trigeminal nerve preservation rates were 37%, 97%, and 98%, respectively [75]. Lastly, with regard to the number of sessions and outcomes, Meijer and colleagues treated 80 patients with a fractionated schedule (20–25 Gy in five fractions) and 49 patients in a single fraction (10 or 12.5 Gy) [65]. Tumor control, facial nerve preservation, and hearing preservation rates at 5 years were similar for the two groups. Interestingly, patients receiving the hypofractionated regimen had a significantly higher trigeminal nerve preservation rate (98% vs. 92%).

Comparing Radiosurgery and Radiotherapy

Currently, data from prospective, randomized studies directly comparing the outcomes following the two methods do not exist, which is partly attributed to physician bias or patient expectations that influence treatment decision, thereby rendering enrollment very challenging [60, 76]. Comparisons across different studies are even more difficult given the wide variety of definitions of tumor control and hearing preservation (the Gardner-Robertson hearing classification scale is less often used by fractionated groups). Though each technique has distinct technical properties and radiobiologic benefits, there is little evidence on the superiority of one technique over the other (Table 10.1).

Andrews and colleagues retrospectively compared 125 patients and found equivalent tumor control (98% vs. 97%) and preservation of CN V (95% vs. 93%) and VII (98% vs. 98%) function between radiosurgery (12 Gy) and fractionated radiotherapy (50 Gy) [76]. Hearing preservation was significantly lower in the radiosurgery group (33% vs. 81% at a median follow-up of 41 and 38 weeks, respectively). In a similar fashion, Combs and colleagues compared 191 patients who were treated with LINAC-based single-dose radiosurgery (≤13 Gy) versus fractionated stereotactic radiotherapy (57.6 Gy) and observed comparable tumor control (96% vs. 96%) and hearing preservation (78% vs. 78%) rates at a median follow-up of 75 months [60].

In regard to hearing preservation, the most satisfactory results have been achieved with stereotactic fractionated radiotherapy, with the majority of studies reporting 61–98% hearing preservation rate after a total dose of 40–57.6 Gy at a median follow-up ranging from 1.6 to 9 years [72]. However, more long-term follow-up data are needed before conclusions are made. Thomas and colleagues reported a delay in sensorineural hearing loss following fractionated radiotherapy occurring with a latency of 1.5–5 years [71]. Interestingly, in the study by Combs and colleagues, the majority of hearing detriment was observed at 6–10 months after treatment [60].

Proton Beam Therapy

Proton beam therapy has been employed for the treatment of VS as well. Its highly conformal properties and rapid dose fall-off in combination with minimal exit dose offer an appealing advantage over photon-based systems, which is particularly beneficial in the treatment of intracranial targets surrounded by sensitive critical structures, including the cochlea.

Proton beam therapy has been utilized in several delivery schemes, including single-fraction, hypofractionated, and fractionated approaches. For example, Bush and colleagues administered 54 and 60 cobalt-Gy equivalents (cGye) in 30–33 fractions for patients with and without useful hearing (Gardner-Robertson class I–II vs. III–V), respectively [77]. Tumor control rates have been reported to range from 84% to 100% at a mean follow-up of 34–60 months [77–80]. Cranial nerve function rates were excellent as well; studies have reported trigeminal and facial nerve preservation rates of 89–100% and 91–100%, respectively. Finally, hearing results are less satisfactory. Based on these early experiences, hearing preservation rates were 31–42%, which might be attributed to the small proportion of patients presenting with useful hearing.

In summary, the theoretical advantages of proton beam therapy should be weighed against its much higher cost; until firmer evidence is established, its application for the treatment of patients with VS will be fairly limited.

Risk of Secondary Malignancy

Risk of malignant transformation is exceedingly rare, and only case reports exist in the literature after an interval of 5–30-years of follow-up [81–83]. According to an institutional review by Rowe and colleagues of 5000 patients treated with SRS over 30,000 patient-years of follow-up, a single new brain astrocytoma was detected, which is lower than the anticipated number of 2.47 cases based on population statistics. Given that SRS typically delivers radiation in a single fraction to a small target and regional tissue volume, which is more likely to lead to cell death than cell transmutation, the risk of delayed malignancy is very small [84]. The risk theoretically might be higher with fractionated external beam radiotherapy as radiation is delivered in more sessions but still remains extremely small.

Summary

The guideline panel of the Congress of Neurological Surgeons recently released its recommendations on the management of acoustic neuromas with radiation [20]. According to the guideline panel, it is recommended that doses less than 13 Gy should be used in single-fraction stereotactic radiosurgery schemes to facilitate hearing preservation and minimize new onset or worsening of preexisting cranial nerve deficits [20]. Additionally, the report highlighted that follow-up imaging should be obtained at regular intervals after SRS based on "clinical indications, a patient's personal circumstances, or institutional protocols" [20]. Currently, there is not sufficient evidence to support the superiority of radiosurgery over radiotherapy with respect to tumor control rates. Therefore, future prospective trials are needed to provide firm evidence on the optimal use of the various radiation modalities, ideally leading to an appropriate individualized management algorithm for patients with VS.

Microsurgery

Microsurgical resection combined with sophisticated cranial nerve monitoring has been a widely accepted option for the treatment of VS with varying degrees of hearing loss. Microsurgical approaches to acoustic tumors can be grouped into three broad categories: retrosigmoid, translabyrinthine, and middle fossa approaches, each with its own advantages and disadvantages. Some surgeons prefer a single technique to remove all types of tumors regardless of size and related symptoms. Others tailor their approach based on tumor characteristics, patient's preference/expectations, and audiologic parameters [85–87].

One of the earliest documentations of VS resection is attributed to Annandale in 1895, who attempted a unilateral suboccipital approach [88, 89]. In 1904, Parry described a middle fossa approach to the vestibulocochlear complex for the surgical management of a patient with tinnitus and vertigo [90]. In 1912, Franciscus H. Quix published the first translabyrinthine resection as part of a two-stage procedure [91]; the approach was later popularized by William House [92]. As previously detailed, Harvey Cushing and Walter Dandy contributed greatly to the advancement of the surgical treatment of VS [4, 89, 93, 94].

As Gonzalez and Spetzler highlight, the internal auditory canal (IAC) may be accessed through different approaches that are based on distinct trajectories [95]. The retrosigmoid is the most common one, as it is the approach that most neurosurgeons are familiar with, allowing for exposure of the IAC in an angle parallel to the petrous surface. On the other hand, the translabyrinthine approach is ideal for tumors confined to the IAC or when they extend laterally beyond the "accessible" region, after the posterior lip of the IAC has been drilled [95]. It is generally preferred when hearing is severely compromised (Gardner-Robertson class III or IV) or is not an issue because of tumor size (usually larger than 2 cm) [95, 96]. Finally, compared to the other two, the middle fossa approach offers satisfactory exposure of the IAC and its contents, including the facial (all segments) and superior vestibular nerves, through a superior trajectory. It is primarily employed for small lesions confined to the IAC, or less than 1 cm in posterior fossa diameter, particularly when preservation of hearing is desired.

Complete surgical removal is the best answer for long-term recurrence-free outcomes. Nakatomi and colleagues also showed the extent of resection to be the strongest predictor of recurrence, with patients treated with STR having a nearly 11-fold greater risk of recurrence compared to those who underwent gross total resection (GTR) [97]. Specifically, recurrence-free survival rates at 10 and 15 years were estimated to be 82% and 73% for GTR compared to 17% and 8% for STR, respectively [97]. Comparably, a study by Jacob and colleagues revealed a 13-fold higher risk of recurrence for STR than near total resection (NTR), with the median to recurrence following NTR being 124 months compared to 32 months after STR [98]. The authors concluded that complete resection should be the primary goal of microsurgery and less than complete resection should be based on intraoperative impression, on the grounds of potential neurological deficit due to "continued dissection of adherent disease" [98]. In addition, a review of the literature by Yamakami and colleagues demonstrated 0–2% recurrence with long-term follow-up when the majority of tumors were completely removed [99]. Significantly higher rate was observed in only one small study with 33 patients in which 69% had a subtotal removal and 20% had a recurrence. More recently, a preliminary report of the Acoustic Neuroma Subtotal Resection Study (prospective, multicenter, nonrandomized cohort study) revealed three-times higher risk of recurrence in patients with vestibular schwannoma ≥2.5 cm who had STR compared to GTR and NTR [100].

Hearing Results

Often, the most important factor determining the surgical approach is preoperative hearing status. Reported rates of hearing preservation after retrosigmoid or middle fossa approaches range from 17% to 88% [101, 102]. Generally, the average risk of serviceable hearing loss correlates with tumor size, with the risk increasing with increasing tumor size. Additionally, the extension of the tumor to the fundus of the IAC and cochlear aperture is a negative predictor of ability to remove the tumor and preserve useful hearing. The considerable variety in audiologic criteria used renders the comparability of hearing outcomes across studies difficult [23, 102, 103]. At a minimum, useful hearing requires speech discrimination scores greater than 50% and a pure tone average sufficient for amplification (typically >50 dB).

Facial Nerve Outcomes

Preservation of facial nerve function is one of the important drivers of surgical success from the patient's perspective. Although not directly life-threatening, facial nerve palsy can be life-altering, particularly in cases of minimal postoperative recovery of function. Excellent rates of facial nerve function preservation can be achieved with all three surgical approaches [101, 102, 104–106]. The middle fossa approach is associated with worse facial nerve outcomes than the retrosigmoid approach based on directly comparative studies [102, 105]. It should be noted that facial nerve outcomes worsen as tumor size increases [107]. For tumors larger than 2.5 cm, the rates for both translabyrinthine and retrosigmoid approaches range from 50% to 94%, with functional "good" results from 20% to 80% [108].

In an attempt to preserve facial nerve function, many surgeons will opt for STR or NTR followed by radiosurgery either primarily or because of tumor remnant growth. According to recently published guidelines, more than 90% of patients maintain normal or near normal facial function, rates better than those reported for GTR (31.4–92.8%) [109]. In the Acoustic Neuroma Subtotal Resection Study, good facial nerve function (House-Brackmann grade I and II) was achieved in 67% immediately and 81% at 1 year [100]. Furthermore, immediate facial nerve function (House-Brackmann grade I/II) was associated with smaller preoperative tumor diameter and volume as well as a larger percentage of the tumor left behind [100].

Cerebrospinal Fluid Leakage

Cerebrospinal fluid (CSF) leakage is the most common complication associated with VS surgery [32]. Reported rates are highly variable in the literature, ranging from more than 20% to as low as 0%, depending on the approach, surgeons' experience, operative time, and patient's body mass index [110–112]. In the largest study to date, Alattar and colleagues queried a statewide administrative database and found an incidence of readmission with CSF leak of 3.5% among 6820 patients with VS treated between 1995 and 2010 [113]. Significant factors found to be independently associated with readmission for CSF leak were male sex, obesity, teaching-hospital status, and hospital case volume. Regardless of the approach, the meticulous surgical technique is critical in reducing the risk of CSF leakage. Careful application of bone wax to exposed air cells and packing autologous fat or muscle is now standard [114]. More recently, hydroxyapatite bony replacement and tissue glues have been proposed as well; however, their effectiveness is not well established, and they may present a higher risk of infection [87, 115].

Patient Reported Quality of Life

Given the increasingly important role of patient reported outcomes in healthcare quality measurement, there have been a rising number of publications investigating patient's health-related quality of life (QOL), symptom-associated disability, and treatment satisfaction using subjective instruments

[116–119]. This increase is particularly relevant to the study of VS because the focus of treatment has shifted from survival to improvement in patient functionality, symptoms, and well-being. To date, the only validated instrument specifically designed for patients with sporadic VS is the Penn Acoustic Neuroma QOL (PANQOL) questionnaire [120].

To date, only four prospective observational studies have been published looking at patients' QOL following different treatment modalities [121–124]. Pollock and colleagues as well as Myrseth and colleagues demonstrated more favorable outcomes for radiosurgery compared to surgical resection, whereas Di Maio observed similar trends in QOL following observation, radiation therapy, or surgery after a mean follow-up period of 31.8 months [121, 123, 124]. Finally, Breivik and colleagues reported a statistically significant, albeit small, improvement in vertigo and balance but no change in tinnitus comparing radiosurgery to microsurgery and observation after a median observation period of 43 months [122].

Carlson and colleagues investigated long-term QOL in VS patients managed with microsurgery, stereotactic radiosurgery, and observation in two tertiary academic referral centers in the United States and Western Europe. Mean interval between treatment and survey was 7.7 years. Interestingly, microsurgical management was found to be associated with the greatest decrease in health-related QOL measurements. Furthermore, patients who underwent microsurgery had significantly lower PANQOL total score by 8–11% compared with those managed with stereotactic radiosurgery or observation, respectively. The questionnaire domains in which the largest differences were observed included facial function (13–14%), balance (10–19%), and pain (19–30%) [125]. In another large-scale study by Soulier and colleagues, patients with tumors ≤10 mm in size under observation reported significantly higher total PANQOL score compared to the radiosurgical and microsurgical groups at a mean follow-up of 4 years [126].

In addition, we recently analyzed QOL data from 143 patients enrolled in a prospective, international study [127]. GTR was achieved in 122 patients while the remaining had STR. Interestingly, we found GTR to be associated with better QOL at a mean follow-up of 7.7 years after surgery across all three measures used (i.e., Short Form-36, PROMIS-10, and PANQOL, even after adjusting for baseline and outcome differences thereby indicating that there is a psychological advantage to patient reported well-being when the entire tumor is removed).

Yet, it should be noted that several of the reported differences in QOL might not represent significant changes from the patient's perspective. Carlson and colleagues published the minimum clinically important thresholds for the PANQOL domain and total scores and found that they exceeded the differences reported in prior studies, which based conclusions on QOL benefit among VS treatment modalities on statistical significance alone [128].

Conclusions

Significant advances have been made in the past three decades in the management of VS. Currently, three options exist: observation, stereotactic radiosurgery/radiotherapy, and microsurgical resection. Observation may be offered to patients with small lesions and minor symptoms while stereotactic radiation/radiosurgery is a good option for tumors up to 3 cm in size. Comparable tumor control rates have been demonstrated using the different radiation modalities. Contemporary single-session radiosurgery schemes allow for hearing preservation rates greater than 60% in short-term follow-up and a risk of facial weakness of approximately 1%. Surgery remains a commonly employed treatment, particularly in patients with large tumors causing brainstem compression or progressive neurological symptoms.

References

1. Ballance SCA. Some points in the surgery of the brain and its membranes. London: Macmillan; 1908.
2. Koerbel A, Gharabaghi A, Safavi-Abbasi S, Tatagiba M, Samii M. Evolution of vestibular schwannoma surgery: the long journey to current success. Neurosurg Focus. 2005;18:e10.
3. Krause F. Discussion of von Eiselsberg's paper. Tr Int Cong Med Lond VII. 1913;214.
4. Cushing H. Tumors of the nervus acusticus and the syndrome of the cerebellopontile angle. Philadelphia: W.B. Saunders; 1917.
5. Cushing H. Further concerning the acoustic neuromas. Laryngoscope. 1921;31:209–28.
6. Dandy WE. An operation for the total extirpation of tumors in the cerebello-pontine angle. A preliminary report. Bull Johns Hopkins Hosp. 1922;33:344–5.
7. Dandy WE, Others. An operation for the total removal of cerebellopontine (acoustic) tumors. Surg Gynecol Obstet. 1925;41:129–48.
8. Dandy WE. Removal of cerebellopontile (acoustic) tumors through a unilateral approach. Arch Surg. 1934;29:337–44.
9. Dandy WE. Results of removal of acoustic tumors by the unilateral approach. Arch Surg. 1941;42:1026–33.
10. Leksell L. A note on the treatment of acoustic tumours. Acta Chir Scand. 1971;137:763–5.
11. Flickinger JC, Lunsford LD, Linskey ME, Duma CM, Kondziolka D. Gamma knife radiosurgery for acoustic tumors: multivariate analysis of four year results. Radiother Oncol. 1993;27:91–8.
12. Smouha EE, Yoo M, Mohr K, Davis RP. Conservative management of acoustic neuroma: a meta-analysis and proposed treatment algorithm. Laryngoscope. 2005;115:450–4.
13. Yoshimoto Y. Systematic review of the natural history of vestibular schwannoma. J Neurosurg. 2005;103:59–63.
14. Hajioff D, Raut VV, Walsh RM, et al. Conservative management of vestibular schwannomas: third review of a 10-year prospective study. Clin Otolaryngol. 2008;33:255–9.
15. Malhotra PS, Sharma P, Fishman MA, et al. Clinical, radiographic, and audiometric predictors in conservative management of vestibular schwannoma. Otol Neurotol. 2009;30:507–14.

16. Hoistad DL, Melnik G, Mamikoglu B, Battista R, O'Connor CA, Wiet RJ. Update on conservative management of acoustic neuroma. Otol Neurotol. 2001;22:682–5.
17. Shin YJ, Fraysse B, Cognard C, et al. Effectiveness of conservative management of acoustic neuromas. Am J Otol. 2000;21:857–62.
18. Stangerup S-E, Caye-Thomasen P. Epidemiology and natural history of vestibular schwannomas. Otolaryngol Clin N Am. 2012;45:257–68.
19. Pullicino R, Radon M, Biswas S, Bhojak M, Das K. A review of the current evidence on gadolinium deposition in the brain. Clin Neuroradiol. 2018;28:159–69. https://doi.org/10.1007/s00062-018-0678-0.
20. Olson JJ, Kalkanis SN, Ryken TC. Congress of neurological surgeons systematic review and evidence-based guidelines on the treatment of adults with vestibular schwannomas: executive summary. Neurosurgery. 2018;82:129–34.
21. Van Gompel JJ, Patel J, Danner C, et al. Acoustic neuroma observation associated with an increase in symptomatic tinnitus: results of the 2007–2008 Acoustic Neuroma Association survey. Collections. 2013;118:864–8.
22. Stangerup S-E, Thomsen J, Tos M, Cayé-Thomasen P. Long-term hearing preservation in vestibular schwannoma. Otol Neurotol. 2010;31:271–5.
23. Balkany TA, Gates GA, Goldenberg RA, et al. Committee on Hearing and Equilibrium guidelines for the evaluation of hearing preservation in acoustic neuroma (vestibular schwannoma). Otolaryngol Head Neck Surg. 1995;113:179–80.
24. Kirchmann M, Karnov K, Hansen S, Dethloff T, Stangerup S-E, Caye-Thomasen P. Ten-year follow-up on tumor growth and hearing in patients observed with an intracanalicular vestibular schwannoma. Neurosurgery. 2017;80:49–56.
25. Flint D, Fagan P, Panarese A. Conservative management of sporadic unilateral acoustic neuromas. J Laryngol Otol. 2005;119:424–8.
26. Telian SA. Management of the small acoustic neuroma: a decision analysis. Am J Otol. 1994;15:358–65.
27. Murphy ES, Suh JH. Radiotherapy for vestibular schwannomas: a critical review. Int J Radiat Oncol Biol Phys. 2011;79:985–97.
28. Link MJ, Driscoll CLW, Foote RL, Pollock BE. Radiation therapy and radiosurgery for vestibular schwannomas: indications, techniques, and results. Otolaryngol Clin N Am. 2012;45:353–66.
29. Kondziolka D, Lunsford LD, McLaughlin MR, Flickinger JC. Long-term outcomes after radiosurgery for acoustic neuromas. N Engl J Med. 1998;339:1426–33.
30. Chopra R, Kondziolka D, Niranjan A, Lunsford LD, Flickinger JC. Long-term follow-up of acoustic schwannoma radiosurgery with marginal tumor doses of 12 to 13 Gy. Int J Radiat Oncol Biol Phys. 2007;68:845–51.
31. Hasegawa T, Fujitani S, Katsumata S, Kida Y, Yoshimoto M, Koike J. Stereotactic radiosurgery for vestibular schwannomas: analysis of 317 patients followed more than 5 years. Neurosurgery. 2005;57:257–65.
32. Pollock BE, Lunsford LD, Kondziolka D, et al. Outcome analysis of acoustic neuroma management: a comparison of microsurgery and stereotactic radiosurgery. Neurosurgery. 1995;36:215–24.
33. Friedman RA, Kesser B, Brackmann DE, Fisher LM, Slattery WH, Hitselberger WE. Long-term hearing preservation after middle fossa removal of vestibular schwannoma. Otolaryngol Head Neck Surg. 2003;129:660–5.
34. Régis J, Pellet W, Delsanti C, et al. Functional outcome after gamma knife surgery or microsurgery for vestibular schwannomas. J Neurosurg. 2013;119:1091–100.
35. Yang I, Sughrue ME, Han SJ, et al. A comprehensive analysis of hearing preservation after radiosurgery for vestibular schwannoma. J Neurosurg. 2010;112:851–9.
36. Kano H, Kondziolka D, Khan A, Flickinger JC, Lunsford LD. Predictors of hearing preservation after stereotactic radiosurgery for acoustic neuroma. J Neurosurg. 2009;111:863–73.
37. Hasegawa T, Kida Y, Kato T, Iizuka H, Yamamoto T. Factors associated with hearing preservation after Gamma Knife surgery for vestibular schwannomas in patients who retain serviceable hearing. J Neurosurg. 2011;115:1078–86.
38. Hasegawa T, Kida Y, Kato T, Iizuka H, Kuramitsu S, Yamamoto T. Long-term safety and efficacy of stereotactic radiosurgery for vestibular schwannomas: evaluation of 440 patients more than 10 years after treatment with Gamma Knife surgery. J Neurosurg. 2013;118:557–65.
39. Carlson ML, Jacob JT, Pollock BE, et al. Long-term hearing outcomes following stereotactic radiosurgery for vestibular schwannoma: patterns of hearing loss and variables influencing audiometric decline. J Neurosurg. 2013;118:579–87.
40. Williams BJ, Xu Z, Salvetti DJ, McNeill IT, Larner J, Sheehan JP. Gamma Knife surgery for large vestibular schwannomas: a single-center retrospective case-matched comparison assessing the effect of lesion size. J Neurosurg. 2013;119:463–71.
41. Chan AW, Black P, Ojemann RG, et al. Stereotactic radiotherapy for vestibular schwannomas: favorable outcome with minimal toxicity. Neurosurgery. 2005;57:60–70.
42. Wise SC, Carlson ML, Tveiten ØV, et al. Surgical salvage of recurrent vestibular schwannoma following prior stereotactic radiosurgery. Laryngoscope. 2016;126:2580–6.
43. Coughlin AR, Willman TJ, Gubbels SP. Systematic review of hearing preservation after radiotherapy for vestibular schwannoma. Otol Neurotol. 2018;39:273–83.
44. Hasegawa T, Kida Y, Kobayashi T, Yoshimoto M, Mori Y, Yoshida J. Long-term outcomes in patients with vestibular schwannomas treated using gamma knife surgery: 10-year follow up. J Neurosurg. 2005;102:10–6.
45. Jacob JT, Pollock BE, Carlson ML, Driscoll CLW, Link MJ. Stereotactic radiosurgery in the management of vestibular schwannoma and glomus jugulare: indications, techniques, and results. Otolaryngol Clin N Am. 2015;48:515–26.
46. Jacob JT, Carlson ML, Schiefer TK, Pollock BE, Driscoll CL, Link MJ. Significance of cochlear dose in the radiosurgical treatment of vestibular schwannoma: controversies and unanswered questions. Neurosurgery. 2014;74:466–74.
47. Massager N, Nissim O, Delbrouck C, et al. Irradiation of cochlear structures during vestibular schwannoma radiosurgery and associated hearing outcome. J Neurosurg. 2007;107:733–9.
48. Friedman WA, Bradshaw P, Myers A, Bova FJ. Linear accelerator radiosurgery for vestibular schwannomas. J Neurosurg. 2006;105:657–61.
49. Foote KD, Friedman WA, Buatti JM, Meeks SL, Bova FJ, Kubilis PS. Analysis of risk factors associated with radiosurgery for vestibular schwannoma. J Neurosurg. 2001;95:440–9.
50. Spiegelmann R, Lidar Z, Gofman J, Alezra D, Hadani M, Pfeffer R. Linear accelerator radiosurgery for vestibular schwannoma. J Neurosurg. 2001;94:7–13.
51. Combs SE, Thilmann C, Debus J, Schulz-Ertner D. Long-term outcome of stereotactic radiosurgery (SRS) in patients with acoustic neuromas. Int J Radiat Oncol Biol Phys. 2006;64:1341–7.
52. Fukuoka S, Takanashi M, Hojyo A, Konishi M, Tanaka C, Nakamura H. Gamma knife radiosurgery for vestibular schwannomas. Prog Neurol Surg. 2009;22:45–62.
53. Iwai Y, Yamanaka K, Kubo T, Aiba T. Gamma knife radiosurgery for intracanalicular acoustic neuromas. J Clin Neurosci. 2008;15:993–7.
54. Kalogeridi M-A, Georgolopoulou P, Kouloulias V, Kouvaris J, Pissakas G. Long-term results of LINAC-based stereotac-

tic radiosurgery for acoustic neuroma: the Greek experience. J Cancer Res Ther. 2009;5:8–13.
55. Kim K-M, Park C-K, Chung H-T, Paek SH, Jung H-W, Kim DG. Long-term outcomes of gamma knife stereotactic radiosurgery of vestibular schwannomas. J Korean Neurosurg Soc. 2007;42:286–92.
56. Myrseth E, Moller P, Pedersen P-H, Vassbotn FS, Wentzel-Larsen T, Lund-Johansen M. Vestibular schwannomas: clinical results and quality of life after microsurgery or gamma knife radiosurgery. Neurosurgery. 2005;56:927–35.
57. Prasad D, Steiner M, Steiner L. Gamma surgery for vestibular schwannoma. J Neurosurg. 2000;92:745–59.
58. Unger F, Walch C, Schröttner O, Eustacchio S, Sutter B, Pendl G. Cranial nerve preservation after radiosurgery of vestibular schwannomas. Acta Neurochir Suppl. 2002;84:77–83.
59. Linskey ME, Flickinger JC, Lunsford LD. Cranial nerve length predicts the risk of delayed facial and trigeminal neuropathies after acoustic tumor stereotactic radiosurgery. Int J Radiat Oncol Biol Phys. 1993;25:227–33.
60. Combs SE, Welzel T, Schulz-Ertner D, Huber PE, Debus J. Differences in clinical results after LINAC-based single-dose radiosurgery versus fractionated stereotactic radiotherapy for patients with vestibular schwannomas. Int J Radiat Oncol Biol Phys. 2010;76:193–200.
61. Murphy ES, Barnett GH, Vogelbaum MA, et al. Long-term outcomes of Gamma Knife radiosurgery in patients with vestibular schwannomas. J Neurosurg. 2011;114:432–40.
62. Wallner KE, Sheline GE, Pitts LH, Wara WM, Davis RL, Boldrey EB. Efficacy of irradiation for incompletely excised acoustic neurilemomas. J Neurosurg. 1987;67:858–63.
63. Maire J-P, Huchet A, Milbeo Y, et al. Twenty years' experience in the treatment of acoustic neuromas with fractionated radiotherapy: a review of 45 cases. Int J Radiat Oncol Biol Phys. 2006;66:170–8.
64. Fuss M, Debus J, Lohr F, et al. Conventionally fractionated stereotactic radiotherapy (FSRT) for acoustic neuromas. Int J Radiat Oncol Biol Phys. 2000;48:1381–7.
65. Meijer OWM, Vandertop WP, Baayen JC, Slotman BJ. Single-fraction vs. fractionated linac-based stereotactic radiosurgery for vestibular schwannoma: a single-institution study. Int J Radiat Oncol Biol Phys. 2003;56:1390–6.
66. Selch MT, Pedroso A, Lee SP, et al. Stereotactic radiotherapy for the treatment of acoustic neuromas. J Neurosurg. 2004;101:362–72.
67. Combs SE, Volk S, Schulz-Ertner D, Huber PE, Thilmann C, Debus J. Management of acoustic neuromas with fractionated stereotactic radiotherapy (FSRT): long-term results in 106 patients treated in a single institution. Int J Radiat Oncol Biol Phys. 2005;63:75–81.
68. Kalapurakal JA, Silverman CL, Akhtar N, Andrews DW, Downes B, Thomas PR. Improved trigeminal and facial nerve tolerance following fractionated stereotactic radiotherapy for large acoustic neuromas. Br J Radiol. 1999;72:1202–7.
69. Andrews DW, Werner-Wasik M, Den RB, et al. Toward dose optimization for fractionated stereotactic radiotherapy for acoustic neuromas: comparison of two dose cohorts. Int J Radiat Oncol Biol Phys. 2009;74:419–26.
70. Koh E-S, Millar B-A, Menard C, et al. Fractionated stereotactic radiotherapy for vestibular schwannoma: single institutional experience at the Princess Margaret Hospital. Radiother Oncol. 2005;76:S29.
71. Thomas C, Di Maio S, Ma R, et al. Hearing preservation following fractionated stereotactic radiotherapy for vestibular schwannomas: prognostic implications of cochlear dose. J Neurosurg. 2007;107:917–26.
72. Jian BJ, Kaur G, Sayegh ET, Bloch O, Parsa AT, Barani IJ. Fractionated radiation therapy for vestibular schwannoma. J Clin Neurosci. 2014;21:1083–8.
73. Litre F, Rousseaux P, Jovenin N, et al. Fractionated stereotactic radiotherapy for acoustic neuromas: a prospective monocenter study of about 158 cases. Radiother Oncol. 2013;106:169–74.
74. Aoyama H, Onodera S, Takeichi N, et al. Symptomatic outcomes in relation to tumor expansion after fractionated stereotactic radiation therapy for vestibular schwannomas: single-institutional long-term experience. Int J Radiat Oncol Biol Phys. 2013;85:329–34.
75. Nguyen T, Duong C, Sheppard JP, et al. Hypo-fractionated stereotactic radiotherapy of five fractions with linear accelerator for vestibular schwannomas: a systematic review and meta-analysis. Clin Neurol Neurosurg. 2018;166:116–23.
76. Andrews DW, Suarez O, Goldman HW, et al. Stereotactic radiosurgery and fractionated stereotactic radiotherapy for the treatment of acoustic schwannomas: comparative observations of 125 patients treated at one institution. Int J Radiat Oncol Biol Phys. 2001;50:1265–78.
77. Bush DA, Mcallister CJ, Loredo LN, Johnson WD, Slater JM, Slater JD. Fractionated proton beam radiotherapy for acoustic neuroma. Neurosurgery. 2002;50:270–5.
78. Harsh GR, Thornton AF, Chapman PH, Bussiere MR, Rabinov JD, Loeffler JS. Proton beam stereotactic radiosurgery of vestibular schwannomas. Int J Radiat Oncol Biol Phys. 2002;54:35–44.
79. Vernimmen FJAI, Mohamed Z, Slabbert JP, Wilson J. Long-term results of stereotactic proton beam radiotherapy for acoustic neuromas. Radiother Oncol. 2009;90:208–12.
80. Weber DC, Chan AW, Bussiere MR, et al. Proton beam radiosurgery for vestibular schwannoma: tumor control and cranial nerve toxicity. Neurosurgery. 2003;53:577–88.
81. Tanbouzi Husseini S, Piccirillo E, Taibah A, Paties CT, Rizzoli R, Sanna M. Malignancy in vestibular schwannoma after stereotactic radiotherapy: a case report and review of the literature. Laryngoscope. 2011;121:923–8.
82. Fusco DJ, Williamson R, Yanamadala V, Eschbacher J, Porter R, Weisskopf P. Malignant transformation of a vestibular schwannoma following gamma knife radiosurgery: case report and review of the literature. J Neurol Surg B Skull Base. 2012;73:A293.
83. Niranjan A, Kondziolka D, Lunsford LD. Neoplastic transformation after radiosurgery or radiotherapy: risk and realities. Otolaryngol Clin N Am. 2009;42:717–29.
84. Kondziolka D, Mousavi SH, Kano H, Flickinger JC, Lunsford LD. The newly diagnosed vestibular schwannoma: radiosurgery, resection, or observation? Neurosurg Focus. 2012;33:E8.
85. Wiet RJ, Mamikoglu B, Odom L, Hoistad DL. Long-term results of the first 500 cases of acoustic neuroma surgery. Otolaryngol Head Neck Surg. 2001;124:645–51.
86. Sanna M, Taibah A, Russo A, Falcioni M, Agarwal M. Perioperative complications in acoustic neuroma (vestibular schwannoma) surgery. Otol Neurotol. 2004;25:379–86.
87. Bambakidis NC, Megerian CA, Spetzler RF. Surgery of the cerebellopontine angle. Shelton, CT: PMPH-USA; 2009.
88. Ramsden RT. A brilliant surgical result, the first recorded: Annandale's case, 3 May 1895. J Laryngol Otol. 1995;109:369–73.
89. Olson JJ, Kalkanis SN, Ryken TC. Congress of neurological surgeons systematic review and evidence-based guidelines on the treatment of adults with vestibular schwannomas: introduction and methods. Neurosurgery. 2018;82:135.
90. Parry RH. A case of tinnitus and vertigo treated by division of the auditory nerve. J Laryngol Otol. 1904;19:402–6.
91. Quix FH. Ein Fall von translabyrintharisch operiertem Tumor acusticus. Verh Dtsch Otol Ges. 1912;21:245–55.
92. House WF. Transtemporal bone microsurgical removal of acoustic neuromas. Report of cases. Arch Otolaryngol. 1964;80:617–67.

93. Dandy WE, et al. An operation for the total removal of cerebellopontine (acoustic) tumors. Surg Gynecol Obstet. 1925;41:129–48.
94. Dandy WE. Removal of cerebellontine (acoustic) tumors through a unilateral approach. Arch Surg. 1934;29:337–44.
95. Gonzalez LF, Lekovic GP, Porter RW, Syms MJ, Daspit CP, Spetzler RF. Surgical approaches for resection of acoustic neuromas. Barrow Q. 2004;20:1–11.
96. Day JD, Chen DA, Arriaga M. Translabyrinthine approach for acoustic neuroma. Neurosurgery. 2004;54:391–6.
97. Nakatomi H, Jacob JT, Carlson ML, et al. Long-term risk of recurrence and regrowth after gross-total and subtotal resection of sporadic vestibular schwannoma. J Neurosurg. 2017;19:1–7.
98. Jacob JT, Carlson ML, Driscoll CL, Link MJ. Volumetric analysis of tumor control following subtotal and near-total resection of vestibular schwannoma. Laryngoscope. 2016;126:1877–82.
99. Yamakami I, Uchino Y, Kobayashi E, Yamaura A. Conservative management, gamma-knife radiosurgery, and microsurgery for acoustic neurinomas: a systematic review of outcome and risk of three therapeutic options. Neurol Res. 2003;25:682–90.
100. Monfared A, Corrales CE, Theodosopoulos PV, et al. Facial nerve outcome and tumor control rate as a function of degree of resection in treatment of large acoustic neuromas: preliminary report of the acoustic neuroma subtotal resection study (ANSRS). Neurosurgery. 2016;79:194–203.
101. Mangham CA Jr. Retrosigmoid versus middle fossa surgery for small vestibular schwannomas. Laryngoscope. 2004;114:1455–61.
102. Sanna M, Khrais T, Russo A, Piccirillo E, Augurio A. Hearing preservation surgery in vestibular schwannoma: the hidden truth. Ann Otol Rhinol Laryngol. 2004;113:156–63.
103. Samii M, Matthies C. Management of 1000 vestibular schwannomas (acoustic neuromas): hearing function in 1000 tumor resections. Neurosurgery. 1997;40:248–62.
104. McElveen JT Jr, Belmonte RG, Fukushima T, Bullard DE. A review of facial nerve outcome in 100 consecutive cases of acoustic tumor surgery. Laryngoscope. 2000;110:1667–72.
105. Colletti V, Fiorino F. Middle fossa versus retrosigmoid-transmeatal approach in vestibular schwannoma surgery: a prospective study. Otol Neurotol. 2003;24:927–34.
106. Arts HA, Telian SA, El-Kashlan H, Thompson BG. Hearing preservation and facial nerve outcomes in vestibular schwannoma surgery: results using the middle cranial fossa approach. Otol Neurotol. 2006;27:234–41.
107. Fenton JE, Chin RY, Fagan PA, Sterkers O, Sterkers JM. Predictive factors of long-term facial nerve function after vestibular schwannoma surgery. Otol Neurotol. 2002;23:388–92.
108. Lanman TH, Brackmann DE, Hitselberger WE, Subin B. Report of 190 consecutive cases of large acoustic tumors (vestibular schwannoma) removed via the translabyrinthine approach. J Neurosurg. 1999;90:617–23.
109. Hadjipanayis CG, Carlson ML, Link MJ, et al. Congress of neurological surgeons systematic review and evidence-based guidelines on surgical resection for the treatment of patients with vestibular schwannomas. Neurosurgery. 2018;82:E40–3.
110. Copeland WR, Mallory GW, Neff BA, Driscoll CLW, Link MJ. Are there modifiable risk factors to prevent a cerebrospinal fluid leak following vestibular schwannoma surgery? J Neurosurg. 2015;122:312–6.
111. Murphy ME, McCutcheon BA, Kerezoudis P, et al. Morbid obesity increases risk of morbidity and reoperation in resection of benign cranial nerve neoplasms. Clin Neurol Neurosurg. 2016;148:105–9.
112. Selesnick SH, Liu JC, Jen A, Carew JF. Management options for cerebrospinal fluid leak after vestibular schwannoma surgery and introduction of an innovative treatment. Otol Neurotol. 2004;25:580–6.
113. Alattar AA, Hirshman BR, McCutcheon BA, et al. Risk factors for readmission with cerebrospinal fluid leakage within 30 d of vestibular schwannoma surgery. Neurosurgery. 2018;82:630–7. https://doi.org/10.1093/neuros/nyx197.
114. Isaacson JE. Radiologic follow-up after vestibular schwannoma surgery. Otol Neurotol. 2005;26:552.
115. Costantino PD, Hiltzik DH, Sen C, et al. Sphenoethmoid cerebrospinal fluid leak repair with hydroxyapatite cement. Arch Otolaryngol Head Neck Surg. 2001;127:588–93.
116. Gauden A, Weir P, Hawthorne G, Kaye A. Systematic review of quality of life in the management of vestibular schwannoma. J Clin Neurosci. 2011;18:1573–84.
117. Gouveris HT, Mann WJ. Quality of life in sporadic vestibular schwannoma: a review. ORL J Otorhinolaryngol Relat Spec. 2010;72:69–74.
118. Martin HC, Sethi J, Lang D, Neil-Dwyer G, Lutman ME, Yardley L. Patient-assessed outcomes after excision of acoustic neuroma: postoperative symptoms and quality of life. J Neurosurg. 2001;94:211–6.
119. Nicoucar K, Momjian S, Vader J-P, De Tribolet N. Surgery for large vestibular schwannomas: how patients and surgeons perceive quality of life. J Neurosurg. 2006;105:205–12.
120. Shaffer BT, Cohen MS, Bigelow DC, Ruckenstein MJ. Validation of a disease-specific quality-of-life instrument for acoustic neuroma: the Penn Acoustic Neuroma Quality-of-Life Scale. Laryngoscope. 2010;120:1646–54.
121. Di Maio S, Akagami R. Prospective comparison of quality of life before and after observation, radiation, or surgery for vestibular schwannomas. J Neurosurg. 2009;111:855–62.
122. Breivik CN, Varughese JK, Wentzel-Larsen T, Vassbotn F, Lund-Johansen M. Conservative management of vestibular schwannoma—a prospective cohort study: treatment, symptoms, and quality of life. Neurosurgery. 2012;70:1072–80.
123. Myrseth E, Møller P, Pedersen P-H, Lund-Johansen M. Vestibular schwannoma: surgery or gamma knife radiosurgery? A prospective, nonrandomized study. Neurosurgery. 2009;64:654–63.
124. Pollock BE, Driscoll CLW, Foote RL, et al. Patient outcomes after vestibular schwannoma management: a prospective comparison of microsurgical resection and stereotactic radiosurgery. Neurosurgery. 2006;59:77–85.
125. Carlson ML, Tveiten OV, Driscoll CL, Goplen FK. Long-term quality of life in patients with vestibular schwannoma: an international multicenter cross-sectional study comparing microsurgery, stereotactic radiosurgery. J Neurosurg. 2015;122:833–42.
126. Soulier G, van Leeuwen BM, Putter H, et al. Quality of life in 807 patients with vestibular schwannoma: comparing treatment modalities. Otolaryngol Head Neck Surg. 2017;157:92–8.
127. Link MJ, Lund-Johansen M, Lohse CM, et al. Quality of life in patients with vestibular schwannomas following gross total or less than gross total microsurgical resection: should we be taking the entire tumor out? Neurosurgery. 2018;82:541–7.
128. Carlson ML, Tveiten ØV, Yost KJ, Lohse CM, Lund-Johansen M, Link MJ. The minimal clinically important difference in vestibular schwannoma quality-of-life assessment: an important step beyond P < .05. Otolaryngol Head Neck Surg. 2015;153:202–8.

11 Translabyrinthine Approach

Sarah Mowry, Maroun T. Semaan, Cliff A. Megerian, Thomas Ostergard, and Nicholas C. Bambakidis

Following its revival by Dr. William House, the translabyrinthine approach (TL) has become a workhorse technique, especially in patients with significant preoperative hearing loss. Dr. House collaborated with William E. Hitselberger and showcased the synergy that can be obtained with a multidisciplinary skull-base surgical team [1]. This model of collaboration between otologists and neurosurgeons has become commonplace and has arguably served as a model for anterior skull-base surgery teams.

S. Mowry
Division of Otology/Neurotology, Department of Otolaryngology—Head and Neck Surgery, University Hospitals Cleveland Medical Center, Case Western Reserve University, Cleveland, OH, USA

M. T. Semaan
Otolaryngology—Otology, University Hospitals Cleveland Medical Center, Cleveland, OH, USA

C. A. Megerian
University Hospitals Health System, Department of Otolaryngology-Head and Neck Surgery, Department of Neurological Surgery, Case Western Reserve University School of Medicine, Cleveland, OH, USA

T. Ostergard
Carolina Neurosurgery and Spine Associates, Greensboro, NC, USA

N. C. Bambakidis (✉)
Neurological Surgery, The Neurological Institute, University Hospitals of Cleveland, Case Western Reserve University School of Medicine, Cleveland, OH, USA
e-mail: Nicholas.Bambakidis2@UHhospitals.org

Preoperative Evaluation

The standard evaluation of a patient with an acoustic neuroma begins with a targeted history and physical examination. The most common presentation associated with acoustic neuroma is hearing loss, which is typically gradual but can occur suddenly [2]. Other common symptoms include high-pitched tinnitus, disequilibrium, headache, and facial numbness from compression of nerves adjacent to the tumor. Although disequilibrium, ataxia, headaches, nausea, and vomiting are rare at presentation, attention must be paid to these symptoms, which may be signs of hydrocephalus and brainstem compression [3, 4]. At presentation, most patients have a completely normal examination but harbor complaints of unilateral sensorineural hearing loss. The most common presenting signs associated with large tumors include an abnormal corneal reflex, nystagmus, facial hypesthesia, and imbalance. Facial palsy, abnormal eye movements, and papilledema are less common and mostly seen in patients with a large tumor associated with hydrocephalus.

When paralysis results from surgery, the House-Brackmann scale is usually used to grade recovery of facial nerve function [5]. However, the scale has been used preoperatively in an effort to quantify preexisting paralysis caused by a tumor. Most patients present with normal facial nerve function and minor hearing complaints. However, an increasing number of acoustic neuromas are now detected incidentally before patients become symptomatic due to improvements in imaging [6].

Because subjective hearing loss and tinnitus are the most common symptoms associated with an underlying acoustic neuroma, most patients go to an otolaryngologist for audiometric testing. Detection of a unilateral sensorineural hearing loss usually triggers imaging studies [6, 7]. The initial screening tool is usually a pure-tone audiogram, which typically establishes a pattern of asymmetric sensorineural hearing loss common in patients with an acoustic neuroma. A difference in hearing of 10–15 dB between ears at two different frequencies is considered significant asymmetry and may

N. C. Bambakidis et al. (eds.), *Surgery of the Cerebellopontine Angle*, https://doi.org/10.1007/978-3-031-12507-2_11

indicate underlying pathology [6, 8]. A speech discrimination test should be performed in conjunction with the pure-tone audiogram. Speech discrimination may be reduced disproportionately to the pure-tone loss. Therefore, a difference of 15–20% between ears should raise suspicion of a retrocochlear problem [6]. Silverstein and colleagues reported a combination of the two hearing tests, which was modified by Gardener and Robertson to classify hearing loss. Twelve percent of patients with acoustic neuromas lack hearing loss [9]. Neurodiagnostic auditory brainstem testing can also be used to diagnose acoustic neuromas, but this modality is less sensitive than magnetic resonance imaging (MRI), particularly for detecting small tumors [10].

The current gold standard for diagnostic imaging of acoustic neuromas is gadolinium-enhanced MRI, which has a sensitivity of 98% and a specificity of almost 100% [11]. Acoustic neuromas are often isodense to the brain and brightly enhancing. Furthermore, cystic degeneration or, rarely, hemorrhage may be detected [12].

Patient Selection

When surgical excision is indicated, the choice of surgical approach should be tailored to each patient. The most important factors in choosing a surgical approach are the patient's preoperative hearing function, tumor size, and tumor location. Simply put, the translabyrinthine approach should strongly be considered when patients do not have serviceable hearing or when an alternative approach is very unlikely to preserve hearing function. This decision becomes more complicated in patients with contralateral hearing loss or neurofibromatosis type 2 (NF2).

When considering hearing function, it is important to review the audiometric data for both ears. Serviceable hearing can be defined using the 50/50 rule or 70/30 rule. The 50/50 rule translates to a pure-tone average greater than 50 dB, a word recognition score greater than 50%, or both. The 50/50 rule is the more relaxed of the two criteria. The 70/30 rule should be reserved for considering patients with coexisting contralateral hearing loss of patients with NF2.

With consideration given to hearing preservation, tumor size and location can help guide the choice of surgical approach. When performed properly, the translabyrinthine approach allows for the resection of large tumors. However, as tumor size increases, brainstem compression becomes more likely and can be more difficult to address through a translabyrinthine approach. For extremely large tumors, the translabyrinthine approach can be combined with other approaches to increase the size of the exposure.

The patient's anatomy should be carefully studied to examine the size of the operative corridor when performing a translabyrinthine approach. The locations of the sigmoid sinus and jugular bulb should be assessed as these form the borders of the approach. An anteriorly located sigmoid sinus can narrow the size of the operative corridor. However, it is usually less limiting than a high-riding jugular bulb, which approaches the inferior aspect of the internal acoustic canal (IAC). A high-riding jugular bulb can prevent the goal of 270° exposure of the IAC and significantly narrow the operative corridor.

While techniques have been described to mobilize the dural venous sinuses, it is likely better to avoid this issue if an alternative surgical approach is viable. Of note, when a high-riding jugular bulb leads to selection of a retrosigmoid approach, its course should still be carefully noted. The jugular bulb can rarely rise above the level of the IAC, which likely increases the risk of injury when maximizing the anterior and inferior margins of a retrosigmoid craniotomy. The degree of temporal bone pneumatization should also be carefully reviewed as hyperpneumatization likely increases the risk of postoperative cerebrospinal (CSF) leak.

The translabyrinthine approach offers a number of benefits that explain its wide use among skull-base surgeons. The facial nerve is identified early in the approach and likely explains why this approach has the lowest incidence of postoperative facial nerve dysfunction [13–19]. There is less cerebellar retraction and often a lower duration of intradural dissection. Drilling is performed prior to dural opening, preventing bone dust from entering the cisternal spaces. The incision is more anterior, which reduces the amount of muscular dissection. These differences likely explain why patients undergoing a translabyrinthine exposure have the shortest hospital stay and lowest incidence of postoperative headache. Aside from loss of hearing, there is also likely a higher rate of postoperative CSF leak in translabyrinthine approaches.

Surgical Procedure

The TL approach is performed with the patient under general endotracheal anesthesia. Long-acting muscle relaxants are avoided because the facial nerve is monitored routinely in all cases. Pneumatic compression stockings are used before anesthesia is induced to avoid deep vein thrombosis of the lower extremities. Due to the length of the procedure and the possibility of administering mannitol, a urinary catheter is placed.

A C-shaped incision is placed 4–5 cm behind the postauricular sulcus, extending just above the auricle and just below the mastoid tip (Fig. 11.1a). The periosteum is incised in a T-shaped fashion, creating three musculoperiosteal flaps. The trifurcation is marked with colored sutures, which help the surgeon to replace the flaps during closure (Fig. 11.1b). When making the inferior periosteal cut, care should be taken to avoid injuring the facial nerve as it exits the stylomastoid foramen.

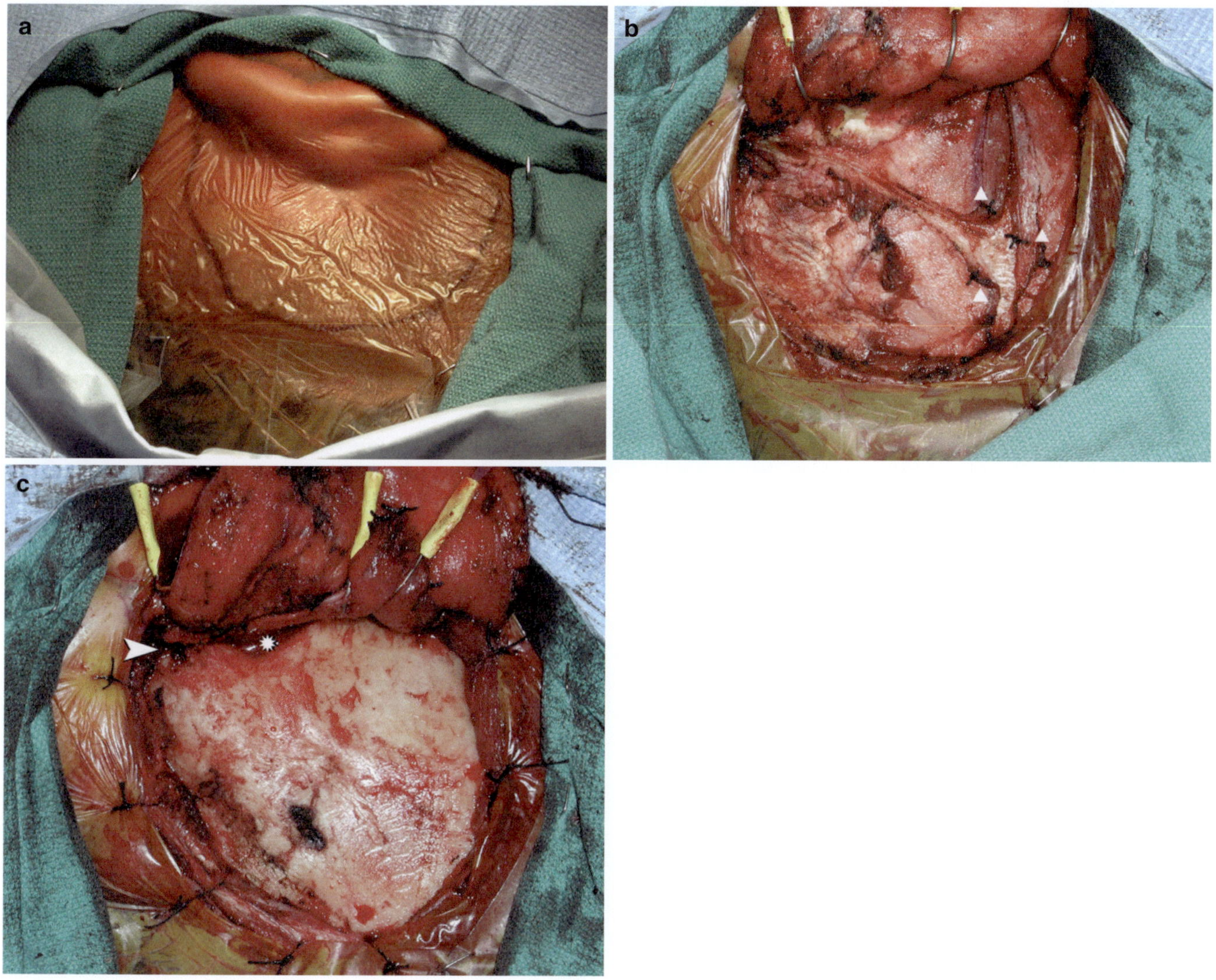

Fig. 11.1 (**a**) A right-sided surgical incision is outlined. (**b**) The skin flap is reflected forward. The musculoperiosteal layer is incised in a "T." The trifurcation is marked by three black stitches (white triangles). (**c**) The musculoperiosteal layers have been elevated and sutured to skin edges. The anterior flap is sutured to the skin flap and reflected forward. The arrow points to the mastoid tip and the asterisk indicates the external auditory canal

Bleeding from the mastoid emissary vein should be anticipated while elevating the periosteum and controlled with bone wax. While this brisk bleeding is often concerning to the early surgical trainee, its occurrence is welcome to provide a landmark for the transverse-sigmoid sinus junction. The anterior flap is sutured to the C-shaped skin flap, and both are retracted anteriorly with skin hooks (Fig. 11.1c). This maneuver provides an excellent exposure without the need for self-retaining retractors and avoids increasing the depth of the surgical field unnecessarily [20].

Cortical landmarks should be identified to orient the surgeon. The floor of the middle fossa can be estimated by the temporal line, which provides a superior boundary for the petrous bone. The posterior aspect of cortical bone forming the external acoustic canal can be estimated by the spine of Henle, which provides an anterior boundary. The sigmoid sinus is the posterior boundary in the mastoidectomy, but it lacks a consistent surface landmark. Its location is represented by a line drawn between the spine of Henle and the temporal line. These three lines mark the suprameatal triangle (also known as Macewen's triangle).

Troughs are drilled along the three lines of the suprameatal triangle. As the anatomy is appreciated during drilling, these lines should be saucerized and maximally widened to prevent narrowing of the surgical corridor. First, the superior trough is extended superiorly above the temporal line to identify the dense cortical bone of the mastoid tegmen. This cortical bone can be followed inferiorly and medially to expose the mastoid tegmen.

Attention is then turned to the anterior boundary of the suprameatal triangle. The anterior mastoid is drilled until the external auditory canal (EAC) becomes eggshell thin. The boundary of the EAC and mastoid tegmen are connected anteriorly toward the root of the zygoma. The posterior border is defined by exposing the sigmoid sinus, which allows for the identification and deepening of the sino-dural angle. It is important to expose the dura of the posterior fossa at least 1–2 cm past the sigmoid sinus, which allows for retraction of the sigmoid sinus if necessary.

As the bone over the sino-dural angle is deepened, Koerner's septum is opened as the antrum is entered. The opening in the antrum is widened until it connects with the cortex of the EAC. The surface of the lateral semicircular canal should be seen as this bone is thinned. The digastric ridge is then identified by further opening the mastoid tip. This important landmark points anteriorly to the stylomastoid foramen, where the mastoid segment of the facial nerve can be identified (Fig. 11.2a).

The labyrinthectomy can usually be completed before the sigmoid sinus, and the dura of the middle and posterior fossae is decompressed. The labyrinthectomy is begun by blue-lining the superior aspect of the horizontal semicircular canal. A cup is then developed within the otic capsule bone superior to the bisected horizontal semicircular canal. At this point, the inferior half of the horizontal semicircular canal is kept intact to protect the tympanic segment of the facial nerve, which lies immediately inferior to it (Fig. 11.2b).

The labyrinthectomy continues by widening the cup to involve the superior and posterior semicircular canals. The crus commune is identified, and the posterior semicircular canal is followed to the ampullated end. The canal and surrounding bone must be visualized at all times because the ampullated end of the posterior canal lies medial to the vertical segment of the facial nerve. The medial aspect of the facial nerve can be injured with the drill if care is not taken during this step. If the facial nerve has not already been identified and skeletonized, care must be taken to avoid drilling under the

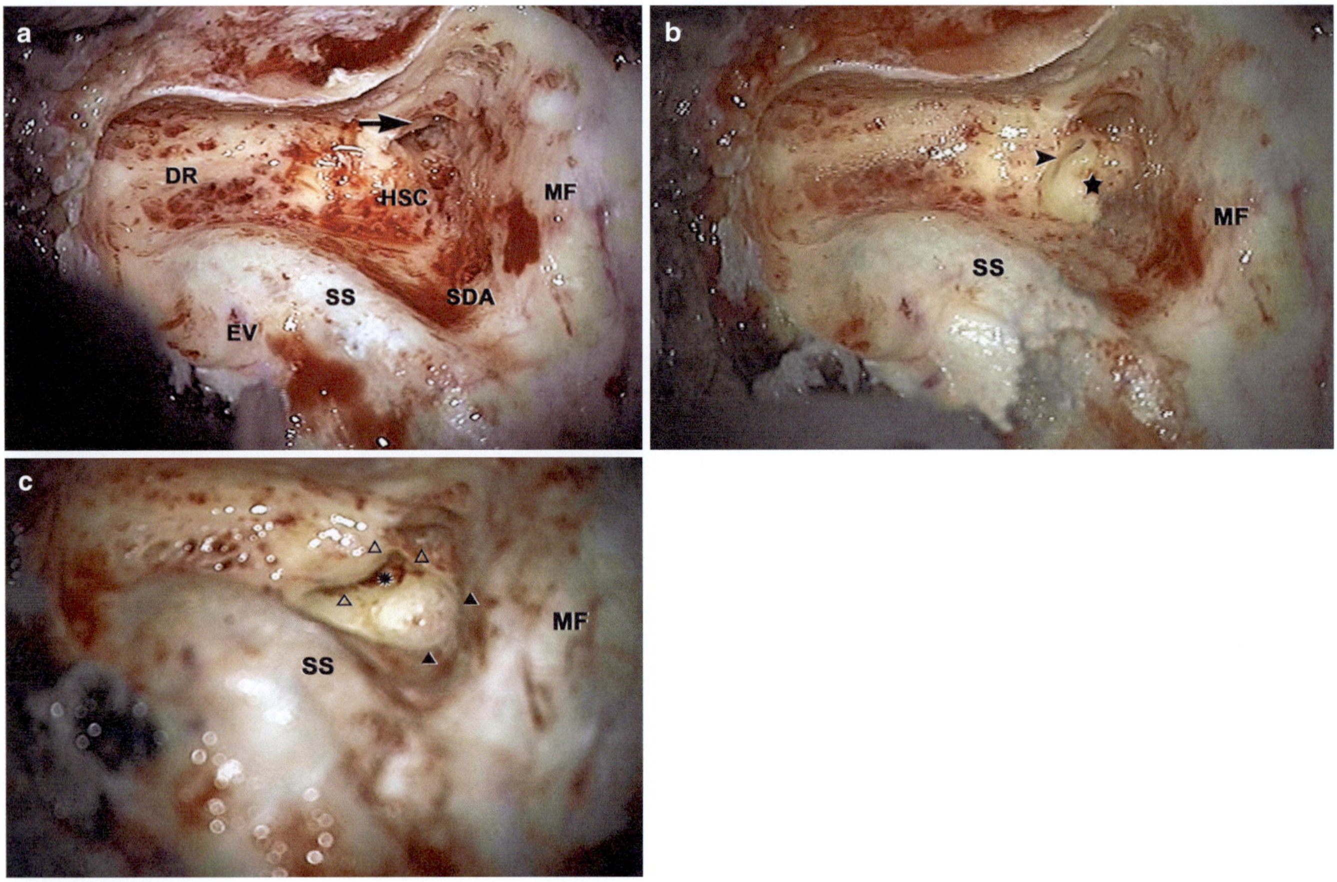

Fig. 11.2 (**a**) A complete mastoidectomy has been performed. The middle fossa (MF) and sigmoid sinus (SS) are identified. The sinodural angle (SDA) is widely open. The mastoid emissary vein (EV) is outlined. The digastric ridge (DR) and the horizontal semicircular canal (HSC) are identified. The incus is also identified (arrow). (**b**) The labyrinthectomy is started. The horizontal semicircular canal is bisected, and the superior half has been removed. The black arrowhead points to the bisected horizontal semicircular canal. A cup within the otic capsule bone is developed superior to the horizontal semicircular canal (black star). (**c**) The labyrinthectomy is completed. The vestibule is opened (black asterisk). The ampullated end of the three semicircular canals is opened (open triangles). The outline of the superior semicircular canal is marked by black triangles

bony shelf that usually develops as the posterior canal is followed inferiorly. This bony shelf should be removed gently by drilling parallel to the facial nerve. This strategy provides clear visualization of the entire drill bit at all times.

The three ampullated ends of the semicircular canals and the bone covering the vestibule are opened, and the neuroepithelial tissue is removed (Fig. 11.2c). The ampullated end of the superior semicircular canal should be preserved as a landmark for the superior vestibular nerve. The sigmoid sinus is decompressed as is the dura of the middle and posterior fossae, both medially and laterally to the sigmoid sinus, and all bone is removed. This step can usually be achieved by thinning the bone with a diamond drill. A dural elevator is used to dissect the dura from the bone, and a pair of rongeurs is used to remove the separated bone. As bone removal over the posterior fossa dura continues medially, the vestibular aqueduct and the beginning of the endolymphatic sac are encountered and divided.

Further medial dissection identifies the porus of the IAC. It is important to remember that the axis of the IAC is almost the same as that of the external auditory canal. Laterally, the fundus of the IAC is near the medial wall of the vestibule. Medially, however, considerable bone needs to be removed to expose the IAC at the porus appropriately and to identify both its superior and inferior borders.

Once the porus is identified, two troughs are created, one superior and the other inferior to the IAC (Fig. 11.3a). The inferior limit of the IAC is identified by drilling the retrofacial air cells between the presumed location of the IAC superiorly and the jugular bulb, which marks the inferior limit of the dissection. As the drilling continues medially and anteriorly, the cochlear aqueduct is identified. This important landmark usually marks the medial limit of dissection to avoid injuring the lower cranial nerves. During resection of small and medium-sized tumors, opening the cochlear aqueduct usually causes leakage of CSF. The aqueduct may be obstructed by large tumors. The superior trough is created by removing bone between the dura of the middle fossa and the superior border of the IAC.

The ampulla of the superior semicircular canal serves as a landmark for the superior vestibular nerve and the superior border of the most lateral extent of the IAC. As dissection continues anteriorly and laterally, care is taken to avoid injuring the facial nerve, which can be identified in its labyrinthine segment at this location. The bone overlying the porus and IAC is thinned and removed completely (Fig. 11.3b). When the troughs are created correctly, more than 270 degrees of the circumference of the IAC are exposed. It is important for the bone to be removed to the anterior border of the superior portion of the porus, particularly in larger tumors. Doing so optimizes exposure and facilitates dissection of the facial nerve in this area.

Finally, the inferior and superior vestibular nerves are identified at the fundus of the IAC with the transverse crest between the two nerves. The facial nerve is separated from the superior vestibular nerve at the fundus of the IAC by a vertical bony crest (Bill's bar).

Before the dura is opened, all air cell tracts should be sealed with bone wax to avoid postoperative leakage of CSF. Furthermore, the aditus ad antrum is sealed with periosteal tissue both lateral and medial to the incus, and then bone wax is applied (Fig. 11.3b).

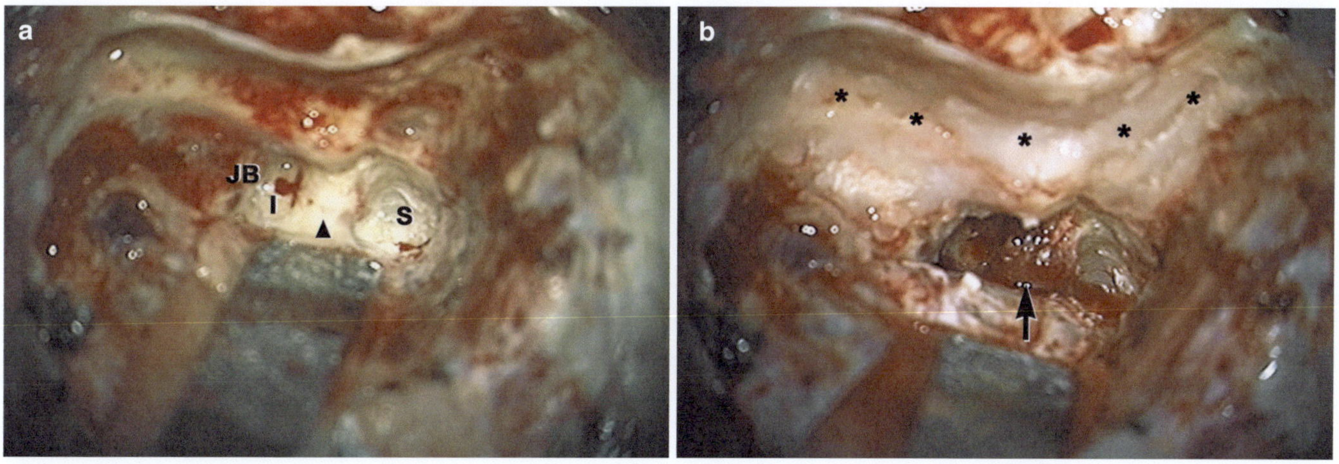

Fig. 11.3 (**a**) The dura of the middle and posterior fossae is decompressed. The jugular bulb (JB), which serves as the inferior limit of the dissection, is identified. An inferior trough (I) and a superior trough (S) are created to outline the internal auditory canal (black triangle). (**b**) The inferior and superior troughs are well developed, and all bone is removed from the posterior fossa, middle fossa, and internal auditory canal. All air cells within the external auditory canal and in the retrofacial tract and zygomatic root are sealed with bone wax (black asterisks). Periosteal tissue is used to plug the aditus, and bone wax is used to seal that area. The internal auditory canal is decompressed (black arrow)

Tumor Dissection

Once drilling of the temporal bone is complete, microsurgical dissection of the tumor from the seventh and eighth nerve complex can begin. Typically, the eggshell-thin bony covering over dura of the middle and posterior cranial fossae has been removed as has the bone covering the entire posterior two-thirds of the IAC from Bill's bar to the porus acusticus [21].

During any surgery involving the cerebellopontine angle (CPA), continuous intraoperative monitoring of the facial nerve is crucial. Multiple studies have shown that intraoperative monitoring of the facial nerve improves outcomes [4, 22–28]. We find that frequent testing of the areas where tumor is attached is essential for safe resection. The signal from the facial nerve may change during tumor dissection or manipulation, brain retraction, or irrigation of the tumor bed.

After the dura is opened (Fig. 11.4a), the diagnosis of a facial nerve schwannoma/neuroma is excluded via facial nerve stimulation and clear visualization of a normal facial nerve anterior and superior to the tumor mass and superior vestibular nerve complex. If the presumed vestibular schwannoma is actually a facial nerve schwannoma, it is our opinion that resection should not be attempted unless the preoperative facial function is abnormal. We have found that the decompression associated with the surgical approach itself provides extra room for future schwannoma growth and often preserves normal facial function for many years.

Bill's bar and intraoperative facial nerve stimulation are used to identify the facial nerve at the distal IAC, which is then carefully separated from the superior vestibular nerve (Fig. 11.4b–d). One advantage of the TL approach is that access to the CPA is shifted anteriorly compared with the suboccipital approach. Therefore, less retraction of the cerebellum is necessary [7]. The extent of the tumor and the involvement of neural structures are assessed (Fig. 11.5a). Depending on the size and extent of the adhesions to the facial nerve, the tumor may need to be debulked before

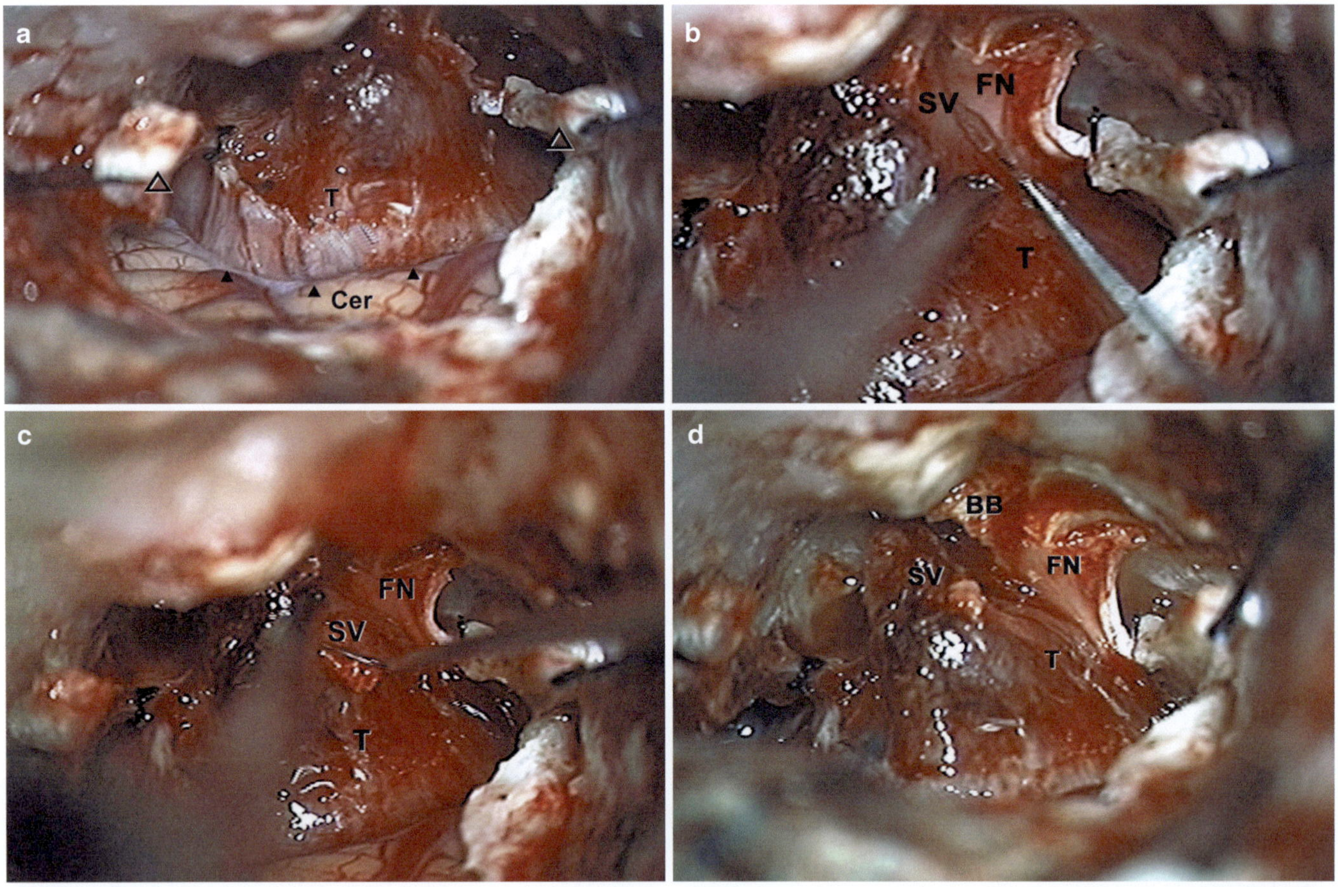

Fig. 11.4 (**a**) The dura is opened, and dural flaps are retained with dural stitches (open triangles). The tumor (T) is exposed. The cerebellum (CER) can be seen. The solid black triangles point to the interface between the tumor and cerebellum. (**b**) The facial nerve (FN) is identified. The edge of the facial nerve is confirmed using facial nerve stimulation. The plane between the facial nerve and the superior vestibular nerve (SV) is developed using sharp dissection. (**c**) The superior vestibular nerve is avulsed from its attachment away from the facial nerve using a right-angled instrument. (**d**) The superior vestibular nerve and the facial nerve are separated by Bill's bar (BB). The plane between the facial nerve and superior vestibular nerve is well developed in the lateral part of the internal auditory canal

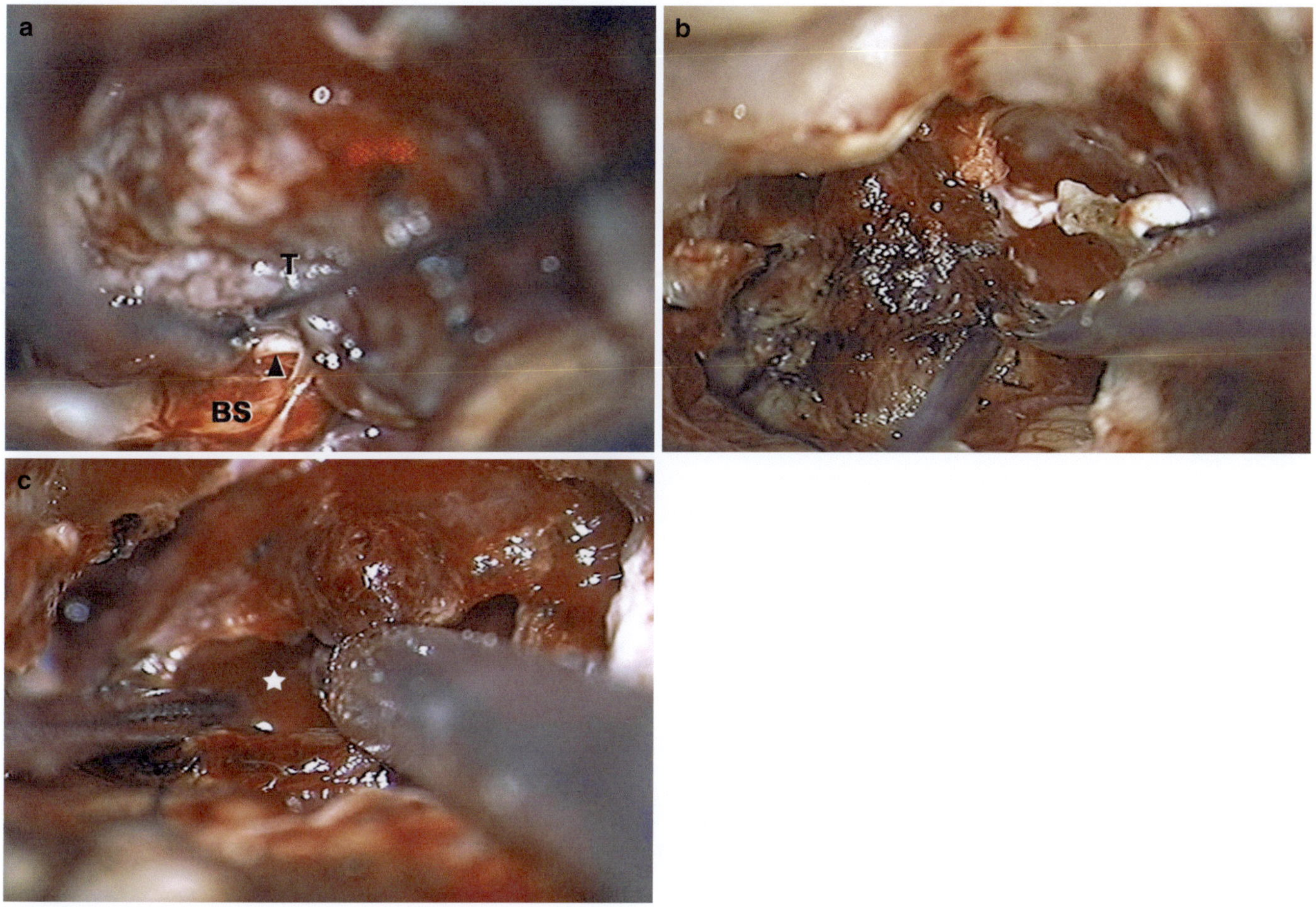

Fig. 11.5 (**a**) The inferior and medial poles of the tumor (T) are dissected. The facial nerve (black arrowhead) is identified, if possible, at the root entry zone at the brainstem (BS). (**b**) After the facial nerve is identified both laterally and medially, the tumor debulking is started. The posterior surface of the tumor is cauterized, and a piece of the tumor is removed and sent for biopsy. (**c**) Tumor debulking continues. A Cavitron ultrasonic surgical aspirator (CUSA) is used to evacuate the contents of the tumor. The remaining tumor cavity is visible (white star)

microdissection proceeds (Fig. 11.5b). When debulking is indicated, we prefer ultrasonic aspiration and typically have this tool available for every case (Fig. 11.5c). After the tumor capsule is opened and debulked or when the tumor is less than 2 cm and debulking is unnecessary, the mass is separated from the facial nerve (Fig. 11.6a–c).

We prefer sharp medial-to-lateral dissection of the tumor to minimize trauma to the nerves and brainstem. Use of electrocautery should be minimized by the use of thrombin-soaked Gelfoam®. When necessary, bipolar cautery should be used on a very low setting. The labyrinthine artery almost invariably runs between the seventh and eighth cranial nerves, and care must be exerted to avoid injuring the vessel inadvertently.

Complete tumor resection is always attempted. However, especially in patients with prior radiation, a portion of the tumor capsule can be very adherent to the facial nerve. We prefer to leave a patient with a small part of a benign tumor capsule than with facial palsy. This decision can be difficult to make intraoperatively and relies on the surgeon's judgment and experience. When considering leaving tumor behind, it should be remembered that when only a small portion of the tumor capsule remains, the risk of tumor recurrence is minimal [29].

After the tumor is removed, the surgical field is gently irrigated and meticulous hemostasis is maintained. A large piece of temporalis fascia is harvested and draped over the posterior aspect of the external auditory canal and aditus to provide an additional layer of protection against CSF leakage. The dura is approximated using a 4–10 Nurolon® suture (Fig. 11.7a). Subcutaneous fat is harvested through an incision in the left lower abdominal quadrant. This step is usually performed after the tumor has been dissected to minimize the time between harvesting the fat and using it to fill the defect.

The fat is cut into strips and kept in an antibiotic solution until it is used. The first fat strip is placed to cover the defect in the dura. It is tied in place using the tail of the suture used to approximate the dural flaps (Fig. 11.7b). This maneuver helps seal the dural defect and prevents the fat from being

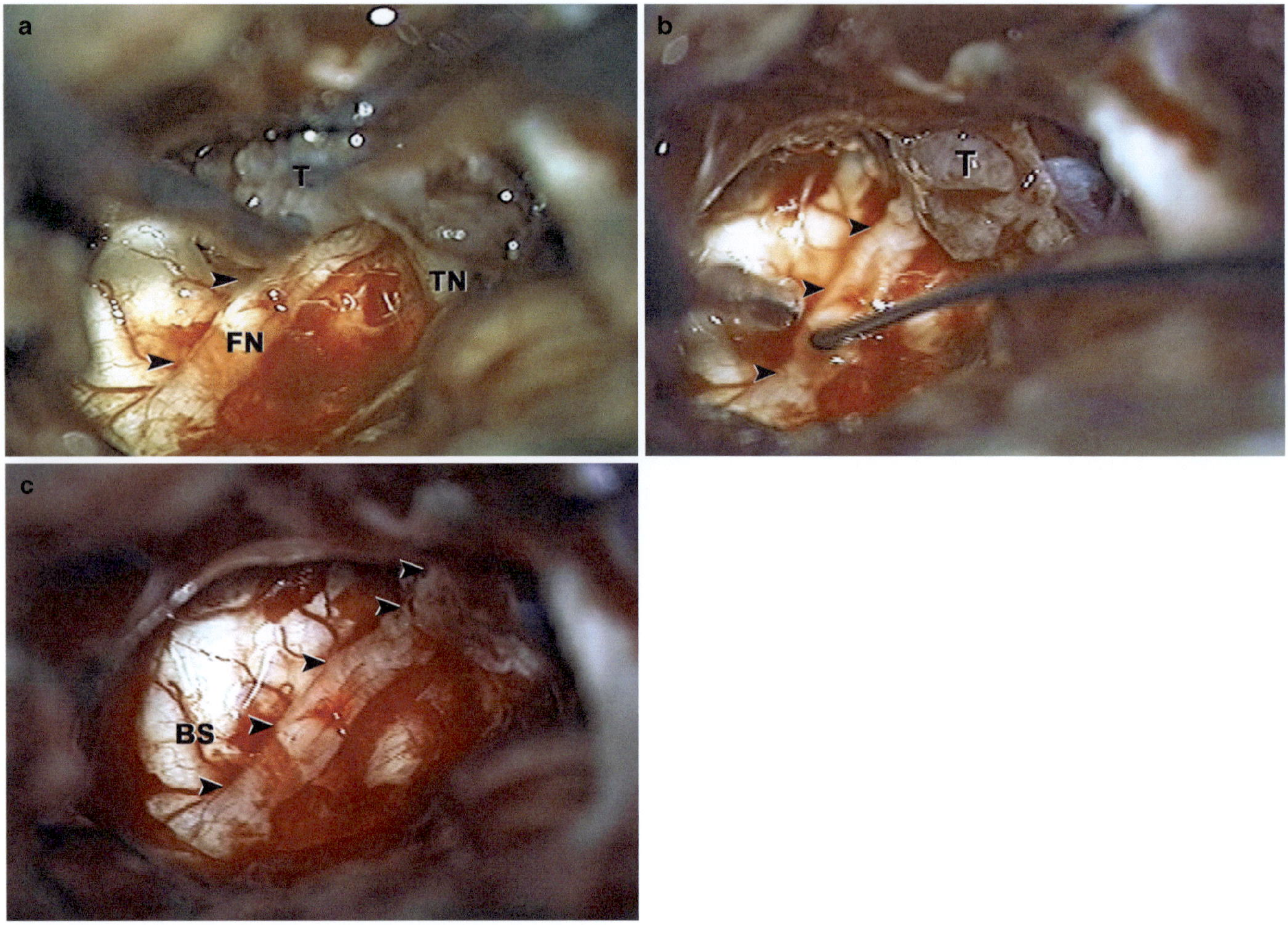

Fig. 11.6 (**a**) As tumor removal continues, the facial nerve (FN) becomes more apparent. The black arrowheads point to the course of the facial nerve from the root entry zone passing laterally. The trigeminal nerve (TN) can be seen at the superior pole of the tumor (T). (**b**) Intermittently, the responsiveness of the facial nerve (black arrowheads) to stimulation is confirmed during dissection. A small tumor remnant (T) is still visible. (**c**) Tumor removal is complete. The entire course of the facial nerve from the brainstem (BS) is visible (black arrowheads)

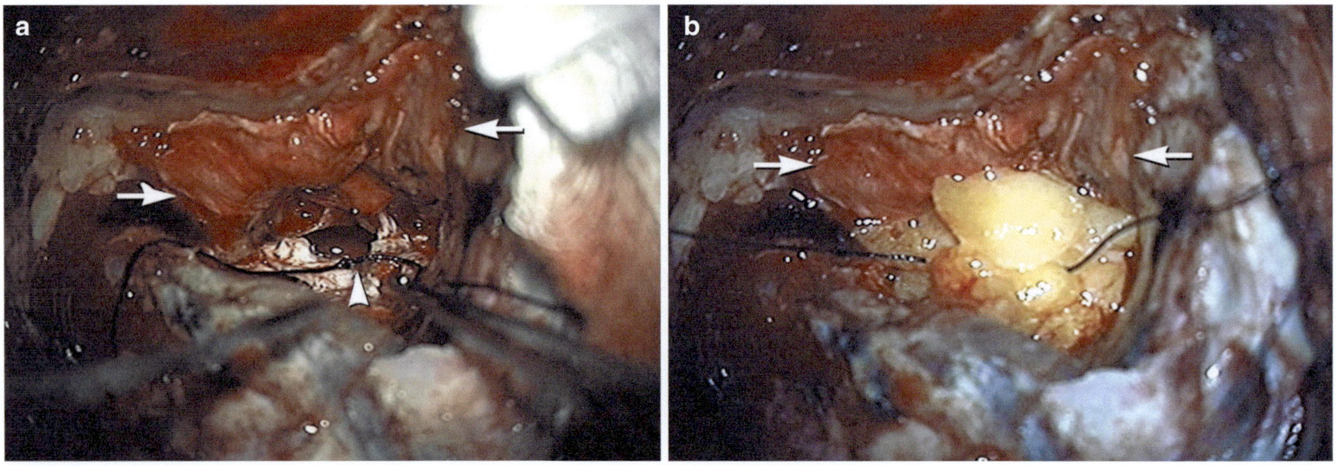

Fig. 11.7 (**a**) During closure, the dural flaps are approximated using 4-0 dural sutures (white triangle). A large piece of temporalis fascia is harvested and draped over the posterior external auditory canal wall and the mastoid antrum (white arrows) as an additional layer of protection against CSF leakage. (**b**) A strip of abdominal fat is placed within the dural defect, and the dural stitch is tied over the fat strip to fix it in place. The temporalis fascia (white arrows) is draped over the posterior canal wall and mastoid antrum

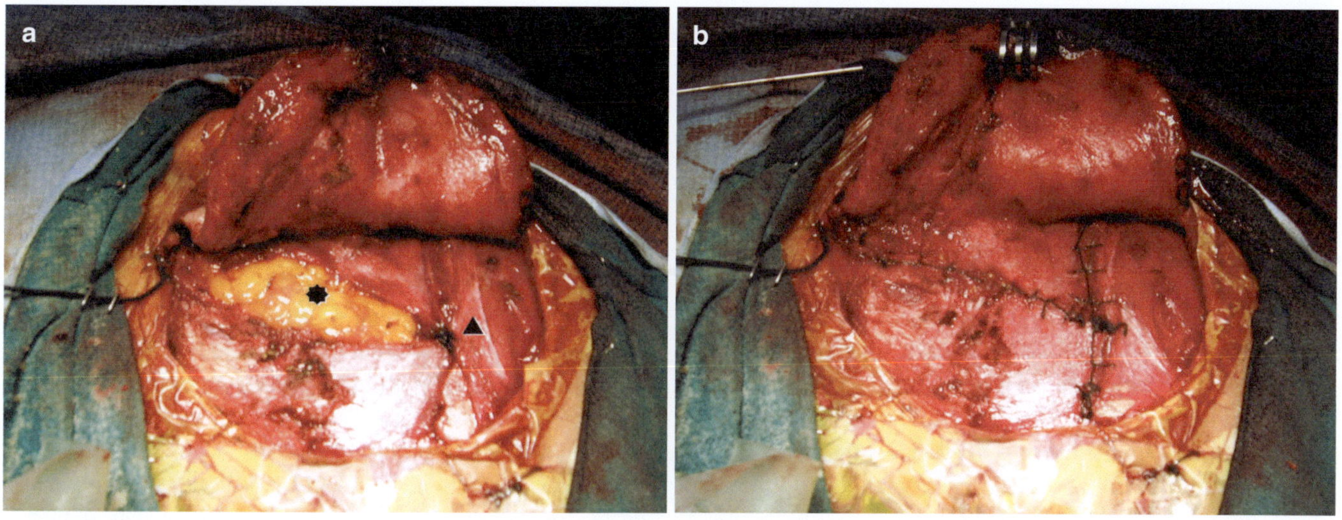

Fig. 11.8 (**a**) The musculoperiosteal layer is closed. The trifurcation, marked by the sutures, is reapposed (black triangle). Fat (black asterisk) is visible within the mastoid cavity and craniectomy defect. (**b**) The musculoperiosteal layer is closed completely in a watertight fashion

dislodged laterally or into the CPA. Several fat strips are used to fill the defect in the bone completely to the level of the periosteum. Tissue glue can also be applied to supplement the closure if suspicion of a potential leak is high. Other authors have advocated the use of hydroxyapatite bone cement in addition to adipose tissue to reconstruct the bony defect and to prevent CSF leakage [7]. Careful attention to occluding the mastoid air cells with bone wax also decreases the likelihood of the patient developing a CSF leak.

The musculoperiosteal layer is closed using 3-0 Vicryl sutures (Fig. 11.8a). If the flaps are elevated appropriately at the beginning of the procedure and kept well hydrated throughout the case, this layer often can be closed in a watertight fashion (Fig. 11.8b). Several 3-0 Vicryl® sutures are used to obliterate the dead space between the skin flap and the musculoperiosteal layer. A watertight closure of the skin incision follows. Finally, a light mastoid pressure dressing is applied.

Complications

The most dreaded complication of any CPA tumor surgery is injury to the surrounding vasculature, especially injury to the anterior inferior cerebellar artery or brainstem, which can cause a stroke. Fortunately, this risk, which is minimized by a good exposure, meticulous technique, and the experience of the skull-base team, is rare.

The most routinely feared complication of the translabyrinthine approach is injury to the facial nerve. Patients and nursing staff should be educated about delayed facial weakness, which can follow normal immediate postoperative facial function, which is usually attributed to nerve edema. When facial nerve integrity has been confirmed by nerve stimulation with good parameters, most patients recovered normal or near-normal facial function [30, 31]. We typically give patients three doses of dexamethasone in the first 24 h after surgery; we then discontinue it unless a delayed facial nerve palsy occurs. There has been continued publication of data that quantifies the high risk of poor wound healing and infection when postoperative glucocorticoids are used.

Other complications include aseptic or bacterial meningitis, CSF leakage, hematomas, transient or permanent neurologic deficits, and standard postoperative risks such as deep venous thrombosis, pneumonia, and cardiac complications. Reported rates of meningitis range from 1.6% to 4% [32–36], and reported rates of CSF leakage range from 1.4% to 8% [13, 16, 33, 34, 37]. With large tumors, the risk of CSF leakage is closer to 15% [32, 35]. When leaks do occur, CSF diversion with lumbar drainage for 3 or 4 days is our initial treatment. In our experience, CSF leaks requiring permanent CSF diversion are usually due to elevated intracranial pressure.

Outcomes

For tumors removed through the TL approach, the most current otolaryngological and neurosurgical texts cite the rate of operative mortality at less than 1% and perhaps as low as 0.1–0.2%, even with large tumors [12]. There was only 1 death in an Italian series of 175 patients with tumors at least 3 cm [16].

Recurrence rates after TL operations are low. Shelton reported five recurrences in a series of 1668 TL resections of acoustic neuromas [38]. Thedinger and colleagues reported a recurrence rate of 0.5% in 999 patients with acoustic or glomus jugulare tumors [39]. After a mean follow-up of

11 years, Schmerber and colleagues reported no cases of recurrences in 91 patients with acoustic tumors [40]. Despite the past criticism that the TL approach is inappropriate for most large tumors, other authors have concluded that total tumor removal is possible in most patients, regardless of the size of their tumor [32]. However, as expected, the risk of complications increases as the size of the tumor increases.

The main outcome measures of the TL approach are the extent of tumor resection and postoperative facial nerve function.

Comparison of outcomes between different surgical approaches in vestibular schwannoma surgery is complicated by multiple biases. Significant selection bias is present as certain tumor characteristics favor one surgical approach over another. For example, small, intracanalicular tumors are much more likely to be removed via the middle fossa approach. Surgeons also frequently have an intrinsic preference for one approach over another due to training and experience.

When reviewing the literature, a "good" facial nerve function outcome is a House-Brackmann grade I or II. Good facial nerve outcomes occur in 97–100% of patients with isolated intracanalicular tumors, in 92.5–95% of those with tumors smaller than 2 cm, and in 63% of those with tumors larger than 2 cm [21, 41–44]. Briggs and colleagues reported that 90% of their patients with tumors smaller than 2 cm had grade 1 or 2 function [13]. Mass and colleagues found that 76% of 258 patients undergoing the TL approach had grade I or II facial function 1 year after follow-up [33]. However, this study included 29 patients with tumors larger than 35 mm. Delayed facial nerve palsy appearing more than 72 h after surgery had been reported [45]. Its incidence is estimated at 5%, but most patients regain their immediate postoperative baseline within a few months. In our experience, delayed facial palsy that persists longer than expected is attributable to postoperative edema.

An important consideration before any surgical intervention is the patient's perception of outcome compared with standard rates of improvement reported in the literature. Ryzenman and colleagues analyzed the self-reports of 1595 patients who underwent acoustic neuroma surgery via any surgical approach [46]. Postoperatively, 45% of the patients reported worsened facial weakness after surgery. However, 70% were "quite a bit" or "very much" content with their quality of life. Similarly, Martin and colleagues analyzed the self-reports of 76 patients who underwent TL resection of acoustic tumors performed by the same surgical team [47]. The quality of life subjectively reported by the patients was reduced compared with their objective results. We believe that the key to matching patients' expectations to any objective outcomes starts with consistent preoperative counseling in a multidisciplinary (neurosurgery and otolaryngology) skull-base clinic.

Postoperative Care

Similar to the other phases of treatment, postoperative care is performed jointly by the neurosurgery and otology services. Patients are admitted to the neurosurgical intensive care unit overnight for the performance of frequent neurologic exams. Patients spend the first night on the neurosurgical service and are then transferred to the otology service. If there are new neurologic deficits or other concerns, an immediate postoperative computed tomography (CT) scan is performed. Otherwise, the patient is closely monitored clinically until the postoperative MRI is obtained. Unless a new deficit is present, minimal steroids are used and rapidly tapered. Patients appear to have less postoperative nausea than in the retrosigmoid approach, likely due to complete obliteration of the labyrinthine structures. Unless there is a concern for venous compromise, intravenous fluids are only continued until patients tolerate appropriate oral fluid intake.

The other phases of care are similar to the modern postoperative care of patients following craniotomy. Mobilization is performed as soon as it is tolerated, preferably starting as soon as the patient is recovered from anesthesia. Aside from the multiple known benefits of mobilization, this also encourages early discontinuation of urinary catheters. The patient's diet is similarly advanced as soon as he or she is recovered from anesthesia. Prevention of deep vein thrombosis begins with sequential compression devices, which are placed before induction in the operating room. Chemoprophylaxis is added on the morning of postoperative day 2 and continued until discharge. A mastoid dressing is placed in the operating room and removed on postoperative day 2. When available, patients benefit from specialized nursing staff that frequently cares for patients following skull-base surgery. At our institution, this tailored care allows for patients with lumbar subarachnoid drains to leave the intensive care unit and still be cared for by nurses with experience in managing CSF drains.

Patients are usually discharged on the morning of postoperative day 3 and are seen in clinic at 2 weeks for suture removal. They are seen again at 6 weeks and—provided there are no concerns—at 1 year with repeat MRI to evaluate for recurrence. In patients with known residual tumor following surgery, a 2-year MRI is used to confirm a lack of progression, followed by a 5-year MRI to confirm stability [40].

The management of postoperative facial weakness deserves special attention. Patients should be counseled regarding the possibility for immediate and delayed facial weakness. Corneal protection is important for any patient with incomplete eye closure (lagophthalmos). Patients with concomitant V1 dysfunction should be counseled to be extra vigilant. Common methods of corneal protection include hourly administration of lubricating drops with nightly lubricating ointment. Lubricating drops should be preservative-free as frequent administration of preservatives can disrupt the tear film and promote inflammation. Methods of temporary eye closure include eyelid taping, patch placement, and temporary tarsorrhaphy. For long-term lagophthalmos, gold weight implantation is frequently used.

Conclusions

The TL approach is a versatile surgical tool for the removal of acoustic tumors. Close cooperation is needed between members of the neurosurgical and neuro-otological team to achieve good results.

References

1. House WF, Hitselberger WE. Transtemporal bone microsurgical removal of acoustic neuromas. Tumors of the cerebellopontine angle. Arch Otolaryngol. 1964;80:720–31.
2. Hol MK, Bosman AJ, Snik AF, et al. Bone-anchored hearing aids in unilateral inner ear deafness: an evaluation of audiometric and patient outcome measurements. Otol Neurotol. 2005;26:999–1006.
3. Harner SG, Laws ER Jr. Clinical findings in patients with acoustic neurinoma. Mayo Clin Proc. 1983;58:721–8.
4. Harner SG, Daube JR, Ebersold MJ, Beatty CW. Improved preservation of facial nerve function with use of electrical monitoring during removal of acoustic neuromas. Mayo Clin Proc. 1987;62:92–102.
5. House JW, Brackmann DE. Facial nerve grading system. Otolaryngol Head Neck Surg. 1985;93:146–7.
6. Ho SY, Kveton JF. Acoustic neuroma. Assessment and management. Otolaryngol Clin N Am. 2002;35:393–404, viii.
7. Day JD, Chen DA, Arriaga M. Translabyrinthine approach for acoustic neuroma. Neurosurgery. 2004;54:391–5.
8. Greenberg MS. Tumors. In: Handbook of neurosurgery. New York: Thieme; 2006.
9. Silverstein H, McDaniel A, Norrell H, Haberkamp T. Hearing preservation after acoustic neuroma surgery with intraoperative direct eighth cranial nerve monitoring: part II. A classification of results. Otolaryngol Head Neck Surg. 1986;95:285–91.
10. El Kashlan HK, Eisenmann D, Kileny PR. Auditory brain stem response in small acoustic neuromas. Ear Hear. 2000;21:257–62.
11. House JW, Waluch V, Jackler RK. Magnetic resonance imaging in acoustic neuroma diagnosis. Ann Otol Rhinol Laryngol. 1986;95:16–20.
12. Sampath P, Long DM. Acoustic neuroma. In: Winn HR, editor. Youmans neurological surgery. 5th ed. Philadelphia: Saunders; 2004. p. 1147–68.
13. Briggs RJ, Fabinyi G, Kaye AH. Current management of acoustic neuromas: review of surgical approaches and outcomes. J Clin Neurosci. 2000;7:521–6.
14. Karpinos M, Teh BS, Zeck O, et al. Treatment of acoustic neuroma: stereotactic radiosurgery vs. microsurgery. Int J Radiat Oncol Biol Phys. 2002;54:1410–21.
15. Mamikoglu B, Esquivel CR, Wiet RJ. Comparison of facial nerve function results after translabyrinthine and retrosigmoid approach in medium-sized tumors. Arch Otolaryngol Head Neck Surg. 2003;129:429–31.
16. Sanna M, Russo A, Taibah A, et al. Enlarged translabyrinthine approach for the management of large and giant acoustic neuromas: a report of 175 consecutive cases. Ann Otol Rhinol Laryngol. 2004;113:319–28.
17. Anderson DE, Leonetti J, Wind JJ, et al. Resection of large vestibular schwannomas: facial nerve preservation in the context of surgical approach and patient-assessed outcome. J Neurosurg. 2005;102:643–9.
18. Tringali S, Bertholon P, Chelikh L, et al. Hearing preservation after modified translabyrinthine approach performed to remove a vestibular schwannoma. Ann Otol Rhinol Laryngol. 2004;113:152–5.
19. Patni AH, Kartush JM. Staged resection of large acoustic neuromas. Otolaryngol Head Neck Surg. 2005;132:11–9.
20. Sanna M, Caylan R. Atlas of acoustic neurinoma microsurgery. Stuttgart: Thieme; 1998.
21. Brackmann DE, Crawford JV, Green JD. Cerebellopontine angle tumors. In: Bailey BJ, Johnson JT, Newlands SD, editors. Head and neck surgery—otolaryngology. 4th ed. Philadelphia: Lippincott Williams & Wilkins; 2006. p. 2207–30.
22. Hammerschlag PE, Cohen NL. Intraoperative monitoring of facial nerve function in cerebellopontine angle surgery. Otolaryngol Head Neck Surg. 1990;103:681–4.
23. Benecke JE Jr, Calder HB, Chadwick G. Facial nerve monitoring during acoustic neuroma removal. Laryngoscope. 1987;97:697–700.
24. Kwartler JA, Luxford WM, Atkins J, Shelton C. Facial nerve monitoring in acoustic tumor surgery. Otolaryngol Head Neck Surg. 1991;104:814–7.
25. Nissen AJ, Sikand A, Welsh JE, et al. A multifactorial analysis of facial nerve results in surgery for cerebellopontine angle tumors. Ear Nose Throat J. 1997;76:37–40.
26. Uziel A, Benezech J, Frerebeau P. Intraoperative facial nerve monitoring in posterior fossa acoustic neuroma surgery. Otolaryngol Head Neck Surg. 1993;108:126–34.
27. Silverstein H, Rosenberg SI, Flanzer J, Seidman MD. Intraoperative facial nerve monitoring in acoustic neuroma surgery. Am J Otol. 1993;14:524–32.
28. Kartush JM, Lundy LB. Facial nerve outcome in acoustic neuroma surgery. Otolaryngol Clin N Am. 1992;25:623–47.
29. El Kashlan HK, Zeitoun H, Arts HA, et al. Recurrence of acoustic neuroma after incomplete resection. Am J Otol. 2000;21:389–92.
30. Isaacson B, Kileny PR, El Kashlan HK. Prediction of long-term facial nerve outcomes with intraoperative nerve monitoring. Otol Neurotol. 2005;26:270–3.
31. Megerian CA, McKenna MJ, Ojemann RG. Delayed facial paralysis after acoustic neuroma surgery: factors influencing recovery. Am J Otol. 1996;17:630–3.
32. Mamikoglu B, Wiet RJ, Esquivel CR. Translabyrinthine approach for the management of large and giant vestibular schwannomas. Otol Neurotol. 2002;23:224–7.
33. Mass SC, Wiet RJ, Dinces E. Complications of the translabyrinthine approach for the removal of acoustic neuromas. Arch Otolaryngol Head Neck Surg. 1999;125:801–4.
34. Rodgers GK, Luxford WM. Factors affecting the development of cerebrospinal fluid leak and meningitis after translabyrinthine acoustic tumor surgery. Laryngoscope. 1993;103:959–62.
35. Lanman TH, Brackmann DE, Hitselberger WE, Subin B. Report of 190 consecutive cases of large acoustic tumors (vestibular schwannoma) removed via the translabyrinthine approach. J Neurosurg. 1999;90:617–23.
36. Sluyter S, Graamans K, Tulleken CA, Van Veelen CW. Analysis of the results obtained in 120 patients with large acoustic neuromas

surgically treated via the translabyrinthine-transtentorial approach. J Neurosurg. 2001;94:61–6.
37. Khrais TH, Falcioni M, Taibah A, et al. Cerebrospinal fluid leak prevention after translabyrinthine removal of vestibular schwannoma. Laryngoscope. 2004;114:1015–20.
38. Shelton C. Unilateral acoustic tumors: how often do they recur after translabyrinthine removal? Laryngoscope. 1995;105:958–66.
39. Thedinger BA, Glasscock ME III, Cueva RA, Jackson CG. Postoperative radiographic evaluation after acoustic neuroma and glomus jugulare tumor removal. Laryngoscope. 1992;102:261–6.
40. Schmerber S, Palombi O, Boubagra K, et al. Long-term control of vestibular schwannoma after a translabyrinthine complete removal. Neurosurgery. 2005;57:693–8.
41. Jain Y, Falcioni M, Agarwal M, et al. Total facial paralysis after vestibular schwannoma surgery: probability of regaining normal function. Ann Otol Rhinol Laryngol. 2004;113:706–10.
42. Kaylie DM, Gilbert E, Horgan MA, et al. Acoustic neuroma surgery outcomes. Otol Neurotol. 2001;22:686–9.
43. Darrouzet V, Martel J, Enee V, et al. Vestibular schwannoma surgery outcomes: our multidisciplinary experience in 400 cases over 17 years. Laryngoscope. 2004;114:681–8.
44. Wiet RJ, Mamikoglu B, Odom L, Hoistad DL. Long-term results of the first 500 cases of acoustic neuroma surgery. Otolaryngol Head Neck Surg. 2001;124:645–51.
45. Grant GA, Rostomily RR, Kim DK, et al. Delayed facial palsy after resection of vestibular schwannoma. J Neurosurg. 2002;97:93–6.
46. Ryzenman JM, Pensak ML, Tew JM Jr. Facial paralysis and surgical rehabilitation: a quality of life analysis in a cohort of 1,595 patients after acoustic neuroma surgery. Otol Neurotol. 2005;26:516–21.
47. Martin HC, Sethi J, Lang D, et al. Patient-assessed outcomes after excision of acoustic neuroma: postoperative symptoms and quality of life. J Neurosurg. 2001;94:211–6.

Hearing Rehabilitation Following Acoustic Neuroma Surgery

12

Cameron C. Wick, Nedim Durakovic, Jacques A. Herzog, and Craig A. Buchman

Hearing loss is the most frequent symptom caused by vestibular schwannomas [1]. Aside from the rare tumor that presents itself for a hearing-preservation surgery, the majority of tumors will likely result in deafness of the affected ear regardless of the intervention modality. The natural history of hearing in observed tumors also predicts eventual decline [2]. Hearing loss attributed to vestibular schwannomas remains a primary driver for poor quality of life in this patient population [3, 4].

The auditory system is designed for hearing from two ears (binaural hearing). When bilateral input is lost, patients suffer from poor sound localization and speech discrimination in noise. The following text will review the audiologic disadvantages of single-sided deafness and the evolution of hearing rehabilitation following vestibular schwannoma surgery.

Unilateral Hearing Loss

The auditory system is designed for binaural input. When one ear suffers from hearing loss, it manifests as difficulty with sound localization and speech recognition, particularly in the presence of background noise. The clinical impact of unilateral hearing loss is dependent on the patient's daily listening environment. For instance, children in a noisy classroom often have a background signal-to-noise ratio (SNR) of 2–9 dB. Children with severe-to-profound unilateral hearing loss in that environment have a 22–35% of chance of repeating a grade and a 12–41% chance of requiring additional educational support [5–7]. Unilateral hearing loss in children is an independent risk factor for poor language comprehension and oral expression scores [8]. Adults with unilateral hearing loss are also subject to the negative psychological and social consequences of this handicap. Recurring adult themes include anxiety about potential hearing loss in the contralateral ear, strong negative emotions including embarrassment and frustration, and negative coping strategies such as withdrawal from social engagements [9]. In a survey of 51 patients who had undergone cerebellopontine angle surgery, the postoperative decreased quality of life strongly correlated with their unilateral profound hearing loss [10].

The audiologic benefits of binaural hearing are based on the principles of binaural summation, binaural squelch, and the head shadow effect. Together these phenomena allow the brain to detect subtle interaural time and intensity differences that facilitate sound localization and improved hearing in noise. Binaural summation occurs when sound is captured from each ear independently and integrated along the auditory pathway. This integration process results in an internal amplification of 4–6 dB [11].

Binaural squelch refers to a patient's ability to listen only to the sound of interest when additional sound sources are present. For instance, honing in during a conversation amidst a loud background environment such as a cocktail party, thus named the cocktail party effect. Binaural squelch also occurs as sound is transmitted along the subcortical and cortical auditory pathways. The threshold benefit of binaural squelch is modest, with only a 1–2 dB increase, but the ability to understand speech at a lower SNR (i.e., loud environment) is significant [12, 13].

Sound travels as an energy wave through space. In the binaural condition, the energy waves arrive at each ear with a slightly different time and intensity. The interaural time difference (ITD) and interaural level difference (ILD) are critical for sound localization. High-frequency sounds, which have wavelengths that are shorter than the circumference of the skull, are subject to further modification secondary to head interference. The interference accentuates the ILD and creates a head shadow effect. For high frequencies, the head shadow effect can result in a 15–20 dB ILD, while lower frequencies have only a 5 dB ILD. Together, binaural sum-

C. C. Wick (✉) · N. Durakovic · J. A. Herzog · C. A. Buchman
Department of Otolaryngology—Head and Neck Surgery, Washington University School of Medicine, St. Louis, MO, USA
e-mail: cameron.wick@wustl.edu

N. C. Bambakidis et al. (eds.), *Surgery of the Cerebellopontine Angle*, https://doi.org/10.1007/978-3-031-12507-2_12

mation, binaural squelch, and the head shadow effect enable patients to localize sound and improve speech comprehension in noise. Without binaural input these elements are lost, thus creating the difficulties seen among patients who suffer from unilateral hearing loss.

Hearing Rehabilitation

Hearing rehabilitation options are dependent on the status of a patient's external ear, cochlea, and cochlear nerve. Some tumors may present with characteristics favorable for a hearing preservation surgical approach. These factors include tumors that originate from the superior vestibular nerve, the presence of cerebrospinal fluid between the lateral tumor edge and the cochlea (i.e., fundal cap), and small tumor size [14–16]. In patients with hearing preserved after surgery, amplification of the operative ear depends solely on the amount of residual hearing that remains after the procedure. The American Academy of Otolaryngology-Head and Neck Surgery (AAO-HNS) and the Gardner-Robertson (GR) hearing classification systems both designate serviceable hearing as greater than 50% on speech discrimination testing and less than 50 dB pure tone average (Table 12.1) [17, 18]. Good hearing (AAO-HNS Class A) may not require additional amplification, while compromised but preserved hearing (AAO-HNS Classes B and C) will likely benefit from a traditional hearing aid. Patients with a speech discrimination less than 50% (AAO-HNS Class D) have a less predictable response to amplification in the affected ear. Some patients may be bothered by poor clarity from the amplification, while others may appreciate improved sound localization from the bilateral input. If some degree of hearing persists, then at least a hearing aid trial should be considered before moving to the single-sided deafness rehabilitation options.

Table 12.1 Classification systems for vestibular schwannoma audiometric outcomes. American Academy of Otolaryngology-Head and Neck Surgery (AAO-HNS) class A and Gardner-Robertson (GR) class I represent good hearing that may not require additional amplification. Serviceable hearing is defined as equal or better to AAO-HNS class B or GR class II hearing

Hearing classification schemes		
	Pure tone average (dB)	Speech discrimination (%)
AAO-HNS		
A	≤30	>70
B	>30 and ≤50	≥50
C	>50	≥50
D	Any level	<50
Gardner-Robertson		
I	0–30	70–100
II	31–50	50–69
III	51–90	5–49
IV	>91	1–4
V	Not testable	0

In traditional cerebellopontine angle surgery where hearing is not preserved, the external ear and cochlea remain intact but the cochlear nerve is damaged secondary to the tumor or tumor resection. This creates a unilateral, profound sensorineural hearing loss with no ability to rehabilitate using a traditional hearing aid or cochlear implant (CI). Therefore, the mainstays of auditory rehabilitation in this patient population have focused on bringing sound from the deafened ear over to the healthy ear.

Contralateral Routing of Signal

The concept of bringing noise from a deafened ear to the better ear via modified hearing aids connected with a "sound tube" was first suggested in 1960 [19]. In 1964, Harry Teder, while working at Telex, created a patent that coined the term contralateral routing of sound (CROS), and by 1965 Harford and Barry introduced the first CROS hearing aid [20]. This device consisted of a microphone attached to eyeglasses on the hearing impaired side. The microphone detected sound from the deafened side and transmitted it via a wire that ran across the eyeglass frame into a hearing aid placed in the better hearing ear. The classic CROS scenario implies normal hearing in the contralateral ear. Harford and Barry also developed a Bi-CROS system in which sound presented on the side of the better hearing ear could also be amplified if that ear had hearing loss. This basic construct of a microphone on the deafened ear connected via a wire to a hearing aid on the better hearing ear, with or without the eyeglasses, remained in place until 2004. While this version of the CROS was a useful option for patients with monaural hearing, the wire attachment was bulky, and patients disliked the blocked feeling, termed occlusal effect, of having a hearing aid placed in the ear canal of a normal hearing ear [21].

In 2004, Siemens developed the first wireless CROS device, called the e2e Wireless®, which has since become the industry standard and has improved patient satisfaction [22]. Directional microphones and improved processing strategies have also improved performance [23]. However, the wireless adaptation does not eliminate the occlusal effect or the perceived cosmetic aspect of wearing bilateral hearing devices. Additionally, insurance coverage in the United States for hearing aids, including the CROS system, is sporadic, and the out-of-pocket expense can be a barrier to access. Still, the noninvasive nature of the device makes it a logical first step for patients entertaining the idea of hearing rehabilitation following lateral skull base surgery.

The first goal of a CROS device is to enhance the SNR, thus improving speech clarity in background noise. The SNR is particularly problematic when the primary speech signal and background noise are spatially separated. If the speaker is talking into the deafened ear with a CROS device in place, the device has the potential to increase clarity of the spoken word by creating an artificial head shadow effect and lowering the speech reception threshold of the spoken word [24, 25]. Conversely, if the ambient noise is presented to the deafened side with a CROS device, there is potential for degradation of speech intelligibility secondary to enhancement of the background noise [25–27].

The second goal of a CROS device is to provide sound awareness on the deafened side. Because CROS aids do not restore the ITD, ILD, and natural head shadow effect, they will not enable the precise localization that is seen with binaural hearing. However, CROS users should have an improved ability to tell from which side of the body sound originates. In a sample of 21 patients with unilateral hearing loss, only 10% could correctly identify which side of their body a sound originated from prior to using a CROS aid. After 4 weeks of use, that sound awareness improved to over 40% [25]. Older CROS aids focused on transmission of high-frequency sound (above 1000 Hz) that is associated with the head shadow effect. Modern CROS processors can transmit the full bandwidth of sound, and this has potential for further improvement in sound awareness on the deafened side but still lacks the ability to precisely localize a noise [27].

Osseointegrated Hearing Implants

The skull's density enables an alternative method for stimulation of the contralateral ear. Bone conduction has an interaural attenuation of 5 dB or less. Therefore, rather than transmitting sound via air like a traditional hearing aid, osseoconductive devices vibrate the skull, which carries the sound through the densely packed bone and into the inner ear. Osseoconductive hearing devices were proposed as early as Roman antiquity. In the eighteenth and nineteenth centuries, crude devices made of wood, metal, or glass were constructed but ultimately failed due to poor sound attenuation through the scalp or discomfort when they were applied to teeth [28].

Pioneering work from Brånemark in Sweden around 1965 revolutionized bone anchored devices. Working with titanium dental implants, his group discovered that osteocytes in direct contact with titanium adhere via a process called osseointegration. This discovery led to titanium's wide utilization in dental and craniofacial reconstructions [29, 30]. Then in 1977, Brånemark's partner, Anders Tjellström, recognized the potential for osseointegrated titanium to conduct sound, paving the way for modern osseoconductive device systems. Tjellström was the first to place a percutaneous abutment attached to a titanium implant in the mastoid bone [31]. A modified hearing aid that vibrates rather than produces sound waves in the air could then be attached to the abutment and propagate sound energy via the skull and into a healthy cochlea. Tjellström's initial patients all had chronic ear disease that prohibited traditional hearing aid placement. After 5 years, the benefit persisted and patient satisfaction remained high, which led to an entire field of osseointegrated hearing devices [32]. The bone anchored hearing aid (BAHA®) device became commercially available in 1987, and it was approved for conductive hearing loss by the U.S. Food and Drug Administration (FDA) in 1996. The initial American experience in forty patients with chronic ear disease mirrored the positive results reported by Tjellström [33]. As of 2010, more than 80,000 osseointegrated devices have been implanted worldwide. In 2002, the FDA approved the BAHA for the indication of single-sided deafness (SSD), and since then Ponto® has also become commercially available.

Osseointegrated devices do require surgical implantation. The surgical steps have evolved considerably. The titanium implant is placed into the mastoid bone approximately 5.5 cm behind the external auditory canal. Initially, the titanium implant was placed at a separate stage to facilitate osseointegration without any load-bearing forces. This technique is still sometimes used in young children or temporal bones that have received radiation, but in general both the titanium implant and its percutaneous abutment can be implanted in a single procedure [34]. The soft-tissue work has also evolved. Initially, no soft tissue reduction was performed, but some patients experienced adverse skin reactions. In an effort to reduce skin reaction, surgeons began thinning the subcutaneous tissue around the abutment. The original soft tissue reduction technique described by the Nijmegen group called for a linear incision, wide soft tissue reduction, and then the implant placed in the middle of the incision [35, 36]. Additional modifications, such as a semicircular skin incision with the implant punched through the base of the pedicle (U-graft technique) or use of a dermatome, were also suggested [37]. Recently, a minimally invasive Ponto surgery (MIPS) technique has been described that forgoes any skin incision and allows placement of the implant through a 5-mm hole created with a skin punch [38]. In general, the surgical techniques have trended toward a single-stage procedure with less need for soft reduction and more emphasis placed on proper skin handling with minimal cauterization. The osseointegration process takes time, and initial protocols suggested waiting 3 months to ensure proper healing before activation with the vibrating hearing aid. Evidence suggests that earlier activation is safe, with most centers loading the implant 6–8 weeks after implantation. Some data also suggest earlier loading may be feasible [39].

Major surgical complications following implantation of an osseointegrated device are rare. Potential injury to the dura or a dural venous sinus is mitigated by drilling the osseous well in a stepwise fashion and confirming that healthy bone is present at the depth of the well prior to implant placement. Two cases of intracerebral abscess following implantation have been reported [40, 41]. Failure of osseointegration is a relatively rare event and can be precipitated by trauma, infection, prior radiation, or improper technique that results in osteocyte death secondary to overheating. The rate of implant extrusion is 3–4% [42–44].

Soft tissue adverse events are unfortunately more common with most reports suggesting a rate between 8.7% and 13%, but some studies suggest the rate is 30% or higher [42, 44]. The skin reactions can be classified according to the Holgers grading system (Table 12.2) [45]. The majority of skin reactions are mild (Holgers grade 1 or 2) and can be treated with topical steroids or topical antibiotics. The presence of granulation tissue (Holgers grade 3) can be addressed with silver nitrate cauterization or the addition of oral antibiotics. More serious infections (Holgers grade 4) may require removal of the abutment or resection of overgrown skin. The rate of revision surgery is from 7% to 12% and is typically due to skin overgrowth (Fig. 12.1) [42, 44].

In an effort to limit the adverse events associated with a percutaneous implant, two modifications have been introduced. The first variation is a transcutaneous magnet that employs the same titanium implant placed during a traditional osseointegrated implant; but rather than attaching a percutaneous abutment, there is a subcutaneous magnet attached to the implant. The magnet is then coupled to a device that rests on the skin. The device vibrates, and that vibration is transmitted to the subcutaneous magnet and then to the titanium implant. This type of transcutaneous model has the benefit of no abutment protruding through the skin. Despite this, the large magnets needed to couple with the external vibrating bone conduction hearing aid can still produce skin related complications [46]. Furthermore, the sound energy has to pass through the soft tissue of the scalp (i.e., transcutaneous), which causes approximately 10 dB of sound attenuation.

Table 12.2 Holgers grading system for soft tissue reactions around percutaneous osseointegrated devices

Scale	Description
0	No irritation
1	Slight redness
2	Red and moist without granulation tissue
3	Red and moist with granulation tissue
4	Removal of skin-penetrating implant necessary due to infection

The second variation is a direct-drive bone conduction system. As of 2020, there are two FDA-approved direct-drive bone conduction systems, specifically MED-EL's Bonebridge® and Cochlear Corporation's Osia®. Their utility in unilateral hearing loss is still being studied but should mirror the previously described pros/cons [47]. There are some differences in how these devices function. For instance, the Bonebridge® involves drilling a well in the mastoid cavity to house a floating-mass transducer (FMT). The FMT attaches to the cortical mastoid bone via two titanium screws. An external processor with two microphones connects to the internal receiver via a magnet. Sound received by the external processor is sent to the internal receiver, which drives the FMT to vibrate skull [48]. This design has the advantage of requiring a smaller magnet, and it eliminates soft tissue attenuation. The surgical steps are slightly more complex secondary to the larger space needed to hold the FMT, and its utilization following lateral skull base

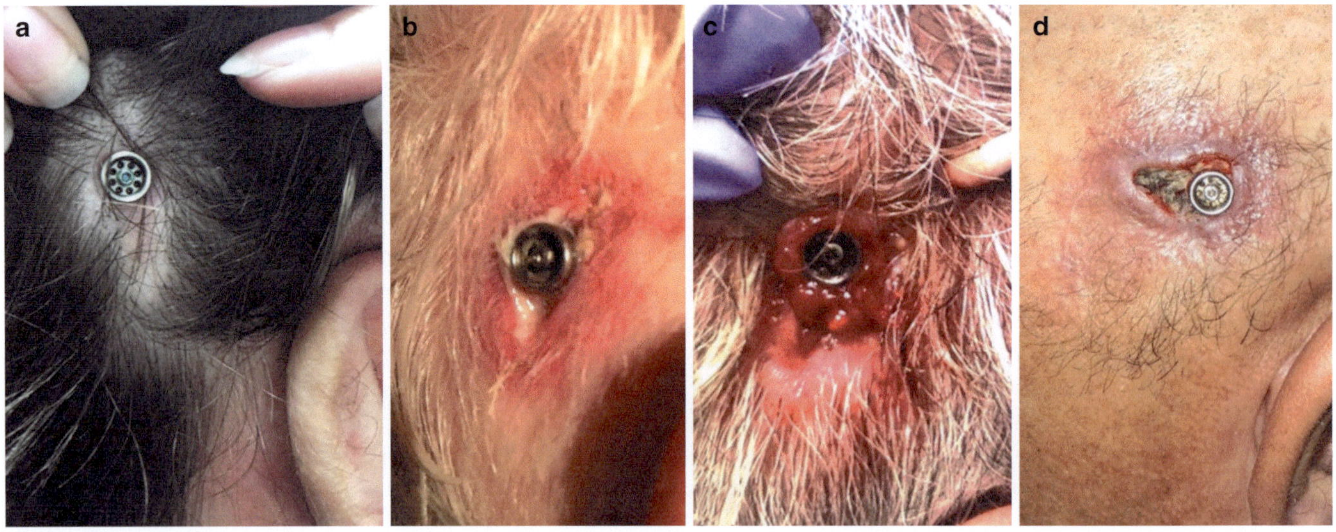

Fig. 12.1 Percutaneous osseointegrated device examples. All cases depict a right ear. (**a**) Healthy appearance of a percutaneous abutment (Holger Grade 0). (**b**) Erythema and moisture around the abutment indicative of a soft tissue infection (Holger Grade 2). (**c**) Robust granulation tissue around the abutment (Holger Grade 3). (**d**) Wound breakdown and granulation tissue following application of silver nitrate (Holger Grade 3)

surgery has not been widely reported. Rather than using a FMT, the Cochlear Corporation's Osia® implant uses a titanium screw identical to the implant used with their BAHA® system. Attached to a titanium screw is a piezoelectric driver that rests under the skin and drives the bone conduction. Both the direct-drive bone conduction system and the transcutaneous magnet system should be used with caution if future magnetic resonance imaging (MRI) is necessary to monitor cerebellopontine angle or intracranial pathology. Both devices have a large metallic artifact secondary to the size of the FMT and internal magnet [49].

Other nonsurgical forms of osseoconductive hearing aids exist but have shown varied commercial success. Bone conduction hearing aids, attached with a headband or a soft elastic band, are available. One more innovative device is the SoundBite®. This system had a behind-the-ear microphone that sent a wireless signal to a transducer that was attached to a molar as a dental appliance. The transducer vibrated the tooth to take advantage of the tooth's inherent osseointegration. Despite early studies showing high patient satisfaction and a global hearing benefit, the start-up company that developed the product filed for bankruptcy in 2015 [50]. Another nonsurgical alternative osseoconductive hearing aid is the TransEar®. This system also has a behind-the-ear microphone, but it is attached via a wire to a custom-fit ear mold that houses an oscillator. The oscillator vibrates the osseous external auditory canal, sending a transcranial signal to the better hearing ear. The TransEar also has had limited commercial success due to patient discomfort from the oscillator and poor hearing results [51].

The potential benefits of an osseointegrated device for unilateral hearing loss following vestibular schwannoma surgery are the same as the CROS hearing aid, specifically improved hearing in noise and sound awareness on the deafened side. Like CROS hearing aids, osseointegrated devices will not restore sound localization because it does not create binaural hearing. An additional benefit of osseointegrated devices compared to CROS is the lack of occlusal effect on the better hearing ear as well as the lack of needing to wear bilateral hearing aids. These benefits must be weighed against the need for a surgery and the possible skin-related complications [24].

The modest hearing benefits of osseointegrated devices for unilateral hearing loss have been documented both subjectively and objectively. In a survey of 139 patients following translabyrinthine resection of a vestibular schwannoma, patients that chose to be implanted with an osseointegrated device had a 17.4% improvement on the Background Noise subscale of the Abbreviated Profile of Hearing Aid Benefit (APHAB) questionnaire. Additionally, they reported an 11.6% improvement on the Ease of Communication subscale and a 13.2% improvement on the Reverberation subscale [52]. A systematic review analyzing 14 studies with 296 unilateral hearing loss patients demonstrated overall improvement with speech discrimination in noise and improved quality of life [53].

When choosing between osseointegrated device and CROS, individual interpretation of the previously discussed advantages and disadvantages must be considered. Trials of the CROS device and a bone conduction hearing aid are recommended so that patients can make an informed decision with appropriate expectations [54]. New techniques of simulating the bone conduction system with real ear measures have the potential to improve fitting parameters and patient satisfaction [55–57].

From an audiologic standpoint, many studies have tried to compare the results of osseointegrated devices and CROS. However, these studies are underpowered, lack randomization, and introduce selection bias as all osseointegrated device patients chose to undergo surgical intervention to address their hearing loss. In 2006, Baguley and colleagues performed a meta-analysis on four prospective studies with 47 patients comparing CROS versus BAHA [58–61]. In this analysis, the BAHA significantly outperformed CROS on all APHAB subscales (Ease of Communication, Reverberation, Background Noise, and Aversiveness of Sounds) [62]. Studies that are more recent have failed to replicate the superiority of osseointegrated devices, citing similar audiometric advantages with both systems [63–65]. In general, when patients are presented with all options following vestibular schwannoma surgery, only 30–50% will ultimately choose to be implanted with an osseointegrated device [52, 54, 63].

The limitations of either an osseointegrated device or a CROS are its inability to restore the ITD and ILD, which results in poor sound localization and limited ability to improve hearing in noise. Individuals with a unilateral hearing loss will function best if they can control their environment to limit the SNR or place the important sound source close to their better hearing ear. An osseointegrated device or a CROS may even be detrimental if it amplifies unfavorable background noise rather than the speaker of interest. In those listening environments, the patient may benefit from temporary removal of the device to prevent a masking phenomenon of the better hearing ear.

Auditory Brainstem Implants

A small subset of patients will present with bilateral profound sensorineural hearing loss accompanied by damaged cochleae or cochlear nerves that prohibit hearing rehabilitation with CROS, BAHA, or cochlear implantation. This clinical scenario most commonly occurs in the setting of neurofibromatosis type 2 (NF2) but may also be applicable for sporadic vestibular schwannomas in an only hearing ear. The auditory brainstem implant (ABI) was developed as a means of bypassing the cochlea and cochlear nerve to directly stimulate the auditory pathway at the cochlear nucleus.

The first ABI was placed by Drs. William House and William Hitselberger in 1979 for a patient with NF2 who lost all hearing following vestibular schwannoma removal in her only hearing ear [66]. Twenty years after placement, this rudimentary paired ball electrode device continued to provide the patient with improved lip-reading ability and environmental sound detection. Since this first case, more than 1000 ABIs have been implanted worldwide, and many device modifications have attempted to improve cochlear nucleus stimulation.

In 2000, Cochlear Corporation first received FDA approval to implant patients 12 years and older with NF2 using the Nucleus 24 ABI® device. (MED-EL also makes an ABI device, but it is not FDA-approved.) Both manufacturers have adapted their CI software platforms for the electrical stimulation required for their ABI products. The latest version of Cochlear Corporation's ABI is the Nucleus ABI54®. This device that includes an external component consisting of a behind-the-ear microphone, speech processor, and transmitter coil sends a digital signal to a receiver-stimulator implanted beneath the scalp. The signal is then transmitted to the ABI electrode paddle, which has 21 individual platinum disks that contact the cochlear nucleus. The paddle is covered by a polyethylene terephthalate (PET) mesh that promotes fibrous ingrowth and long-term device fixation along the dorsolateral brainstem (Fig. 12.2) [67].

Placement of the ABI targets the cochlear nucleus complex, which lies at the dorsal pontomedullary junction located along the lateral recess at the floor of the fourth ventricle. The cochlear nucleus is not visible on the surface of the brainstem, so its location must be approximated by nearby landmarks. Access to this area is usually achieved during vestibular schwannoma resection, classically through a translabyrinthine approach. The vestibulocochlear nerve, glossopharyngeal nerve, and choroid plexus serve as important landmarks for ABI placement. In large tumors, the brainstem anatomy and vestibulocochlear nerve may be distorted. By tracing the glossopharyngeal nerve superiorly to the choroid plexus, the lateral aperture of the lateral recess (foramen of Luschka) is identified. With gentle posterior and superior retraction of the choroid plexus, the lateral recess can be opened to allow placement of the ABI paddle in proximity of the cochlear nucleus (Fig. 12.3) [68]. During this dissection, it is important to be aware of cardiac and cranial nerve monitoring (VII, VIII, IX, X, XI) because surgical dissection or stimulation can result in bradycardia or hemodynamic instability.

The ABI is placed on the surface of the cochlear nucleus complex, which is a structure with several distinct subunits that carry different auditory processing functions. The main subunits are the dorsal and ventral cochlear nuclei. In brief, the ventral cochlear nucleus serves as the primary relay center for afferent auditory input and maintains the tonotopic organization started in the cochlea—this is the primary ABI target. The dorsal cochlear nucleus receives afferent input but also efferent input that facilitates complex auditory processing. In an attempt to better access the different cochlear nucleus subunits, a penetrating auditory brainstem implant (PABI) was designed. This design had penetrating microelectrodes emanating from the traditional ABI surface paddle. Ultimately, the PABI design failed to improve cochlear nucleus stimulation. Results showed no improvement in speech perception, with less than 25% of the penetrating electrodes producing auditory sensation compared with 60% of the surface electrodes [69].

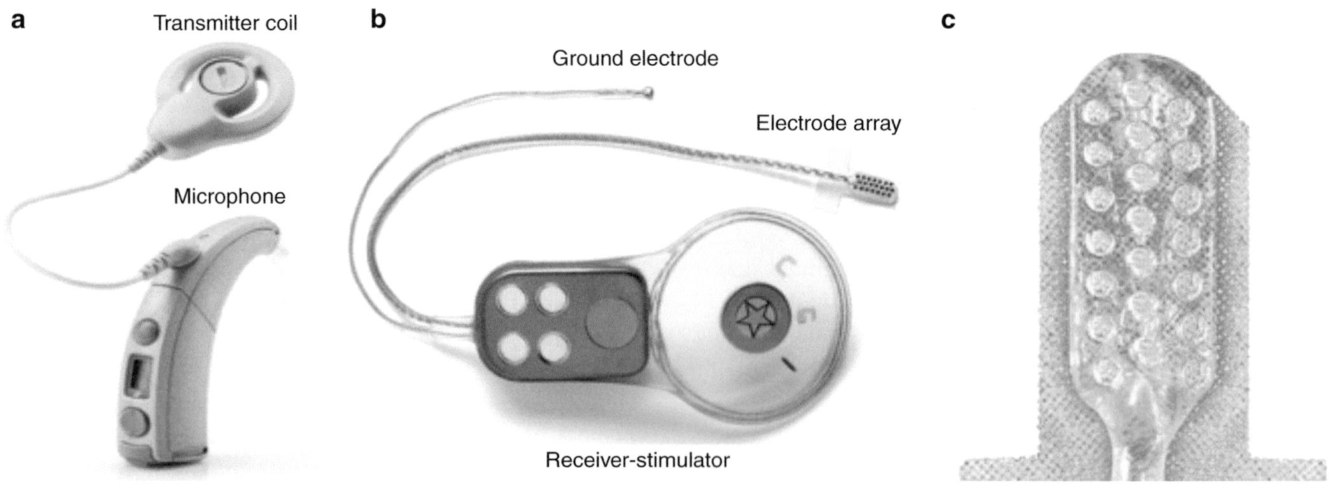

Fig. 12.2 Cochlear Corporation's auditory brainstem implant system. (**a**) The behind-the-ear component contains two microphones and a speech processor attached to an external transmitter coil. (**b**) The internal receiver-stimulator gets the signal from the external transmitter coil and sends it down the electrode array. (**c**) The electrode array ends in a paddle containing 21 platinum disk contacts. The back side of the paddle is coated with a PET mesh to prevent future movement

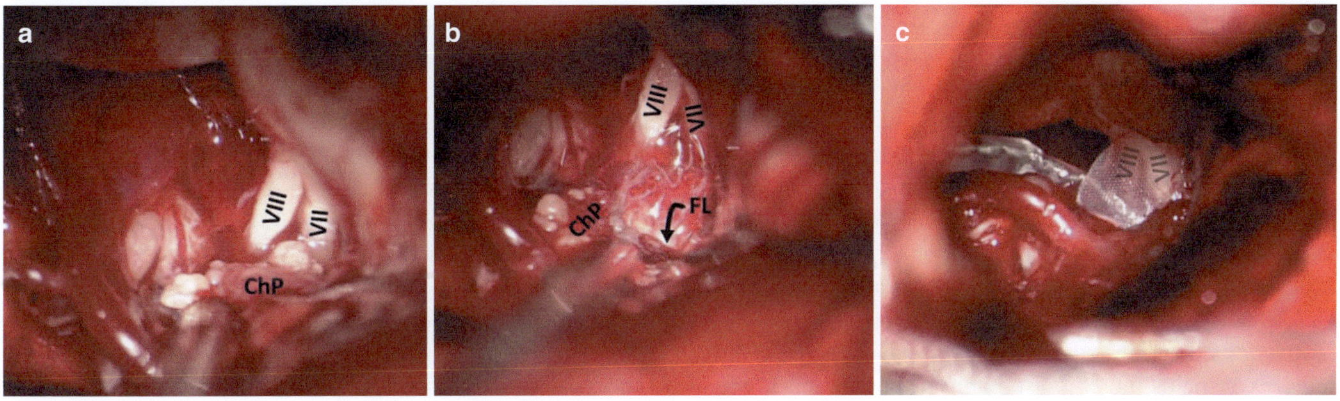

Fig. 12.3 Intraoperative photos of a right-sided auditory brainstem implant (ABI). The fourth ventricle connects to the cerebellopontine cistern via the lateral recess. The lateral aperture of the lateral recess is termed the foramen of Luschka (FL). (**a**) The choroid plexus (ChP) is a key landmark for identification of the lateral recess. (**b**) With the choroid plexus retracted, the opening of the FL becomes apparent. (**c**) The ABI is placed into the lateral recess so that its platinum contacts face the dorsolateral surface of the pontomedullary junction. The vestibulocochlear nerve (VIII) and facial nerve (VII) are labeled

Like the PABI, the auditory midbrain implant (AMI) was another experimental device hoping to overcome some of the challenges associated with cochlear nucleus stimulation. The target for the AMI is further rostral along the auditory pathway at the inferior colliculus. The implant is a penetrating electrode array placed in the midbrain. The device continues to undergo modifications, but to date it remains an experimental option for NF2 patients [70].

With more than 1000 patients implanted with ABIs, primarily for hearing loss due to NF2, the expected auditory outcomes include environmental sound awareness and assistance with lip-reading. Only a small subset of patients will obtain open-set word understanding. Some factors responsible for the outcome variability include tumor growth that distorts the brainstem anatomy, ABI electrode positioning, imprecise cochlear nucleus stimulation, and surgical trauma [71]. A 2014 consensus statement evaluated 84 NF2 patients with ABIs to identify several factors associated with improved outcomes. Overall, 26 of 84 (31%) patients achieved open-set sentence scores greater than 30%. The surgical factors thought to portend a good outcome included the use of a semi-sitting surgical position and early cutting of the vestibulocochlear nerve near the brainstem to minimize transfer of electrocautery excitotoxicity to the cochlear nucleus during tumor dissection. In addition, patient factors like duration of preoperative deafness correlated with performance. Among excellent performers, the ability to identify eleven distinct pitches predicted a greater than 80% open-set speech recognition without background noise [72]. Another cohort of 23 NF2 patients with ABI showed that 19 (83%) continued to use their device after implantation while 8 of 23 (35%) patients achieved speech perception and only 4 (17%) patients could use the telephone [71].

In general, ABI placement does not increase the risk of complications during vestibular schwannoma surgery. Potential complications include cerebrospinal fluid (CSF) leak, meningitis, cranial neuropathy, hydrocephalus, stroke, and even death while device-specific complications include device failure, extrusion, migration, and nonauditory stimulation. In a review of 61 patients undergoing ABI, Otto and colleagues identified two patients with CSF leaks (3.3%) and one with meningitis (1.6%). Electrode migration occurred in one (1.6%) patient and failure to produce useful auditory sensation occurred in six (9.8%) patients demonstrating the importance of accurate device position. No serious consequences of nonauditory stimulation occurred, but 24% of tested electrodes could not be used due to these stimuli. The deactivated electrodes generally were located at either the proximal or distal end of the electrode paddle; nonauditory sensations included tingling, altered vision, and dizziness [73]. The risk of CSF leak does require particular diligence during closure because the ABI can serve as a wick for CSF into the mastoid or soft tissue.

Given the low complication rate and preference to avoid additional surgery, many centers use the concept of a "sleeper" ABI when planning auditory rehabilitation for NF2 patients. These situations are unique in that patients have bilateral vestibular schwannomas and eventual bilateral deafness is expected. Therefore, an ABI can be placed during the first tumor removal despite still having useful hearing in the contralateral ear. Then, if hearing in the contralateral ear is lost or surgical intervention requires sacrifice of that cochlear nerve, the previously placed ABI can be activated. ABI placement at the time of large tumor removal or with brainstem compression can be technically difficult, so the "sleeper" approach also creates an extra opportunity for accurate ABI placement.

Cochlear Implantation

Surgical priorities for vestibular schwannoma microsurgery continue to evolve as the operative morbidity declines. Early surgical techniques focused on lowering the disconcertingly high mortality rate. The next iteration of advances reduced major perioperative morbidities such as facial nerve paralysis and CSF leaks. Finally, optimization of hearing preservation outcomes based on various patient and tumor factors yields fairly predictive surgical outcomes. Despite these innovations, hearing can be lost even when cochlear nerve integrity remains intact, presumably from vascular insult to the cochlea or trauma to the cochlear nerve.

In the early 1990s, studies by Cueva and colleagues, Kartush and colleagues, and Vrabec colleagues demonstrated that, after labyrinthectomy or vestibular schwannoma microsurgery, a preserved cochlear nerve could transmit an auditory signal despite complete loss of hearing [74–76]. These studies performed transtympanic promontory stimulation to identify positive auditory responses as well as distinct auditory pitch perception. Positive responses could be achieved at 9 months after initial surgery and were comparable to responses achieved by CI candidates. These findings were supported by temporal bone studies of patients after labyrinthectomy that revealed spiral ganglion cell survival years after surgery [77]. If spiral ganglion cells can survive and the cochlear nerve integrity is maintained, then the possibility of cochlear implantation exists.

As early as 1992, several case reports showed the feasibility of a staged cochlear implantation after labyrinthectomy or removal of a vestibular schwannoma, with an intact cochlear nerve [78–82]. These studies confirmed that the auditory pathway could transmit an electrical signal despite postoperative hearing loss and that cochlear ossification did not always occur, thus allowing CI placement. In 1995, Arriaga and colleagues reported the first cases of a simultaneous CI performed during translabyrinthine vestibular schwannoma removal. This patient's tumor was in his only hearing ear [83]. Intraoperative promontory stimulation was not performed. At 10 months, the patient was still using the CI with enhanced lip-reading ability. Some authors advocate simultaneous CI and tumor removal in an effort to minimize delays in auditory rehabilitation, reduce the number of surgical procedures, and avoid potential cochlear obstruction if ossification occurs [84].

Recently, several case series have demonstrated that either staged or simultaneous cochlear implantation is safe and feasible for hearing rehabilitation as long as the cochlea is patent and the cochlear nerve is intact. Many patients can achieve improved sound awareness and open-set speech, but the results are more variable than traditional CI candidates [85–87]. A recent prospective study evaluated simultaneous cochlear implantation and translabyrinthine tumor resection for sporadic vestibular schwannomas. All seven patients had preservation of the cochlear nerve and five of seven (71%) had auditory precepts with CI activation. In regard to the five patients, at 1 month their sound localization improved from 78° ± 13°, with the CI off to 41° ± 9° with the CI on. This improvement in sound localization is a distinct benefit over the hearing rehabilitation with CROS or BAHA. Additionally, the five patients in this study also demonstrated modest improvement in speech understanding and tinnitus reduction [88].

If the cochlear nerve is preserved and a CI is placed, one potential concern is the sustainability of the benefits, particularly in patients with NF2 who are susceptible to distorted brainstem anatomy, tumor recurrence, or new tumor growth. Neff and colleagues reported on six patients with NF2 who had undergone tumor resection with CI placement and had long-term follow-up with a mean of 7.9 years (range: 5–13 years). In all but one patient, the benefit from CI was maintained, and five of six (83%) patients were still able to use a telephone with their CI devices [89]. Although continued long-term follow-up is needed, no case reports have been published in which a CI had to be removed due to tumor re-growth. Additionally, tumor surveillance by MRI is improved by newly expanded FDA guidelines, allowing 1.5–3 T strength MRI depending on the CI device manufacturer. CI magnets do produce artifact that may distort surveillance of the cerebellopontine angle. Placement of the internal receiver-stimulator in a more superior position and use of reformatted coronal and sagittal views can help mitigate this distortion. In a retrospective review of 34 ears undergoing a 1.5 T MRI scan with a CI in place secured by a firm head wrap, the authors found the ipsilateral cerebellopontine angle could be visualized without difficulty in 94% of cases. However, there was a 15% risk of magnet movement even with the use of a head wrap [90]. Clearly, caution must be used in device selection when considering postoperative tumor surveillance.

In conclusion, management of vestibular schwannomas has made great strides in patient safety and decreased morbidity. Still, the loss of hearing is an inevitable fate for many patients with a vestibular schwannoma and has a significant impact on patients' quality of life. The most common hearing rehabilitation options, CROS and BAHA, can improve sound awareness and speech in noise but fail to restore the audiologic benefits of binaural hearing. If the cochlea is accessible and the cochlear nerve is intact, then CI has the potential to restore binaural function. If no cochlear nerves are viable, then an ABI can provide sound detection to improve lip-reading abilities and, in rare cases, even open-set speech.

References

1. Matthies C, Samii M. Management of 1000 vestibular schwannomas (acoustic neuromas): clinical presentation. Neurosurgery. 1993;40:1–10.
2. Stangerup SE, Thomsen J, Tos M, Cayé-Thomasen P. Long-term hearing preservation in vestibular schwannoma. Otol Neurotol. 2010;31:271–5.
3. Wiegand D, Fickel V. Acoustic neuroma, the patient's perspective: subjective assessment of symptoms, diagnosis, therapy, and outcome in 541 patients. Laryngoscope. 1989;99:179–87.
4. Tos T, Cayé-Thomasen P, Stangerup S, et al. Patients' fears, expectations and satisfactions in relation to management of vestibular schwannoma: a comparison of surgery and observation. Acta Otolaryngol. 2003;123:600–5.
5. Bess F, Tharpe A. Unilateral hearing impairment in children. Pediatrics. 1984;74:2016–216.
6. Keller W, Bundy R. Effects of unilateral hearing loss upon educational achievement. Child Care Health Dev. 1980;6:93–100.
7. Oyler R, Oyler A, Matkin N. Unilateral hearing loss: demographics and educational impact. Lang Speech Hear Serv Sch. 1988;19:201–10.
8. Lieu JEC, Tye-Murray N, Karzon RK, Piccirillo JF. Unilateral hearing loss is associated with worse speech-language scores in children. Pediatrics. 2010;125:e1348–55.
9. Lucas L, Katiri R, Kitterick PT. The psychological and social consequences of single-sided deafness in adulthood. Int J Audiol. 2018;57:21–30.
10. Subramaniam K, Eikelboom RH, Eager KM, Atlas MD. Unilateral profound hearing loss and the effect on quality of life after cerebellopontine angle surgery. Otolaryngol Head Neck Surg. 2005;133:339–46.
11. Mencher GT, Davis A. Bilateral or unilateral amplification: is there a difference? A brief tutorial. Int J Audiol. 2006;45:S3–11.
12. Snik A, Agterberg M, Bosman A. How to quantify binaural hearing in patients with unilateral hearing using hearing implants. Audiol Neurotol. 2015;20:44–7.
13. Killion M. SNR loss: "I can hear what people say, but I can't understand them". Hear Rev. 1997;4:8–14.
14. Shelton C, Brackmann DE, House WF, Hitselberger WE. Acoustic tumor surgery. Prognostic factors in hearing conservation. Arch Otolaryngol Head Neck Surg. 1989;115:1213–6.
15. Dubrulle F, Ernst O, Vincent C, Vaneecloo F, Lejeune J, Lemaitre L. Cochlear fossa enhancement at MR evaluation of vestibular schwannoma: correlation with success at hearing-preservation surgery. Radiology. 2000;215:458–62.
16. Kutz JW, Scoresby T, Isaacson B, et al. Hearing preservation using the middle fossa approach for the treatment of vestibular schwannoma. Neurosurgery. 2012;70:334–40.
17. Committee on hearing and equilibrium guidelines for the evaluation of hearing preservation in acoustic neuroma (vestibular schwannoma): American Academy of Otolaryngology—Head and Neck Surgery Foundation, INC. Otolaryngol Head Neck Surg. 1995;113:179–80.
18. Gardner G, Roberston J. Hearing preservation in unilateral acoustic neuroma surgery. Ann Otol Rhinol Laryngol. 1988;97:55–66.
19. Fowler E. Bilateral hearing aids for monaural total deafness. Arch Otolaryngol. 1960;72:41–2.
20. Harford E, Barry J. A rehabilitative approach to the problem of unilateral hearing impairment; the contralateral routing of signals (CROS). J Speech Hear Dis. 1965;30:121–38.
21. Aufricht H. A follow-up study of the CROS hearing aid. J Speech Hear Dis. 1972;37:113–7.
22. Herbig R, Barthel R, Branda E. A history of e2e wireless technology. Hear Rev. 2014;21:34–7.
23. Valente M, Oeding K. Evaluation of a BICROS System with a directional microphone in the receiver and transmitter. J Am Acad Audiol. 2015;26:856–71.
24. Bishop CE, Eby TL. The current status of audiologic rehabilitation for profound unilateral sensorineural hearing loss. Laryngoscope. 2010;120:552–6.
25. Ryu NG, Moon IJ, Byun H, et al. Clinical effectiveness of wireless CROS (contralateral routing of offside signals) hearing aids. Eur Arch Oto-Rhino-Laryngol. 2015;272:2213–9.
26. Lotterman S, Kasten R. Examination of the CROS type hearing aid. J Speech Hear Res. 1971;14:416–20.
27. Lin LM, Bowditch S, Anderson MJ, May B, Cox KM, Niparko JK. Amplification in the rehabilitation of unilateral deafness: speech in noise and directional hearing effects with bone-anchored hearing and contralateral routing of signal amplification. Otol Neurotol. 2006;27:172–82.
28. Mudry A, Tjellström A. Historical background of bone conduction hearing devices and bone conduction hearing aids. Adv Otorhinolaryngol. 2011;71:1–9.
29. Brånemark P, Adell R, Breine U, Hansson B, Lindström J, Ohlsson A. Intra-osseous anchorage of dental prostheses. Experimental studies. Scand J Plast Reconstr Surg. 1969;3:81–100.
30. Albrektsson T, Brånemark P, Hansson H, Lindström J. Osseointegrated titanium implants. Requirements for ensuring long-lasting, direct bone-to-implant anchorage in man. Acta Orthop Scand. 1981;52:155–70.
31. Tjellström A, Lindström J, Hallen O, Albrektsson T, Brånemark P. Osseointegrated titanium implant in the temporal bone. A clinical study on bone-anchored hearing aids. Am J Otol. 1981;2:304–10.
32. Tjellström A, Rosenhall J, Lindström O, Hallen T, Albrektsson T, Brånemark P. Five-year experience with skin-penetrating bone-anchored implants in the temporal bone. Acta Otolaryngol. 1983;95:568–75.
33. Lustig LR, Arts H, Brackmann DE, et al. Hearing rehabilitation using the BAHA bone-anchored hearing aid: results in 40 patients. Otol Neurotol. 2001;22:328–34.
34. Tjellström A, Granstrom G. One stage procedure to establish osseointegration. A zero to five years follow-up report. J Laryngol Otol. 1995;109:593–8.
35. Myalnus E, Cremers C. A one-stage surgical procedure for placement of percutaneous implants for the bone-anchored hearing aid. J Laryngol Otol. 1994;108:1031–5.
36. De Wolf MJF, Hol MKS, Huygen PLM, Mylanus EAM, Cremers CWRJ. Clinical outcome of the simplified surgical technique for BAHA implantation. Otol Neurotol. 2008;29:1100–8.
37. Stalfors J, Tjellström A. Skin reactions after BAHA surgery: a comparison between the U-graft technique and the BAHA dermatome. Otol Neurotol. 2008;29:1109–14.
38. Calon TGA, van Hoof M, van den Berge H, et al. Minimally Invasive Ponto Surgery compared to the linear incision technique without soft tissue reduction for bone conduction hearing implants: study protocol for a randomized controlled trial. Trials. 2016;17:1–11.
39. McLarnon CM, Johnson I, Davison T, et al. Evidence for early loading of osseointegrated implants for bone conduction at 4 weeks. Otol Neurotol. 2012;33:1578–82.
40. Scholz M, Eufinger H, Anders A, et al. Intracerebral abscess after abutment change of a bone anchored hearing aid (BAHA). Otol Neurotol. 2003;24:896–9.
41. Tjellström A, Niparko JK. Intracerebral abscess after BAHA abutment change. Otol Neurotol. 2005;26:552–3.
42. House JW, Kutz JW Jr. Bone-anchored hearing aids: incidence and management of postoperative complications. Otol Neurotol. 2007;28:213–7.
43. Shirazi MA, Marzo SJ, Leonetti JP. Perioperative complications with the bone-anchored hearing aid. Otolaryngol Head Neck Surg. 2006;134:236–9.

44. Hobson JC, Roper AJ, Andrew R, Rothera MP, Hill P, Green KM. Complications of bone-anchored hearing aid implantation. J Laryngol Otol. 2010;124:132–6.
45. Holgers K, Tjellström A, Bjursten L, Erlandsson B. Soft tissue reactions around percutaneous implants: a clinical study of soft tissue conditions around skin-penetrating titanium implants for bone-anchored hearing aids. Am J Otol. 1988;9:56–9.
46. Dimitriadis PA, Farr MR, Allam A, Ray J. Three year experience with the cochlear BAHA attract implant: a systematic review of the literature. BMC Ear Nose Throat Disord. 2016;16:1–8.
47. Laske RD, Röösli C, Pfiffner F, Veraguth D, Huber AM. Functional results and subjective benefit of a transcutaneous bone conduction device in patients with single-sided deafness. Otol Neurotol. 2015;36:1151–6.
48. Sprinzl G, Lenarz T, Ernst A, et al. First European multicenter results with a new transcutaneous bone conduction hearing implant system: short-term safety and efficacy. Otol Neurotol. 2013;34:1076–83.
49. Steinmetz C, Mader I, Arndt S, Aschendorff A, Laszig R, Hassepass F. MRI artefacts after Bonebridge implantation. Eur Arch Oto-Rhino-Laryngol. 2014;271:2079–82.
50. Gurgel RK, Shelton C. The SoundBite hearing system: patient-assessed safety and benefit study. Laryngoscope. 2013;123:2807–12.
51. Battista RA, Mullins K, Wiet RM, Sabin A, Kim J, Rauch V. Sound localization in unilateral deafness with the Baha or TransEar device. JAMA Otolaryngol Head Neck Surg. 2013;139:64–70.
52. House JW, Kutz JW, Chung J, Fisher LM. Bone-anchored hearing aid subjective benefit for unilateral deafness. Laryngoscope. 2010;120:601–7.
53. Kim G, Ju HM, Lee SH, Kim HS, Kwon JA, Seo YJ. Efficacy of bone-anchored hearing aids in single-sided deafness: a systematic review. Otol Neurotol. 2017;38:473–83.
54. Siau D, Dhillon B, Andrews R, Green KMJ. Bone-anchored hearing aids and unilateral sensorineural hearing loss: why do patients reject them? J Laryngol Otol. 2015;129:321–5.
55. Laitakari K, Löppönen H, Salmivalli A, Sorri M. Objective real ear measurements of bone-conduction hearing aid performance. Scand Audiol. 1995;24:53–6. http://www.ncbi.nlm.nih.gov/pubmed/7761800. Accessed 5 Jun 2018.
56. Håkansson B, Carlsson P. Skull simulator for direct bone conduction hearing devices. Scand Audiol. 1989;18:91–8. http://www.ncbi.nlm.nih.gov/pubmed/2756338. Accessed 5 Jun 2018.
57. Valente M, Oeding K, Brockmeyer A, Smith S, Kallogjeri D. Differences in word and phoneme in quiet, sentence recognition in noise and subjective outcomes between manufacturer first fit and bone-anchored device programmed to DSL I/O. J Am Acad Audiol. 2018;29:706–21.
58. Wazen J, Spitzer J, Ghossaini S, et al. Transcranial contralateral cochlear stimulation in unilateral deafness. Otolaryngol Head Neck Surg. 2003;129:248–54.
59. Hol M, Bosman A, Snik A, Mylanus E, Cremers C. Bone-anchored hearing in unilateral inner ear deafness: a study of 20 patients. Audiol Neurotol. 2004;9:274–81.
60. Bosman A, Hol M, Snik A, Mylanus E, Cremers C. Bone-anchored hearing aids in unilateral inner ear deafness. Acta Otolaryngol. 2003;123:258–60.
61. Niparko JK, Cox KM, Lustig LR. Comparison of the bone anchored hearing aid implantable hearing device with contralateral routing of offside signal amplification in the rehabilitation of unilateral deafness. Otol Neurotol. 2003;24:73–8.
62. Baguley DM, Bird J, Humphriss RL, Prevost AT. The evidence base for the application of contralateral bone anchored hearing aids in acquired unilateral sensorineural hearing loss in adults. Clin Otolaryngol. 2006;31:6–14.
63. Hol MKS, Kunst SJW, Snik AFM, Cremers CWRJ. Pilot study on the effectiveness of the conventional CROS, the transcranial CROS and the BAHA transcranial CROS in adults with unilateral inner ear deafness. Eur Arch Oto-Rhino-Laryngol. 2010;267:889–96.
64. Snapp HA, Holt FD, Liu X, Rajguru SM. Comparison of speech-in-noise and localization benefits in unilateral hearing loss subjects using contralateral routing of signal hearing AIDS or bone-anchored implants. Otol Neurotol. 2017;38:11–8.
65. Finbow J, Bance M, Aiken S, Gulliver M, Verge J, Caissie R. A comparison between wireless CROS and bone-anchored hearing devices for single-sided deafness: a pilot study. Otol Neurotol. 2015;36:819–25.
66. House WF, Hitselberger WE. Twenty-year report of the first auditory brain stem nucleus implant. Ann Otol Rhinol Laryngol. 2001;110:103–4.
67. Shannon RV, Fayad J, Moore J, et al. Auditory brainstem implant: II. Postsurgical issues and performance. Otolaryngol Head Neck Surg. 1993;108:634–42.
68. Abe H, Rhoton AL. Microsurgical anatomy of the cochlear nuclei. Neurosurgery. 2006;58:728–39.
69. Otto SR, Shannon RV, Wilkinson EP, et al. Audiologic outcomes with the penetrating electrode auditory brainstem implant. Otol Neurotol. 2008;29:1147–54.
70. Lim HH, Lenarz T. Auditory midbrain implant: research and development towards a second clinical trial. Hear Res. 2015;322:212–23.
71. Sanna M, Di Lella F, Guida M, Merkus P. Auditory brainstem implants in NF2 patients. Otol Neurotol. 2012;33:154–64.
72. Behr R, Colletti V, Matthies C, et al. New outcomes with auditory brainstem implants in NF2 patients. Otol Neurotol. 2014;35:1844–51.
73. Otto SR, Brackmann DE, Hitselberger WE, Shannon RV, Kuchta J. Multichannel auditory brainstem implant: update on performance in 61 patients. J Neurosurg. 2002;96:1063–71.
74. Kartush JM, Linstrom CJ, Graham MD, Kulick KC, Bouchard KR. Promontory stimulation following labyrinthectomy: implications for cochlear implantation. Laryngoscope. 1990;100:5–9.
75. Cueva RA, Thedinger BA, Harris JP, Glasscock ME. Electrical promontory stimulation in patients with intact cochlear nerve and anacusis following acoustic neuroma surgery. Laryngoscope. 1992;102:1220–4.
76. Vrabec JT, Lambert PR, Arts HA, Ruth RA. Promontory stimulation following translabyrinthine excision of acoustic neuroma with preservation of the cochlear nerve. Am J Otol. 1995;16:643–7. http://www.ncbi.nlm.nih.gov/pubmed/8588670. Accessed 23 May 2018.
77. Chen DA, Linthicum FH, Rizer FM. Cochlear histopathology in the labyrinthectomized ear: implications for cochlear implantation. Laryngoscope. 1988;98:1170–2. http://www.ncbi.nlm.nih.gov/pubmed/3185070. Accessed 23 May 2018.
78. Hoffman RA, Kohan D, Cohen NL. Cochlear implants in the management of bilateral acoustic neuromas. Am J Otol. 1992;13:525–8. http://www.ncbi.nlm.nih.gov/pubmed/1449178. Accessed 23 May 2018.
79. Pensak ML, Tew JM, Keith RW, Vanloveren HR. Management of the acoustic neuroma in an only hearing ear. Skull Base Surg. 1991;1:93–6. http://www.ncbi.nlm.nih.gov/pubmed/17170828. Accessed 23 May 2018.
80. Tono T, Ushisako Y, Morimitsu T. Cochlear implantation in an intralabyrinthine acoustic neuroma patient after resection of an intracanalicular tumor. Adv Otorhinolaryngol. 1997;52:155–7. http://www.ncbi.nlm.nih.gov/pubmed/9042475. Accessed 23 May 2018.
81. Zwolan TA, Shepard NT, Niparko JK. Labyrinthectomy with cochlear implantation. Am J Otol. 1993;14:220–3. http://www.ncbi.nlm.nih.gov/pubmed/8372917. Accessed 23 May 2018.
82. Hulka GF, Bernard EJ, Pillsbury HC. Cochlear implantation in a patient after removal of an acoustic neuroma. The implications of magnetic resonance imaging with gadolinium on patient management. Arch Otolaryngol Head Neck Surg. 1995;121:465–8.

83. Arriaga MA, Marks S. Simultaneous cochlear implantation and acoustic neuroma resection: imaging considerations, technique, and functional outcome. Otolaryngol Head Neck Surg. 1995;112:325–8.
84. Roehm PC, Clair JM-S, Jethanamest D, et al. Auditory rehabilitation of patients with neurofibromatosis Type 2 by using cochlear implants. J Neurosurg. 2011;115:827–34.
85. Carlson ML, Breen JT, Driscoll CL, et al. Cochlear implantation in patients with neurofibromatosis type 2: variables affecting auditory performance. Otol Neurotol. 2012;33(5):853–62.
86. Lloyd SK, Glynn FJ, Rutherford SA, et al. Ipsilateral cochlear implantation after cochlear nerve preserving vestibular schwannoma surgery in patients with neurofibromatosis type 2. Otol Neurotol. 2014;35(1):43–51.
87. Lassaletta L, Aristegui M, Medina M, et al. Ipsilateral cochlear implantation in patients with sporadic vestibular schwannoma in the only or best hearing ear and in patients with NF2. Eur Arch Oto-Rhino-Laryngol. 2016;273(1):27–35.
88. Rooth MA, Dillon MT, Brown KD. Prospective evaluation of patients undergoing translabyrinthine excision of vestibular schwannoma with concurrent cochlear implantation. Otol Neurotol. 2017;38:1512–6.
89. Neff BA, Wiet RM, Lasak JM, et al. Cochlear implantation in the neurofibromatosis type 2 patient: long-term follow-up. Laryngoscope. 2007;117(6):1069–72.
90. Carlson ML, Neff BA, Link MJ, et al. Magnetic resonance imaging with cochlear implant magnet in place. Otol Neurotol. 2015;36(6):965–71.

Acoustic Neuroma Surgery: Retrosigmoid Techniques

13

Justin M. Moore, Robert K. Jackler, and Griffith R. Harsh IV

The last century has seen great strides in the accurate diagnosis and microsurgical management of acoustic neuroma (AN), with improvements in mortality rate and preservation of both facial nerve function and hearing [1]. Acoustic neuromas were among the earliest intracranial lesions to be anatomically localized on the basis of symptoms [2, 3]. The first reported surgical attempt was by Charles McBurney, who opened the suboccipital plate with a chisel in 1881 but was forced to abort the case following excessive cerebella swelling [4]. Early surgical attempts were heroic interventions of last resort in moribund patients and were associated with surgical mortality rates of up to 78% [5]. With developments in surgical technique and sterility, Harvey Cushing reported a mortality rate of 4% in 1931 [6]. Walter Dandy further advanced the field using ventriculographic and pneumoencephalographic imaging and a unilateral suboccipital craniotomy [7, 8]. With such advancements, complete tumor excision became more commonplace and rates of anatomic preservation of the facial nerve approached 65% in 1941 [9–11].

William House introduced the operating microscope to acoustic neuroma surgery in 1961 and advocated that each operation be performed by a team of a neurosurgeon and neuro-otologist [12]. Elliott and McKissock in 1954 were the first to report hearing preservation following a retrosigmoid (RS) resection of an AN [13]. Subsequently, surgeons have focused on the extent of resection and avoidance of facial weakness and hearing loss—factors critical to a patient's choice among management options of clinical and radiographic monitoring, three surgical approaches, and stereotactic irradiation. This chapter will focus on the indications, predictive factors, classification, microsurgical technique, and outcomes for a retrosigmoid approach to an AN resection.

Pathology and Pathophysiology

The pathophysiology of ANs in relation to hearing is comprehensively explored in Chap. 12, while the biology and genetics are covered in Chap. 9. Briefly, mechanisms of cranial nerve dysfunction, including hearing loss, can be categorized as compressive, infiltrative, ischemic, or a combination of these. Although the vast majority of ANs arises from the vestibular divisions of the eighth cranial nerve, infiltration of the cochlear nerve is common even in cases with small tumors, good preoperative hearing, and unremarkable intraoperative appearance [14, 15].

Preservation of the cranial nerves requires a functional, anatomically continuous nerve with an adequate vascular supply. Tumor exposure, cerebellar retraction, or dissection of the tumor from adjacent normal structures can disrupt a nerve's continuity, function, or vascularity [16]. Sekiya and Moller demonstrated in a primate model that avulsion of the internal auditory artery in the cerebellopontine angle (CPA) could result in hearing loss [17]. In canine models, either mechanical nerve distortion or vasospasm from vascular manipulation alters brainstem auditory potentials [18, 19] and produces demyelination and thrombosis of the vasa nervorum [19]. The occasional spontaneous recovery of cochlear nerve function weeks to months after its loss during

J. M. Moore
Neurosurgery, Skull-Base Neuro-Oncology, Beth Israel Deaconess Medical Center, Harvard Medical School, Boston, MA, USA
e-mail: jmoore4@bidmc.harvard.edu

R. K. Jackler (✉)
Department of Otolaryngology—Head and Neck Surgery, Department of Neurosurgery, Department of Surgery, Stanford University School of Medicine, Stanford, CA, USA
e-mail: jackler@stanford.edu

G. R. Harsh IV
Department of Neurological Surgery, UC Davis Health and School of Medicine, UC Davis Comprehensive Cancer Center, Center for Skull Base Surgery, Sacramento, CA, USA

N. C. Bambakidis et al. (eds.), *Surgery of the Cerebellopontine Angle*, https://doi.org/10.1007/978-3-031-12507-2_13

surgery may represent resolution of a neural conduction defect caused by ischemia, mechanical retraction, or a combination of both [16].

The cranial nerves, particularly the cochlear nerve, can be injured by traction on the nerve from sustained cerebellar retraction, which may be required in a retrosigmoid approach to large tumors. Traction injury to the nerve fibers occurs at mechanically weak sections, such as the Obersteiner–Redlich zone of transition from Schwann cell sheath to glial cell coverage, which lacks the reinforcing endoneurium of the distal nerve [20]. Furthermore, in the case of the cochlear nerve, the fragile small fibers located laterally at the modiolus are prone to avulsion from the base of the cochlea, evident intraoperatively as sudden loss or prolonged latency of wave V of the auditory brainstem response (ABR) despite preservation of wave I following cerebellar retraction [21].

Meticulous surgical technique is required at all times. Sharp dissection can partially or completely divide the nerve. Blunt dissection can stretch, shear, or avulse vital nerve components or blood vessels. Electrocauterization can cause thermal injury to the cochlear or facial nerve or its blood supply and should be avoided in its proximity. Preservation of the vascularity of a cranial nerve is often key to maintenance of function. Drilling away the posterior wall of the internal auditory canal (IAC) in the retrosigmoid approach can inadvertently damage the inner ear either directly or by thermal conduction. Opening into the bony labyrinth can also compromise hearing, an outcome prevented in some cases by early recognition and closure of the opening with bone wax, particularly if the fenestration occurs at the convexity of a semicircular canal. Hearing preservation is much less likely if either the cochlea or vestibule is transgressed.

ABR findings can help differentiate true neural injury from cochlear injury. In cochlear nerve injury, wave I of the ABR is preserved, but injury to the cochlear nerve itself affects all waves of the ABR. Isolated cochlear injury is confirmed postoperatively by the ability to activate the cochlear nerve electrically by stimulating the promontory despite clinical deafness [22].

Investigation

Audiometry

The quality of a patient's hearing is a major consideration in choice of treatment of an acoustic neuroma. Given the high dependence of postoperative hearing on preoperative hearing, outcomes for all treatment strategies, both interventional and observational, are stratified according to preoperative hearing level [23, 24]. Thus, accurate preoperative assessment of hearing is critical.

A patient's hearing quality is usually described in terms of thresholds for hearing pure tones and accuracy in speech discrimination. The unit of measurement for sound pressure is the decibel (dB), which is based on a logarithmic ratio. In pure-tone audiometry, the pure-tone average (PTA) is the mean threshold for sound detection (dB) at the octave frequencies of 250, 500, 1000, 2000, 4000, and 8000 Hz. Occasionally, interoctave frequencies of 3000 Hz and 6000 Hz are also used. Zero decibel is the lowest amplitude of sound detected by an ideal ear. Normal thresholds fall between 0 and 25 dB for all frequencies. The standard audiogram represents a graph of the perception threshold (dB) as a function of frequencies (Hz) tested. The frequencies most needed for speech lie between 500 and 3000 Hz. One hearing classification system based on dB level includes normal hearing (0–25 dB) and mild (25–40 dB), moderate (40–60 dB), severe (60–80 dB), and profound (>80 dB) hearing loss.

Speech audiometry evaluates the relative clarity or "usefulness" of the patient's hearing of speech. Word recognition is tested using a standardized list of 25–50 single-syllable words "phonetically balanced" to represent the relative frequency of sounds in the language being tested. The word recognition score (WRS) is the percentage of words the patient is able to repeat correctly.

The combination of PTA and speech reception threshold is highly informative about the usefulness of a patient's speech, the etiology of hearing loss, and potential therapeutic interventions. For example, patients with poor pure-tone thresholds but relatively preserved word recognition should respond well to hearing aids because they can still process amplified speech in a meaningful way. However, patients with favorable pure-tone thresholds but poor word discrimination may not benefit from amplification because of perceived distortion. This is often the case in patients with neural hearing losses caused by retrocochlear pathology such as an AN; the resulting disordered firing of the cochlear nerve both raises perception thresholds and disproportionately limits understanding by impairing sound processing. Traditionally, a WRS higher than 50% is thought to be required for effective use of hearing aids. A simplistic WRS model includes class 1 (100–70%), class 2 (69–50%), class 3 (49–1%), and class 4 (0%) word recognition [25, 26].

Classification

The classification scheme of Gardner and Robertson, which combines PTA and WRS, was used by many early studies of acoustic neuromas (Table 13.1) [27]. It has been supplanted by a scheme developed by the American Academy of

Table 13.1 Gardner–Robertson hearing classification

Grade[a]	Description	PTA or SRT (dB)[b]	WRS
I	Good	0–30	70–100
II	Serviceable	31–50	50–69
III	Nonserviceable	51–90	5–49
IV	Poor	>91–max loss	1–4
V	None	No response	No response

PTA pure-tone average, *SRT* speech reception threshold, *WRS* word recognition score
[a] If PTA/SRT score and WRS do not qualify for the same class, use the class appropriate for poorer of the two scores
[b] Use better score of either PTA or SRT

Table 13.2 American Academy of Otolaryngology-Head and Neck Surgery (AAO-HNS)

Class[a]	Description	PTA or SRT (dB)[b]	WRS
A	Good	0–30	70–100
B	Serviceable	31–50	50–69
C	Nonserviceable	>51	>50
D	Poor	>51	<50

PTA pure-tone average, *SRT* speech reception threshold, *WRS* word recognition score
[a] If PTA/SRT score and WRS do not qualify for the same class, use the class appropriate for poorer of the two scores
[b] Use better score of either PTA or SRT

Otolaryngology-Head and Neck Surgery (AAO-HNS) (Table 13.2) [28]. AAO-HNS class A and B hearing correspond to Gardner–Robertson grade I and II hearing. However, the AAO-HNS class C and D place a greater emphasis on the WRS and thus provide greater insight into a patient's potential to benefit from hearing aids.

More recently, guidelines elucidating the minimum standard for reporting hearing loss have been published by the AAO-HNS hearing committee in an attempt to improve data comparison between studies and enable pooling of data for meta-analysis [29]. These guidelines recommend the use of preintervention and postintervention scattergrams, which plot WRS along the *x*-axis and PTA along the *y*-axis, enabling a granular display of hearing outcomes at the individual patient level. Importantly, the PTA is calculated using 0.5-, 1-, 2-, and 3-kHz air conduction thresholds, and the WRS is presented at up to 40 dB sensation level of maximum comfortable loudness [29].

Definition of Success

Comparisons of hearing outcomes from managing ANs have long been confounded by investigators' inadequate characterization of initial hearing [23], use of different hearing classification systems, and employment of varying definitions of useful hearing and, thus, of rates of successful hearing preservation. This discrepancy has been recognized in both the otolaryngology and neurosurgical literature. In 2012, the hearing committee of the AAO-HNS produced an updated set of reporting standards, which have been outlined in the previous section [29]. More recent consistent use of current classification systems utilizing PTA and WRS has facilitated more meaningful analysis of outcome.

For vestibular schwannoma management, the 2018 guidelines of the Congress of Neurological Surgeons propose that useful (or serviceable) hearing be defined as a WRS of greater than 50% and a PTA or speech response threshold of less than 50 dB, which is equivalent to AAO-HNS class A or B and Gardner–Robertson score of grade I or II [23]. However, these scales must be used cautiously. The AN patient who has a good WRS in the quiet may still complain of substantial impairment of speech understanding in noise. Furthermore, the usefulness of a specific level of hearing in a tumor-affected ear also depends on the quality of hearing in the contralateral ear. In general, if hearing in the affected ear has perception thresholds in the speech frequencies more than 30 dB above or if WRS is more than 30% below those of the contralateral ear, hearing in the affected ear contributes little to the patient's speech comprehension. This 30/30 criterion for useful hearing is used by clinicians who counsel patients about treatment options and expectations. In the future, it may be more appropriate to present data according to a change in PTA and WRS over time, with use of visual aids such as scattergrams, and to include metrics that have improved correlation with the real-world impact of hearing loss, such as speech recognition in noise and associated quality-of-life surveys [30].

Auditory Brainstem Responses

ABRs are the most sensitive and specific audiologic tests for the diagnosis of ANs and were used extensively prior to magnetic resonance imaging (MRI). Among patients with documented ANs, 20–30% have lost all ipsilateral ABR waves, 10–20% have only wave I, 40–60% have all waves but the latency of wave V is increased, and 10–15% have normal waveforms [31]. However, the technique suffers from a rate of false-negatives of approximately 15%, but this rate can range from 33% for intracanalicular tumors to 4% for larger lesions [31–33]. Rates of false-positives (an abnormal ABR when no AN is present) are much higher, exceeding 80% in some series [34–36].

ABRs also may be prognostic for hearing preservation. One study of 286 patients correlated preserved hearing with lower mean interwave V latencies (0.51 vs 0.7 ms for those with no postoperative hearing) and absolute wave V latencies (5.35 vs 5.96 ms) on preoperative ABR [37]. Another study of 107 patients found that rates of hearing preservation were significantly higher if the preoperative ABR had good morphology (63% vs 48% in those with poor ABR morphology) and a wave III (66.7% vs 33.3% with no wave III) [38]. Matthies and Samii classified preoperative ABRs into five types: B1–B5. Types B1 and B2 contained waves I, III, and V with variable latencies [39, 40]. Patients with a wave III (types B1–B2) had a higher rate of hearing preservation than patients without wave III (types B3–B5). Aihara and colleagues found that an interaural difference of wave V latency (IT5) of less than 1.12 ms was prognostic of useful postoperative hearing [41].

Otoacoustic Emissions

Some hearing loss from an AN or its treatment involves loss of cochlear function, some of which may reflect disruption of its vascular supply [42]. Otoacoustic emissions (OAEs) emanate from the cochlea's outer hair cells. Preserved OAEs may indicate preserved cochlear function and encourage hearing preservation strategies. Although several studies have examined OAEs in AN patients, only a few patients both lack an ABR and yet have intact OAEs that meet the criteria predictive of potential hearing preservation [43–45]. Ferber-Viart and colleagues found that OAEs were a significant predictor of hearing preservation, but Brackmann and colleagues failed to identify a significant correlation. Further studies are needed to fully evaluate the role of OAEs in AN surgery [37, 38]. Another study found that preoperative transient otoacoustic emission was a favorable prognostic indicator of preservation of useful hearing preservation after surgery [46].

Vestibular Testing

Electronystagmography (ENG) is frequently abnormal in AN patients. The caloric response stimulates the lateral semicircular canal, which is innervated by the superior vestibular nerve (SVN). An absent caloric response may indicate injury to the superior vestibular nerve (SVN) by a tumor originating from either vestibular nerve. Ninety-eight percent of patients with an AN originating from the superior vestibular nerve show a reduced caloric response compared with 60% of those with a tumor from the inferior vestibular nerve (IVN) [47]. Furthermore, those with an AN arising from the SVN had significantly less postoperative hearing loss, likely because the SVN is less intimately related anatomically with the cochlear nerve and the internal auditory artery than is the IVN [36, 48, 49]. Three recent studies have failed to demonstrate ENG as a significant prognostic factor in hearing preservation, likely because ENG is not specific for the nerve of origin [37, 50, 51]. Therefore, we do not routinely order caloric testing.

Radiology

Imaging of the CPA and the AN is covered comprehensively in Chap. 3. The discussion here focuses on imaging characteristics important to hearing conservation microsurgery.

MRI Screening: When to Do It?

Whether all patients with otherwise unexplained asymmetrical hearing loss should undergo MRI screening for a potential AN is controversial. In a retrospective cohort comparison study of more than 400 patients with asymmetrical hearing loss, Gimsing and colleagues found an interaural asymmetry of perception threshold of greater than 15 dB at two contiguous frequencies (between 2000 and 8000 Hz), an interaural asymmetry of WRS of greater than 20%, unilateral deafness, an interaural asymmetry of perception threshold of greater than 20 dB at two contiguous frequencies, or unilateral tinnitus that had the highest sensitivity for identifying an AN. Another retrospective study of more than 200 patients found an interaural asymmetry of greater than 15 dB at 3000 Hz provided the highest positive likelihood ratio (2.91) for the presence of an AN [52, 53]. Guidelines of the Congress of Neurological Surgeons recommend that greater than 10 dB asymmetry at two or more contiguous frequencies or greater than 15 dB at any single frequency warrants MRI [54].

Imaging Characteristics

Contrast-enhanced MRI is the imaging modality of choice for ANs. Key features can confirm the expected diagnosis, guide the choice of approach, and help assess risks of complications. For instance, far-lateral extension of a tumor in the IAC raises concern that all of the tumor may not be removed by a retrosigmoid exposure without increased risk of hearing loss [55]. In most retrosigmoid approaches, exposure of the lateral third of the canal risks injury to the otic capsule and thereby reduces the chances of hearing preservation [56–58].

In a cadaveric study, high-resolution computed tomography (CT)-based frameless navigation (with or without endoscope) further facilitated lateral access; whether outcomes in patients improve remains to be shown [59]. Gerganv and colleagues found that a shorter distance between the lateral tumor margin and fundus significantly correlated with worse hearing outcomes [60]. Another study found incomplete obliteration of the IAC to be a positive predictor of serviceable hearing after surgery [61]. Lateral intracanalicular extension of tumor can also challenge a middle fossa approach in which the lateral 25% of the IAC may be obscured by the overhang of the transverse crest [62].

Anterior extension, including erosion of the anterior bony wall of the IAC, is unfavorable for facial nerve outcome and likely associated with significant tumor compression of the cochlear nerve and possibly hearing loss [63]. Similarly, tumor prolapsed laterally into the cochlear modiolus eliminates the chance of hearing preservation.

As previously mentioned, the origin of the tumor from the superior or inferior vestibular nerve is significant for preserving both hearing and facial nerve function [48]. The intimate relationship between inferior vestibular nerve tumors and the cochlear nerve and internal auditory artery reduces the likelihood of hearing conservation [64]. These tumors also tend to deflect the facial nerve superiorly, leaving it in a less favorable position for a middle fossa approach. We routinely use coronal MRI to determine the tumor's location relative to the transverse crest because this relationship has practical implications for selecting a surgical approach. The optimal MRI sequence for visualizing cranial nerves is a high-resolution T2-weighted MRI; however, improved definition of nerves utilizing tractography is an area under active investigation [55, 65, 66].

The size and location of the tumor are major considerations in the choice of surgical approach. Intracanalicular tumors can be managed via either the middle fossa or retrosigmoid approaches. The middle fossa approach probably provides the best chance of hearing conservation in small tumors. However, it often requires significant manipulation of the facial nerve situated between the surgeon and the tumor, carrying higher risk of facial nerve dysfunction, particularly for a tumor from the SVN [62, 67].

In tumors with a CPA component of 0–15 mm in diameter, the middle fossa approach is associated with a relatively high rate of transient facial nerve dysfunction, but long-term results are similar to those of the retrosigmoid approach [67, 68]. In tumors with CPA components of 10–18 mm in diameter, the hearing conservation rate via the middle fossa approach was only 34% compared with 63% for tumors with less than 10 mm extension into the CPA, while long-term facial nerve outcomes were worse [69]. Similarly, a meta-analysis of surgical approach for an AN found that hearing preservation rates were similar for middle fossa and retrosigmoid approaches to tumors more than 1.5 cm in diameter, but facial nerve dysfunction was significantly higher with the middle fossa approach [67]. Informed patient participation in the choice of approach is essential because different patients may weigh the relative importance of hearing and facial function differently.

In patients with serviceable hearing and tumors with 10–25 mm diameter extension into the CPA, a retrosigmoid approach is preferred if the lateral third of the IAC is free of tumor. Hearing preservation rates are low in tumors with a CPA extension greater than 25 mm [70]. Yet, it is still reasonable to attempt hearing conservation via the retrosigmoid approach in these cases, particularly if the patient has excellent preoperative hearing and the extension of the tumor into the IAC is limited.

Complications

The complication profile associated with the retrosigmoid approaches will be considered here with a focus on hearing preservation. In contemporary acoustic neuroma surgery, facial nerve injury is uncommon, and the risk of permanent severe or total paralysis is below 10%. This risk is greater for large tumors [67]. Facial nerve outcomes of translabyrinthine and retrosigmoid approaches are generally comparable, although a meta-analysis suggested that a retrosigmoid approach results in better facial nerve outcomes than translabyrinthine or middle fossa approaches for tumors greater than 3 cm and significantly better outcomes than the middle fossa approach for intracanicular tumors [67]. Others have found that the middle fossa approach has a higher incidence of transient weakness for tumors with less than 10 mm extension into the CPA and of permanent weakness for tumors with 10–18 mm CPA extension [68, 69]. Therefore, if hearing preservation is to be attempted, we prefer the retrosigmoid approach for all tumors with more than 10 mm extension into the CPA.

Persistent postoperative headache can be a significant morbidity. Headache is more common with the retrosigmoid approach; in one study, postoperative headache was 3.8 times higher after a retrosigmoid than after a translabyrinthine approach. It may persist for 6 months after surgery [32, 67, 71]. Its cause is not completely clear. The risk of headache associated with postoperative aseptic meningitis can be reduced by limiting dissemination of and thoroughly removing intradural bone dust that results from drilling open the IAC. Replacement of the suboccipital bone plate and a curvilinear incision have been advocated to reduce postoperative headaches [48, 72–81].

Retraction of the cerebellum during the retrosigmoid approach can injure it; encephalomalacia in the lateral 1–2 cm of the hemisphere is sometimes seen on T2-weighted MRI after surgery. Most patients have no symptoms. If the injury extends more deeply, a prolonged ataxia may result.

In our experience, efforts to spare the cochlear nerve in hearing preservation approaches increase operative time and the risks of postoperative vestibular dysfunction and tumor recurrence. However, a study of more than 700 patients found that the middle fossa approach was associated with a higher risk of recurrence than retrosigmoid and translabyrinthine approaches whose risks were similar [76]. The increased vestibular dysfunction likely reflects abnormal signals from vestibular nerve remnants, which may slow vestibular compensation. Tumors can recur from a small fragment left in the fundus [77]. The chances of recurrence are higher with the middle fossa approach than with the other two. The relative risk of recurrence after retrosigmoid and translabyrinthine approaches is controversial. Recurrence after a retrosigmoid approach may be more common when dissection of the lateral third of the IAC is blinded by the preserved otic capsule [56–58, 62, 76]. Although the endoscope is routinely used in some centers to inspect the distal IAC for residual tumor, there is minimal evidence that this reduces recurrence [78, 79]. In our experience, it is often difficult to use angled endoscopes in such a small area without risking injury to the facial nerve and difficult to discern tumor from nerve and in the fundus.

Operative Techniques

Choice among operative approaches should consider numerous factors, including whether hearing preservation is to be attempted, the size of the tumor, its radiological characteristics, potential complications, and patient preferences. The comparison of operative strategies is considered in detail in Chap. 5. The focus of this chapter will be the surgical nuances of the retrosigmoid approach.

Retrosigmoid Approach

The retrosigmoid approach takes a suboccipital intradural route between the posterior petrous face and the lateral cerebellum to the CPA and IAC. It is perhaps the most versatile of all approaches to the CPA as it may be used both in hearing preservation procedures and for large tumors in which hearing preservation is not a consideration [67]. The following steps are critical.

Patient Position and Monitoring

After general anesthesia is induced, arterial and bladder catheters are inserted. A prophylactic antibiotic (cefuroxime 2 g, intravenous [IV]) is typically given. Electrodes for monitoring cranial nerves (V, VII, IX, XI) and earphones and electrodes for monitoring ABR are placed (when ABR is being monitored). Care should be taken to isolate the external auditory canal and insure that the sterilizing solution does not compromise hearing assessment.

The patient is placed in the supine-lateral position, and the ipsilateral shoulder is elevated on a folded blanket. The head is turned away from the side of the lesion, ideally 20° beyond lateral, while the neck is flexed 20°, and the vertex is angled inferiorly 10° to place the retromastoid region uppermost in the surgical field. Some surgeons use rigid head fixation (e.g., a Mayfield head holder), but it is unnecessary unless navigation is to be used. The left lower quadrant of the abdomen is prepared in a sterile fashion and draped in anticipation of harvesting a fat graft. The surgeon stands or sits at the head of the operative table. To confirm awareness of the surgical plan by the entire team, a "team time-out" is performed prior to the incision.

Incision

The retromastoid region is shaved, prepared, and draped in sterile fashion. The incision is designed to expose bone overlying retrosigmoid dura from the origin of the sigmoid sinus from the transverse sinus to just above the jugular bulb. The course of the transverse sinus is approximated by a horizontal depression in the skull, immediately above the superior occipital line, extending laterally from just above the inion to the asterion, just above and posterior to the top of the pinna. The course of the sigmoid sinus can be approximated by the vertical prominence of the posterior aspect of the mastoid superior to the digastric groove. A 6-cm vertical incision is marked parallel and 1 cm posteromedial to the vertical prominence from 2 cm above to 4 cm below the horizontal depression (Fig. 13.1). Curving the ends of the incision slightly can be useful in patients with bulky necks by enabling greater retraction of the scalp flap. Before the marked line is incised, it is injected with local anesthetic (lidocaine 1% with 1/100,000 epinephrine).

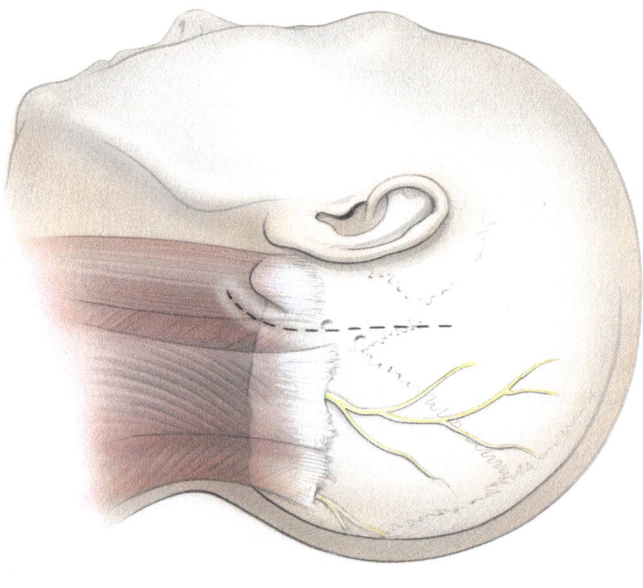

Fig. 13.1 The incision is made in the retromastoid region. Placing the incision in a relatively anterior position minimizes trauma to the nuchal musculature and the occipital nerve. (Reproduced from Jackler RK [90] with permission, copyright © 2007 RK Jackler, MD)

Soft Tissue Dissection

The incision extends through skin, galea, and suboccipital fascia and muscle down to the bone. Inferiorly, special care is taken to avoid injuring a vertebral artery passing anomalously above the foramen magnum. To minimize devascularization and facilitate closure, we advocate minimal use of the monopolar cautery until the muscle layer is reached. The soft tissue is elevated from underlying bone to expose the posterior mastoid anterolaterally and 3 cm of suboccipital bone posteromedially from just above the level of the transverse sinus to below the suboccipital convexity. Ideally, a periosteal elevator is used to minimize muscle trauma and thermal injury. The Apfelbaum modification of a suboccipital self-retaining retractor is placed.

Craniotomy

A single burr hole is drilled just medial and inferior to the asterion, which overlies the transition of the transverse sinus to the sigmoid sinus, a point approximated by the intersection of the vertical retromastoid line and transverse depression. The dura is carefully cleared from the bone using a Penfield dissector #3. A craniotomy 3–4 cm high and 2–3 cm wide (depending on the size of the tumor) is opened immediately inferior to the transverse sinus and posterior to the sigmoid sinus. Residual bone covering the posterior aspect of the sigmoid sinus is drilled away to increase the anterolateral exposure (Fig. 13.2). Doing so usually requires isolation, coagulation, and division of a prominent emissary vein entering the midportion of the sigmoid sinus. Particularly for large tumors, bone removal should extend below the convexity of the suboccipital bone to facilitate access to the cisterna magna. The margins of the craniotomy should be coated with bone wax, particularly occluding any opened mastoid air cells.

Dural Opening

The dural incision runs from the superolateral corner to the midline of the craniotomy. It proceeds inferiorly in a vertical line before turning inferolaterally to the inferior-lateral corner, thereby creating a rhomboid-shaped flap based anteriorly. Tack-up sutures pull the flap taut anterolaterally, partially rotating the posterior margin of the sigmoid sinus forward. Alternatively, a posteriorly based dural incision can be made to allow the flap to be held under the retractor (Fig. 13.3). An additional incision from the inferoposterior corner of the durotomy to the inferoposterior corner of the craniotomy frees an inferior triangle of dura, which can be retracted inferiorly to provide access to the cisterna magna. Prompt elevation of the cerebellar tonsil (using a Teflon-coated retractor) and opening of the arachnoid of the cisterna magna (using a No. 11 blade) under direct vision with a microscope permit drainage of cerebrospinal fluid and decompression of the posterior fossa—a maneuver particularly important with large tumors.

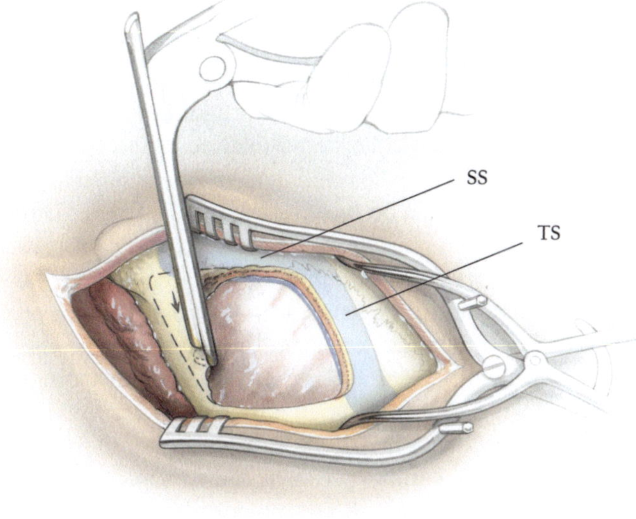

Fig. 13.2 A single burr hole is drilled just medial and inferior to the asterion. A craniotomy is opened immediately inferior to the transverse sinus and posterior to the sigmoid sinus. Any residual bone covering the posterior aspect of the sigmoid sinus is removed using a combination of rongeur and drill to increase the anterolateral exposure. *SS* sigmoid sinus, *TS* transverse sinus. (Reproduced from Jackler RK [90] with permission, copyright © 2007 RK Jackler, MD)

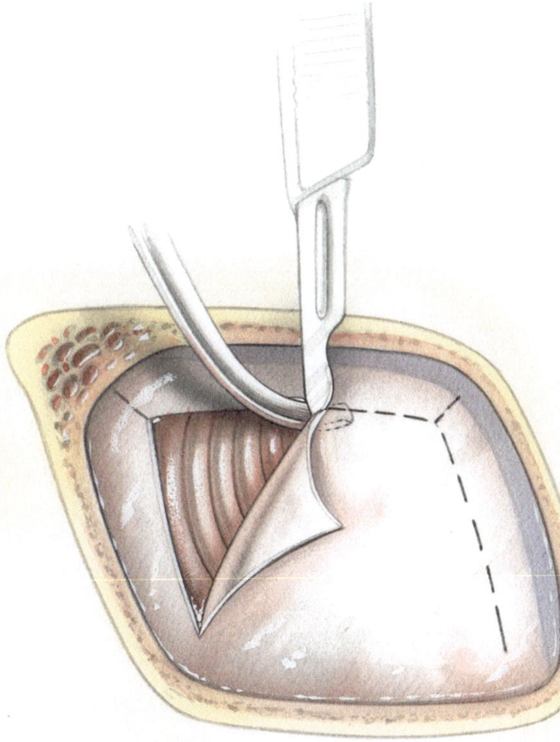

Fig. 13.3 The dura is incised about 5 mm from the edge of the craniotomy to facilitate its suture closure. Relaxing incisions are created to define small dural flaps, which are tacked up with small sutures. (Reproduced from Jackler RK [90] with permission, copyright © 2007 RK Jackler, MD)

Retraction

The approach to the tumor at the meatus and in the CPA is along the anterolateral surface of the cerebellar hemisphere and middle cerebellar peduncle. Arachnoid of the posterior aspect of the central CPA cistern is incised to allow a 5/8-in.-wide retractor blade to be positioned so that the lateral cerebellar hemisphere can be elevated from the posterior petrous face. Adaptic™, a nonadherent material, is placed between the cerebellum and the blade to protect the cerebellum and enhance hemostasis. The retractor is positioned just dorsal to the interface of the posterolateral convexity of the tumor with the middle cerebellar peduncle. The arachnoid just superior to the nerves of the jugular foramen is divided to allow their relaxation inferiorly, away from the inferior pole of the tumor. A similar division of arachnoid superiorly allows the superior pole of the tumor to be separated from the petrosal vein, which should be preserved (Fig. 13.4).

Identification of Nerves at Brainstem

Early identification of the eighth and seventh cranial nerves proximally at the brainstem is helpful to their preservation. If the tumor is large enough to completely obscure the seventh and eighth cranial nerves at the brainstem, it must first be partially debulked as described below. In other cases, the proximal nerves can be found beneath the inferior pole of the tumor. A tuft of choroid plexus at the foramen of Luschka lying just inferior to the flocculus is often a helpful landmark [64]. It lies just posterior to the origin of the ninth cranial nerve from the brainstem. The entry of the eighth cranial nerve into the brainstem is about 4 mm superior and 2 mm posterior to the origin of the ninth cranial nerve. The seventh cranial nerve exits the brainstem at a point in line with the origins of the glossopharyngeal and vagal nerves, 2 mm anterior and inferior to the entrance of the eighth cranial nerve [80].

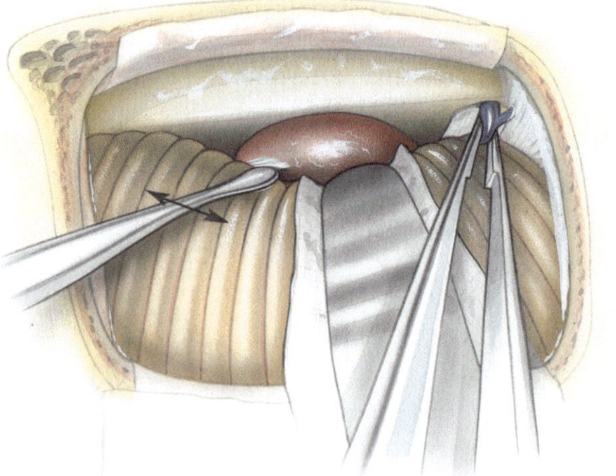

Fig. 13.4 An Apfelbaum retractor is used as the base of a retractor arm that supports the malleable blade. The blade is positioned over the lateral aspect of the cerebellum over a strip of Adaptic™. The lateral lobe of the cerebellum and the flocculus is then elevated off the tumor to expose the posterior aspect of its extracanalicular portion. The petrosal vein (also known as Dandy's vein) should be preserved. If needed for large tumors, it may be controlled with bipolar cauterization. (Reproduced from Jackler RK [90] with permission, copyright © 2007 RK Jackler, MD)

Electrophysiologic stimulation can confirm the identity of the nerve. The main stem of the anterior inferior cerebellar artery (AICA) usually passes laterally below the facial and vestibular nerves at the brainstem, but it can pass above or, rarely, between them [81]. Usually a moderately sized vein of the pontomedullary sulcus, sometimes accompanied by a twig of the rostral branch of the AICA, passes between them. Aggressive bipolar coagulation in the area should be avoided lest either nerve be injured.

The facial nerve almost always passes anterior to the tumor. Its course can be estimated from the initial direction of the nerve along the brainstem, but its subsequent path to the meatus cannot be reliably predicted as inferior (immediately lateral beneath the lower pole), intermediate (obliquely across the midportion of the tumor), or superior (up along the brainstem and then lateral to the anterior part of the upper pole). It rarely passes through the tumor and almost never lies posterior to the tumor [81]. Nonetheless, electrophysiologic simulation should always be performed prior to incising the pseudocapsule to exclude a possible posterior location, during general debulking to exclude potentially injurious penetration of the anterior pseudocapsule, and when tracing the nerve during its dissection from the pseudocapsule.

The cochlear nerve typically passes along the anterior aspect of the lower third of the tumor. Its preservation is best attempted by dissecting tumor away from any uninvolved nerve at the inferior pole. Often the cochlear component is not distinct from residual uninvolved vestibular nerve throughout the dissection. Instead, the tumor's smooth surface—evident as it is separated from the chalice of expanded uninvolved nerves—serves to reassure that the cochlear nerve, passing even more anterior, is being preserved. Such a strategy is also more likely to preserve the critical microvascular supply to the nerve and inner ear.

Removal of CPA Tumor

The arachnoid covering the posterolateral aspect of the tumor is swept posteriorly from the petrous face back over the tumor to the cerebellum. Preservation of this arachnoid plane permits extra-arachnoidal resection of tumor and greatly facilitates dissection of the tumor pseudocapsule from cerebellum, middle cerebellar peduncle, brainstem, and cranial nerves.

Removal of a CPA tumor begins with internal debulking. Risk of injury to the facial and cochlear nerves is minimized by entry into the posterior aspect of the tumor after electrophysiological screening for the facial nerve. The pseudocapsule is incised after bipolar coagulation and after the tumor within it is morselized and removed. This intratumoral debulking relaxes the pseudocapsule, encourages its separation from the facial nerve, and permits rotation of more of the tumor into direct surgical access without excessive manipulation of the facial nerve. Iterative internal tumor debulking, dissection of the pseudocapsule away from uninvolved nerves, and trimming freed tumor reduce the tumor to a thin plaque along the facial and cochlear nerves.

The larger the tumor, the greater is the risk of traumatic or ischemic injury to the cranial nerves or brainstem [82]. In this circumstance, the facial and cochlear nerves are likely to be elongated and attenuated and more vulnerable to injury. Therefore, dissection must be meticulous. The facial nerve is particularly vulnerable when it takes a long superior course along the brainstem before turning back inferiorly and laterally to cross to the meatus. Occasionally, a small plaque of tumor wedged at the apex of this hairpin turn must be left to avoid injuring the nerve.

Larger tumors are more likely to compress the brainstem and breach its arachnoidal protection. On preoperative T2-weighted MRI, this scenario is often apparent as brainstem edema. However, the brainstem's surface is usually remarkably tolerant of careful microdissection of the tumor's pseudocapsule. Such dissection must be performed with great care to avoid diverging from the surface of the tumor into neural tissue. This risk is greatest at points where the tumor attaches to the brainstem, usually corresponding to small arteries or veins bridging between tumor and brainstem [83]. Veins leaving the tumor and arteries branching solely to tumor should be isolated from the brainstem, coagulated, and divided. Bleeding caused by inadvertent rupture of such small vessels often stops with time and gentle pressure. Consequently, patience is preferable to aggressive efforts at coagulation, which might injure the brainstem or nerves [84]. Any attachment to larger, more proximal branches of the AICA and, with much larger tumors, to the superior cerebellar, posterior inferior cerebellar, basilar, and vertebral arteries must be identified and carefully freed [85]. Incorporation of such an artery within the tumor is another indication for leaving a small plaque of residual tumor.

Opening the Posterior Wall of the IAC

The IAC portion of the tumor can be exposed by drilling away the bone from its posterior wall. The IAC can be drilled early after cerebellar retraction or later after the CPA component of tumor has been retracted. When possible, we prefer to drill the IAC early, before dissection of arachnoid planes in the CPA. Doing so helps minimize the spread of bone dust into the cistern and may reduce the incidence of aseptic meningitis and postoperative headache. The definitive identification of the facial nerve in the IAC may also help during subsequent dissection of the CPA component. With larger tumors, the CPA component may be debulked to obtain sufficient access to the posterior petrous face prior to IAC drilling.

The location of the porus acusticus can be palpated with a ball hook, as can that of the operculum endolymphatic sac, which represents the origin of the vestibular aqueduct. The axis of the IAC extends from the porus to just superior to the operculum. The dura over the petrous face is carefully incised along this line to avoid cutting the endolymphatic sac. Superior and inferior dural flaps are retracted to expose the bone posterior to the IAC (Fig. 13.5). The superior flap is

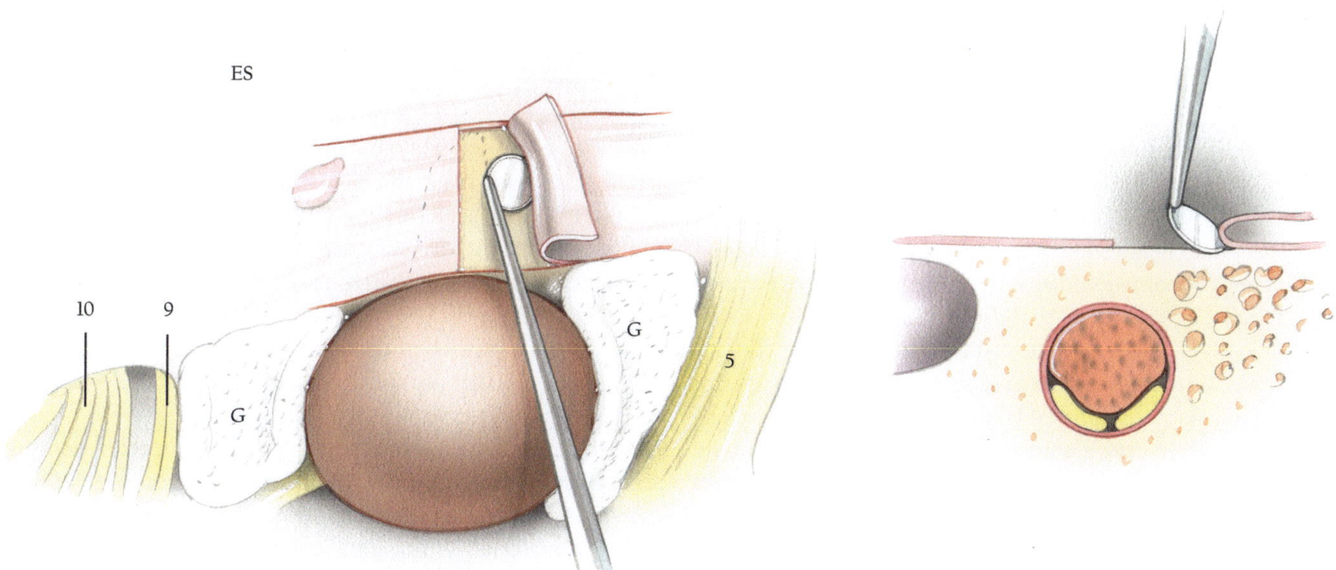

Fig. 13.5 To expose the IAC component of the tumor, the posterior osseous wall of the canal must be opened. With larger tumors, this aspect of the procedure is performed after the CPA component is debulked. To expose the bone overlying the IAC, dural flaps are elevated anteriorly and posteriorly. Preserving the dural flaps provides a purchase for suture closure of the defect at the end of the procedure. Before bone removal, Gelfoam® (G) is placed in the posterior fossa to confine the spread of bone dust within the subarachnoid space. 10 = vagus nerve; 9 = glossopharyngeal nerve; ES = endolymphatic sac; 5 = trigeminal nerve. (Reproduced from Jackler RK [90] with permission, copyright © 2007 RK Jackler, MD)

Fig. 13.6 (**a**) A cutting bur is used to rapidly drill a trough to the level of the IAC dura. (**b**) Diamond burs are then used to excavate troughs anterior and posterior to the IAC. Approximately two-thirds of its circumference is exposed to allow the IAC to be in high relief. It is particularly important to funnel the porus acusticus widely to avoid overhangs that might obscure the tumor–facial nerve interface as it angulates sharply into the CPA. (Reproduced from Jackler RK [90] with permission, copyright © 2007 RK Jackler, MD)

elevated to the tentorium. Doing so often entails sacrifice of the subarcuate artery, a branch of the AICA. This sacrifice is generally well tolerated as this artery is usually an end artery into the surrounding bone [64]. The inferior flap is elevated off the endolymphatic sac and to the superior margin of the jugular foramen. Gelfoam® is packed around the tumor to limit the spread of bone dust.

Bone removal commences with a 3 mm cutting bur at the porus to identify the posteromedial dura of the IAC. A 3-mm and then a 2-mm diamond bur is used to define the IAC further. The endolymphatic aqueduct is a useful landmark for the lateral extent of safe bone removal. Drilling through the endolymphatic aqueduct risks injury to the underlying crus commune and subsequent irreversible inner ear damage.

Troughs are drilled superior and inferior to the medial IAC to facilitate tumor exposure and resection. The jugular bulb may be immediately inferior to the IAC and, in some cases, may overlap its posterior face, which may obstruct exposure in an anatomic variant called a high-riding jugular bulb. The surgeon should review the patient's preoperative images to be alert to this possibility and to avoid injury to the jugular bulb. The dura of the IAC is opened along its axis with a No. 11 blade or a myringotomy knife, and superior and inferior flaps are created (Fig. 13.6). Given the variability of the facial nerve's course, the nerve stimulator should be used before the dura is incised to prevent inadvertent sharp injury to the nerve.

Removal of Intracanalicular Tumor

Once the dura of the IAC is incised and the contents of the canal are exposed, tumor removal can begin. The nerves are identified using the landmarks and features discussed above. Given the posterior exposure of the IAC, the vestibular nerves and tumor are encountered first. At the lateral end of the canal's opening, the facial nerve is sought just anterior to the superior vestibular nerve. The plane between the facial nerve and tumor is developed, and the cochlear nerve is identified just anterior to the inferior vestibular nerve. Careful debulking of tumor allows additional neural exposure. The portion of the vestibular nerve of tumor origin continuous with tumor is divided and dissected from the remainder of that nerve as well as from the other vestibular nerve, facial nerve, and cochlear nerve. Special effort must be made to verify removal of all lateral tumor extending deeply toward the fundus. This far-lateral dissection must sometimes be performed without the benefit of direct visualization; a small endoscope may permit a more definitive view of the distal canal. Small, cupped micro-instruments passed gently along the facial nerve are used to palpate osseous landmarks (such as the transverse crest) and to retrieve any residual tumor.

The initial dissection within the IAC usually proceeds laterally to medially. However, as noted below, the direction of dissection is not as important as its delicacy. Critical issues include avoiding traction on tumor tissue or on any nerve that might result in stretch of cochlear or facial fibers anchored at the meatus (commonly) or fundus as well as identifying and preserving the internal auditory artery. The dissection is continued through the meatus and along the superior petrous face to join that from the CPA. Once the removal of the tumor is complete, the facial nerve can be stimulated to ensure functionality; stimulus at 0.1 mA predicts good facial nerve outcome [86].

Closure

Closure begins with verification of hemostasis with the patient's blood pressure at normal levels and with a Valsalva maneuver. Irrigation of the microscopic field flushes debris from the subarachnoid space. The drilled petrous surfaces of the IAC are coated with bone wax to obliterate any opened mastoid air cells. Subcutaneous fat from the abdomen is placed over the nerves in the IAC and covered by a piece of Surgicel® to hold it in place. Sometimes, a single suture (4-0 nylon) can be placed to appose the dural flaps of the posterior petrous face over the fat graft. The cerebellar retractor is removed, and the cortex of the hemisphere is inspected for bleeding. The dura is closed in watertight fashion, using a graft or muscle patch as needed. The margins of the craniotomy are again waxed. The bone plate is secured with titanium miniplates. Suboccipital muscle and fascia and galea flaps are sutured, and the skin is stapled.

Microsurgical Dissection

Microsurgical dissection of the tumor can be difficult, and certain challenges are common to all approaches. Removal of tumor remnant from the proximal acousticofacial bundle represents one such challenge. The remaining nerves are often compressed and distorted into a shape that resembles a tulip or wine chalice surrounding the tumor remnant. Usually, the remaining vestibular nerve is posterior, the cochlear nerve is more inferior, and the facial nerve is anterior. The tumor can often be separated from the more substantial facial nerve before it is dissected from the cochlear nerve. Preservation of any uninvolved vestibular nerve often helps during dissection. The margin of the tumor is not a true capsule. Rather, it is a pseudocapsule formed by peripheral tumor cells arranged more compactly and more tangentially to the tumor surface compared with central tumor cells [87]. Because peripheral tumor cells can adhere to attenuated nerves, this final stage of dissection must be extremely delicate.

Often, partial rotation of the tumor and nerves can optimize the orientation of the dissection plane. Turning the plane to enable multiple approaches for dissection can help. The direction of dissection is less important than minimizing the traction on the nerves. Fine blunt dissection along a cleavage plane with a small disk dissector is useful. This maneuver can stabilize the nerve, while gentle traction of the tumor is maintained with a small suction. A broad plane of dissection is always desirable and is best maintained by sweeping the dissector delicately over as much of the surface of the tumor interface as possible. When the correct plane is maintained, the tumor's pseudocapsule appears smooth.

Loss of the correct plane can result in tiny remnants of tumor against nerve. These tumor plaques often infiltrate where fine vessels bridge tumor and nerve. They can become progressively thicker if dissection continues in a false plane. The correct plane can be regained either by sharply dividing the inciting attachment and elevating the plaque or by dissecting at another edge of the tumor. Remaining nerves should be inspected closely for residual tumor fragments. Small bleeding points along the facial or cochlear nerves should not be coagulated; thrombin-impregnated Gelfoam® pledgets, gentle pressure, and patience are preferable.

Intraoperative Monitoring

Intraoperative monitoring of cranial nerve function was introduced by Delgado and colleagues in the 1970s and is now standard procedure in most operating rooms [88, 89]. While it has primarily been aimed at helping identify and preserve cranial nerves, there is increasing interest in using it as a electroprognostic marker for early postoperative counseling of patients and in timing facial reanimation [90, 91]. The recent guidelines for AN surgery released by the Congress of Neurological Surgeons have recommended the use of intraoperative eighth cranial nerve monitoring in AN surgery [91]. This chapter specifically focuses on monitoring for hearing preservation. The first and most common method is recording of ABRs. The measurement of direct cochlear nerve action potentials (CNAPs), electrocochleography (ECoG), and evoked OAEs are other potential options.

Intraoperative ABR recording uses headphones within the ear canal to deliver a repetitive click stimulus to the ear. Electrodes over the mastoid and scalp then measure the electrical response of the inner ear, cochlear nerve, and brainstem. By averaging the response over time, distinct waves (I–V) can be recorded, providing information on the integrity of the auditory pathway. Despite the use of high stimulus rates, more than 1 min may be needed to obtain a reproducible waveform. A stimulus intensity of 95 dB is used to maintain an adequate signal-to-noise ratio. An ABR from the contralateral ear serves as a control and as a monitor for generalized effects such as anesthesia and temperature [92]. Clinically, the amplitude and latency of waves I, III, and V are monitored. Although each wave is generated from numerous sources, it is useful to consider wave I as arising from the distal eighth cranial nerve, wave III from the superior olivary complex, and wave V from the inferior colliculus [93]. Harper found significant improvement in hearing preservation rates for small tumors (less than 11 mm) using monitoring, with the presence of waves I and V being a positive predictor variable (with 67% likelihood of useful hearing preservation) [94].

In a review of intraoperative ABR changes in 201 patients undergoing AN resection, the risk of deafness associated with temporary loss of either wave I, III, or V was 11–14%. The risk associated with permanent loss of any of these waves was 65–78% [39]. The disappearance of waves I and III usually preceded the disappearance of wave V. The disappearance of wave III was the earliest and most sensitive sign. Neu and colleagues classified intraoperative ABR into four prognostic patterns [95]. Hearing was preserved in all patients with a stable wave V (pattern 1), whereas all patients with an abrupt loss of ABR (pattern 2) lost hearing. An irreversible loss of either wave I or wave V (pattern 3) was associated with eventual postoperative hearing loss. Patients with reversible ABR changes (pattern 4) had variable outcomes. Despite correlations between intraoperative ABR changes and postoperative hearing, some surgeons believe that changes in the ABR lack specificity. A major deficiency is that the lengthy acquisition times may not give sufficient warning to enable surgeons to take corrective action if the nerve is in danger.

The direct measurement of CNAPs using an electrode adjacent to the cochlear nerve in the operative field allows reproducible waveform averages to be obtained within seconds, compared with as long as 1 min for ABR averaging [92]. Both monopolar and bipolar electrodes are placed at the root entry zone of the eighth cranial nerve or more distally in the IAC. Amplitude and latency variability are measured continually during surgical maneuvers that put the nerve at risk. Advantages of CNAP over conventional ABR include near real-time feedback to the surgeon, easier identification of waveforms, and reliable responses even when conventional ABR is lost or deformed [96]. In one study, CNAP waveforms could be recorded in 92% of patients, whereas ABR could be obtained in only 48% of patients undergoing hearing conservation surgery [97]. The first positive peak (N1) in the CNAP waveform is generated by the cochlear nerve, and the latency is similar to that of wave II on the ABR [98]. Either decreased amplitude or increased latency of N1 can signify injury to the eighth cranial nerve [99, 100]. At the end of surgery, the presence of the N1 waveform in the CNAP is prognostically significant. In one review, no patient lacking N1 had postoperative hearing, whereas 79% of patients with N1 had measurable hearing [101]. Piccirillo and colleagues found that patients with tumors smaller than 1.5 cm and normal preoperative hearing were more likely to have AAO-HNS class A hearing; however the presence of CNAP did not ensure a good hearing outcome [102].

The primary disadvantage of the CNAP is that it reflects the integrity of the cochlear nerve only to the point where the electrode is placed. It does not give information about the integrity of the auditory pathway downstream, as does the ABR. With large tumors, the root entry zone of the cochlear nerve may be inaccessible until some tumor has been removed. In cases where the root entry zone is inaccessible, the electrode can be placed extradurally against the bone of the IAC and adjacent to the cochlear nerve [103]. CNAP recordings are highly dependent on electrode position; therefore, care must be taken during manipulations that might displace the electrode. With care, the electrode and wire can be placed outside the path of microsurgical instruments.

ECoG, another near-field technique, also can be used to record cochlear microphonic (CM) potential and summating potential (SP). CM potentials are generated by cochlear outer hair cells, and the SP represents a depolarization of the hair cells. The SP is a presynaptic response, whereas the CNAP is a postsynaptic response [92]. When ECoG and CNAP are used together, the site of damage can be localized to the cochlea or the eighth cranial nerve. However, use of ECoG alone is limited. ECoG potentials can persist for some time despite complete division of the eighth cranial nerve [104].

Several studies have compared the utility of these various intraoperative monitoring techniques. Battista and colleagues retrospectively reviewed 66 patients who underwent either ABR, ECoG, or CNAP monitoring during hearing conservation surgery [105]. Postoperatively, they found serviceable hearing in 24% of patients with ABR monitoring, 17% with ECoG monitoring, and 40% with CNAP monitoring. However, these differences did not reach statistical significance. In a review of 77 patients by Danner and colleagues, CNAP monitoring was associated with a significantly higher rate of measurable postoperative hearing than ABR (64% vs 41%) and was highest in tumors smaller than 1.5 cm [106]. However, when only serviceable hearing was considered, there was no statistically significant difference (43% vs 27%). Colletti and Fiorino found that patients monitored with ABR and CNAP had a significantly better postoperative PTA than those monitored with ABR alone (54.1 dB vs 82.5 dB) [107]. Unfortunately, data regarding the WRS or percentage of patients with serviceable hearing were not given.

Facial nerve monitoring is almost universal in AN microsurgical procedures. Lenarz and Ernest reported improved facial nerve function in both immediate and long-term (1 year) outcomes, particularly in larger tumors (>1.5 cm in diameter) with 87% of monitored patients having a House–Brackmann grade I–III immediate result compared to 74% of unmonitored patients [108]. A retrospective analysis in patients undergoing both translabyrinthine and retrosigmoid approaches found similar results in 121 patients [109]. In view of these findings, recent guidelines from the Congress of Neurological Surgeons have recommended the use of facial nerve monitoring [91].

Hearing Results

The success of hearing preservation surgery varies widely, and confounding factors and bias must be considered when comparing different surgical approaches and techniques (Table 13.3). Guidelines from the Congress of Neurological Surgeons found that the probability of maintaining serviceable hearing for small to medium tumors (<2 cm in diameter)

Table 13.3 Results of hearing preservation studies

Study	Number of patients with serviceable hearing	Approach	Tumor size (cm)[a]	AAO-HNS Class A + B[b] No (%)
Glasscock et al. [112]	136	38 MF, 98 RS	<1.5	37 (27)
Brookes and Woo [113]	17	RS	<1.0	9 (53)
Arriaga et al. [110]	26	RS	Mean = 1.66	14 (54)
	34	MF	Mean = 0.72	24 (71)
Slattery et al. [50]	143	MF	Mean = 1.2	74 (52)
Irving et al. [68]	25	MF	IC	11 (44)
	20	MF	0.1–1.0	12 (60)
	5	MF	1.1–2.0	1 (20)
	17	RS	IC	2 (12)
	12	RS	0.1–1.0	3 (25)
	21	RS	1.1–2.0	3 (14)
Satar et al. [69]	104	MF	IC–0.9	57 (62)
	47	MF	1–1.8	15 (33)
Rohit et al. [114]	107	59 MF, 48 RS	<1.5	34 (32)
Arts et al. [111]	62	MF	0.3–1.8	45 (73)
Grayeli et al. [115]	44	RS/MF	<1.5	25 (57)
Quist et al. [116]—immediate	49	MF	NR	27 (55)
Quist et al. [116]—5-year follow-up	16	MF	NR	12 (75)
Sughrue [117]	702	RS	NR	330 (47)
Yamakami et al. [118]	36	RS	<1.5	26 (72)
Mazzoni et al. [119]	189	RS	>3.2	47 (25)
Di Maio et al. [120]	28	RS	>3.0	6 (21%)
Hilton et al. [121]	78	MF	NR	51 (65%)
Maw et al. [122]	33	RS	<3.0	38%
Chee et al. [123]	126	RS	<2.0	43 (34%)
Lee [124]	59	RS	<3.0	11 (19)
Kaylie et al. [125]	27	RS	<4.0	8 (29)
Ferber-Viart [38]	86	RS	>4.0	47 (55)
Gormley [126]	69	RS	<3.9 cm	38%
Post et al. [127]	46	RS	0.9–4.0	18 (39%)
Rowed [128]	26	RS	IC	50%
Samii [129]	16	RS	IC	56%
Colletti [107]	25	RS	0.4–1.2	57 (%) (A, B, C)
Nonaka [130]	170	RS	<2.0	82.8%
Sameshima [131]	82	RS	<1.5	73.2%
Sanna et al. [132]	107	RS		54.2%
				Hannover Class[c] (H1 + H2)
Samii and Matthies [133]	29	RS	T1[d]	6 (21)
	96	RS	T2[d]	25 (26)
	249	RS	T3[d]	39 (16)
				Gardner–Robertson Grade I + II
Cohen et al. [134]	128	RS	<0.5	32 (37)[e]
			0.6–1.0	32 (34)[e]
			1.1–1.5	38 (24)[e]
			>1.5	26 (11)[e]
Dornhoffer et al. [51]	65	MF	<0.5	39 (60)[e]
	11	MF	0.5–1.0	7 (64)[e]
	17	MF	1.0–1.5	8 (47)[e]
Betchen et al. [135]	142	RS	0.4–4.0[f]	43 (30)[e]
Rowed and Nedzelski [128]	26	RS	IC	13 (50)[g]
	68	RS	0.4–1.5	20 (29)[g]
Lin [136]	113	RS	<2.0	30 (27), 18 (16) at 9.5 years
Goel et al. [137]	42	RS	>2.5	13 (31)
Fischer et al. [138]	22	RS	>3.0 to <1.0	12 (55)

IC intracanalicular, *MF* middle fossa, *RS* retrosigmoid

Note: Selected studies using the middle fossa approach are included in the table for comparison

Modified with permission from Jackler RK and Driscoll CLW [139]

[a] Tumor size includes posterior fossa component except when indicated

[b] AAO-HNS classification system

[c] New Hannover classification system

[d] T1 = intrameatal; T2 = intrameatal and extrameatal; T3 = filling the cerebellopontine angle

[e] Pure-tone average <50 dB and word recognition >50%

[f] Size range of tumors with preserved hearing

[g] Pure-tone average <50 dB and word recognition >60%

following microsurgical resection was between 25% and 50% at 2, 5, and 10 years postoperatively [23]. For patients with AAO-HNS class A or Gardner–Robertson grade I, 2-year and 5-year probabilities of serviceable hearing were 50–75%, dropping to 25–50% at 10 years [23].

Factors with a heavy impact on hearing outcome postoperatively include preoperative serviceable hearing, size (particularly less than 15 mm in diameter), and a distal internal auditory cerebrospinal fluid cap, while age and sex were not strong predictors [23]. Other factors that confound comparison of results among series include differing restrictions on tumor location, surgical approaches, metrics of hearing results, classification systems, and definitions of success.

The highest rates of hearing preservation have generally been reported with small tumors treated via the middle fossa approach [67–69, 110, 111]. In the most favorable conditions, the rate of preservation of useful hearing surpasses 50%. The middle fossa approach, however, has three disadvantages. Firstly, exposure of the CPA component of the tumor is limited. Secondly, in contrast to the translabyrinthine approach, the lateral IAC may require blind dissection. Thirdly, compared with other approaches, the facial nerve is at increased risk of permanent palsy if the cisternal tumoral component is more than 1.0 cm in diameter [62, 67, 69].

Overall hearing preservation rates via the retrosigmoid approach tend to be lower than those after a middle fossa approach for smaller tumors (less than 15 mm in diameter) [67]. However, a direct comparison controlling for tumor size and preoperative hearing status is difficult. In one series, as many as 25% of patients retained serviceable hearing after the retrosigmoid approach for tumors less than 20 mm in diameter [68]. Hearing preservation rates are diminished when the cisternal tumoral component is more than 20 mm in diameter [128, 133, 134, 140].

Which Approach?

A recent review found hearing preservation rates of 18.9–77% with the middle fossa approach with a facial nerve preservation rate of 50–86%. The retrosigmoid approach also had excellent hearing preservation rates of between 11% and 68% with a higher facial preservation rate (59–98.7%) [25, 130, 131, 133, 141–145]. Recent consensus guidelines found either approach was reasonable for hearing preservation [146]. When choosing the approach for a particular patient, overall success rates are not as important as individual prognostic factors. For example, a patient with a small tumor, minimal IAC involvement, excellent preoperative hearing, and a normal ABR will likely have a 50% chance of retaining hearing regardless of whether the middle fossa or retrosigmoid approach is used. Colletti and colleagues found that tumors less than 3 mm from the IAC fundus had higher preservation rates with a middle fossa approach while, for those with more medial location, the middle fossa approach was not superior to a retrosigmoid approach [147]. Conversely, patients lacking these favorable characteristics will likely have poor results. Given that only a small fraction of patients with ANs are candidates for hearing preservation and the probability of success is limited, one can estimate that only 5% of patients with ANs will have useful hearing in the tumor ear after surgery. In comparison, a recent review of the literature found similar facial nerve preservation rates for retrosigmoid (36–95%) and translabyrinthine (29–89%) approaches [146].

Attempts at hearing preservation surgery are encouraged for patients with good preoperative hearing (class A or B) and tumors less than 20 mm in diameter [146]. Using a retrosigmoid approach, Sameshima found a hearing preservation rate of 73.2% in tumors less than 15 mm in diameter, and Nonaka and colleagues reported hearing preservation rates of approximately 83% for tumors less than 20 mm in diameter [130, 131]. At a mean follow-up of 18 months, Grayeli and colleagues found a hearing preservation rate of 57% in patients who presented with serviceable hearing [115]. An attempt at hearing preservation may be warranted for even large tumors. In patients with tumors larger than 30 mm in diameter and serviceable hearing preoperatively, Di Maio and colleagues found that 21% had serviceable hearing following RS surgery [120].

Follow-Up and Long-Term Outcomes

Imaging

Protocols for postoperative imaging stipulate different intervals between scans and lengths of follow-up depending on tumor, patient, and surgical factors. In a study of 299 patients for whom gross total resection of tumor was achieved, Bennett and colleagues found just 3 patients with nodular enhancement on MRI at 1 and 5 years; 2 of these were the only patients who developed recurrence [148]. Similarly, low recurrence rates were found in a translabyrinthine series by Tysome and colleagues: of 314 patients, 97% had no recurrence at 2 years, while 8 had linear enhancement at 2 years, none of whom progressed over 5–15 years [149]. One patient with nodular enhancement at 2 years had tumor progression. In a study of 50 patients, Arlt and colleagues found that 2 of 22 patients had recurrence after gross total resection at approximately 3.5 years, while 9 of 28 patients had recurrence after subtotal resection [150]. Recent guidelines recommend that baseline MRI be obtained within the first year following surgery, with annual or biannual imaging for at least 5 years [55]. If the patient develops nodular enhancement, more frequent imaging is indicated [55].

Hearing

Even after initially successful hearing preservation surgery, both pure-tone thresholds and speech discrimination can deteriorate over time. In 14 of 25 patients operated on via the middle fossa route, the average speech reception threshold loss was 12 dB, and the average loss of speech discrimination was 25% over a mean follow-up of 8.1 years [49]. A different study assessed preservation of serviceable hearing in 35 patients with Gardner–Robertson grade I and II hearing after a retrosigmoid approach over an average of 7 years. Overall, 30 patients (86%) maintained serviceable hearing, 5 patients (14%) dropped to class 3 or 4, and 3 patients (9%) increased from a class 3 into the serviceable range [135]. Similar rates of long-term hearing deterioration, ranging from 22% to 36% over 5 years, have been reported by others [79, 151]. Another retrospective study found 27% of patients had serviceable hearing in the immediate postoperative period, but this number dropped to 16% over 10 years of follow-up [136]. In contrast, in a study of patients under 40 years of age, Sughrue and colleagues found that, if patients had preserved hearing postoperatively, no patient progressed to nonserviceable hearing even after 10 years [152]. Similarly, in a study of 15 patients who had preserved hearing postoperatively, Yamakami and colleagues found that 12 patients (80%) maintained serviceable hearing after 7 years [118]. Another study found that, for tumors less than 20 mm in diameter and serviceable hearing prior to surgery, rates of continued serviceable hearing at 2, 5, and 10 years are 47%, 45%, and 43%, respectively [23].

Long-Term Risk of Recurrence

In a study of 299 patients who underwent gross total resection, Bennett and colleagues found only 2 patients (0.67%) developed recurrence [148]. Similarly, another study found only 1 patient of 314 developed recurrence following gross total resection [149]. However, in 203 patients, Carlson and colleagues found that subtotal resection increased future recurrence 16-fold [153]. Bloch and colleagues found that the recurrence rate of near total and subtotal resection over 3 years in 79 patients was 3% and 32%, respectively [154]. Another study of 20 subtotal resected tumors found only 1 recurrence over a mean follow-up of 5 years [155]. A recent study on a patient with unilateral AN who underwent a retrosigmoid approach found that there was a significant recurrence rate in subtotal resected ANs, with a recurrence-free survival rate at 5, 10, 15, and 20 years of 93%, 78%, 68%, and 51%, respectively [156]. Even in gross total resection, recurrence-free survival for 5, 10, 15, and 20 years was 96%, 82%, 73%, and 56%, respectively, while subtotal resection had 5-, 10-, and 15-year recurrence-free survival of 47%, 17%, and 8%, respectively [156]. A recent report evaluating large ANs (>2.5 cm), where residual tumor was treated with radiation, found that the likelihood of regrowth was three times higher in subtotal resection and radiation when compared to gross total or near total resection, with similar facial nerve outcomes between the groups [157]. Overall, there appears to be a low risk of recurrence over the first 5 years following gross total resection. Because the risk is higher after subtotal resection, patients with incomplete tumor removal should be followed for decades.

References

1. McRackan TR, Brackmann DE. Historical perspective on evolution in management of lateral skull base tumors. Otolaryngol Clin N Am. 2015;48(3):397–405.
2. Stevens G. A case of tumor of the auditory nerve occupying the fossa for the cerebellum. Arch Otolaryngol. 1879;8:171–6.
3. Toynbee J. Neuroma of the auditory nerve. Trans Path Soc Lond. 1853;4:259–60.
4. McBurney C, Starr M. A contribution to cerebral surgery: diagnosis, localization and operation for removal of three tumors of the brain: with some comments upon the surgical treatment of brain tumors. Am J Med Sci. 1893;55:361–87.
5. von Eiselsberg A. Uber die chirurgische Behandlung der Hirntumoren. Trans Int Congr Med. 1913;7:203–7.
6. Cushing H. The acoustic tumors. In: Intracranial tumours. Springfield, IL: Charles C. Thomas; 1932.
7. Dandy WE. Ventriculography following the injection of air into the cerebral ventricles. Ann Surg. 1918;68(1):5–11.
8. Machinis TG, Fountas KN, Dimopoulos V, Robinson JS. History of acoustic neurinoma surgery. Neurosurg Focus. 2005;18(4):e9.
9. Dandy W. Results of removal of acoustic tumors by the unilateral approach. AMA Arch Surg. 1941;42:1026–33.
10. Cairns H. Acoustic neuroma of the right cerebellopontine angle: spontaneous recovery from postoperative facial palsy. Proc R Soc Med. 1931;25:35–40.
11. Olivecrona H. Acoustic tumours. J Neurol Psychiatry. 1940;3(2):141–6.
12. Hitselberger WE, House WF. Surgical approaches to acoustic tumors. Arch Otolaryngol Chic Ill 1960. 1966;84(3):286–91.
13. Elliott FA, McKissock W. Acoustic neuroma; early diagnosis. Lancet Lond Engl. 1954;267(6850):1189–91.
14. Neely JG. Is it possible to totally resect an acoustic tumor and conserve hearing? Otolaryngol Head Neck Surg. 1984;92(2):162–7.
15. Neely JG. Hearing conservation surgery for acoustic tumors—a clinical-pathologic correlative study. Am J Otol. 1985;(Suppl):143–6.
16. Kveton JF. Delayed spontaneous return of hearing after acoustic tumor surgery: evidence for cochlear nerve conduction block. Laryngoscope. 1990;100(5):473–6.
17. Sekiya T, Møller AR. Effects of cerebellar retractions on the cochlear nerve: an experimental study on rhesus monkeys. Acta Neurochir. 1988;90(1–2):45–52.
18. Sekiya T, Iwabuchi T, Kamata S, Ishida T. Deterioration of auditory evoked potentials during cerebellopontine angle manipulations. An interpretation based on an experimental model in dogs. J Neurosurg. 1985;63(4):598–607.
19. Sekiya T, Møller AR. Cochlear nerve injuries caused by cerebellopontine angle manipulations. An electrophysiological and morphological study in dogs. J Neurosurg. 1987;67(2):244–9.
20. Sekiya T, Møller AR, Jannetta PJ. Pathophysiological mechanisms of intraoperative and postoperative hearing deficits in cerebellopontine angle surgery: an experimental study. Acta Neurochir. 1986;81(3–4):142–51.

21. Jackler R, Pfister M. Acoustic neuroma. In: Jackler and Brackman (eds) Neurotology. 2nd ed. Philadelphia: Mosby; 2005. p. 727–82.
22. Lambert PR, Ruth RA, Thomas JF. Promontory electrical stimulation in postoperative acoustic tumor patients. Laryngoscope. 1992;102(7):814–9.
23. Carlson ML, Vivas EX, McCracken DJ, Sweeney AD, Neff BA, Shepard NT, et al. Congress of Neurological Surgeons systematic review and evidence-based guidelines on hearing preservation outcomes in patients with sporadic vestibular schwannomas. Neurosurgery. 2018;82(2):E35–9.
24. Stangerup S-E, Caye-Thomasen P. Epidemiology and natural history of vestibular schwannomas. Otolaryngol Clin N Am. 2012;45(2):257–268, vii.
25. Meyer TA, Canty PA, Wilkinson EP, Hansen MR, Rubinstein JT, Gantz BJ. Small acoustic neuromas: surgical outcomes versus observation or radiation. Otol Neurotol. 2006;27(3):380–92.
26. Stangerup S-E, Caye-Thomasen P, Tos M, Thomsen J. Change in hearing during "wait and scan" management of patients with vestibular schwannoma. J Laryngol Otol. 2008;122(7):673–81.
27. Gardner G, Robertson JH. Hearing preservation in unilateral acoustic neuroma surgery. Ann Otol Rhinol Laryngol. 1988;97(1):55–66.
28. Committee on Hearing and Equilibrium guidelines for the evaluation of hearing preservation in acoustic neuroma (vestibular schwannoma). American Academy of Otolaryngology-Head and Neck Surgery Foundation, INC. Otolaryngol Head Neck Surg. 1995;113(3):179–80.
29. Gurgel RK, Jackler RK, Dobie RA, Popelka GR. A new standardized format for reporting hearing outcome in clinical trials. Otolaryngol Head Neck Surg. 2012;147(5):803–7.
30. Oghalai JS, Jackler RK. New web-based tool for generating scattergrams to report hearing results. Otolaryngol Head Neck Surg. 2016;154(6):981.
31. Fraysse B, Fraysse M, Bounaix M. Acoustic neuroma with normal ABR. In: Tos M, Thomsen J (eds) Proceeding of the first international conference on acoustic neuroma. Amsterdam: Kugler; 1992. p. 91–5.
32. Ruckenstein MJ, Cueva RA, Morrison DH, Press G. A prospective study of ABR and MRI in the screening for vestibular schwannomas. Am J Otol. 1996;17(2):317–20.
33. Wilson DF, Hodgson RS, Gustafson MF, Hogue S, Mills L. The sensitivity of auditory brainstem response testing in small acoustic neuromas. Laryngoscope. 1992;102(9):961–4.
34. Weiss MH, Kisiel DL, Bhatia P. Predictive value of brainstem evoked response in the diagnosis of acoustic neuroma. Otolaryngol Head Neck Surg. 1990;103(4):583–5.
35. Walsted A, Kisiel K, Salomon G. Auditory brainstem response in the diagnosis of acoustic neuroma. In: Tos M, Thomsen J (eds) Proceeding of the first international conference on acoustic neuroma. Amsterdam: Kugler; 1992. p. 77–81.
36. Olsson J, Barrs D, Krueger W, Gibbons D. Use of receiver operating curves in the design of diagnostic strategies for retrocochlear lesions. In: Tos M, Thomsen J (eds) Proceeding of the first international conference on acoustic neuroma. Amsterdam: Kluger; 1992.
37. Brackmann DE, Owens RM, Friedman RA, Hitselberger WE, De la Cruz A, House JW, et al. Prognostic factors for hearing preservation in vestibular schwannoma surgery. Am J Otol. 2000;21(3):417–24.
38. Ferber-Viart C, Laoust L, Boulud B, Duclaux R, Dubreuil C. Acuteness of preoperative factors to predict hearing preservation in acoustic neuroma surgery. Laryngoscope. 2000;110(1):145–50.
39. Matthies C, Samii M. Management of vestibular schwannomas (acoustic neuromas): the value of neurophysiology for intraoperative monitoring of auditory function in 200 cases. Neurosurgery. 1997;40(3):459–66; discussion 466–8.
40. Matthies C, Samii M. Management of vestibular schwannomas (acoustic neuromas): the value of neurophysiology for evaluation and prediction of auditory function in 420 cases. Neurosurgery. 1997;40(5):919–29; discussion 929–30.
41. Aihara N, Murakami S, Takemura K, Yamada K. Interaural difference of wave V predicting postoperative hearing in Gardner-Robertson class II acoustic neuroma patients. J Neurol Surg B Skull Base. 2013;74(5):274–8.
42. Babbage MJ, Feldman MB, O'Beirne GA, Macfarlane MR, Bird PA. Patterns of hearing loss following retrosigmoid excision of unilateral vestibular schwannoma. J Neurol Surg B Skull Base. 2013;74(3):166–75.
43. Filipo R, Delfini R, Fabiani M, Cordier A, Barbara M. Role of transient-evoked otoacoustic emissions for hearing preservation in acoustic neuroma surgery. Am J Otol. 1997;18(6): 746–9.
44. Telischi F. An objective method of analyzing cochlear versus noncochlear patterns of distortion-product otoacoustic emissions in patients with acoustic neuromas. Laryngoscope. 2000;110(4):553–62.
45. Prasher DK, Tun T, Brookes GB, Luxon LM. Mechanisms of hearing loss in acoustic neuroma: an otoacoustic emission study. Acta Otolaryngol (Stockh). 1995;115(3):375–81.
46. Kim AH, Edwards BM, Telian SA, Kileny PR, Arts HA. Transient evoked otoacoustic emissions pattern as a prognostic indicator for hearing preservation in acoustic neuroma surgery. Otol Neurotol. 2006;27(3):372–9.
47. Linthicum F. Electronystagmography findings in patients with acoustic tumors. Semin Hear. 1983;4:47–53.
48. Borgmann H, Lenarz T, Lenarz M. Preoperative prediction of vestibular schwannoma's nerve of origin with posturography and electronystagmography. Acta Otolaryngol (Stockh). 2011;131(5):498–503.
49. Shelton C, Brackmann DE, House WF, Hitselberger WE. Acoustic tumor surgery. Prognostic factors in hearing conversation. Arch Otolaryngol Head Neck Surg. 1989;115(10):1213–6.
50. Slattery WH, Brackmann DE, Hitselberger W. Middle fossa approach for hearing preservation with acoustic neuromas. Am J Otol. 1997;18(5):596–601.
51. Dornhoffer JL, Helms J, Hoehmann DH. Hearing preservation in acoustic tumor surgery: results and prognostic factors. Laryngoscope. 1995;105(2):184–7.
52. Saliba I, Martineau G, Chagnon M. Asymmetric hearing loss: rule 3,000 for screening vestibular schwannoma. Otol Neurotol. 2009;30(4):515–21.
53. Saliba I, Bergeron M, Martineau G, Chagnon M. Rule 3,000: a more reliable precursor to perceive vestibular schwannoma on MRI in screened asymmetric sensorineural hearing loss. Eur Arch Oto-Rhino-Laryngol. 2011;268(2):207–12.
54. Sweeney AD, Carlson ML, Shepard NT, McCracken DJ, Vivas EX, Neff BA, et al. Congress of Neurological Surgeons systematic review and evidence-based guidelines on otologic and audiologic screening for patients with vestibular schwannomas. Neurosurgery. 2018;82(2):E29–31.
55. Dunn IF, Bi WL, Mukundan S, Delman BN, Parish J, Atkins T, et al. Congress of Neurological Surgeons systematic review and evidence-based guidelines on the role of imaging in the diagnosis and management of patients with vestibular schwannomas. Neurosurgery. 2018;82(2):E32–4.
56. Domb GH, Chole RA. Anatomical studies of the posterior petrous apex with regard to hearing preservation in acoustic neuroma removal. Laryngoscope. 1980;90(11 Pt 1):1769–76.
57. Kartush JM, Telian SA, Graham MD, Kemink JL. Anatomic basis for labyrinthine preservation during posterior fossa acoustic tumor surgery. Laryngoscope. 1986;96(9 Pt 1):1024–8.

58. Laine T, Johnsson LG, Palva T. Surgical anatomy of the internal auditory canal. A temporal bone dissection study. Acta Otolaryngol (Stockh). 1990;110(1–2):78–84.
59. Pillai P, Sammet S, Ammirati M. Image-guided, endoscopic-assisted drilling and exposure of the whole length of the internal auditory canal and its fundus with preservation of the integrity of the labyrinth using a retrosigmoid approach: a laboratory investigation. Neurosurgery. 2009;65(6 Suppl):53–9; discussion 59.
60. Gerganov V, Nouri M, Stieglitz L, Giordano M, Samii M, Samii A. Radiological factors related to pre-operative hearing levels in patients with vestibular schwannomas. J Clin Neurosci. 2009;16(8):1009–12.
61. Mohr G, Sade B, Dufour J-J, Rappaport JM. Preservation of hearing in patients undergoing microsurgery for vestibular schwannoma: degree of meatal filling. J Neurosurg. 2005;102(1):1–5.
62. Driscoll CL, Jackler RK, Pitts LH, Banthia V. Is the entire fundus of the internal auditory canal visible during the middle fossa approach for acoustic neuroma? Am J Otol. 2000;21(3):382–8.
63. Wong RH, Copeland WR, Jacob JT, Sivakanthan S, Van Gompel JJ, van Loveren H, et al. Anterior extension of tumor is as important as tumor size to facial nerve outcome and extent of resection for vestibular schwannomas. J Neurol Surg B Skull Base. 2017;78(6):473–80.
64. Rhoton AL. The cerebellopontine angle and posterior fossa cranial nerves by the retrosigmoid approach. Neurosurgery. 2000;47(3 Suppl):S93–129.
65. Gerganov VM, Giordano M, Samii M, Samii A. Diffusion tensor imaging-based fiber tracking for prediction of the position of the facial nerve in relation to large vestibular schwannomas. J Neurosurg. 2011;115(6):1087–93.
66. Taoka T, Hirabayashi H, Nakagawa H, Sakamoto M, Myochin K, Hirohashi S, et al. Displacement of the facial nerve course by vestibular schwannoma: preoperative visualization using diffusion tensor tractography. J Magn Reson Imaging JMRI. 2006;24(5):1005–10.
67. Ansari SF, Terry C, Cohen-Gadol AA. Surgery for vestibular schwannomas: a systematic review of complications by approach. Neurosurg Focus. 2012;33(3):E14.
68. Irving RM, Jackler RK, Pitts LH. Hearing preservation in patients undergoing vestibular schwannoma surgery: comparison of middle fossa and retrosigmoid approaches. J Neurosurg. 1998;88(5):840–5.
69. Satar B, Jackler RK, Oghalai J, Pitts LH, Yates PD. Risk-benefit analysis of using the middle fossa approach for acoustic neuromas with >10 mm cerebellopontine angle component. Laryngoscope. 2002;112(8 Pt 1):1500–6.
70. Yates PD, Jackler RK, Satar B, Pitts LH, Oghalai JS. Is it worthwhile to attempt hearing preservation in larger acoustic neuromas? Otol Neurotol. 2003;24(3):460–4.
71. Levo H, Pyykkö I, Blomstedt G. Postoperative headache after surgery for vestibular schwannoma. Ann Otol Rhinol Laryngol. 2000;109(9):853–8.
72. Soumekh B, Levine SC, Haines SJ, Wulf JA. Retrospective study of postcraniotomy headaches in suboccipital approach: diagnosis and management. Am J Otol. 1996;17(4):617–9.
73. Schessel DA, Rowed DW, Nedzelski JM, Feghali JG. Postoperative pain following excision of acoustic neuroma by the suboccipital approach: observations on possible cause and potential amelioration. Am J Otol. 1993;14(5):491–4.
74. Harner SG, Beatty CW, Ebersold MJ. Headache after acoustic neuroma excision. Am J Otol. 1993;14(6):552–5.
75. Harner SG, Beatty CW, Ebersold MJ. Impact of cranioplasty on headache after acoustic neuroma removal. Neurosurgery. 1995;36(6):1097–9; discussion 1099–100.
76. Sughrue ME, Kaur R, Rutkowski MJ, Kane AJ, Kaur G, Yang I, et al. Extent of resection and the long-term durability of vestibular schwannoma surgery. J Neurosurg. 2011;114(5):1218–23.
77. Roberson JB, Brackmann DE, Hitselberger WE. Acoustic neuroma recurrence after suboccipital resection: management with translabyrinthine resection. Am J Otol. 1996;17(2):307–11.
78. Kumon Y, Kohno S, Ohue S, Watanabe H, Inoue A, Iwata S, et al. Usefulness of endoscope-assisted microsurgery for removal of vestibular schwannomas. J Neurol Surg B Skull Base. 2012;73(1):42–7.
79. McKennan KX. Endoscopy of the internal auditory canal during hearing conservation acoustic tumor surgery. Am J Otol. 1993;14(3):259–62.
80. Rhoton AL. Microsurgical anatomy of the brainstem surface facing an acoustic neuroma. Surg Neurol. 1986;25(4):326–39.
81. Sampath P, Rini D, Long DM. Microanatomical variations in the cerebellopontine angle associated with vestibular schwannomas (acoustic neuromas): a retrospective study of 1006 consecutive cases. J Neurosurg. 2000;92(1):70–8.
82. Sampath P, Holliday MJ, Brem H, Niparko JK, Long DM. Facial nerve injury in acoustic neuroma (vestibular schwannoma) surgery: etiology and prevention. J Neurosurg. 1997;87(1):60–6.
83. Ojemann RG. Management of acoustic neuromas (vestibular schwannomas) (honored guest presentation). Clin Neurosurg. 1993;40:498–535.
84. Samii M, Gerganov V, Samii A. Improved preservation of hearing and facial nerve function in vestibular schwannoma surgery via the retrosigmoid approach in a series of 200 patients. J Neurosurg. 2006;105(4):527–35.
85. Martin RG, Grant JL, Peace D, Theiss C, Rhoton AL. Microsurgical relationships of the anterior inferior cerebellar artery and the facial-vestibulocochlear nerve complex. Neurosurgery. 1980;6(5):483–507.
86. Silverstein H, Willcox TO, Rosenberg SI, Seidman MD. Prediction of facial nerve function following acoustic neuroma resection using intraoperative facial nerve stimulation. Laryngoscope. 1994;104(5 Pt 1):539–44.
87. Kuo TC, Jackler RK, Wong K, Blevins NH, Pitts LH. Are acoustic neuromas encapsulated tumors? Otolaryngol Head Neck Surg. 1997;117(6):606–9.
88. Sughrue ME, Yang I, Rutkowski MJ, Aranda D, Parsa AT. Preservation of facial nerve function after resection of vestibular schwannoma. Br J Neurosurg. 2010;24(6):666–71.
89. Delgado TE, Bucheit WA, Rosenholtz HR, Chrissian S. Intraoperative monitoring of facila muscle evoked responses obtained by intracranial stimulation of the facila nerve: a more accurate technique for facila nerve dissection. Neurosurgery. 1979;4(5):418–21.
90. National Institutes of Health Consensus Development Conference Statement on acoustic neuroma, December 11–13, 1991. The Consensus Development Panel. Arch Neurol. 1994;51(2):201–7.
91. Vivas EX, Carlson ML, Neff BA, Shepard NT, McCracken DJ, Sweeney AD, et al. Congress of Neurological Surgeons systematic review and evidence-based guidelines on intraoperative cranial nerve monitoring in vestibular schwannoma surgery. Neurosurgery. 2018;82(2):E44–6.
92. Yingling C, Ashram Y. Intraoperative monitoring of cranial nerves in skull base surgery. In: Jackler RK, Brackmann DE, editors. Neurotology. 2nd ed. Philadelphia: Elsevier Mosby; 2005. p. 958–93.
93. Legatt AD. Mechanisms of intraoperative brainstem auditory evoked potential changes. J Clin Neurophysiol. 2002;19(5):396–408.
94. Harper CM, Harner SG, Slavit DH, Litchy WJ, Daube JR, Beatty CW, et al. Effect of BAEP monitoring on hearing preservation during acoustic neuroma resection. Neurology. 1992;42(8):1551–3.

95. Neu M, Strauss C, Romstöck J, Bischoff B, Fahlbusch R. The prognostic value of intraoperative BAEP patterns in acoustic neurinoma surgery. Clin Neurophysiol. 1999;110(11):1935–41.
96. Matthies C, Samii M. Direct brainstem recording of auditory evoked potentials during vestibular schwannoma resection: nuclear BAEP recording. Technical note and preliminary results. J Neurosurg. 1997;86(6):1057–62.
97. Jackson LE, Roberson JB. Acoustic neuroma surgery: use of cochlear nerve action potential monitoring for hearing preservation. Am J Otol. 2000;21(2):249–59.
98. Møller AR, Jannetta PJ, Sekhar LN. Contributions from the auditory nerve to the brain-stem auditory evoked potentials (BAEPs): results of intracranial recording in man. Electroencephalogr Clin Neurophysiol. 1988;71(3):198–211.
99. Møller AR. Monitoring auditory function during operations to remove acoustic tumors. Am J Otol. 1996;17(3):452–60.
100. Cueva RA, Morris GF, Prioleau GR. Direct cochlear nerve monitoring: first report on a new atraumatic, self-retaining electrode. Am J Otol. 1998;19(2):202–7.
101. Zappia JJ, Wiet RJ, O'Connor CA, Martone L. Intraoperative auditory monitoring in acoustic neuroma surgery. Otolaryngol Head Neck Surg. 1996;115(1):98–106.
102. Piccirillo E, Hiraumi H, Hamada M, Russo A, De Stefano A, Sanna M. Intraoperative cochlear nerve monitoring in vestibular schwannoma surgery—does it really affect hearing outcome? Audiol Neurootol. 2008;13(1):58–64.
103. Roberson J, Senne A, Brackmann D, Hitselberger WE, Saunders J. Direct cochlear nerve action potentials as an aid to hearing preservation in middle fossa acoustic neuroma resection. Am J Otol. 1996;17(4):653–7.
104. Silverstein H, McDaniel A, Wazen J, Norrell H. Retrolabyrinthine vestibular neurectomy with simultaneous monitoring of eighth nerve and brain stem auditory evoked potentials. Otolaryngol Head Neck Surg. 1985;93(6):736–42.
105. Battista RA, Wiet RJ, Paauwe L. Evaluation of three intraoperative auditory monitoring techniques in acoustic neuroma surgery. Am J Otol. 2000;21(2):244–8.
106. Danner C, Mastrodimos B, Cueva RA. A comparison of direct eighth nerve monitoring and auditory brainstem response in hearing preservation surgery for vestibular schwannoma. Otol Neurotol. 2004;25(5):826–32.
107. Colletti V, Fiorino FG. Advances in monitoring of seventh and eighth cranial nerve function during posterior fossa surgery. Am J Otol. 1998;19(4):503–12.
108. Lenarz T, Ernst A. Intraoperative facial nerve monitoring in the surgery of cerebellopontine angle tumors: improved preservation of nerve function. ORL J Oto-Rhino-Laryngol Relat Spec. 1994;56(1):31–5.
109. Silverstein H, Rosenberg SI, Flanzer J, Seidman MD. Intraoperative facial nerve monitoring in acoustic neuroma surgery. Am J Otol. 1993;14(6):524–32.
110. Arriaga MA, Luxford WM, Berliner KI. Facial nerve function following middle fossa and translabyrinthine acoustic tumor surgery: a comparison. Am J Otol. 1994;15(5):620–4.
111. Arts HA, Telian SA, El-Kashlan H, Thompson BG. Hearing preservation and facial nerve outcomes in vestibular schwannoma surgery: results using the middle cranial fossa approach. Otol Neurotol. 2006;27(2):234–41.
112. Glasscock ME, Hays JW, Minor LB, Haynes DS, Carrasco VN. Preservation of hearing in surgery for acoustic neuromas. J Neurosurg. 1993;78(6):864–70.
113. Brookes GB, Woo J. Hearing preservation in acoustic neuroma surgery. Clin Otolaryngol Allied Sci. 1994;19(3):204–14.
114. Rohit, Piccirillo E, Jain Y, Augurio A, Sanna M. Preoperative predictive factors for hearing preservation in vestibular schwannoma surgery. Ann Otol Rhinol Laryngol. 2006;115(1):41–6.
115. Grayeli AB, Kalamarides M, Ferrary E, Bouccara D, El Gharem H, Rey A, et al. Conservative management versus surgery for small vestibular schwannomas. Acta Otolaryngol (Stockh). 2005;125(10):1063–8.
116. Quist TS, Givens DJ, Gurgel RK, Chamoun R, Shelton C. Hearing preservation after middle fossa vestibular schwannoma removal: are the results durable? Otolaryngol Head Neck Surg. 2015;152(4):706–11.
117. Sughrue ME, Yang I, Aranda D, Kane AJ, Parsa AT. Hearing preservation rates after microsurgical resection of vestibular schwannoma. J Clin Neurosci. 2010;17(9):1126–9.
118. Yamakami I, Ito S, Higuchi Y. Retrosigmoid removal of small acoustic neuroma: curative tumor removal with preservation of function. J Neurosurg. 2014;121(3):554–63.
119. Mazzoni A, Zanoletti E, Calabrese V. Hearing preservation surgery in acoustic neuroma: long-term results. Acta Otorhinolaryngol Ital. 2012;32(2):98–102.
120. Di Maio S, Malebranche AD, Westerberg B, Akagami R. Hearing preservation after microsurgical resection of large vestibular schwannomas. Neurosurgery. 2011;68(3):632–40; discussion 640.
121. Hilton CW, Haines SJ, Agrawal A, Levine SC. Late failure rate of hearing preservation after middle fossa approach for resection of vestibular schwannoma. Otol Neurotol. 2011;32(1):132–5.
122. Maw AR, Coakham HB, Ayoub O, Butler SR. Hearing preservation and facial nerve function in vestibular schwannoma surgery. Clin Otolaryngol Allied Sci. 2003;28(3):252–6.
123. Chee GH, Nedzelski JM, Rowed D. Acoustic neuroma surgery: the results of long-term hearing preservation. Otol Neurotol. 2003;24(4):672–6.
124. Lee SH, Willcox TO, Buchheit WA. Current results of the surgical management of acoustic neuroma. Skull Base. 2002;12(4):189–95.
125. Kaylie DM, Gilbert E, Horgan MA, Delashaw JB, McMenomey SO. Acoustic neuroma surgery outcomes. Otol Neurotol. 2001;22(5):686–9.
126. Gormley WB, Sekhar LN, Wright DC, Kamerer D, Schessel D. Acoustic neuromas: results of current surgical management. Neurosurgery. 1997;41(1):50–8; discussion 58–60.
127. Post KD, Eisenberg MB, Catalano PJ. Hearing preservation in vestibular schwannoma surgery: what factors influence outcome? J Neurosurg. 1995;83(2):191–6.
128. Rowed DW, Nedzelski JM. Hearing preservation in the removal of intracanalicular acoustic neuromas via the retrosigmoid approach. J Neurosurg. 1997;86(3):456–61.
129. Samii M, Matthies C, Tatagiba M. Intracanalicular acoustic neurinomas. Neurosurgery. 1991;29(2):189–98; discussion 198–9.
130. Nonaka Y, Fukushima T, Watanabe K, Friedman AH, Sampson JH, Mcelveen JT, et al. Contemporary surgical management of vestibular schwannomas: analysis of complications and lessons learned over the past decade. Neurosurgery. 2013;72(2 Suppl Operative):ons103–15; discussion ons115.
131. Sameshima T, Fukushima T, McElveen JT, Friedman AH. Critical assessment of operative approaches for hearing preservation in small acoustic neuroma surgery: retrosigmoid vs middle fossa approach. Neurosurgery. 2010;67(3):640–4; discussion 644–5.
132. Sanna M, Khrais T, Russo A, Piccirillo E, Augurio A. Hearing preservation surgery in vestibular schwannoma: the hidden truth. Ann Otol Rhinol Laryngol. 2004;113(2):156–63.
133. Samii M, Matthies C. Management of 1000 vestibular schwannomas (acoustic neuromas): hearing function in 1000 tumor resections. Neurosurgery. 1997;40(2):248–60; discussion 260–2.
134. Cohen NL, Lewis WS, Ransohoff J. Hearing preservation in cerebellopontine angle tumor surgery: the NYU experience 1974-1991. Am J Otol. 1993;14(5):423–33.
135. Betchen SA, Walsh J, Post KD. Long-term hearing preservation after surgery for vestibular schwannoma. J Neurosurg. 2005;102(1):6–9.

136. Lin VYW, Stewart C, Grebenyuk J, Tsao M, Rowed D, Chen J, et al. Unilateral acoustic neuromas: long-term hearing results in patients managed with fractionated stereotactic radiotherapy, hearing preservation surgery, and expectantly. Laryngoscope. 2005;115(2):292–6.
137. Goel A, Sekhar LN, Langheinrich W, Kamerer D, Hirsch B. Late course of preserved hearing and tinnitus after acoustic neurilemoma surgery. J Neurosurg. 1992;77(5):685–9.
138. Fischer G, Fischer C, Rémond J. Hearing preservation in acoustic neurinoma surgery. J Neurosurg. 1992;76(6):910–7.
139. Jackler RK, Driscoll CLW. Tumors of the ear and temporal bone. Philadelphia: Lippincott Williams & Wilkins; 2000.
140. Sanna M, Zini C, Gamoletti R. Hearing preservation: a critical review of the literature. In: Tos M, Thomsen J (eds) Proceeding of the first international conference on acoustic neuroma. Amsterdam: Kluger; 1992. p. 631–8.
141. Hillman T, Chen DA, Arriaga MA, Quigley M. Facial nerve function and hearing preservation acoustic tumor surgery: does the approach matter? Otolaryngol Head Neck Surg. 2010;142(1):115–9.
142. Kanzaki J, Ogawa K, Inoue Y, Shiobara R. Hearing preservation surgery in acoustic neuroma patients with normal hearing. Skull Base Surg. 1997;7(3):109–13.
143. Rabelo de Freitas M, Russo A, Sequino G, Piccirillo E, Sanna M. Analysis of hearing preservation and facial nerve function for patients undergoing vestibular schwannoma surgery: the middle cranial fossa approach versus the retrosigmoid approach—personal experience and literature review. Audiol Neurootol. 2012;17(2):71–81.
144. Yang J, Grayeli AB, Barylyak R, Elgarem H. Functional outcome of retrosigmoid approach in vestibular schwannoma surgery. Acta Otolaryngol (Stockh). 2008;128(8):881–6.
145. Baumann I, Polligkeit J, Blumenstock G, Mauz P-S, Zalaman IM, Maassen MM. Quality of life after unilateral acoustic neuroma surgery via middle cranial fossa approach. Acta Otolaryngol (Stockh). 2005;125(6):585–91.
146. Hadjipanayis CG, Carlson ML, Link MJ, Rayan TA, Parish J, Atkins T, et al. Congress of Neurological Surgeons systematic review and evidence-based guidelines on surgical resection for the treatment of patients with vestibular schwannomas. Neurosurgery. 2018;82(2):E40–3.
147. Colletti V, Fiorino F. Is the middle fossa approach the treatment of choice for intracanalicular vestibular schwannoma? Otolaryngol Head Neck Surg. 2005;132(3):459–66.
148. Bennett ML, Jackson CG, Kaufmann R, Warren F. Postoperative imaging of vestibular schwannomas. Otolaryngol Head Neck Surg. 2008;138(5):667–71.
149. Tysome JR, Moffat DA. Magnetic resonance imaging after translabyrinthine complete excision of vestibular schwannomas. J Neurol Surg B Skull Base. 2012;73(2):121–4.
150. Arlt F, Trantakis C, Seifert V, Bootz F, Strauss G, Meixensberger J. Recurrence rate, time to progression and facial nerve function in microsurgery of vestibular schwannoma. Neurol Res. 2011;33(10):1032–7.
151. Atlas MD, Harvey C, Fagan PA. Hearing preservation in acoustic neuroma surgery: a continuing study. Laryngoscope. 1992;102(7):779–83.
152. Sughrue ME, Kaur R, Rutkowski MJ, Kane AJ, Yang I, Pitts LH, et al. A critical evaluation of vestibular schwannoma surgery for patients younger than 40 years of age. Neurosurgery. 2010;67(6):1646–53; discussion 1653–4.
153. Carlson ML, Van Abel KM, Driscoll CL, Neff BA, Beatty CW, Lane JI, et al. Magnetic resonance imaging surveillance following vestibular schwannoma resection. Laryngoscope. 2012;122(2):378–88.
154. Bloch DC, Oghalai JS, Jackler RK, Osofsky M, Pitts LH. The fate of the tumor remnant after less-than-complete acoustic neuroma resection. Otolaryngol Head Neck Surg. 2004;130(1):104–12.
155. Kemink JL, Langman AW, Niparko JK, Graham MD. Operative management of acoustic neuromas: the priority of neurologic function over complete resection. Otolaryngol Head Neck Surg. 1991;104(1):96–9.
156. Nakatomi H, Jacob JT, Carlson ML, Tanaka S, Tanaka M, Saito N, et al. Long-term risk of recurrence and regrowth after gross-total and subtotal resection of sporadic vestibular schwannoma. J Neurosurg. 2017;19:1–7.
157. Monfared A, Corrales CE, Theodosopoulos PV, Blevins NH, Oghalai JS, Selesnick SH, et al. Facial nerve outcome and tumor control rate as a function of degree of resection in treatment of large acoustic neuromas: preliminary report of the Acoustic Neuroma Subtotal Resection Study (ANSRS). Neurosurgery. 2016;79(2):194–203.

14 Acoustic Neuroma Surgery: Middle Fossa Approach

Daniel Q. Sun and Bruce J. Gantz

Introduction

The middle cranial fossa (MCF) approach was first reported in 1904 and then popularized by William House in 1961 for the excision of small intracanalicular vestibular schwannoma (VS) [1]. In contrast to translabyrinthine and retrosigmoid approaches, it offers superior exposure of the distal internal auditory canal (IAC) and identification of the labyrinthine facial nerve that is uninvolved by tumor, without sacrificing hearing. It is a technically challenging procedure due to the lack of reliable landmarks in the middle fossa and that the facial nerve is commonly displaced between the surgeon and the tumor, placing it at additional risk for injury. However, the advent of facial nerve monitoring and steady evolution in technique have rendered it a safe and effective procedure that is ideally suited to the microsurgical excision of a small VS when hearing preservation is an important goal. In discussing hearing outcome, this chapter uses American Academy of Otolaryngology—Head and Neck Surgery (AAO-HNS) and word recognition score (WRS) hearing classification schemes (Fig. 14.1). This chapter focuses on the use of the MCF approach in the treatment of small VS. The surgical management of other surgical pathologies in the temporal bone or cerebellopontine angle (CPA) using an MCF approach or variants thereof, such as extended MCF or transpetrosal approaches, is beyond the scope of this chapter.

D. Q. Sun (✉)
Department of Otorhinolaryngology—Head and Neck Surgery, University of Iowa Hospitals and Clinics, Iowa City, IA, USA
e-mail: dsun8@jhmi.edu

B. J. Gantz
Department of Otolaryngology—Head and Neck Surgery, University of Iowa Hospitals and Clinics, Iowa City, IA, USA

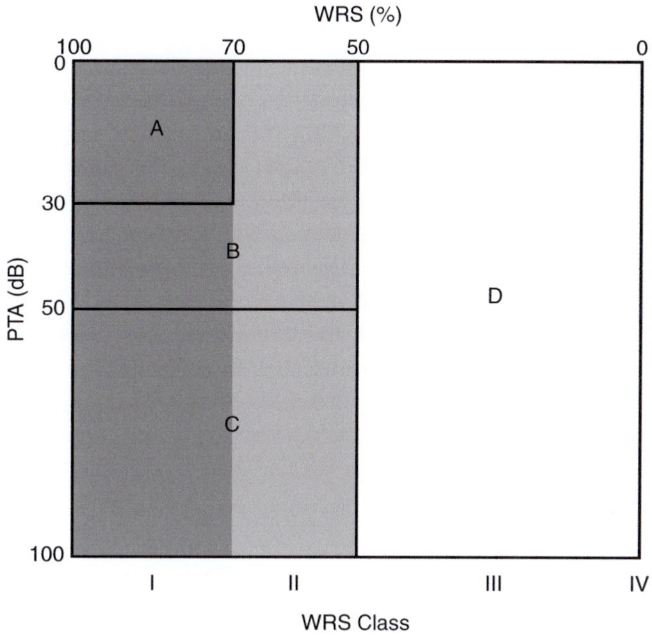

Fig. 14.1 American Academy of Otolaryngology—Head and Neck Surgery (A–D) and word recognition score (WRS) (I–IV) hearing classification criteria. *PTA* pure tone average. (Copyright: Otology & Neurotology)

Surgical Candidacy

At our center, an MCF approach for VS excision is offered to patients 65 years of age or younger, with serviceable hearing, and whose tumors do not contact the brainstem on magnetic resonance (MR) imaging. Intent for hearing preservation is the key indication for microsurgical excision of small VS. The likelihood of hearing preservation with surgical intervention is balanced against the natural history of intracanalicular VS. An observational longitudinal study in a Danish population demonstrated that, after 10 years, 34% and 58% of patients retained at least serviceable hearing as defined by AAO-HNS (A or B) and WRS classes (I or II),

N. C. Bambakidis et al. (eds.), *Surgery of the Cerebellopontine Angle*, https://doi.org/10.1007/978-3-031-12507-2_14

respectively [2]. In addition, while tumor growth occurred in only 37% of patients during the observational period, mean WRS decreased from 63% at diagnosis to 33% at last follow-up even in patients whose tumors did not demonstrate growth. Other observational studies have also elicited similar findings [3, 4]. Furthermore, the subjective importance of residual hearing can vary greatly between patients. For instance, localization ability may still be important in some individuals despite presenting with nonserviceable hearing in the tumor ear. Therefore, it is critical that surgical decision-making be customized to each patient.

MCF surgery is not offered to patients older than 65 years of age due to the risks associated with temporal lobe retraction and thinning dura. While the MCF approach was traditionally described for tumors that are fully contained within the IAC, we have had good success in extending this hearing preservation approach to tumors that extend into the CPA by augmenting the traditional MCF technique with superior petrosal sinus ligation and division, and partial division of the tentorium cerebelli for additional CPA exposure. However, in our experience, hearing preservation via an MCF approach is not a realistic goal for tumors that contact the brainstem. Although the presence of a cerebrospinal fluid (CSF) cap in the lateral IAC has traditionally been used as a favorable prognostic indicator for hearing preservation; available evidence suggests that it has no impact on hearing, and we do not use it as a guide in decision making (Fig. 14.2) [5, 6].

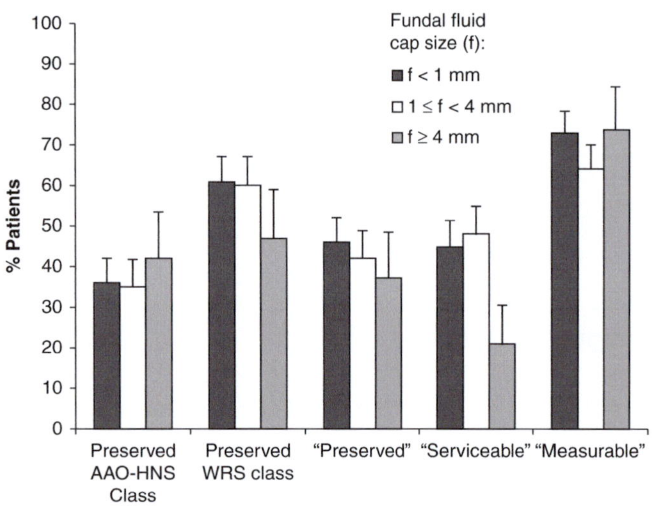

Fig. 14.2 Hearing preservation stratified by fundal fluid size and definition of hearing outcome in a group of 138 patients (mean tumor size: 1 cm) who underwent middle cranial fossa excision for vestibular schwannoma, with hearing preservation intent. "Preserved" was defined as pure tone average (PTA) change ≤15 dB and WRS change ≤15%, "serviceable" was defined as PTA ≤50 dB and word recognition score (WRS) ≥50%, and "measurable" was defined as PTA ≤90 dB and WRS >0%. Error bars: standard error of the mean. (Copyright: Otology & Neurotology)

Surgical Technique

Preoperative Preparation

Preoperative imaging consists of a contrast-enhanced MR imaging scan of the brain and skull base. Imaging is helpful to localize the position of the superior semicircular canal (SSCC) relative to the middle fossa floor; if an MR coronal T2 sequence is not already available, a Stenvers projection plain radiograph of the temporal bone may be obtained. We do not routinely use temporal bone CT or image-guided navigation. General anesthesia and orotracheal intubation are accomplished; thereafter, the bed is rotated 180° for access. Paralytic agents must be reversed before the skin incision is made. A urinary catheter is placed to monitor fluids and diuresis. Hair is shaved approximately 10 cm above and 5 cm behind the ear. The entire side of the head and face are prepared, and EMG needles are placed in the orbicularis oculi and oris muscles for facial nerve monitoring. Standard auditory brainstem-evoked recording electrodes are placed in the right and left mastoid tips and the vertex and forehead (ground), and insert headphones are placed in both external auditory canals. The auditory brainstem response is monitored throughout the procedure. A clear drape is placed over the prepared area to allow visualization of the entire side of the face in the case of monitoring equipment failure. Preoperative medications administered include prophylactic antibiotics, dexamethasone, and mannitol (0.5 g/kg ideal body weight).

Surgical Technique

Several soft tissue approaches are available. We use a posteriorly based skin flap (Fig. 14.3) and an anteriorly based temporalis muscle flap. A large piece of temporalis fascia is harvested and set aside in moist gauze for use at the time of closure. The zygomatic root identifies the floor of the MCF and is the central landmark of the craniotomy. A roughly square craniotomy measuring 4–5 cm on each side is created, using an otologic drill or craniotome. It is important to keep the anterior and posterior borders parallel for stable engagement of the MCF retractor. The bone flap should be elevated with care by use of a blunt dural elevator. Occasionally, the middle meningeal artery is embedded within the bone, requiring bipolar coagulation to free it. The bone flap is wrapped in moist gauze and set aside for use at closure.

Dural elevation from the floor of the MCF is accomplished with a Freer or Joker elevator, always in a posterior-to-anterior direction, which prevents injury to the greater superficial petrosal nerve and (possible dehiscent) geniculate ganglion. The petrous ridge is identified at the posterior mar-

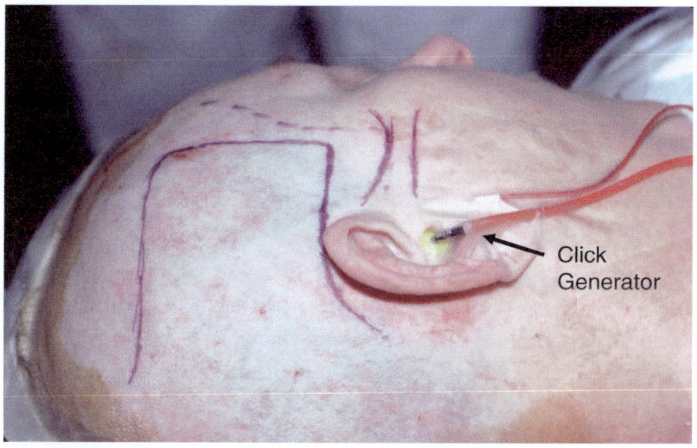

Fig. 14.3 Posteriorly based skin flap for MCF craniotomy. Also shown are the approximate locations of the zygomatic root (center of craniotomy) and frontal branch (dashed line). A click generator in the ear canal is used for intraoperative audiologic monitoring. (Copyright: Authors)

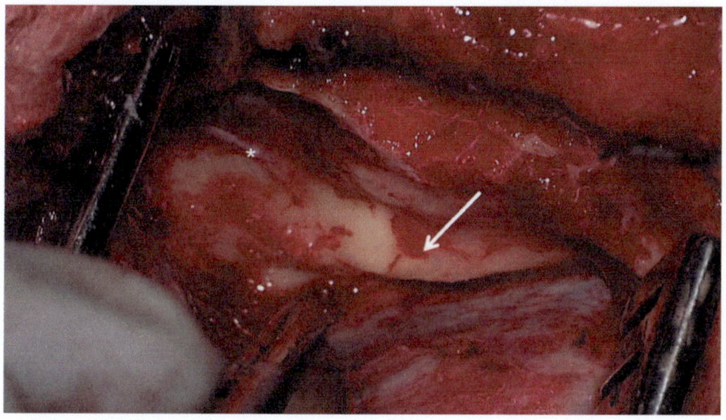

Fig. 14.4 Intraoperative surface anatomy of middle fossa floor showing greater superficial petrosal nerve (*) and arcuate eminence (arrow). Dura of temporal lobe is retracted using the House-Urban retractor engaged at the craniotomy window. (Copyright: Authors)

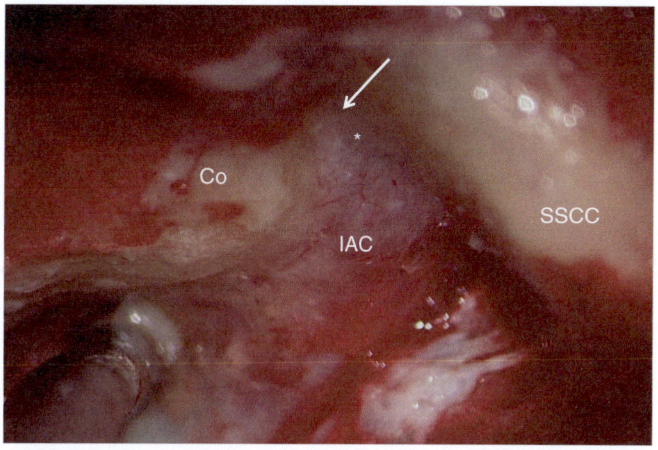

Fig. 14.5 Decompression of internal auditory canal (IAC) is performed using blue-lined superior semicircular canal (SSCC) as a landmark, revealing tumor under IAC dura, labyrinthine segment of facial nerve (arrow), and Bill's bar (*). Note the complete decompression of the posterior trough, creating a corridor for tumor dissection and delivery. *Co* cochlea. (Copyright: Authors)

gin of the craniotomy, and the dura is slowly elevated over the arcuate eminence and meatal plane. Occasionally, a superior canal dehiscence may be present. Dural reflections are cauterized and sharply transected to allow elevation to the anterior petrous ridge. Broad elevation of the dura around both the craniotomy window and the middle fossa floor prevents "bow-stringing" with retraction and thereby reduces pressure exerted on the temporal lobe. Frequently, the middle meningeal artery may need to be divided at the foramen spinosum to provide the broad exposure necessary. Cottonoid sponges can be placed at the anterior and posterior margins of the elevation to help retract the dura during placement of the self-retaining MCF retractor (Fig. 14.4).

Bony dissection of the middle fossa begins with locating the dome of the SSCC within the temporal bone, using preoperative imaging to help gauge its depth below the middle fossa floor and its position relative to the arcuate eminence, both of which can be highly variable. Bone of the middle fossa floor around the arcuate eminence is carefully removed until the dense yellowish bone of the otic capsule is identified; then the dome is thinned further to a "blue line," which is always perpendicular to the petrous ridge. While the relationship between the labyrinth and middle fossa landmarks can be highly variable, the relative location of labyrinthine structures to each other is highly conserved. Therefore, accurately locating the SSCC dome provides a crucial "sign post" for other structures within the temporal bone, such as the cochlea and IAC.

When the location of the superior canal is confirmed, an anterior line 60° to the blue line locates the position of the IAC. The depth of the IAC varies, but drilling medially near the petrous ridge provides the safest method in locating it, which appears pink due to the intracanalicular tumor. The IAC is then followed laterally toward the cochlea, SSCC ampulla, and labyrinthine facial nerve with identification of Bill's bar (Fig. 14.5). Due to the proximity of the cochlea anteriorly and SSCC ampulla posteriorly, only a 90° decompression of the labyrinthine facial nerve can be safely achieved.

Successful facial nerve and hearing outcomes are predicated on achieving the best possible decompression of the IAC to provide room for tumor dissection. To this end, maximum decompression of the posterior trough is especially important, as it becomes the corridor for tumor dissection and delivery. Medially, the posterior trough is decompressed to the dura of the CPA. Laterally, the blue line of the SSCC is used as a guide for the extent of dissection, and the surgeon watches carefully for a blue line on the SSCC ampulla.

After bony dissection is completed, a linear dural opening along the length of the IAC is made using a Beaver 59-10 blade or microscissors to expose the IAC from labyrinthine facial nerve to the CPA. The meatal segment of the facial nerve is usually readily identified in the anterior portion of the IAC and displaced superiorly by the tumor (Fig. 14.6). At this time, a cochlear nerve action potential (CNAP) electrode is placed in the anterior trough between the dura and bone for direct monitoring of CN VIII. Tumor microdissection starts with carefully establishing a dissection plane between the facial nerve and tumor. The superior vestibular nerve is then divided laterally. Using small cup forceps, the tumor is systematically debulked from the posterior trough, which reduces traction on neural structures during tumor manipulation. All dissection proceeds from medial to lateral to avoid traction on the labyrinthine segment of the facial nerve and the modiolus for the cochlear nerve. The inferior vestibular nerve, once visualized, is also disconnected at its lateral extent. As tumor dissection proceeds laterally, the fundus is obscured by the transverse crest and labyrinthine facial nerve. A sinus tympani excavator can be used to gently sweep and deliver tumor from this recess. The cochlear nerve can often be visualized in the lateral IAC (Fig. 14.7).

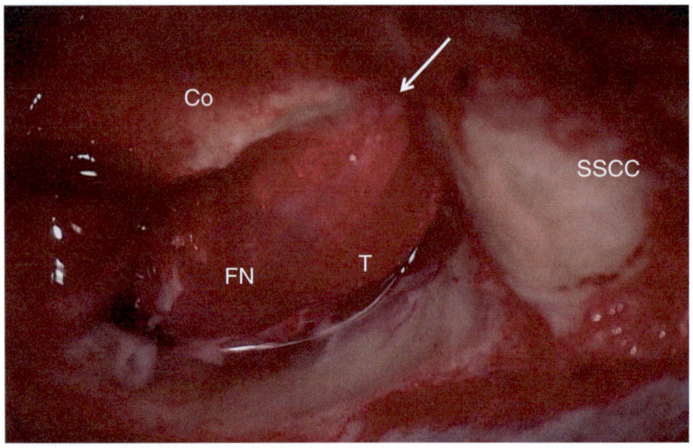

Fig. 14.6 After internal auditory canal (IAC) dura is opened, tumor (T) is seen filling the IAC and displacing the facial nerve (FN) superiorly. *Co* cochlea, *SSCC* superior semicircular canal, arrow = labyrinthine segment of FN. (Copyright: Authors)

To visualize the medial extent of tumors that extend into the CPA, the dural opening may need to be extended medially. If the view is still not adequate, the superior petrosal sinus may be divided by first ligating, with hemoclips placed at points anterior and posterior to the IAC, and then dividing sharply using microscissors (Fig. 14.8). Further division of the tentorium cerebelli may require linear dural incisions over the temporal lobe to expose the free edge of the tentorium. Although complete division of the tentorium requires careful visualization of cranial nerve IV in the incisura medially (Fig. 14.9), doing so is seldom required for VS excision.

During tumor dissection, close communication between the monitoring audiologist and surgeon is critical. At our center, CNAP N1 amplitude is tracked during tumor dissection, and any amplitude attenuation is immediately communicated to the surgeon, who may then reduce any traction on the tumor or change the area of microdissection, for instance. If CNAP monitoring is not available, far-field auditory brainstem response (ABR) may be used instead, although its longer sweep times may not provide real-time feedback of cochlear nerve physiology to the surgeon.

After tumor extirpation, reconstruction can be achieved using only autologous materials. A piece of temporalis muscle or abdominal fat may be harvested to plug the IAC. Exposed air cells in the temporal bone are carefully waxed. The previously harvested fascia is then laid over the middle fossa floor. Dura is then carefully inspected for leaks and hemostasis verified. The craniotomy and soft tissue are then closed in standard fashion. A mastoid-type dressing is applied and no drains are used.

Postoperative Care

Postoperative care includes observation in the intensive care unit overnight, dexamethasone (6 mg every 6 h for 36 h),

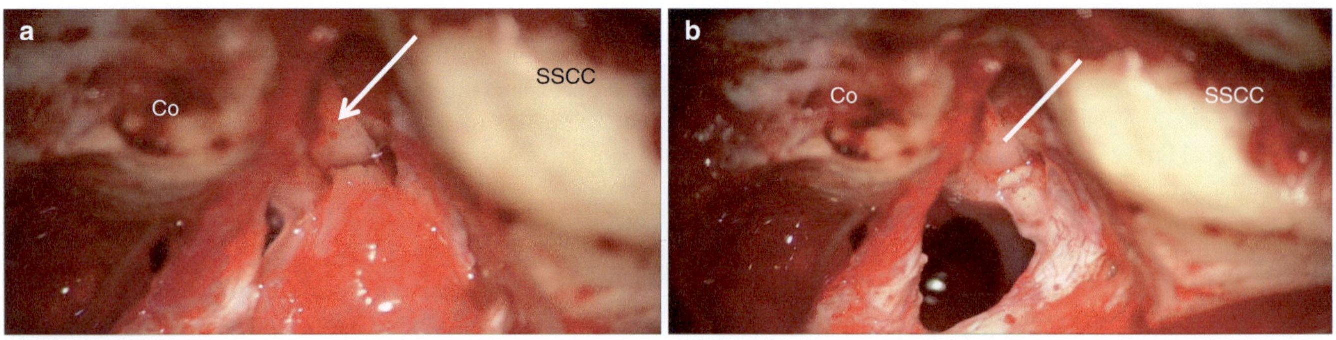

Fig. 14.7 Distal internal auditory canal (IAC) microanatomy is illustrated. (**a**) After division of the superior vestibular nerve, tumor (T) originating from the inferior vestibular nerve is reflected medially, revealing cochlear nerve (arrow). Facial nerve (*) is seen anterior to tumor. (**b**) Facial and cochlear nerves are seen in IAC after tumor removal. *Co* cochlea, *SSCC* superior semicircular canal. (Copyright: Authors)

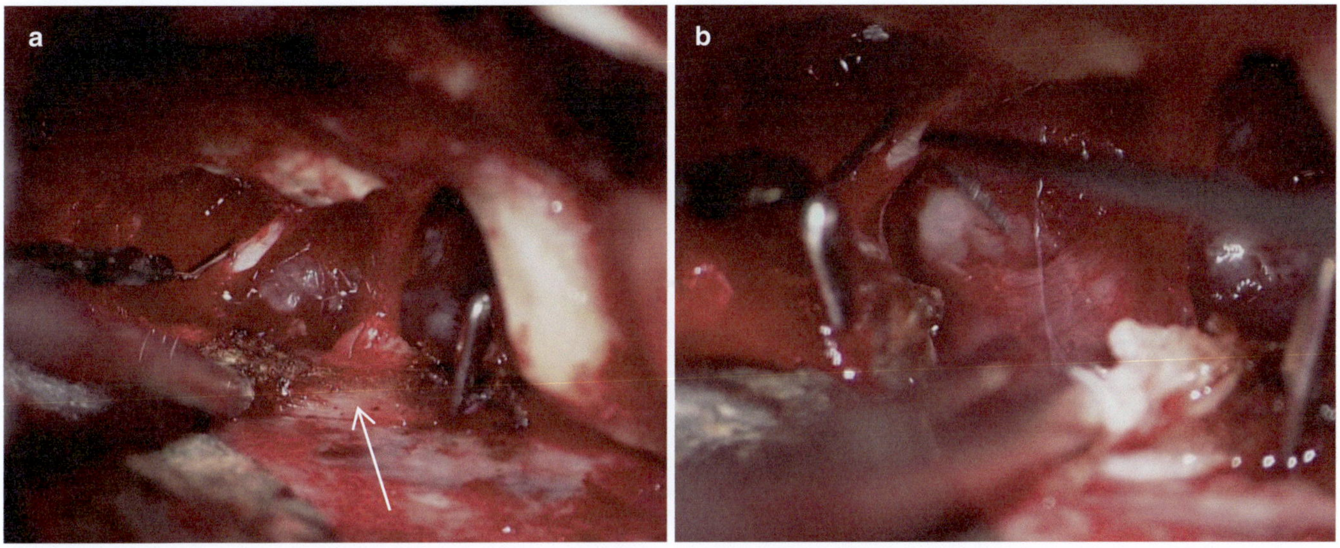

Fig. 14.8 For larger tumors, superior petrosal sinus (SPS) ligation and division may be performed to achieve adequate exposure of the tumor and allow safe microdissection. After the extirpation of tumor from the lateral internal auditory canal, SPS is ligated (**a**) using hemoclips and (**b**) then divided. Following SPS division, the medial extent of tumor is visualized, including its relationship to the cisternal segment of facial nerve. Also pictured is the cochlear nerve action potential electrode placed in the anterior trough. (Copyright: Authors)

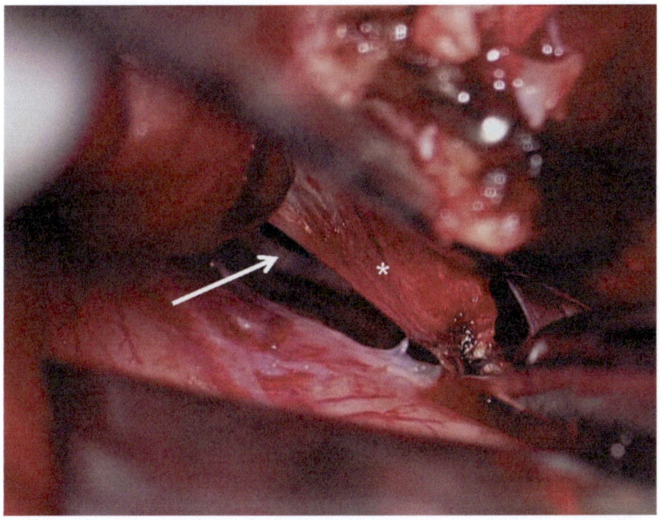

Fig. 14.9 In addition to ligation and division of the superior petrosal sinus, tentorium cerebelli (*) may be divided sharply using microscissors from lateral to medial to provide further exposure of the posterior fossa. However, it is important to identify cranial nerve IV (arrow) in the incisura to avoid injury. (Copyright: Authors)

cefazolin (1 g every 8 h for 36 h), routine neural checks, and limitation of analgesia to codeine. There is typically little postoperative pain, and narcotics stronger than codeine may mask intracranial complications. The patient is transferred to a routine postoperative floor the next morning, encouraged to begin ambulation, and started on a diet as tolerated. Although acute vestibulopathy generally subsides within the first several days after surgery, it may take several weeks for patients to resume their previous activities. Vestibular physical therapy can be helpful for patients whose vestibular compensation may be inadequate. If CSF rhinorrhea occurs, a spinal drain must be placed for 4–5 days. Following this regimen, only very rarely has a patient required surgical closure of the leak.

Complications and Outcomes

Major complications such as stroke, epidural hematoma, seizure, and meningitis are extremely rare in all reported series to date [7, 8]. Rarely, transient aphasia has been observed within the immediate postoperative period, likely associated with temporal lobe retraction of the dominant hemisphere. No permanent deficits have occurred in our experience. CSF leak occurs in 2–7% of patients, depending on the series [7, 9]. Tumor recurrence is extremely rare (<1%) and is related to the extent of resection [7]. While gross total resection is usually possible for small VS, near- or subtotal resections are sometimes performed to maximize facial nerve and hearing outcome, especially in instances where the tumor is found to be very adherent to adjacent structures. In the modern era, facial nerve outcomes have been similarly favorable, with House–Brackmann score 1 or 2 achieved in >95% of patients at 1 year [7, 10, 11].

Due to its ability to provide superior access to the lateral IAC, the MCF approach has become the preferred modality for microsurgical excision of intracanalicular VS, where hearing preservation is a key goal. In a series of 162 patients treated with MCF for VS excision [7], postoperative WRS class I or II hearing was maintained in 78% of patients when

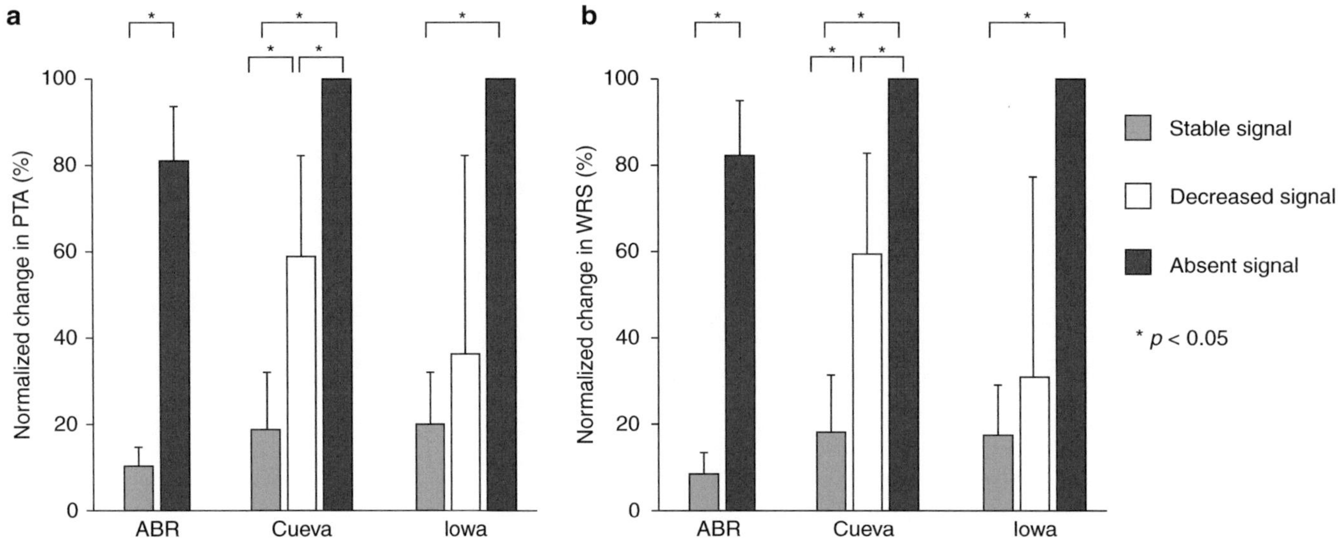

Fig. 14.10 Mean change in postoperative (**a**) pure tone average (PTA) and (**b**) word recognition score (WRS) associated with changes in signal characteristic on auditory brainstem response differential modalities of intraoperative audiologic monitoring in a group of 126 patients who underwent middle cranial fossa excision for vestibular schwannoma. Far-field auditory brainstem response (ABR) and near-field cochlear nerve action potential (CNAP) performed at conclusion of tumor dissection and prior to closure were used for analysis. For far-field ABR, presence or absence of wave V amplitude was assessed; for CNAP electrodes (Cueva or Iowa), N1 amplitude was assessed as stable (same as baseline), decreased, or absent. Changes in PTA and WRS are normalized to the total amount of hearing in the affected ear prior to surgery; 0% and 100% represent preservation and loss of all residual hearing, respectively. Error bars: 95% confidence interval. Intragroup differences analyzed using ANOVA with post-hoc Tukey test. (Copyright: Otology & Neurotology)

tumor size was <1 cm. For those presenting with class I hearing, 70% were able to maintain class I hearing postoperatively. However, the success rate declines significantly when tumor size is larger than 1 cm, where only 42% of patients maintained class I or II hearing postoperatively. These outcomes have been consistently replicated in other studies [11, 12]. Regardless of tumor size, one of the most important factors in achieving good hearing outcome is the degree of adherence between the tumor and adjacent structures in the IAC, which is likely a reflection of the biological behavior of the tumor. As other authors have observed [13], hearing preservation can be successfully achieved in larger tumors that are not highly adherent, whereas it can be difficult if not impossible in highly adherent small tumors. Multiple studies have also demonstrated that preserved hearing after MCF surgery remains durable over time, with some studies reporting follow-up for as long as 10 years [14–16].

At our center, intraoperative audiologic monitoring plays an important role during MCF excision. Both far-field ABR and near-field CNAP play complementary roles before, during, and after tumor excision. A recent study demonstrated that wave V and N1 amplitude changes on ABR and CNAP [17], respectively, immediately after tumor extirpation are associated with postoperative changes in pure tone thresholds and WRS (Fig. 14.10). Using amplitude changes on both ABR and CNAP provided the best prognostic value for detecting postoperative hearing decline, with sensitivity and specificity of 83% and 100%, respectively.

Conclusion

The MCF approach is an important tool in the surgical management of small VS. It has evolved over the previous decades to be a safe and effective treatment option that can offer excellent facial nerve and hearing outcome in appropriate patients. While it is most commonly used for tumors confined to the IAC, those with moderate extension into the CPA can be successfully accessed via augmented techniques such as superior petrosal sinus ligation and division.

References

1. House WF. Surgical exposure of the internal auditory canal and its contents through the middle, cranial fossa. Laryngoscope. 1961;71:1363–85.
2. Kirchmann M, Karnov K, Hansen S, et al. Ten-year follow-up on tumor growth and hearing in patients observed with an intracanalicular vestibular schwannoma. Neurosurgery. 2017;80:49–56.
3. Lin VY, Stewart C, Grebenyuk J, et al. Unilateral acoustic neuromas: long-term hearing results in patients managed with fractionated stereotactic radiotherapy, hearing preservation surgery, and expectantly. Laryngoscope. 2005;115:292–6.
4. Sughrue ME, Kane AJ, Kaur R, et al. A prospective study of hearing preservation in untreated vestibular schwannomas. J Neurosurg. 2011;114:381–5.
5. Sun DQ, Kung RW, Hansen MR, et al. Does a "fundal fluid cap" predict successful hearing preservation in vestibular schwannoma resection via the middle cranial fossa approach? Otol Neurotol. 2018;39:772–7.

6. Goddard JC, Schwartz MS, Friedman RA. Fundal fluid as a predictor of hearing preservation in the middle cranial fossa approach for vestibular schwannoma. Otol Neurotol. 2010;31:1128–34.
7. Meyer TA, Canty PA, Wilkinson EP, et al. Small acoustic neuromas: surgical outcomes versus observation or radiation. Otol Neurotol. 2006;27:380–92.
8. House WF, Shelton C. Middle fossa approach for acoustic tumor removal. Otolaryngol Clin N Am. 1992;25:347–59.
9. Slattery WH 3rd, Brackmann DE, Hitselberger W. Middle fossa approach for hearing preservation with acoustic neuromas. Am J Otol. 1997;18:596–601.
10. Arriaga MA, Luxford WM, Berliner KI. Facial nerve function following middle fossa and translabyrinthine acoustic tumor surgery: a comparison. Am J Otol. 1994;15:620–4.
11. Arts HA, Telian SA, El-Kashlan H, et al. Hearing preservation and facial nerve outcomes in vestibular schwannoma surgery: results using the middle cranial fossa approach. Otol Neurotol. 2006;27:234–41.
12. Shelton C, Brackmann DE, House WF, et al. Middle fossa acoustic tumor surgery: results in 106 cases. Laryngoscope. 1989;99:405–8.
13. Moriyama T, Fukushima T, Asaoka K, et al. Hearing preservation in acoustic neuroma surgery: importance of adhesion between the cochlear nerve and the tumor. J Neurosurg. 2002;97:337–40.
14. Roche JP, Goates AJ, Hasan DM, et al. Treatment of lateral skull base and posterior cranial fossa lesions utilizing the extended middle cranial fossa approach. Otol Neurotol. 2017;38:742–50.
15. Woodson EA, Dempewolf RD, Gubbels SP, et al. Long-term hearing preservation after microsurgical excision of vestibular schwannoma. Otol Neurotol. 2010;31:1144–52.
16. Ahmed S, Arts HA, El-Kashlan H, et al. Immediate and long-term hearing outcomes with the middle cranial fossa approach for vestibular schwannoma resection. Otol Neurotol. 2018;39:92–8.
17. Sun DQ, Sullivan CB, Kung RW, et al. How well does intraoperative audiologic monitoring predict hearing outcome during middle fossa vestibular schwannoma resection? Otol Neurotol. 2018;39:908–15.

Complications and Cranial Nerve Rehabilitation

15

Daniel Jethanamest and J. Thomas Roland Jr.

Advances in microsurgical techniques have reduced the morbidity and mortality in surgery of the cerebellopontine angle (CPA) significantly. Nevertheless, surgical complications involving the intricate neurovascular structures or multiple cranial nerves of the skull base can occur. Surgeons can minimize complications with thorough knowledge of the relevant skull-base anatomy and its relationship to the targeted pathologic lesion, collaboration between members of a skull-base team, careful review of preoperative imaging, the use of intraoperative monitoring techniques, and well executed surgical techniques. Mortality for lesions of the CPA such as vestibular schwannoma (VS) in contemporary series is now very rare, well less than 1%, even for very large tumors [1–3]. This has shifted the focus of further complication prevention to other morbidities such as cerebrospinal fluid (CSF) leaks and the preservation and rehabilitation of cranial nerve dysfunction.

The management of complications begins with careful observation and recognition of common pitfalls in surgery and during the postoperative course. Anticipation of potential complications and prompt diagnosis can often limit the magnitude morbidities and allow for faster recovery. Different pathologic entities of the CPA and each surgical approach can be associated with particular complications. In a retrospective analysis of a large multi-institutional quality improvement database, overall complication rates of VS resection did not differ among transtemporal, retrosigmoid, or middle cranial fossa approaches [4]. While complications can be difficult for both the patient and the surgeon, continuing attentive care is important and may help avoid compounding an existing problem or missing secondary complications.

D. Jethanamest (✉)
Division of Otology and Neurotology, Department of Otolaryngology—Head and Neck Surgery, New York University School of Medicine, New York, NY, USA
e-mail: Daniel.Jethanamest@nyulangone.org

J. Thomas Roland Jr.
Department of Otolaryngology—Head and Neck Surgery, Department of Neurosurgery, New York University School of Medicine, New York, NY, USA

Cerebrospinal Fluid Leak and Meningitis

One of the most frequent complications of CPA surgery is postoperative CSF leak, which may manifest through different routes including through the primary wound, as otorrhea or as rhinorrhea. In a retrospective review of 300 surgical cases (100 of each surgical approach: translabyrinthine, middle fossa, and retrosigmoid), a leak rate of 10–13% was found, and neither approach nor tumor size was a factor in the rate of postoperative CSF leak nor the need for revision surgery [5]. A meta-analysis of 5964 cases similarly found no differences between surgical approaches, with rates of 9.5–10.6% reported [6]. A number of different surgical techniques have been suggested to help reduce the incidence of CSF leak after CPA surgery. Proposed techniques have all reported good outcomes, though preferences and surgical details vary significantly in different authors' hands—for example, in the degree of middle ear and eustachian tube manipulation, use of titanium mesh/hydroxyapatite cement, and obliteration in translabyrinthine approaches [7–10]. Abdominal fat grafting is a commonly used method that has reduced the rate of CSF leak in these surgical techniques, and care should be taken to meticulously close and monitor the donor site for rare but potential wound site morbidities, such as subcutaneous hematoma, which has been reported in approximately 3% of cases [2, 10, 11].

The management of a postoperative CSF leak often utilizes a graduated approach from conservative measures to surgical interventions [12]. Conservative measures may include bed rest, head of bed elevation, acetazolamide, wound oversewing, and pressure dressings. CSF diversion, such as with a lumbar drain, is an additional technique at times employed before pursuing surgical options that may include wound re-exploration, subtotal petrosectomy, or

N. C. Bambakidis et al. (eds.), *Surgery of the Cerebellopontine Angle*, https://doi.org/10.1007/978-3-031-12507-2_15

other transnasal approaches to eustachian tube closure [13, 14]. Infrequently, lumbar drain diversion in the setting of an active CSF leak can result in increasing pneumocephalus, an example of which is shown in a case in Fig. 15.1, which resolved after subtotal petrosectomy and plugging of the eustachian tube.

Meningitis can be a serious and threatening complication of skull-base surgery. Although uncommon overall, the incidence of meningitis seen in a systematic review assessing postoperative CSF leaks noted a significantly higher risk of meningitis in the presence of a leak, occurring in 14% of these cases [6]. Allen and colleagues reported on 508 lateral skull-base procedures, identifying meningitis in 3.1% with a median time from surgery to onset of 12 days and a much higher risk of meningitis in the presence of a CSF leak by a factor of 10.2 [15]. Higher rates of meningitis have been reported, including a 9.2% incidence seen in a series of 500 cases [16].

Many cases of meningitis postoperatively are likely chemical meningitis with symptoms of headache or fever but negative CSF Gram stain and cultures. In a study of 1146 patients investigating the differences between bacterial and chemical meningitis, an overall incidence of meningitis in 4.54% of cases was found [17]. Culture-proven bacterial meningitis was seen in 0.87% and, when combined with strongly suspected bacterial cases, had a total incidence of 1.92%, with the remaining 2.6% of cases suspected to be chemical. The bacterial meningitis cases had significantly higher CSF and serum white blood cell counts and lower CSF glucose. For CPA pathologies, notably epidermoid cysts of the skull base, cyst rupture and exposure of proteinaceous contents to the subarachnoid space may be particularly likely to trigger recurrent episodes of aseptic meningitis [18]. Care should be taken intraoperatively to avoid contamination of the CSF with byproducts such as bone dust from any drilling during skull-base approaches.

Vascular Complications

A vascular injury or complication after skull-base surgery is a dreaded and potentially devastating outcome. Microsurgery in the CPA involves careful dissection of and around critical structures, including segments of the carotid artery, vertebrobasilar system, venous sinuses, jugular bulb, brainstem perforators, and other critical structures. Intraoperative bleeding from vessels or the venous dural sinuses can be controlled with gentle pressure using thrombin-soaked gelatin or other absorbable hemostatic agents external to the vessel, with the goal of controlling bleeding while avoiding vessel occlusion or complete thrombosis.

A postoperative hematoma within the CPA can occur in the early recovery period and can vary greatly from a minor collection to a rapidly evolving and compressive hemorrhage. Larger or threatening hematomas may require immediate surgical evacuation with a thorough inspection of the

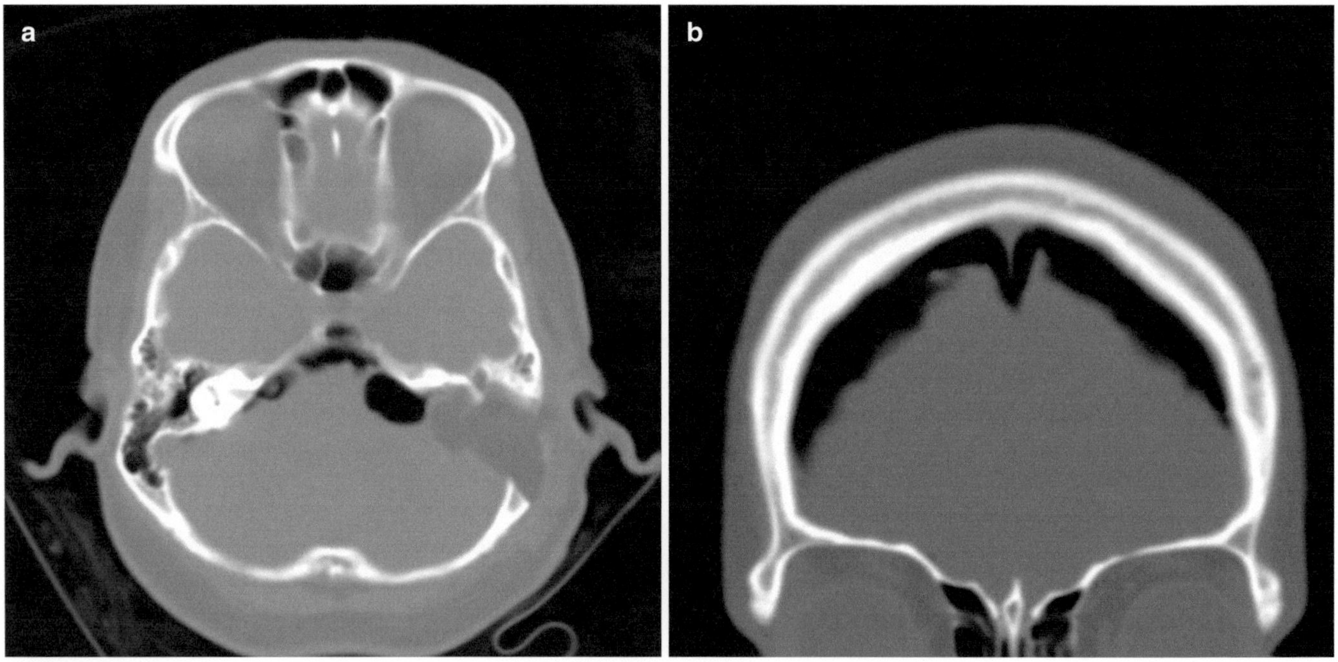

Fig. 15.1 (**a**) Axial and (**b**) coronal computed tomography images after left translabyrinthine approach to resection of a large left-sided vestibular schwannoma, showing worsening pneumocephalus after lumbar cerebrospinal fluid (CSF) diversion for postoperative CSF rhinorrhea. The patient underwent left subtotal petrosectomy with obliteration of the middle ear and plugging of the eustachian tube with resolution of the CSF leak and pneumocephalus

surgical field to identify a source of hemorrhage (Fig. 15.2). Postoperative hemorrhage or hematoma formation is rare, having been reported in approximately 1–3% of cases postoperatively [2, 16, 19].

Portions of the vertebrobasilar arterial system, brainstem perforators, and the anterior inferior cerebellar artery (AICA) in particular are often encountered in surgery of the CPA. The close relationship between branches of the AICA and the seventh and eighth cranial nerves make it a vulnerable structure for many pathologies of the CPA or in some rare cases of an aneurysm of AICA [20]. The labyrinthine or internal auditory artery can be injured, or potentially acute vasospasm may be initiated from surgery, leading to auditory and vestibular symptoms of hearing loss, tinnitus, and vertigo. Occlusion or injury to the AICA can also clinically manifest with other severe neurologic sequelae, including dysarthria, ipsilateral facial palsy, facial sensory loss, Horner's syndrome, dysmetria, contralateral loss of sensation, ipsilateral conjugate lateral gaze palsy, dysphagia, and ipsilateral motor weakness.

The dural venous sinuses and bridging veins are at risk during lateral skull-base surgery, particularly in combined middle and posterior fossa transpetrosal approaches [21]. The anastomotic vein of Labbé can have variable anatomy but bridges the lateral cortical temporal lobe to the transverse sinus and can potentially be the sole route of venous drainage for a large region of the temporal and parietal lobes. Vein of Labbé or other lateral temporal skull-base bridging vein injuries can cause severe neurologic consequences due to temporal lobe ischemia, edema, or infarction, including nausea, vomiting, aphasia, and hemiparesis [22]. Preoperative planning and careful division of the superior petrosal sinus and tentorium a distance from the variable venous bridging anastomoses near the transverse sinus can help to avoid injuries and complications. If the vein is severed intraoperatively, it can be reconstructed or revascularized, such as with a saphenous vein graft [23].

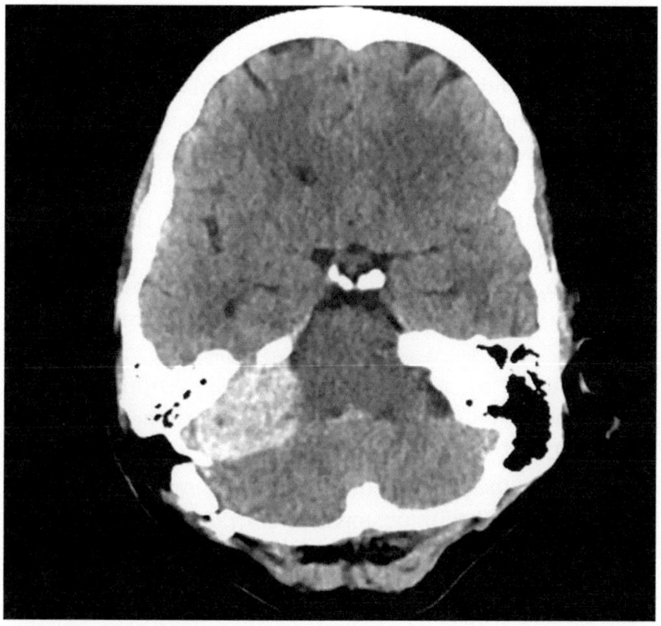

Fig. 15.2 Axial computed tomography image shows a post right-sided cerebellopontine hematoma, in this case requiring surgical evacuation without residual symptoms

Venous Sinus Thrombosis

Lateral skull-base approaches to the CPA involve careful surgical preservation and meticulous handling of the dural venous sinuses. Thrombosis of these venous sinuses resulting in morbidity or mortality is an uncommon but important complication for which to monitor carefully in the postoperative setting (Fig. 15.3). Occluding thromboses can cause slowly progressive symptoms of increased intracranial pressure, headaches, papilledema, visual disturbance, venous infarction, intracranial hemorrhage, seizures, or other focal neurologic deficits. In extremely rare cases, involvement of the superior sagittal sinus can lead to mortality [24].

Retrospective reviews of postoperative sinus thrombosis have reported an incidence ranging from 4.6% to 11.6%, presenting as early as the day of surgery to 40 days postoperatively [25–27]. Ohata and colleagues also noted that two cases of thrombosis were only noted on follow-up imaging 5.4 and 6.4 years postoperatively. Retrospective studies tend to report cases found due to clinical symptoms or intraoperative findings, likely underreporting the true incidence as many cases of smaller or partial thromboses may remain asymptomatic. In a prospective study with planned preoperative and postoperative magnetic resonance venography (MRV) in a series of lateral skull-base cases, 31.9% of patients showed some radiographic signs of at least a partial filling defect, though all of these patients were asymptomatic and none required anticoagulation [28].

Treatment strategies for diagnosed postoperative thromboses vary greatly and are often tailored to the case based upon surgical findings and patient symptoms. Conservative measures including observation, hydration, corticosteroids, and acetazolamide have been used. A much larger body of evidence exists for spontaneous or trauma-induced dural venous thrombosis for which anticoagulation is recommended [29, 30]. However, in the setting of recent intracranial CPA surgery, treatment of dural sinus thrombosis with systemic anticoagulation is weighed against the risks of postoperative intracranial hemorrhage. In some cases with symptom deterioration, other management options available include endovascular therapies, such as thrombolysis or mechanical venous thrombectomy, and CSF diversion, such as a ventriculoperitoneal shunt [31].

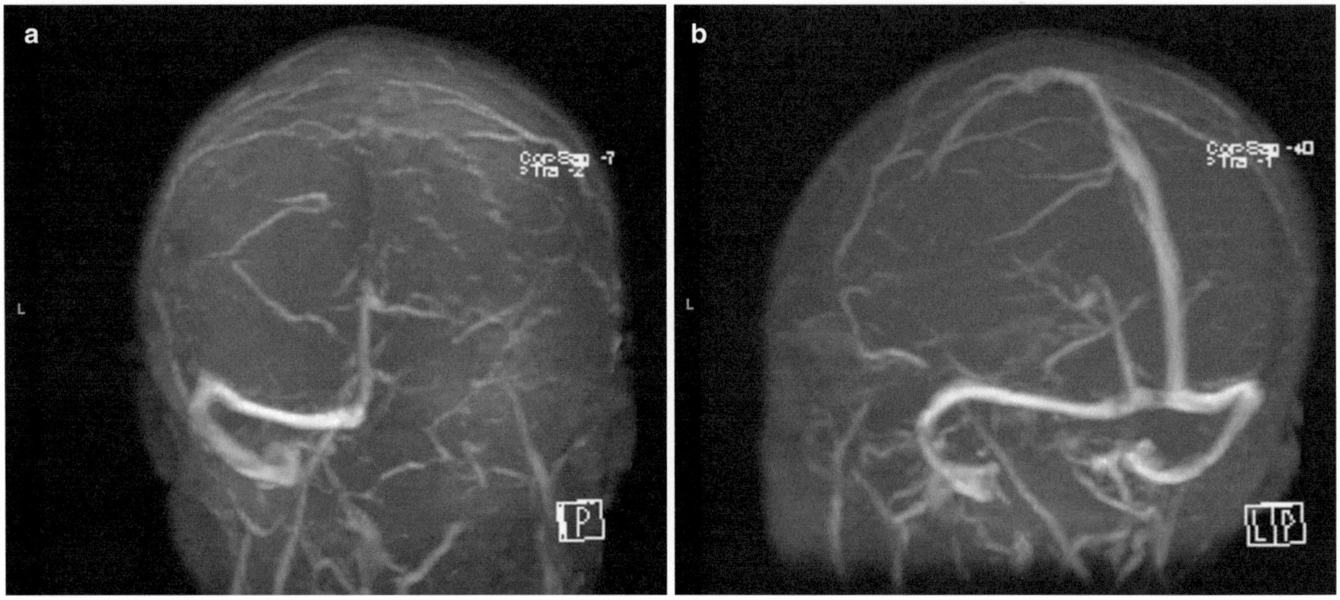

Fig. 15.3 (**a**) Magnetic resonance venography (MRV) after the resection of a right-sided vestibular schwannoma reveals a filling defect extending from a portion of the superior sagittal sinus into the right transverse sinus, sigmoid sinus, and jugular vein. (**b**) A follow-up MRV 1 year later revealed normal flow throughout the dural venous sinus system

Cranial Nerve Dysfunction

Microsurgical approaches to tumors within the CPA strive to provide complete removal of lesions while preserving the multiple cranial nerves that may be locally involved. These nerves may be already affected by the skull-base tumors preoperatively or altered by intraoperative dissection. Hearing loss is a very common presenting symptom of CPA lesions and, when feasible, hearing preservation approaches to save residual hearing and the cochlear nerve are undertaken. Other chapters of this text address hearing preservation and rehabilitation options after lateral skull-base surgery. A review of other potential cranial nerve neuropathies follows.

Vestibular Dysfunction

The vestibular nerves are commonly involved, depending on the nature of the pathologic lesion. In VS surgery, typically already dysfunctional vestibular nerves are sectioned resulting in complete loss of any residual ipsilateral vestibular function. In these cases, improvement in balance and dizziness may require adaptation and vestibular compensation over a significant period of time. Although hearing loss and facial nerve function are deservedly critical considerations in CPA surgery, in VS patients, ongoing dizziness was associated with the greatest reduction in quality-of-life measures [32].

In a study of 48 patients operated on for VS and assessed with vestibular testing and the Dizziness Handicap Inventory, 71% of patients had no change or reported improved equilibrium postoperatively [33]. Preoperative serviceable hearing, cystic transformation, normal cervical vestibular evoked myogenic potentials (cVEMPs), diplopia, or other vestibular syndromes were predictive of having worse equilibrium postoperatively, while having preoperative vestibulopathy (caloric weakness >75%) was a good prognostic factor. Similarly, in another study of 81 patients who had undergone surgery for VS, abnormal preoperative vestibular testing measures—such as caloric weakness, abnormal positional nystagmus, and abnormal vestibulo-ocular reflex (VOR) asymmetry on rotary chair testing—correlated with lower postoperative disability [34]. Patients with preoperative dysfunction may have already completed some degree of compensation compared to patients with normal function who suffer an abrupt change and complete loss of ipsilateral vestibular function in the acute postoperative period. In a review of 210 patients operated on for VS via a retrosigmoid approach, 31% were noted to have dysequilibrium lasting greater than 3 months postoperatively, based upon a retrospective chart review of documentation for recorded symptoms [35]. In a follow-up study by the same group, completed by surveying the patients, 65% reported some degree of persistent dysequilibrium postoperatively [36].

Vestibular rehabilitation is considered beneficial to reduce the duration of symptoms and for overall equilibrium after CPA surgeries that may disturb balance. However, existing reports may not always show the benefit, with noted limitations in selection bias as typically patients with greater struggles with equilibrium are prescribed or choose to pursue vestibular rehabilitation programs while those with no symptoms do not [33]. The use of brief periods of vestibular exercises even in the very early stages of recovery after CPA surgery may be beneficial to postoperative patients [37]. The use of simple VOR exercises and education has also been studied and shown to help improve the rate of compensation in the absence of a formal physical therapy program [38]. Patients receiving therapy have reported a longer time period to ambulate independently, though this may be due to accentuated symptoms in the acute period due to exercises, and 89% of patients reported they felt the exercises to be helpful in regaining their balance [34]. In a prospective randomized controlled trial comparing general instructions to a customized vestibular rehabilitation protocol for 12 weeks, younger patients <50 years improved significantly with either intervention, but patients over the age of 50 years receiving customized vestibular rehabilitation showed improved balance test results compared with those only given general instructions [39].

Facial Nerve

Preservation of facial nerve function is a critical goal in lateral skull-base surgery as facial nerve paresis can be a disfiguring and difficult complication. The facial nerve is most commonly injured at the porous region, and careful avoidance of trauma caused by suction on the nerve is important [40]. Microsurgery for vestibular schwannoma has a varied rate of reported facial nerve preservation. In a series of 162 consecutive patients with small tumors undergoing excision through a middle cranial fossa approach, House–Brackmann (HB) grade I or II was achieved in 97% of cases [41]. In a retrospective review of 410 cases operated on with a variety of approaches, good facial nerve function (HB I or II) was found in 86% of patients immediately postoperatively, and 58.9% of those with initially poor function would go on to improve during follow-up [42]. In 1052 patients with anatomically preserved facial nerves and total tumor removal, 65% maintained HB grade I or II, with another 29.4% with HB grade III [43]. In a prospective cohort including tumors of all sizes, 73% of patients had good facial function at postoperative day 180 [44]. Even for large vestibular schwannomas undergoing surgical resection, good facial nerve function has been reported in up to 88% of patients [45, 46]. In a systematic review of the literature that included an analysis of 11,873 patients, facial nerve preservation (HB I or II) was found in 78–85%, varying by approach. Although rare, in some complex skull-base lesions with significant vascularity, preoperative angiogram, and embolization help reduce blood loss and facilitate surgical resection but carry a small risk of cranial nerve dysfunction, including facial palsy [47, 48].

Delayed Facial Paralysis

In a subset of patients in whom the facial nerve is anatomically preserved and who awaken with good facial nerve function, delayed onset palsy may occur. A wide range of rates of delayed palsy has been reported, with varying definitions regarding the initial postoperative facial function and timing of worsening. A bimodal distribution of cases of delayed onset has been reported—those within the first 2 days and another group a week or more later [49]. In a series of 129 patients undergoing VS resection, a 29% incidence of delayed facial nerve dysfunction was found and primarily occurred within the first few postoperative days [50]. In this series, neurophysiologic stimulation parameters did not differ between patients with delayed palsy and those without. Those with delayed palsies had an excellent prognosis, with 89% recovering to HB grade I or II by 1 year. Similarly, a large series of 255 consecutive patients was evaluated to identify a 24.3% rate of delayed facial paresis occurring at an average of 3.65 postoperative days [51]. The vast majority (90%) ultimately recovered to their initial postoperative HB grade. In a review of 314 consecutive patients, excluding cases of early onset weakness (within 48 h) and counting only delayed facial weakness >72 h postoperatively, a 4.8% rate of delayed facial palsy was found [52]. These patients also had excellent recovery over time, with 93% recovering to HB grade I or II by 1 year. In a review of 489 patients that focused on facial deterioration of at least two HB grades from postoperative days 5 to 30, 16% of cases experienced a delayed weakness.

Viral reactivation is a proposed mechanism for the delayed palsies. In a prospective study of 20 patients undergoing vestibular schwannoma surgery, seven patients developed postoperative delayed facial weakness. Serum IgM titers of herpes simplex 1, herpes simplex 2, and varicella zoster virus were found to be significantly more elevated postoperatively in those with delayed palsies than those without, and IgG titers did not differ significantly [53]. However in another small series in which three patients had serology, IgG had a significant increase without IgM changes [54]. Perioperative administration of famciclovir has been suggested to reduce the risk of delayed facial palsy. Patients undergoing VS surgery who received famciclovir showed potential benefit compared to a historical group without pretreatment [55].

Facial Paralysis and Eye Complications

In cases of facial nerve weakness or paralysis, ocular complications can arise due to weakened musculature as well as potential lacrimal dysfunction from nervus intermedius dysfunction. Lagophthalmos causes poor distribution of tears that may lead to exposure keratitis and corneal injury. In some cases of larger CPA lesions, trigeminal nerve dysfunction with resultant corneal hypoesthesia can further contribute to eye complications. In one review, up to 44% of patients undergoing VS surgery required some form of ophthalmologic procedure postoperatively, though in that series a high rate, 70%, of cases had facial palsy [56]. Patients with trigeminal involvement and corneal hypoesthesia are at highest risk to develop corneal pathology [56, 57]. A more contemporary review of 174 patients undergoing VS resection reported a much lower incidence of the need for ophthalmologic referral (7.6%) and only 5.3% of patients requiring an ophthalmic procedure [58]. Treatment for the eye most commonly includes an upper eyelid loading procedure to address lagophthalmos and potentially a lower eyelid tightening procedure.

Contemporary care of facial nerve paralysis after skull-base surgery has incorporated a wide range of advancements in techniques: free muscle transfer, masseteric to facial nerve transfer or as a source of innervation for microvascular free flaps, cross-face grafting, static procedures, and botulinum toxin injections [59–61]. Advanced techniques in microsurgical excision of lateral skull-base tumors have led to improved facial nerve results. However, in the cases of complete facial paralysis postoperatively, even in the setting of an anatomically preserved facial nerve, early assessment of recovery and consideration of intervention by 6 months may be considered [62]. Facial nerve reanimation is discussed in greater detail in another chapter of this text.

For patients with facial paralysis and a challenging path to recovery, facial nerve rehabilitation therapy in addition to medical and surgical treatment is often utilized. Physical therapy can be applied in various forms including mime therapy, neuromuscular retraining, massage therapy, and mirror feedback for coordination of exercises. These approaches have been utilized to promote function and inhibit or control synkinesis [63, 64]. Specialized therapy can be a useful adjunctive therapy in cases of postoperative facial paralysis and improves patients' quality of life [65, 66].

Lower Cranial Nerves

Extensive lesions of the CPA, such as those involving the jugular foramen, can place the lower cranial nerves at risk during surgery. Pathologies such as meningiomas of the CPA or jugular foramen and other tumors of the jugular foramen, such as paragangliomas or schwannomas of the cranial nerves themselves, may present preoperatively with neural dysfunction and may be challenging or, at times, impossible to excise without changes to lower cranial nerve function (Fig. 15.4).

A high vagal lesion impairs the larynx and pharynx both by the loss of motor function and a loss of sensory innervation. This combination leads to ipsilateral vocal fold paralysis and associated dysphonia as well as dysphagia and a high risk of aspiration. Voice and swallowing dysfunction in the

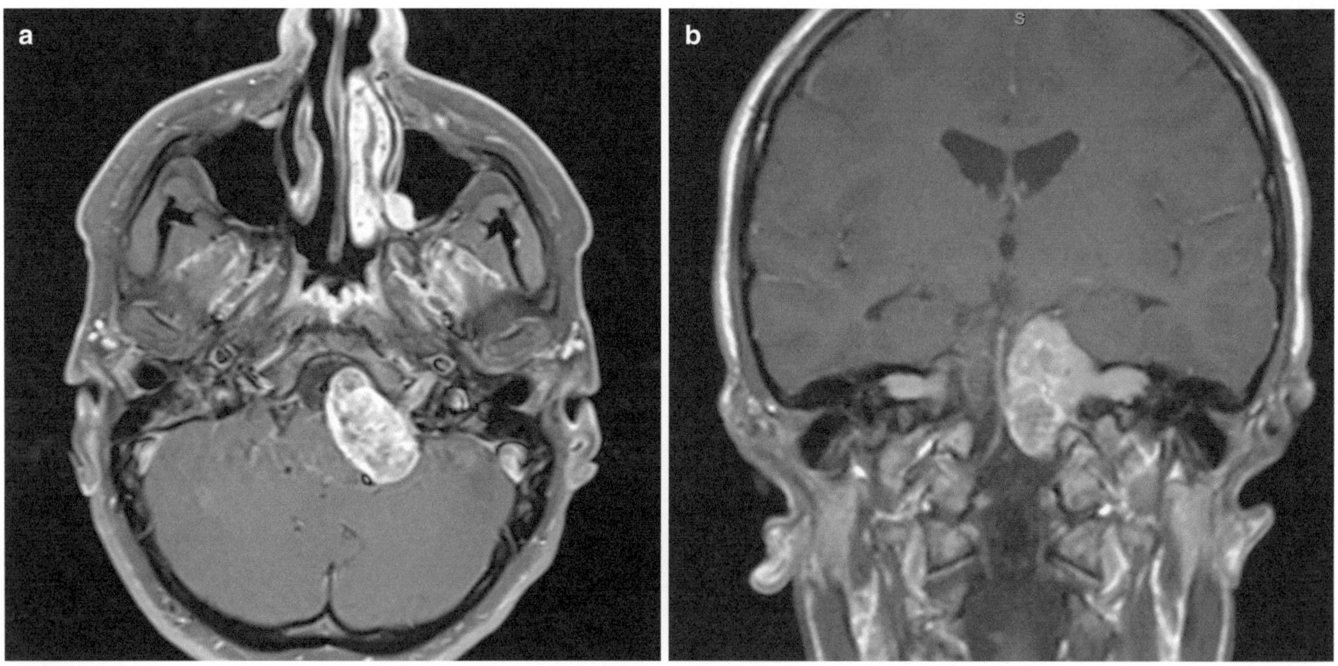

Fig. 15.4 T1 postcontrast magnetic resonance images in the (**a**) axial and (**b**) coronal planes of a patient with neurofibromatosis type 2, with multiple cranial nerve schwannomas, hearing loss, left vocal fold paralysis, and hypoglossal nerve paralysis due to collision tumors involving the left vestibular nerve and lower cranial nerves

immediate postoperative period likely varies based upon particular CPA tumor characteristics and extension but was found in 10% of one series of CPA surgeries [67]. CPA tumor size was found to be an independent risk factor for postoperative vagal palsy. In a series of 50 patients with giant VS, 10% of patients had lower cranial nerve dysfunction preoperatively and 6% developed new dysfunction postoperatively, though most recovered over time [1]. Although the severity of symptoms for a vagal lesion can vary greatly, it appears the timing of onset plays a role. Sudden onset high vagal paralysis, such as that induced as a result of skull-base surgery, is associated with a higher rate of tube feeding in comparison to a more gradual onset of paralysis, such as from progressive tumor effect [68]. Patients with normal function preoperatively and sudden loss of vagal function postoperatively have no time to adapt or modify their swallowing behavior, leading to abrupt dysphagia and the potential need for an alternative route of feeding or other interventions. Palsies induced slowly by tumor growth provide a longer period for compensation and swallowing modification. Surgical resection affecting additional combinations of the lower cranial nerves, including the glossopharyngeal and hypoglossal nerves, or other neurologic changes, such as in cognitive status, may further impair the patient's ability to compensate.

Laryngeal procedures to help address dysphonia and dysphagia include laryngeal framework surgery, such as medialization thyroplasty, or vocal fold injection using a variety of materials. In a review of 35 patients with high vagal lesions due to a variety of causes in addition to skull-base surgery, 14 patients had tracheotomies before any laryngeal interventions, but 11 of these 14 patients were able to be decannulated after laryngeal framework surgery [69]. The procedures included medialization thyroplasty with or without arytenoid adduction or cricopharyngeal myotomies. Most of those patients (94%) had some improvement in aspiration, though 19% continued to require a feeding tube. Fang and colleagues reviewed high vagal lesions also of various causes, including CPA surgery, and found the feeding tube dependency rate improved from 27% to 5.9% after laryngeal interventions. Medialization thyroplasty has been previously suggested to be performed primarily at the time of skull-base surgery to provide immediate improvement and avoid the need for tracheotomy, though other authors note final vocal cord status is difficult to judge immediately and suggest injection laryngoplasty for short-term improvement, with further surgery determined when the cord position is constant [68, 70]. Early arytenoid adduction as the sole method of medialization by postoperative day 2 has also been reported in a series of 26 patients as another option for early rehabilitation. In that group, 62% of patients required a percutaneous feeding tube after skull-base surgery, though all but one was able to resume nutrition by mouth with removal of the feeding tube by 1 year, and 33% of patients required tracheotomy, all of whom were decannulated by 3 months [71].

Headache

Patients with CPA lesions such as VS, even untreated, are more likely than controls with tumors to have severe headache disability, and 60% overall report some degree of headache before treatment [72]. Headache disability outcomes have not been shown to be statistically different between the treatment modalities of observation, stereotactic radiosurgery, and microsurgery.

In studies of CPA surgery approaches, retrosigmoid craniotomy has frequently been identified as having a greater risk of postoperative headache in comparison to other lateral skull-base approaches. In a systematic review of surgery for VS, the retrosigmoid approach was significantly more likely to result in persistent postoperative headache (17.3%) compared to the translabyrinthine (0%) approach but statistically not significantly more than middle cranial fossa cases (8%) [73]. Although most reports describe short-term postoperative headaches, it is possible that long-term outcomes at 1 year may not show significant differences between approaches [74]. Potential causes of this postoperative headache include cervical muscle adhesion and subsequent irritation to exposed dura at the craniotomy site, dural tension, intradural bone dust initiating aseptic meningitis from intradural drilling, and injury to either the lesser or greater occipital nerves from the incision and approach.

To address potential dural adhesions, several authors have reported utilizing replacement of a bone flap or cranioplasty techniques to reduce the incidence or severity of postoperative headache [75–77]. A retrospective review of 565 retrosigmoid approaches to the CPA reported significant differences between the incidence of postoperative headache based on if patients were treated for vestibular nerve section (5%) or removal of VS (54%), suggesting internal auditory canal drilling and dispersed bone dust as the primary difference between those approaches being a significant contributor to the headaches [78]. In addition to intradural drilling, fibrin glue as a cause for aseptic meningitis and tight dural tension from closure has also been considered as factors [79]. The use of Gelfoam to trap residue or bone dust has been advocated as a method to reduce postoperative headaches [80]. Modifications of surgical technique using a curvilinear incision design has also been suggested as a method to avoid occipital nerve injury and headache [81].

For most cases of postoperative headache, simple analgesics such as NSAIDs, COX-2 inhibitors or paracetamol/acetaminophen are effective and used as first-line medical therapy [82]. Sumatriptan has also been described as an effective treatment in a small study that suggested some cases may have pain mediated by the trigeminal nerve [83]. A subset of the patients with postoperative headaches exhibit occipital neuralgia with occipital neuromas or nerve entrapment and may benefit from procedures targeting these pathologies [84]. Many large tumors of the CPA can also cause direct compression or vascular compression of the trigeminal nerve with associated neuralgia. Microsurgical resection of tumors improves trigeminal neuralgia in the majority of these cases and can alleviate facial numbness and paresthesia in some cases [85, 86].

Conclusion

Although microsurgery within the CPA has seen remarkable advancements in surgical technique and intraoperative monitoring, perioperative complications still occur. Management of potential morbidities often begins during preoperative counseling when the risks and possibilities for a given lesion and surgical plan are fully discussed so that patients understand their risks and may be prepared for the unlikely event that complication is encountered. Preoperative dysfunction of cranial nerves can be recognized, and abrupt postoperative neuropathies, such as in the vestibular system and swallowing mechanisms, can benefit from therapy and compensation. Knowledge of the broad range and likelihood of various complications allows for early identification and treatment. Advancements in rehabilitation techniques and improved options for surgical rehabilitation have led to a trend toward early management of some cranial neuropathies, such as facial paralysis and laryngeal dysfunction, to facilitate the return of function and quality of life for patients.

References

1. Samii M, Gerganov VM, Samii A. Functional outcome after complete surgical removal of giant vestibular schwannomas. J Neurosurg. 2010;112(4):860–7.
2. Sanna M, Taibah A, Russo A, Falcioni M, Agarwal M. Perioperative complications in acoustic neuroma (vestibular schwannoma) surgery. Otol Neurotol. 2004;25(3):379–86.
3. McClelland S, Kim E, Murphy JD, Jaboin JJ. Operative mortality rates of acoustic neuroma surgery: a national cancer database analysis. Otol Neurotol. 2017;38(5):751–3.
4. Tolisano AM, Littlefield PD. Adverse events following vestibular schwannoma surgery: a comparison of surgical approach. Otol Neurotol. 2017;38(4):551–4.
5. Becker SS, Jackler RK, Pitts LH. Cerebrospinal fluid leak after acoustic neuroma surgery: a comparison of the translabyrinthine, middle fossa, and retrosigmoid approaches. Otol Neurotol. 2003;24(1):107–12.
6. Selesnick SH, Liu JC, Jen A, Newman J. The incidence of cerebrospinal fluid leak after vestibular schwannoma surgery. Otol Neurotol. 2004;25(3):387–93.
7. Manjila S, Weidenbecher M, Semaan MT, Megerian CA, Bambakidis NC. Prevention of postoperative cerebrospinal fluid leaks with multilayered reconstruction using titanium mesh-hydroxyapatite cement cranioplasty after translabyrinthine resection of acoustic neuroma. J Neurosurg. 2013;119(1):113–20.
8. Cueva RA, Mastrodimos B. Approach design and closure techniques to minimize cerebrospinal fluid leak after cerebellopontine angle tumor surgery. Otol Neurotol. 2005;26(6):1176–81.
9. Merkus P, Taibah A, Sequino G, Sanna M. Less than 1% cerebrospinal fluid leakage in 1,803 translabyrinthine vestibular schwannoma surgery cases. Otol Neurotol. 2010;31(2):276–83.
10. Goddard JC, Oliver ER, Lambert PR. Prevention of cerebrospinal fluid leak after translabyrinthine resection of vestibular schwannoma. Otol Neurotol. 2010;31(3):473–7.
11. Lee EQ, Ruiz R, Lebowitz R, Roland JT, Jethanamest D, Givi B. Donor site complications of free fat transfer in otolaryngologic procedures. Poster presented at 2018 Triological Society Combined Sections Meeting, Scottsdale, AZ, 18 Jan 2018.
12. Mangus BD, Rivas A, Yoo MJ, Alvarez J, Wanna GB, Haynes DS, et al. Management of cerebrospinal fluid leaks after vestibular schwannoma surgery [miscellaneous article]. Otol Neurotol. 2011;32(9):1525–9.
13. Lemonnier LA, Tessema B, Kuperan AB, Jourdy DN, Telischi FF, Morcos JJ, et al. Managing cerebrospinal fluid rhinorrhea after lateral skull base surgery via endoscopic endonasal eustachian tube closure. Am J Rhinol Allergy. 2015;29(3):207–10.
14. Orlandi RR, Shelton C. Endoscopic closure of the eustachian tube. Am J Rhinol. 2004;18(6):363–5.
15. Allen KP, Isaacson B, Kutz JW, Purcell PL, Roland PS. The association of meningitis with postoperative cerebrospinal fluid fistula. J Neurol Surg B Skull Base. 2012;73(6):401–4.
16. Dubey A, Sung W-S, Shaya M, Patwardhan R, Willis B, Smith D, et al. Complications of posterior cranial fossa surgery—an institutional experience of 500 patients. Surg Neurol. 2009;72(4):369–75.
17. Sanchez GB, Kaylie DM, O'Malley MR, Labadie RF, Jackson CG, Haynes DS. Chemical meningitis following cerebellopontine angle tumor surgery. Otolaryngol Head Neck Surg. 2008;138(3):368–73.
18. Samii M, Tatagiba M, Piquer J, Carvalho GA. Surgical treatment of epidermoid cysts of the cerebellopontine angle. J Neurosurg. 1996;84(1):14–9.
19. Slattery WH, Francis S, House KC. Perioperative morbidity of acoustic neuroma surgery. Otol Neurotol. 2001;22(6):895–902.
20. Bambakidis NC, Manjila S, Dashti S, Tarr R, Megerian CA. Management of anterior inferior cerebellar artery aneurysms: an illustrative case and review of literature. Neurosurg Focus. 2009;26(5):E6.
21. Sakata K, Al-Mefty O, Yamamoto I. Venous consideration in petrosal approach: microsurgical anatomy of the temporal bridging vein. Neurosurgery. 2000;47(1):153–61.
22. Lustig LR, Jackler RK. The vulnerability of the vein of Labbé? During combined craniotomies of the middle and posterior fossae. Skull Base Surg. 1998;8(1):1–9.
23. Morita A, Sekhar LN. Reconstruction of the vein of Labbé by using a short saphenous vein bypass graft. Technical note. J Neurosurg. 1998;89(4):671–5.
24. Sawarkar DP, Verma SK, Singh PK, Doddamani R, Kumar A, Sharma BS. Fatal superior sagittal sinus and torcular thrombosis after vestibular schwannoma surgery: report of a rare complication and review of the literature. World Neurosurg. 2016;96:607.e19–24.
25. Keiper GL, Sherman JD, Tomsick TA, Tew JM. Dural sinus thrombosis and pseudotumor cerebri: unexpected complications of suboccipital craniotomy and translabyrinthine craniectomy. J Neurosurg. 1999;91(2):192–7.
26. Moore J, Thomas P, Cousins V, Rosenfeld JV. Diagnosis and management of dural sinus thrombosis following resection of

cerebellopontine angle tumors. J Neurol Surg B Skull Base. 2014;75(6):402–8.
27. Ohata K, Haque M, Morino M, Nagai K, Nishio A, Nishijima Y, et al. Occlusion of the sigmoid sinus after surgery via the presigmoidal-transpetrosal approach. J Neurosurg. 1998;89(4):575–84.
28. Benjamin CG, Sen RD, Golfinos JG, et al. Postoperative sinus thrombosis in the setting of skull base and parasagittal surgery. J Neurosurg. 2018;1–7.
29. Saposnik G, Barinagarrementeria F, Brown RD, Bushnell CD, Cucchiara B, Cushman M, et al. Diagnosis and management of cerebral venous thrombosis: a statement for healthcare professionals from the American Heart Association/American Stroke Association. Stroke. 2011;42(4):1158–92.
30. Ferro JM, Bousser M-G, Canhão P, Coutinho JM, Crassard I, Dentali F, et al. European Stroke Organization guideline for the diagnosis and treatment of cerebral venous thrombosis—endorsed by the European Academy of Neurology. Eur Stroke J. 2017;2(3):195–221.
31. Manzoor NF, Ray A, Singer J, Nord R, Sunshine J, Megerian CA, et al. Successful endovascular management of venous sinus thrombosis complicating trans-labyrinthine removal of vestibular schwanomma. Am J Otolaryngol. 2016;37(4):379–82.
32. Carlson ML, Tveiten ØV, Driscoll CL, Goplen FK, Neff BA, Pollock BE, et al. What drives quality of life in patients with sporadic vestibular schwannoma? Laryngoscope. 2015;125(7):1697–702.
33. Thomeer H, Bonnard D, Franco-Vidal V, Porez F, Darrouzet P, Liguoro D, et al. Prognostic factors of balance quality after transpetrosal vestibular schwannoma microsurgery: an instrumentally and DHI-based prospective cohort study of 48 patients. Otol Neurotol. 2015;36(5):886–91.
34. El-Kashlan HK, Shepard NT, Arts HA, Telian SA. Disability from vestibular symptoms after acoustic neuroma resection. Am J Otol. 1998;19(1):104–11.
35. Driscoll CL, Lynn SG, Harner SG, Beatty CW, Atkinson EJ. Preoperative identification of patients at risk of developing persistent dysequilibrium after acoustic neuroma removal. Am J Otol. 1998;19(4):491–5.
36. Lynn SG, Driscoll CL, Harner SG, Beatty CW, Atkinson EJ. Assessment of dysequilibrium after acoustic neuroma removal. Am J Otol. 1999;20(4):484–94.
37. Herdman SJ, Clendaniel RA, Mattox DE, Holliday MJ, Niparko JK. Vestibular adaptation exercises and recovery: acute stage after acoustic neuroma resection. Otolaryngol Head Neck Surg. 1995;113(1):77–87.
38. Enticott JC, O'Leary SJ, Briggs RJS. Effects of vestibulo-ocular reflex exercises on vestibular compensation after vestibular schwannoma surgery. Otol Neurotol. 2005;26(2):265–9.
39. Vereeck L, Wuyts FL, Truijen S, De Valck C, Van de Heyning PH. The effect of early customized vestibular rehabilitation on balance after acoustic neuroma resection. Clin Rehabil. 2008;22(8):698–713.
40. Tos M, Youssef M, Thomsen J, Turgut S. Causes of facial nerve paresis after translabyrinthine surgery for acoustic neuroma. Ann Otol Rhinol Laryngol. 1992;101(10):821–6.
41. Meyer TA, Canty PA, Wilkinson EP, Hansen MR, Rubinstein JT, Gantz BJ. Small acoustic neuromas: surgical outcomes versus observation or radiation. Otol Neurotol. 2006;27(3):380–92.
42. Nonaka Y, Fukushima T, Watanabe K, Friedman AH, Sampson JH, Mcelveen JT, et al. Contemporary surgical management of vestibular schwannomas: analysis of complications and lessons learned over the past decade. Neurosurgery. 2013;72(2 Suppl Operative):ons103–15; discussion ons115.
43. Falcioni M, Fois P, Taibah A, Sanna M. Facial nerve function after vestibular schwannoma surgery. J Neurosurg. 2011;115(4):820–6.
44. Esquia-Medina GN, Grayeli AB, Ferrary E, Tubach F, Bernat I, Zhang Z, et al. Do facial nerve displacement pattern and tumor adhesion influence the facial nerve outcome in vestibular schwannoma surgery? Otol Neurotol. 2009;30(3):392–7.
45. Roland JT, Fishman AJ, Golfinos JG, Cohen N, Alexiades G, Jackman AH. Cranial nerve preservation in surgery for large acoustic neuromas. Skull Base. 2004;14(2):85–91.
46. Grahnke K, Garst JR, Martin B, Leonetti JP, Anderson DE. Prognostic indices for predicting facial nerve outcome following the resection of large acoustic neuromas. J Neurol Surg B Skull Base. 2017;78(6):454–60.
47. Gaynor BG, Elhammady MS, Jethanamest D, Angeli SI, Aziz-Sultan MA. Incidence of cranial nerve palsy after preoperative embolization of glomus jugulare tumors using Onyx: clinical article. J Neurosurg. 2014;120(2):377–81.
48. Gartrell BC, Hansen MR, Gantz BJ, Gluth MB, Mowry SE, Aagaard-Kienitz BL, et al. Facial and lower cranial neuropathies after preoperative embolization of jugular foramen lesions with ethylene vinyl alcohol. Otol Neurotol. 2012;33(7):1270–5.
49. Sargent EW, Kartush JM, Graham MD. Meatal facial nerve decompression in acoustic neuroma resection. Am J Otol. 1995;16(4):457–64.
50. Lalwani AK, Butt FY, Jackler RK, Pitts LH, Yingling CD. Delayed onset facial nerve dysfunction following acoustic neuroma surgery. Am J Otol. 1995;16(6):758–64.
51. Megerian CA, McKenna MJ, Ojemann RG. Delayed facial paralysis after acoustic neuroma surgery: factors influencing recovery. Am J Otol. 1996;17(4):630–3.
52. Grant GA, Rostomily RR, Kim DK, Mayberg MR, Farrell D, Avellino A, et al. Delayed facial palsy after resection of vestibular schwannoma. J Neurosurg. 2002;97(1):93–6.
53. Gianoli GJ. Viral titers and delayed facial palsy after acoustic neuroma surgery. Otolaryngol Head Neck Surg. 2002;127(5):427–31.
54. Franco-Vidal V, Nguyen D-Q, Guerin J, Darrouzet V. Delayed facial paralysis after vestibular schwannoma surgery: role of herpes viruses reactivation—our experience in eight cases. Otol Neurotol. 2004;25(5):805–10.
55. Brackmann DE, Fisher LM, Hansen M, Halim A, Slattery WH. The effect of famciclovir on delayed facial paralysis after acoustic tumor resection. Laryngoscope. 2008;118(9):1617–20.
56. Rogers NK, Brand CS. Acoustic neuroma and the eye. Br J Neurosurg. 1997;11(4):292–7.
57. Mulhern MG, Aduriz-Lorenzo PM, Rawluk D, Viani L, Eustace P, Logan P. Ocular complications of acoustic neuroma surgery. Br J Ophthalmol. 1999;83(12):1389–92.
58. Gange WS, Kirchner ID, Thompson JA, Hill J, Grahnke K, Ibrahim T, et al. Ophthalmic complications following acoustic neuroma resection. Oper Neurosurg (Hagerstown, Md). 2018;14(1):58–65.
59. Bhama PK, Weinberg JS, Lindsay RW, Hohman MH, Cheney ML, Hadlock TA. Objective outcomes analysis following microvascular gracilis transfer for facial reanimation: a review of 10 years' experience. JAMA Facial Plast Surg. 2014;16(2):85–92.
60. Murphey AW, Clinkscales WB, Oyer SL. Masseteric nerve transfer for facial nerve paralysis: a systematic review and meta-analysis. JAMA Facial Plast Surg. 2018;20(2):104–10.
61. Hontanilla B, Marré D. Comparison of hemihypoglossal nerve versus masseteric nerve transpositions in the rehabilitation of short-term facial paralysis using the Facial Clima evaluating system. Plast Reconstr Surg. 2012;130(5):662e–72e.
62. Albathi M, Oyer S, Ishii LE, Byrne P, Ishii M, Boahene KO. Early nerve grafting for facial paralysis after cerebellopontine angle tumor resection with preserved facial nerve continuity. JAMA Facial Plast Surg. 2016;18(1):54–60.
63. Beurskens CHG, Heymans PG. Physiotherapy in patients with facial nerve paresis: description of outcomes. Am J Otolaryngol. 2004;25(6):394–400.
64. Lindsay RW, Robinson M, Hadlock TA. Comprehensive facial rehabilitation improves function in people with facial paralysis: a

5-year experience at the Massachusetts Eye and Ear Infirmary. Phys Ther. 2010;90(3):391–7.
65. Diels HJ. Facial paralysis: is there a role for a therapist? Facial Plast Surg FPS. 2000;16(4):361–4.
66. Luijmes RE, Pouwels S, Beurskens CHG, Kleiss IJ, Siemann I, Ingels KJAO. Quality of life before and after different treatment modalities in peripheral facial palsy: a systematic review. Laryngoscope. 2017;127(5):1044–51.
67. Best SR, Starmer HM, Agrawal Y, Ward BK, Hillel AT, Chien WW, et al. Risk factors for vagal palsy following cerebellopontine angle surgery. Otolaryngol Head Neck Surg. 2012;147(2):364–8.
68. Fang T-J, Tam Y-Y, Courey MS, Li H-Y, Chiang H-C. Unilateral high vagal paralysis: relationship of the severity of swallowing disturbance and types of injuries. Laryngoscope. 2011;121(2):245–9.
69. Pou AM, Carrau RL, Eibling DE, Murry T. Laryngeal framework surgery for the management of aspiration in high vagal lesions. Am J Otolaryngol. 1998;19(1):1–7.
70. Netterville JL, Jackson CG, Civantos F. Thyroplasty in the functional rehabilitation of neurotologic skull base surgery patients. Am J Otol. 1993;14(5):460–4.
71. Bielamowicz S, Gupta A, Sekhar LN. Early arytenoid adduction for vagal paralysis after skull base surgery. Laryngoscope. 2000;110(3 Pt 1):346–51.
72. Carlson ML, Tveiten ØV, Driscoll CL, Boes CJ, Sullan MJ, Goplen FK, et al. Risk factors and analysis of long-term headache in sporadic vestibular schwannoma: a multicenter cross-sectional study. J Neurosurg. 2015;123(5):1276–86.
73. Ansari SF, Terry C, Cohen-Gadol AA. Surgery for vestibular schwannomas: a systematic review of complications by approach. Neurosurg Focus. 2012;33(3):E14.
74. Ruckenstein MJ, Harris JP, Cueva RA, Prioleau G, Alksne J. Pain subsequent to resection of acoustic neuromas via suboccipital and translabyrinthine approaches. Am J Otol. 1996;17(4):620–4.
75. Wazen JJ, Sisti M, Lam SM. Cranioplasty in acoustic neuroma surgery. Laryngoscope. 2000;110(8):1294–7.
76. Harner SG, Beatty CW, Ebersold MJ. Impact of cranioplasty on headache after acoustic neuroma removal. Neurosurgery. 1995;36(6):1097–9.
77. Schessel DA, Rowed DW, Nedzelski JM, Feghali JG. Postoperative pain following excision of acoustic neuroma by the suboccipital approach: observations on possible cause and potential amelioration. Am J Otol. 1993;14(5):491–4.
78. Jackson CG, McGrew BM, Forest JA, Hampf CR, Glasscock ME, Brandes JL, et al. Comparison of postoperative headache after retrosigmoid approach: vestibular nerve section versus vestibular schwannoma resection. Am J Otol. 2000 May;21(3):412–6.
79. Schaller B, Baumann A. Headache after removal of vestibular schwannoma via the retrosigmoid approach: a long-term follow-up-study. Otolaryngol Head Neck Surg. 2003;128(3):387–95.
80. Catalano PJ, Jacobowitz O, Post KD. Prevention of headache after retrosigmoid removal of acoustic tumors. Am J Otol. 1996;17(6):904–8.
81. Silverman DA, Hughes GB, Kinney SE, Lee JH. Technical modifications of suboccipital craniectomy for prevention of postoperative headache. Skull Base. 2004;14(2):77–84.
82. Rimaaja T, Haanpää M, Blomstedt G, Färkkilä M. Headaches after acoustic neuroma surgery. Cephalalgia Int J Headache. 2007;27(10):1128–35.
83. Levo H, Blomstedt G, Hirvonen T, Pyykkö I. Causes of persistent postoperative headache after surgery for vestibular schwannoma. Clin Otolaryngol Allied Sci. 2001;26(5):401–6.
84. Ducic I, Felder JM, Endara M. Postoperative headache following acoustic neuroma resection: occipital nerve injuries are associated with a treatable occipital neuralgia. Headache. 2012;52(7):1136–45.
85. Liu P, Liao C, Zhong W, Yang M, Li S, Zhang W. Symptomatic trigeminal neuralgia caused by cerebellopontine angle tumors. J Craniofac Surg. 2017;28(3):e256–8.
86. Neff BA, Carlson ML, O'Byrne MM, Van Gompel JJ, Driscoll CLW, Link MJ. Trigeminal neuralgia and neuropathy in large sporadic vestibular schwannomas. J Neurosurg. 2017;127(5):992–9.

Facial Reanimation

16

Tessa A. Hadlock and Nate Jowett

Facial nerve disorders encompass a broad spectrum of dysfunction, ranging from subtle dynamic facial asymmetry to dense flaccid paralysis. Following repair or grafting, the extent of facial nerve regeneration can greatly vary. Restricted movement may result from hypofunction (persistent weakness of facial muscles), hyperfunction (hypertonicity, spasm), aberrant regeneration (synkinesis), or a combination of these states. Facial nerve dysfunction may lead to numerous functional problems including corneal exposure, dry eye, epiphora, oral incompetence, poor manipulation of the food bolus, speech and articulation difficulties, nasal obstruction, and facial pain. Inability to convey emotion through facial expression and the accompanying psychological penalty as well as social isolation have a profound impact on a patient's quality of life. This chapter reviews anatomy of the facial nerve, grading of facial nerve injury, and contemporary surgical and adjunctive techniques for facial reanimation. An algorithm for zonal management of the paralyzed face is provided.

Anatomy of Facial Nerve

A neuron consists of a cell body with dendritic and axonal extensions enclosed by a plasma membrane. Axons are enveloped and supported by Schwann cells, some forming a myelin sheath serving to increase the velocity of action potential propagation. Individual myelinated axons are enclosed within a connective tissue network (the endoneurium) and arranged in groups of fascicles, each of which is surrounded by a distinct perineurium. The fascicles and surrounding perineurium are enclosed by loose areolar tissue containing multiple vascular channels, known as the internal epineurium. The external epineurium encloses all the fascicles and encases the entire peripheral nerve [1]. The mesoneurium consists of loose areolar tissue that extends from the external epineurium, through which segmental blood supply enters the nerve. Peripheral nerve sheaths are well vascularized and include two intracommunicative systems: (1) the perifascicular system, located in the internal epineurium, and (2) the intrafascicular system, located in the endoneurial network of perineurium-enveloped fascicles [2].

Voluntary facial motor function originates from upper motor neurons in the lower portion of the precentral gyrus. The frontotemporal cerebral cortex as well as limbic and basal ganglion sources house central neurons controlling involuntary expression. The facial motor nucleus is located in the ventral aspect of the caudal pons. The dorsal portion of the facial motor nucleus houses neuronal cell bodies controlling the upper third of the face and receives bilateral upper motor neuron input, while the ventral portion controlling the lower two-thirds of the face receives only crossed input [3]. Facial nerve fibers exit the motor nucleus, pass medioventral around the nucleus of the abducens (sixth) cranial nerve, and exit the lateral brainstem near the cerebellopontine junction (Fig. 16.1) [3]. The somatic motor component of the facial nerve exits the pontomedullary junction 1–2 mm anterior to the vestibulocochlear nerve together with the nervus intermedius, which carries the somatic sensory, special sensory, and visceral motor components of the facial nerve. The nerves are loosely joined, devoid of epineurium, and bathed in cerebrospinal fluid within this cisternal segment that spans the 17–24 mm gap between the brainstem and the porus acusticus at the cerebellopontine angle. The meatal segment spans 8–10 mm between the porus acusticus and the meatal foramen; the facial nerve occupies the anterosuperior quadrant of the internal auditory canal (IAC).

The facial nerve assumes its narrowest dimension within the IAC fundus at the meatal foramen, the entrance to the fallopian canal. Herein, the nerve is most susceptible to injury from trauma or inflammation. The fallopian canal,

T. A. Hadlock (✉) · N. Jowett
Department of Otolaryngology—Head and Neck Surgery, Massachusetts Eye and Ear Infirmary, Harvard Medical School, Boston, MA, USA
e-mail: Tessa_Hadlock@meei.harvard.edu

N. C. Bambakidis et al. (eds.), *Surgery of the Cerebellopontine Angle*, https://doi.org/10.1007/978-3-031-12507-2_16

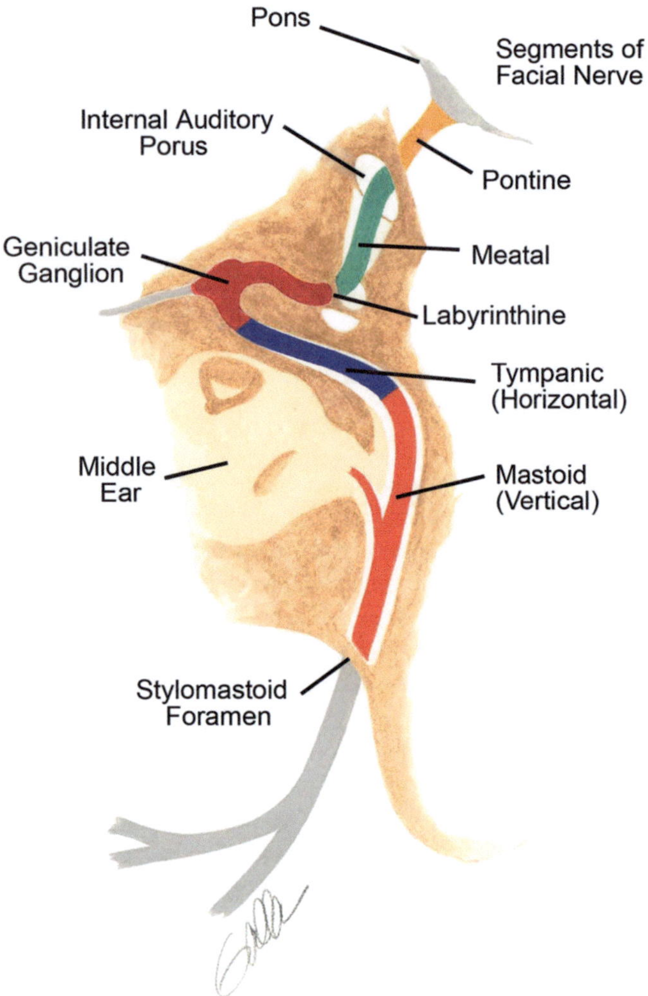

Fig. 16.1 The extramedullary segments of the facial nerve. (Modified with permission from BC Decker Inc., from Nadol JB Jr. [32])

which has the longest bony course of any cranial nerve, is divided into three segments (Fig. 16.1): labyrinthine (3–5 mm), tympanic or horizontal (8–11 mm), and mastoid or vertical (10–14 mm). The labyrinthine segment extends from the fundus of the IAC to the distal portion of the geniculate ganglion. The greater superficial petrosal nerve branches from the geniculate ganglion, carrying preganglionic parasympathetic secretory fibers to the nose, lacrimal gland, and palate. The tympanic segment spans the distal geniculate ganglion where the nerve sharply turns posteriorly (the first genu) to the pyramidal eminence where the nerve sharply turns inferiorly (the second genu). The nerve to stapedius muscle emerges near the second genu. The mastoid segment spans the distance between the second genu and the stylomastoid foramen and has two other branches: the ascending branch of the auricular branch of the vagus nerve (Arnold's nerve) and the chorda tympani. Arnold's nerve provides sensation to the ear canal, tragus, and auricle. The chorda tympani carries preganglionic parasympathetic secretory fibers of the submandibular and sublingual glands as well as sensory taste fibers from the anterior two-thirds of the tongue. The arachnoid pia-dura mater junction typically lies near the fundus of the IAC but may extend as far as the geniculate ganglion. Proximal to this juncture, the facial nerve is unsheathed and bathed in cerebrospinal fluid.

After exiting the stylomastoid foramen, the facial nerve gives off a posterior auricular branch, a motor branch to the posterior belly of the digastric muscle, and a motor branch to the stylohyoid muscle prior to the pes anserinus. The posterior auricular nerve carries motor fibers to the superior and posterior auricular muscles and occipitalis muscles and is thought to supply the skin covering the mastoid process and adjacent parts of the auricle. Though branching patterns are highly variable, the main trunk of the facial nerve often splits into upper and lower divisions that further branch to supply five zones: temporal, zygomatic, buccal, marginal mandibular, and cervical. Though these branches generally innervate separate facial regions, there is significant arborization and redundancy among neighboring territories, especially in the midface.

Nerve Injury Classification

The degree to which a nerve is injured may be classified according to the Sunderland system, which includes five levels of severity (Fig. 16.2) [4]. The Sunderland scale provides a conceptual framework that guides management of nerve injury.

First-Degree Injury

In first-degree injury or neuropraxia, nerve conduction is interrupted at the injury site. Axon continuity is preserved, and there is no Wallerian degeneration. Neuropraxia often results from compression and ischemic insults. The period of denervation is short, and function recovers rapidly and completely.

Second-Degree Injury

In a second-degree injury, axons are disrupted within their endoneurial tubules. The endoneurium, which consists of the basal lamina of the Schwann cells, and a fibrillar reticular lamina with surrounding collagen fibrils, is preserved. Wallerian degeneration occurs distal to the site of injury. The confines of the endoneurial tube accurately guide regenerating axons to their original targets. Functional recovery is complete or near complete.

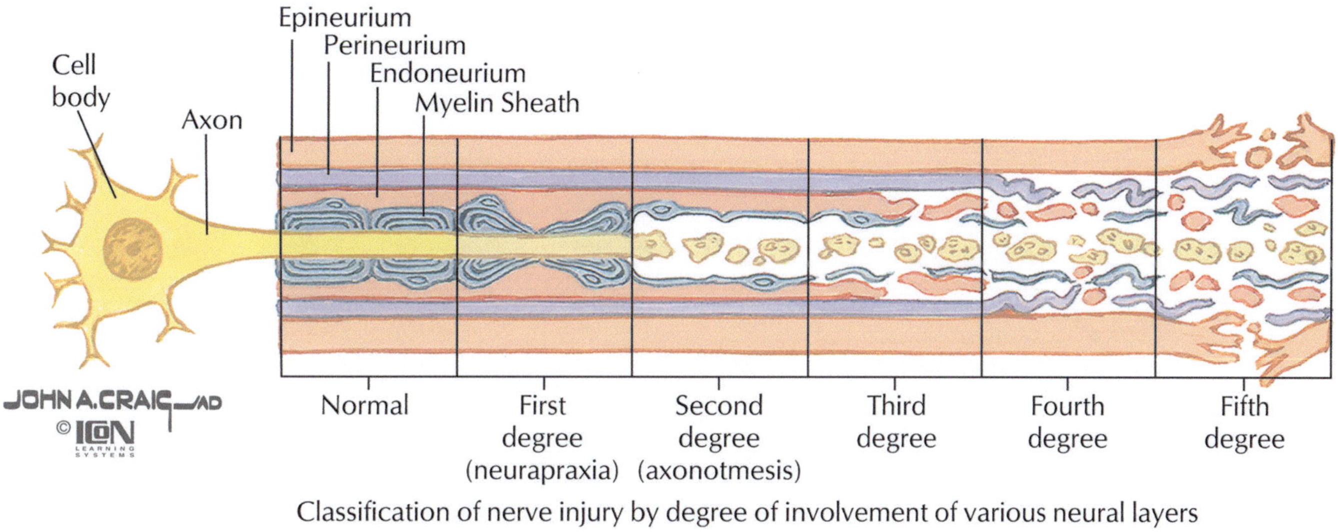

Fig. 16.2 Sunderland classification of degrees of nerve injury based on involvement of the neural layers. (Netter illustration used with permission of Elsevier Inc. All rights reserved)

Third-Degree Injury

At this level of severity, endoneurial disruption occurs without perineurial disruption. Continuity of the endoneurial tube is lost. However, fasciculi remain continuous and their arrangement in the nerve trunk is preserved. This level of injury may result from traction, hemorrhage, edema, vascular stasis, and ischemia. Resulting intrafascicular fibrosis severely impedes the process of regeneration, and extent of functional recovery varies. Endoneurial disruption may result in some aberrant axonal regeneration of axons or ephaptic communication with subsequent development of involuntary and uncoordinated facial movements, known as synkinesis.

Fourth-Degree Injury

This level of injury results in disruption of the endoneurium and perineurium. Only the external epineurium and mesoneurium remain intact. Intraneural fibrosis limits recovery, and pronounced aberrant interfascicular regeneration occurs causing disfiguring facial synkinesis.

Fifth-Degree Injury

At this highest level of injury, also known as neurotmesis, anatomic discontinuity is complete. Minimal to absent recovery occurs without surgical repair. Poor somatotopic fascicular organization of motor axons within the facial nerve results in significant aberrant regeneration and subsequent facial synkinesis despite meticulous repair of main trunk injuries [4–6].

Nerve Repair and Nerve Grafting

When facial nerve discontinuity is encountered, first-line therapy dictates reestablishment of neural continuity between proximal and distal facial nerve stumps. Direct end-to-end repair is preferred where nerve ends may be reapposed without tension; other interposition graft repair is favored [7]. In the setting of facial nerve defects of the fallopian canal, intratemporal rerouting of the nerve by means of mastoidectomy may be employed to facilitate repair and avoid need for interposition grafting [8]. The distal vertical segment of the nerve is amenable to suturing. A defect of the horizontal segment is typically addressed with simple approximation of nerve ends with reinforcement using fibrin glue, collagen, or hemostatic agents. During repair, the operating microscope should be used to evaluate the cut nerve endings. The stumps should be debrided and all devitalized tissue removed, followed by approximation and coaptation of the epineurial sheath. Interfascicular repair has not shown benefit over epineurial repair.

Nerve Grafting

When a tension-free neurorrhaphy cannot be achieved, an autograft is interposed between the proximal and distal endings of the facial nerve. Most often, donor nerve grafts are harvested from the great auricular, sural, or medial antebrachial cutaneous nerves (Fig. 16.3). The great auricular nerve is ideal for repairs that require grafts less than 6 cm long (Fig. 16.3a). A contraindication to its use is the presence of a neurotrophic malignancy. In such cases, the sural (Fig. 16.3b) or medial antebrachial nerve (Fig. 16.3c) is pre-

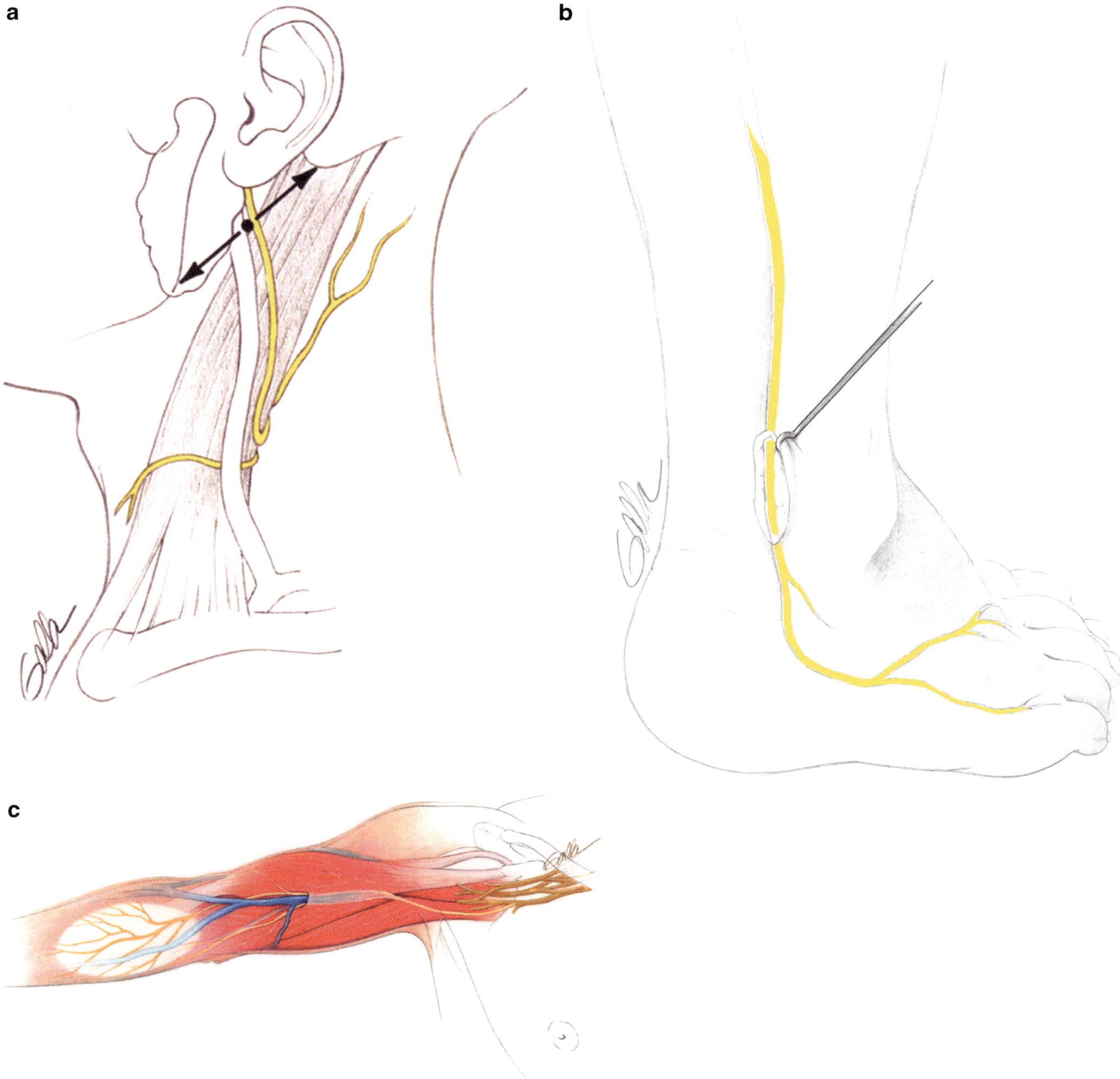

Fig. 16.3 (**a**) The great auricular nerve (yellow) is located on the lateral surface of the sternocleidomastoid muscle at the midpoint (dot) of a line (arrows) drawn between the mastoid tip and the angle of the mandible. (**b**) The sural nerve (yellow) is located in a subcutaneous plane posterior to the lateral fibular malleolus. The nerve runs parallel to the small saphenous vein. (**c**) The medial antebrachial cutaneous nerve arises primarily from the medial cord of the brachial plexus with contributions from the ventral rami of C8 and the first thoracic nerve. As the nerve enters the arm, it lies superficial to the brachial artery near the basilic vein. At the elbow, it divides into posterior and anterior branches that supply sensation to the ulnar aspect of both the flexor and extensor surfaces of the forearm. (Figure **a**, **b** from Nadol JB Jr. [32]. Figure **c** reproduced with permission from Cheney [22] © 2007 Mack L. Cheney, MD)

ferred. The latter is ideally suited for total nerve reconstruction to multiple distal branches. The results of cable grafting can be favorable [9]. The quality and quantity of axonal regrowth are best when repair is executed immediately following nerve injury or intentional resection. Under ideal circumstances, neural reconstruction proceeds in the same operative setting as sacrifice. Factors that lead to poor recovery include wound disruption, infection, or tension on the site of coaptation. In most cases, movement returns within 6–12 months following the reestablishment of neural continuity, depending on the location of the neural repair. Improvement continues to occur over several years.

Facial Reanimation

When neural continuity cannot be reestablished, either due to lack of a proximal stump at the brainstem or due to severe traumatic distortion of temporal bone anatomy, other methods of reestablishing facial balance and movement may be considered. Facial reanimation procedures refer to interventions that restore facial symmetry, resting tone, voluntary and involuntary movement, or a combination thereof. There are several broad categories of facial reanimation techniques, each appropriate to a specific set of clinical, anatomic, or outcome-related circumstances. These techniques include reinnervation techniques, muscle transfers, static procedures, and nonsurgical adjunctive therapy.

Nerve Substitution Techniques

Nerve substitution techniques, also known as nerve transfers, or reinnervation techniques, refer to procedures that provide neural input to the facial musculature via distal facial nerve branches using motor nerves other than the native facial nerve. Nerve transfers may be performed to the main trunk of the facial nerve, with the goal of restoring facial tone and some form of blink, or to more distal facial nerve branches, with the goal of restoring volitional control of specific facial movements such as smile. These techniques are indicated when the proximal facial nerve stump is unavailable but the distal facial nerve and facial musculature are present and functional. For example, resection of a skull base tumor requiring resection of the facial nerve at or near the brainstem may render neurorrhaphy technically infeasible. In this setting, immediate nerve transfer is indicated. Nerve transfers may be appropriate when no discernible facial function is noted 6–12 months following skull base surgery, intracranial injury, and traumatic facial paralysis, where the facial nerve is believed to be anatomically intact. While electrophysiologic demonstration of the lack of reinnervation potentials and the presence of fibrillation potentials at the 12-month mark may confirm persistent and complete denervation, lack of obvious functional recovery by this time period is a sufficient indication for intervention. These findings suggest insufficient regenerative potential from the proximal facial nerve stump and mandate alternative proximal axonal input to the distal facial nerve and facial musculature before atrophy and fibrosis become irreversible. Ongoing debate surrounds optimal timing for reinnervation in flaccid facial paralysis after skull-base surgery, though the most recent data suggest that complete flaccidity after 6 months portends a very poor smile prognosis. Nerve transfers are only indicated where facial muscles are likely to be receptive to reinnervation: typically 2 years from denervation in adults and possibly longer in children.

Hypoglossal–Facial Transfer (Cranial Nerve XII–VII Crossover)

The hypoglossal nerve was historically most often used to reinnervate the distal facial nerve. Its proximity to the extratemporal facial nerve, its dense population of myelinated motor axons, and the relative acceptability of the resultant hemi-tongue weakness made it a logical choice in the past [10–13]. In the classic cranial nerve XII–VII transfer, the entire hypoglossal nerve is transected and reflected upward for direct neurorrhaphy to the facial nerve stump (Fig. 16.4a). Several modifications have been described (Fig. 16.4b, c). In the "split" XII–VII transfer [14], the hypoglossal nerve is incised to a depth of approximately 30% of its caliber, and dissection is performed to elevate a segment that is several centimeters long for coaptation to the facial nerve or its branches (see Fig. 16.4b). This technique is inadvisable as the hypoglossal nerve is monofascicular in its proximal segment, without clear perineurial boundaries between groups of axons to guide dissection.

Another modification, the XII–VII jump graft, is designed to reduce tongue morbidity by avoiding the splicing away of a significant length of the hypoglossal trunk. An end-to-side neurorrhaphy between the hypoglossal nerve and a donor cable graft (usually the great auricular nerve) is sewn to the distal facial trunk (Fig. 16.4c) [15]. This modification is based on improved understanding of the microanatomy of the hypoglossal nerve, which has an interwoven fascicular architecture. Consequently, separating a 30% segment from the main trunk for several centimeters divides a significantly greater number of axons than if the fibers were oriented in parallel [15].

When the facial nerve can be mobilized from the second genu within the temporal bone and reflected inferiorly, removal of the mastoid tip allows direct coaptation of the facial nerve to the hypoglossal nerve, without the need for an interposition graft (Fig. 16.4d) [16]. Elimination of the cable graft provides a regenerative advantage by reducing the neurorrhaphies from two to one. Ongoing additional modifications to further simplify the delivery of axons from the hypoglossal to the distal facial nerve are continuously being devised, though lack of centralized or codified determination of outcomes hinders clear emergence of the superiority of one technique over others.

Surgical Technique

The classic XII–VII transfer is performed via a modified Blair parotidectomy incision. The parotid tail is elevated off the sternocleidomastoid muscle with preservation of the great auricular nerve, and the posterior belly of digastric is identified. Meticulous dissection in the plane between the perichondrium of the ear canal and parotidomasseteric fascia of the posterolateral aspect of the parotid gland is performed to identify the main trunk of the facial nerve, which is then

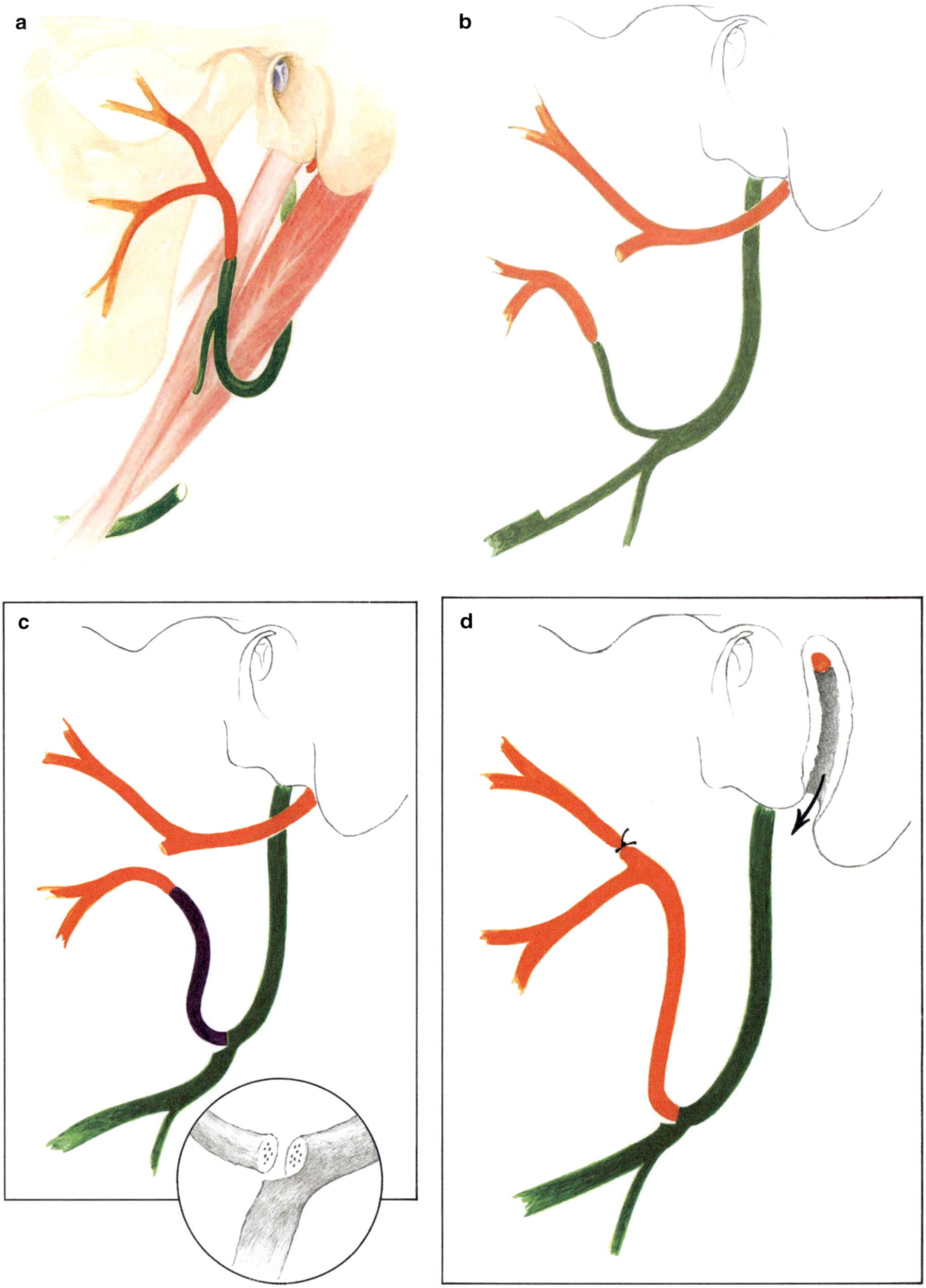

Fig. 16.4 Hypoglossal-facial nerve transfer. Hypoglossal nerve is shown in green; the facial nerve is shown in orange. (**a**) Classic procedure, with the entire hypoglossal nerve transected. (**b**) Modification with 40% segment of nerve secured to lower division. (**c**, left) Jump graft (purple) modification. (Inset) The graft is positioned to capture axons extending from the proximal aspect of the opened hypoglossal nerve. (**d**, right) Reflection of the facial nerve out of the mastoid bone (arrow) to meet the hypoglossal nerve in the neck. (Figure **a**, **b**, and **d** from Nadol JB Jr. [32] with permission from BC Decker Inc. Figure **c** published with permission © Tessa A. Hadlock, MD and Mack L. Cheney, MD)

traced to the pes anserinus. The ascending portion of the hypoglossal nerve is located deep to the posterior belly of the digastric muscle along the medial surface of the internal jugular vein and anterior surface of the internal and external carotid arteries. The nerve is mobilized distally to the branch point of the descendens hypoglossi, with ligation of occipital artery branches. The hypoglossal nerve is transected sharply and reflected superiorly to meet the facial nerve near the stylomastoid foramen. The main trunk of the facial nerve is sharply transected and secured to the hypoglossal nerve with five to seven 10-0 nylon epineurial microsutures under high stereoscopic magnification.

A modification designed to decrease mass movement of the face with XII–VII transfer involves coaptation of the hypoglossal nerve to selective nerve branches, or transection of selected facial nerve branches distal to the point of coaptation. For example, the hypoglossal nerve may be coapted to the inferior division of the facial nerve; alternatively, it may be coapted to the main trunk with transection of the upper division distal to the pes. Alternative reanimation techniques are then used to address the upper face.

The jump graft procedure is also termed the XII–VII side-to-end procedure. The great auricular nerve graft is harvested. The hypoglossal nerve is preserved in continuity once mobilized and an epineurial window made with transection of 30% of hypoglossal axons. Side-to-end coaptation of the graft is made in epineurial fashion, with end-to-end coaptation of the distal graft end to the facial nerve. Alternatively, the proximal facial nerve may be mobilized from the temporal bone, sectioned at the second genu, and transposed down into the neck by removal of the mastoid tip for direct side-to-end coaptation to the hypoglossal nerve.

With a XII–VII transfer, good resting facial tone is achieved in more than 90% of patients. When successful, the transfer allows deliberate facial movement with intentional manipulation of the tongue. However, results are variable. Time from denervation to transfer plays a key role in outcome. Reinnervation must occur within 2 years of injury; otherwise, neuromuscular fibrosis and atrophy progress to a point where meaningful tone and movement cannot be achieved [15].

Two significant drawbacks are associated with the procedure. Many patients experience mass facial movement, and the variable tongue dysfunction has been categorized as "severe" in as many as 25% of patients. Articulation and mastication difficulties are common. The modifications mentioned above are aimed at one or the other of these two problems. The procedure is contraindicated in patients who are likely to develop other cranial neuropathies (i.e., patients with neurofibromatosis type 2) or who have ipsilateral deficits of cranial nerve X. Combined cranial nerve X–XII deficits can lead to profound swallowing dysfunction.

Trigeminal-to-Facial Nerve Transfer

Over the past 5 years, the popularity of the masseteric branch of the trigeminal nerve as a donor source of axons for reinnervation of specific midfacial musculature driving smile has surged [17]. First popularized as a neural source for driving free muscle transfer for facial reanimation, it rapidly gained favor for its ease of access, abundance of motor axons, low donor-site morbidity, and ideal location for direct coaptation to relevant branches of the facial nerve driving smile. Rehabilitation of bite-driven smile is straightforward for most patients. Advances in surgical techniques now allow specific targeting of nerve-to-masseter transfer to distal zygomatic branches of the facial nerve driving smile, with preservation of facial nerve continuity elsewhere. This paradigm shift has led to earlier intervention to optimize outcomes in the setting of persistent flaccid paralysis at 6 months following skull base surgery where facial nerve continuity was preserved, while still allowing for the possibility of recovery of native function by avoidance of main trunk transection. Contrary to the hypoglossal nerve, the nerve-to-masseter does not provide resting tone. Though its use permits reanimation of a powerful smile, the midface remains flaccid at rest. In adults, the technique is best combined with concurrent nerve transfer of the hypoglossal nerve more proximally to the main trunk of the facial nerve to provide facial tone (which can be performed at a later date if native recovery is still possible) or alternatively with cross-face nerve grafting or static suspension of the midface. Results can be expected within 3–5 months and generally are superior to those achieved with muscle transfer (Fig. 16.5).

Surgical Technique

The procedure begins with elevation of a facial flap under the superficial musculo-aponeurotic system (SMAS), directly on the parotido-masseteric fascia. Branches of the facial nerve are identified as they emerge from the parotid gland, and a single large-caliber branch inferior to the zygomatic arch coursing toward the zygomaticus major and minor muscles is isolated. Retrograde dissection toward the upper division of the facial nerve through the parotid gland is carried out until the branching pattern of the upper division is fully appreciated and all other branches are left intact. Dissection proceeds deep to the parotid gland through the masseter muscle, where the nerve is located entering its deep surface. Once identified, the nerve is isolated using a vessel loop and dissected anteriorly as it courses more superficially into the muscle belly. When adequate length for primary coaptation to the recipient facial nerve is exposed, the nerve is transected distally and reflected out of the wound bed, and microsurgical coaptation to the recipient branch of the facial nerve is executed. When possible, proximal superomedial branches of the nerve-to-masseter are preserved during har-

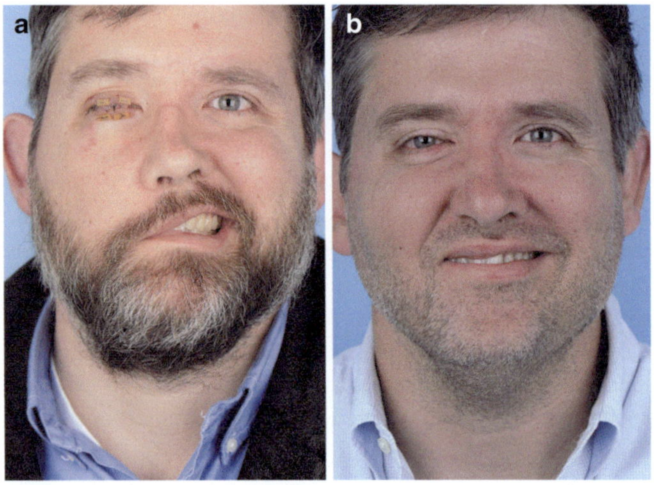

Fig. 16.5 (**a**) Preoperative and (**b**) postoperative view of patient attempting to smile, after complete facial nerve sacrifice at brainstem, with no grafting, followed 12 weeks later by five to seven transfer and two cross-face nerve grafts, one to the eye and one to a midface smile branch. Patient also underwent delayed static suspension

vest to lessen the risk of masseter muscle atrophy and subsequent hollowing of the cheek.

Cranial Nerve VII–VII Cross-Facial Grafting

Another potential source of axons for facial reinnervation is the healthy contralateral facial nerve [18]. It is the only donor source with the potential to reanimate mimetic function, such as spontaneous blink and emotive smile. Because it manifests significant distal arborization, several branches may be sacrificed for use in cross-facial grafting without adversely affecting healthy-side function. Donor branches contain far fewer motor axons than the hypoglossal or masseteric nerves to power the paralyzed side [19]. The use of contralateral facial nerve branches strictly for reinnervation of native facial musculature has largely been replaced by cross-face nerve grafting in conjunction with other reinnervation techniques or in preparation for free-muscle transfer; direct coaptation to branches of the paralyzed side is now thought to be useful only when performed within 3 months of proximal facial nerve sacrifice because of the time required for axons to traverse the face and the sensitivity of paralyzed muscles to denervation time.

Surgical Technique

A preauricular incision is made on the nonparalyzed side. A flap is raised on the parotid-masseteric fascia until the anterior border of the parotid gland is identified. With the guidance of electrical stimulation, the masseter fascia is dissected to identify 5–10 branches of the facial nerve. The 1–3 branches yielding isolated smile or blink movement are

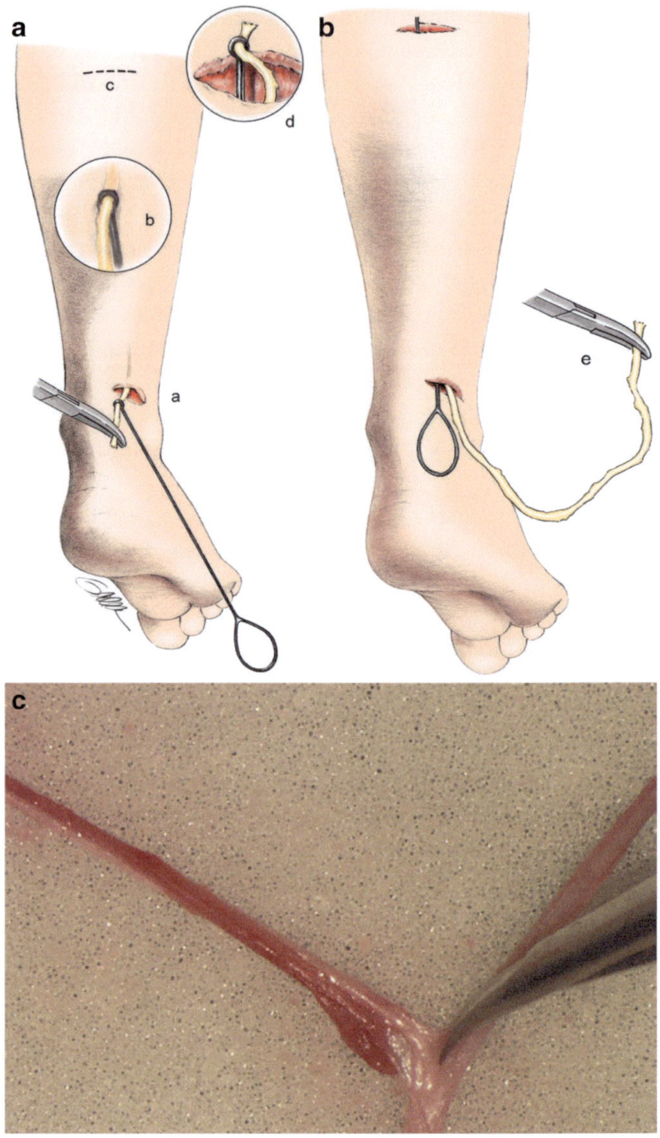

Fig. 16.6 Steps involved in minimally invasive sural nerve harvest. (**A**, a) The sural nerve is identified 1 cm lateral to the lateral malleolus, divided distally and inserted through the islet of the nerve stripper. (b) The nerve stripper is passed superoposteriorly, freeing the nerve from the surrounding subcutaneous fat. (c) When an appropriate length of nerve has been freed from surrounding tissues, a second skin incision is made by palpating the eyelet through the skin. (d) The eyelet of the stripper is delivered through the incision, and the proximal end of the sural nerve is cut, preparing it for removal through the distal incision. (**B**, e) Removal of a 15–20 cm sural nerve graft through the distal incision. Note the avoidance of a long skin incision. (**C**) Intrafascicular dissection of a single sural nerve into two strands, using a microscissors and microscopic magnification. (Published with permission © Tessa A. Hadlock, MD and Mack L. Cheney, MD)

selected as donor branches and transected sharply. A sural nerve graft is harvested from the leg through an open, endoscopic or minimally invasive approach (Fig. 16.6) [17]. The nerve is used either singly or divided into two strands under microscopic guidance if both blink and smile are targeted.

The strands are then tunneled subcutaneously from the donor branches either to the gingivo-buccal sulcus on the paralyzed side (if free tissue transfer is planned) or across into the paralyzed face for direct coaptation, in which case an identical facial nerve dissection is executed on the paralyzed side (direct hookup). In direct hook-up cases, end-to-end neurorrhaphy is performed to recipient smile and/or blink branches. On the donor side, nerve coaptation between the sural nerve and the donor facial nerve branches is performed with 10-0 nylon sutures. Clinically, the growth of axons into the graft is followed by tapping on the graft (Tinel's sign); tingling indicates the presence of regenerating axons. When required, a second-stage free-muscle transfer is performed 6–9 months later (see section "Free-Muscle Transfer" later in this chapter).

Regional Muscle Transfer Techniques

When the distal facial nerve or facial musculature has atrophied or become significantly fibrotic, the delivery of viable motor axons will not yield adequate excursion to create meaningful facial expression. In such cases, transfer of functional innervated musculature into the face offers the only reliable possibility of providing meaningful facial movement. A segment of innervated muscle can be transposed into the appropriate segment of the face from the temporalis, masseter, digastric, or other regional muscles. Alternatively, a muscle segment can be transferred as a free flap from a distant site (gracilis, pectoralis minor, serratus anterior, latissimus dorsi) and reinnervated locally.

Effective rehabilitation requires training and physical therapy to achieve optimal function. The literature supports the concept of neural plasticity; after a certain training period, some patients with trigeminally driven muscle transfers are believed to achieve movement without consciously clenching their teeth [20].

Temporalis Muscle Transfer

The temporalis muscle has historically been employed for reanimation of the smile in patients whose face is chronically paralyzed. The procedure is also useful as an interim therapy when the regenerative potential of the facial nerve is in question (i.e., after skull-base surgery) and during the waiting period for regeneration because it does not interfere with potential facial nerve regeneration [21].

Before proceeding, it is imperative to establish that the muscle and its nerve and vascular supply are intact. Some neurotologic procedures affect these structures, and several congenital facial palsy syndromes are associated with other cranial nerve abnormalities that may affect function of the temporalis muscle. Severe atrophy of the musculature, such as in an edentulous patient, is also a contraindication to temporalis transfer.

Surgical Technique

In the classic description of the procedure (Fig. 16.7), dissection is performed through an incision from the superior temporal line to the attachment of the lobule [22]. Scalp flaps are raised both anteriorly and posteriorly in the subdermal plane, just under the hair follicles. Care is taken to preserve the superficial temporal artery and veins so that the temporoparietal fascial flap (TPFF) can be used to obliterate the donor-site defect. The TPFF is incised posterior to the course of the temporal branch of the facial nerve and reflected from the true temporalis muscular fascia, leaving the TPFF pedicled on its vessels. A flap is raised deep to the subdermal plane from the zygomatic arch to the oral commissure. Some fat is left on the skin flap to avoid direct apposition of the transferred muscle to the overlying skin, which can produce tethering. The skin flap extends medially to the modiolus necessary for adequate coaptation to the transferred muscle.

A 1.5-cm–wide strip of temporalis muscle with its underlying pericranium is elevated from the calvarium. The segment is chosen so that reflection over the zygomatic arch pulls the commissure in a vector appropriate to the patient's smile pattern. The muscle is reflected into the midface and secured with polyglactin sutures to the orbicularis oris. Secure muscle-to-muscle contact is necessary to promote potential neurotization of the orbicularis fibers (Fig. 16.7a). The commissure is deliberately overcorrected so that with relaxation, an appropriate position is achieved. The TPFF is placed into the donor defect, and the incision is closed over a drain (Fig. 16.7b) [21].

Over the past decade, antidromic temporalis transposition has been largely supplanted by orthodromic approaches, where the tendinous attachment of the temporalis muscle is transferred from the coronoid process to the modiolus and nasolabial fold area. This approach avoids the characteristic bulge of the muscle over the zygomatic arch, which is accentuated by the hollowing in the temporal fossa, created by absence of muscle in the original position.

Irrespective of maneuver, the temporalis muscle has been shown to lead to significantly less oral commissure excursion than free muscle, thus in centers where microvascular surgery is widely performed, regional muscle transfer is reserved for patients who are extremely high surgical risks or who have a poor survival prognosis.

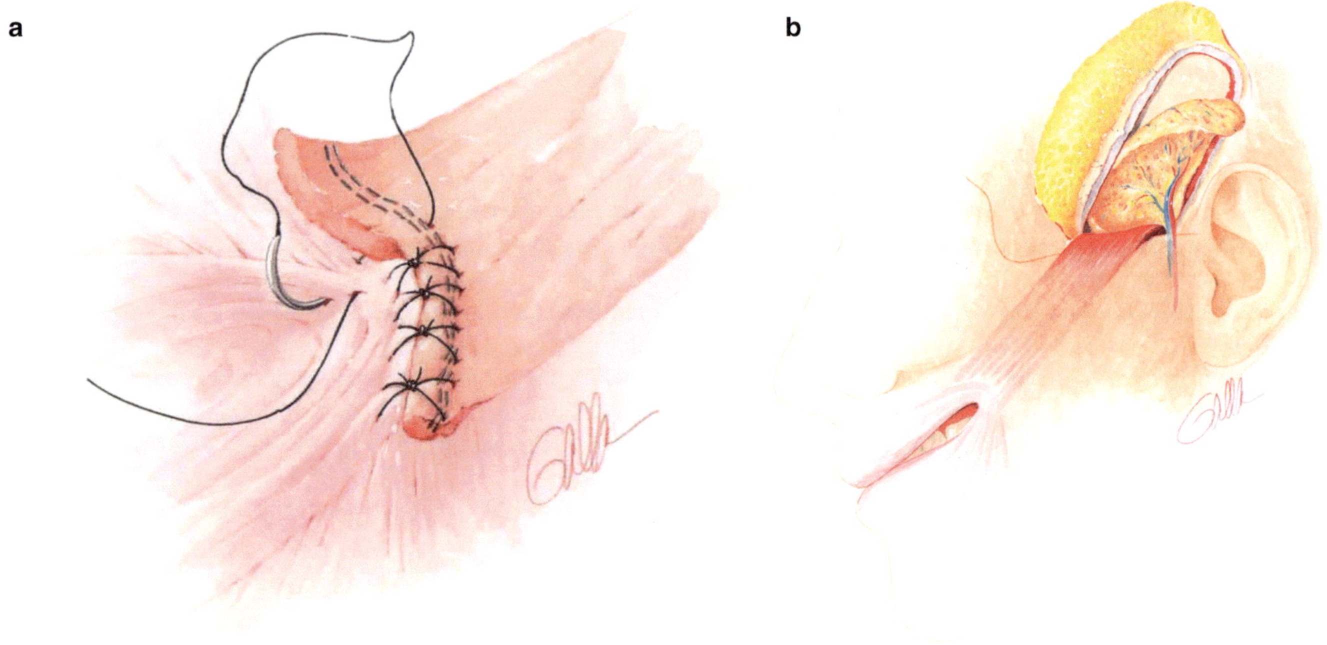

Fig. 16.7 Temporalis muscle transposition. (**a**) Securing the transposed muscle to the orbicularis oris. Note the double staple line and mattress sutures from the temporalis muscle to the modiolus. (**b**) Note the overcorrection of the commissure so that the first molar is visible. (From Nadol JB Jr. [32] with permission from BC Decker Inc.)

Other Regional Muscle Transfers

The masseter muscle transfer, popularized by Rubin and Baker and Conley, can also provide excursion at the oral commissure [23, 24]. The muscle is freed from its mandibular attachments and secured to the lateral aspect of the orbicularis oris, in the same fashion as the temporalis muscle. However, its more lateral vector pull, significant resulting contour defect, and availability of superior options have rendered the procedure obsolete.

The digastric muscle transfer has been described as useful in isolated marginal mandibular nerve injuries for lower lip reanimation. However, it may compromise oral competence in patients with total facial paralysis. In appropriately selected patients with an isolated injury of the marginal mandibular nerve, the procedure may effectively restore depressor function to the lower lip. The procedure involves sectioning the digastric muscle at the junction of the posterior belly and its tendon. The anterior belly and tendon are then freed from surrounding structures and secured to the orbicularis oris along the ipsilateral inferior border (Fig. 16.4). Mylohyoid nerve innervation to the anterior belly can be maintained [25], or the muscle can be driven by a cross-face nerve graft [26].

Other local muscle flaps have been suggested (for example, the innervated platysma musculocutaneous flap [27]) but insufficient numbers of treated patients leave their ultimate utility in question.

Free-Muscle Transfer

Free-muscle transfer may be employed for facial reanimation in several different clinical scenarios. If the proximal facial nerve stump is available but the facial musculature has been resected, a free-muscle flap can be placed in the face and driven by the ipsilateral proximal facial nerve. Patients with congenital facial palsy and those with longstanding facial paralysis or resected or myopathic facial muscle may likewise be good candidates for a free-muscle transfer. The procedure is performed in one or two stages. In the single-stage procedure, the muscle is driven by a branch of the ipsilateral trigeminal nerve (masseteric or deep temporal), while in the two-stage procedure, the muscle is powered by a cross-facial graft (with the first-stage operation performed as described above in the reinnervation section) or is dually innervated by both a cross-facial graft and trigeminal input. The waiting period for axonal extension through the cable graft before muscle transplantation is 6–9 months.

The gracilis muscle was the first muscle used in successful facial reanimation and remains the most popular choice for this purpose [28]. Although modifications involving subsegments of the muscle and alternative neural sources for the graft have been described [29, 30], the muscle implantation procedure is described below.

Surgical Technique

Preoperatively, the vector of the smile on the healthy side (if present) is noted so that it can be emulated on the affected side. The procedure (Fig. 16.8) is begun by harvest of the gracilis muscle from the medial aspect of the thigh. A curvilinear incision is made 1.5 cm posterior to a line connecting the pubic tubercle to the medial condyle of the tibia. The soft tissues are divided until the belly of the gracilis muscle is identified. The vascular pedicle is located entering the deep surface of the muscle, 8–10 cm distal to the pubic tubercle, and followed proximally for 6 cm. The obturator nerve is identified 1–2 cm proximal to the vascular pedicle and similarly traced. The pedicle, nerve, and approximately 40% of the width of the muscle belly are isolated, using a running locked suture at one or both ends to create pseudotendons useful to subsequent inset. The muscle is then thinned *in situ* by removal of approximately 40% of its superficial surface and removed from the surgical bed (Fig. 16.8a) [31].

A preauricular incision is made and extended to immediately below the mandible to identify the facial vessels for microvascular anastomosis. A thick skin flap is raised, exposing the zygomatic arch and malar eminence, and extends medially to expose the orbicularis oris. In the two-stage procedure, the stump of the cross-face nerve graft is identified in the gingivobuccal sulcus for later neurorrhaphy. In single-stage procedures, the masseteric nerve is identified exactly as described in the reinnervation section above. The gracilis muscle is then secured to the modiolus, stretched to its resting tension length, and secured to the temporalis fascia in the appropriate vector. The microvascular anastomoses and neurorrhaphy are performed, and the incisions are closed in layers over suction drainage (Fig. 16.8b). Movement is expected between 3 and 9 months following muscle transfer (Fig. 16.8c, d).

Alternative free-muscle flaps for facial reanimation, including the pectoralis minor, latissimus dorsi, serratus anterior, and abductor hallucis, have been described. The choice of which muscle to employ is based on surgeon experience.

Static and Adjunctive Facial Reanimation

Patients with facial paralysis are best rehabilitated through combinations of static and dynamic modalities. A treatment algorithm (Fig. 16.9) outlining the evaluation and ongoing management of patients with facial paralysis helps to prevent overlooking and thus undermanaging a specific facial zone. Static procedures are directed at specific functional and cosmetic issues, almost all of which are performed as office procedures under local anesthesia. Management options for the eye, which are paramount, include thin-profile, platinum-weight placement (Fig. 16.10) and unilateral correction of brow ptosis (Fig. 16.11). Nasal obstruction from collapse of the nasal valve caused by paralysis of the dilator nares can be addressed with standard or fascia lata nasal valve repair (Fig. 16.12). If oral incompetence is a significant complaint, resection of the lateral lower lip, fascia lata slings, or both can improve cosmesis and competence in this area. Subtle alteration of the nasolabial fold region to correct effacement or hyperprominence can be performed via minor suture-suspension techniques. Chemodenervation with botulinum toxin and aggressive neuromuscular retraining via physical therapy are vital to optimize facial balance.

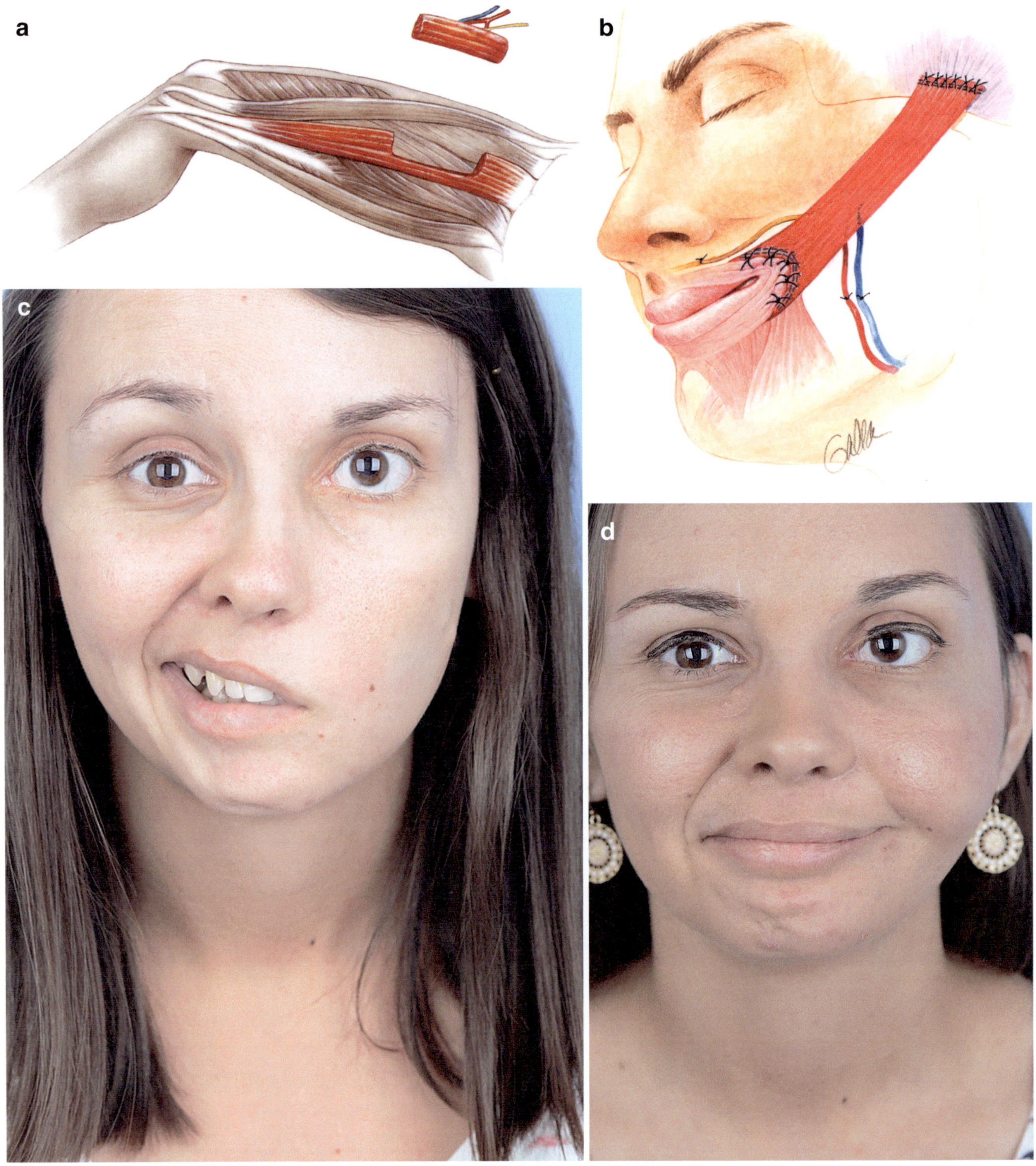

Fig. 16.8 (**a**) The branching pattern of the anterior division of the obturator nerve allows the gracilis muscle to be separated into at least two functional muscular units. A single fascicle usually supplies the anterior 25% of the muscle; the remaining nerve fascicles supply the rest of the muscle. A small portion of the muscle can be harvested with the main vascular pedicle and the fascicle from the anterior branch of the obturator nerve. (**b**) The suture lines can be seen at both ends of the transferred portion of the gracilis muscle. (**c**) Preoperative and (**d**) postoperative views of a patient smiling after gracilis muscle transfer with concomitant static facial suspension. (Figure **a** reproduced with permission from Urken with permission from Cheney et al. [30] © 1995 Mack L. Cheney, MD. Figure **b** from Nadol JB Jr. [32] BC Decker Inc.)

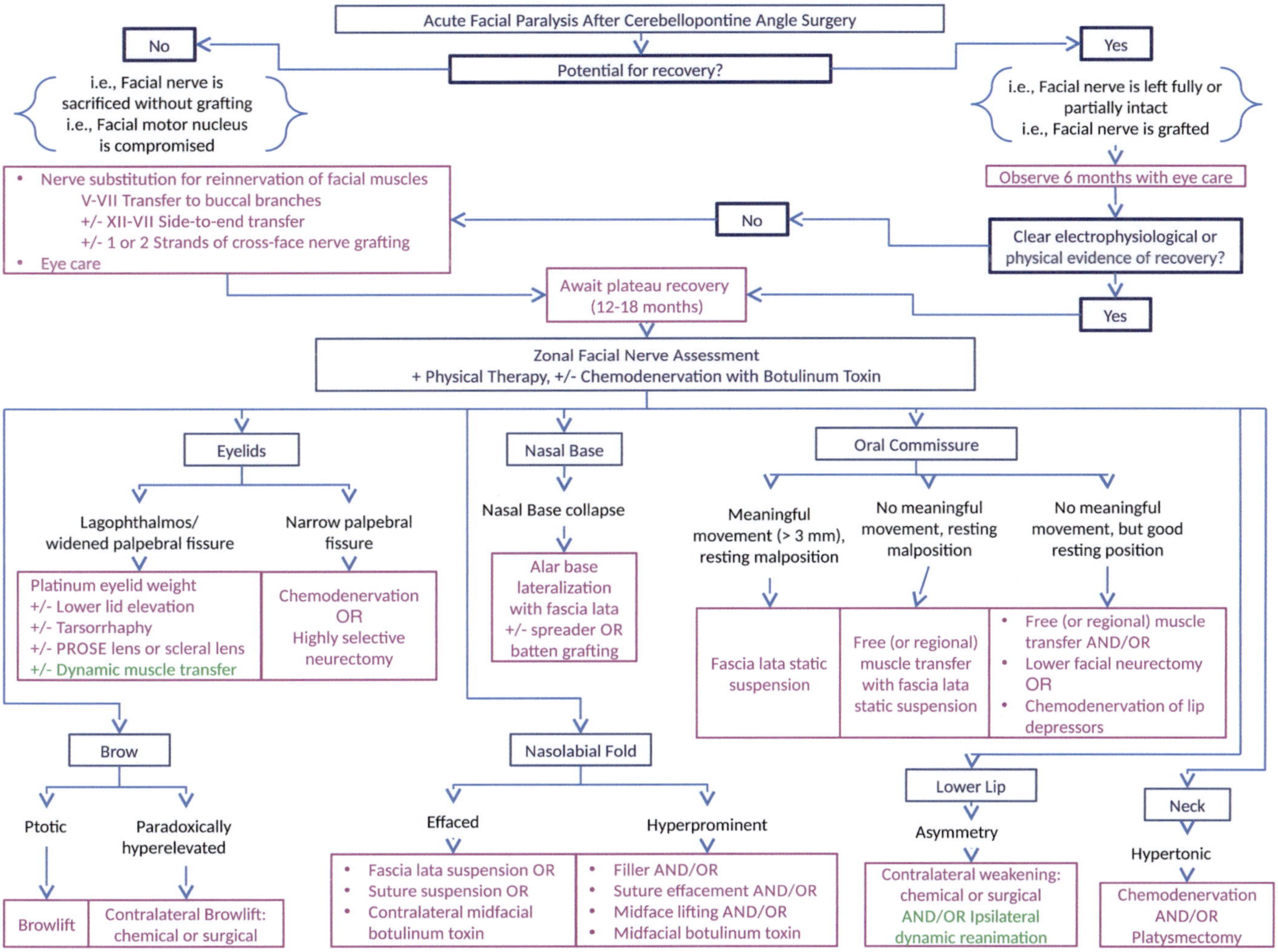

Fig. 16.9 Algorithm for acute facial paralysis after cerebellopontine angle surgery. Blue indicates broader categories, black indicates decision points, pink indicates action and interventions, and green indicates therapy that is not yet mainstream. These interventions are still experimental and describe future directions of treatment

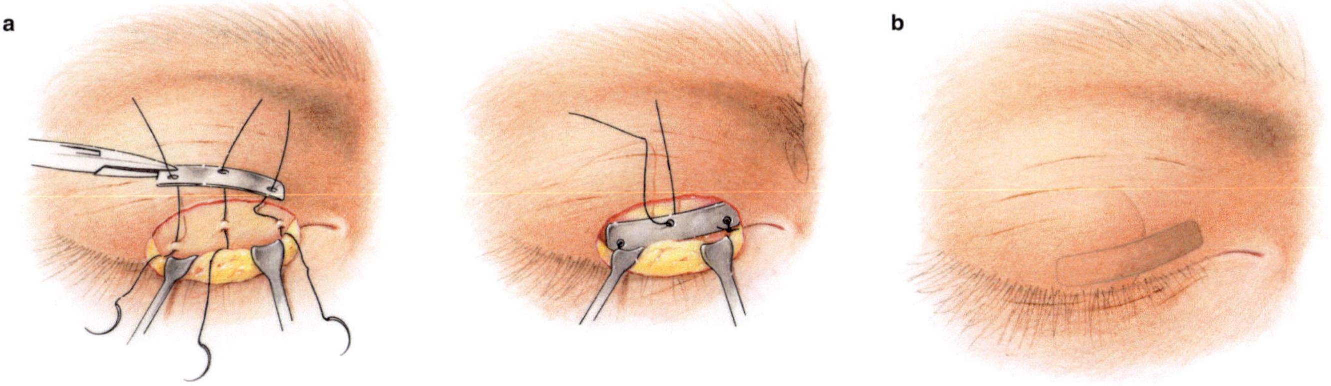

Fig. 16.10 (**a**, left) Implant positioned over tarsal plate. (**a**, right) Implant sutured onto tarsal plate. (**b**) Implant centered between medial and canthal tarsus on eyelid. (Published with permission, © Tessa A. Hadlock, MD and Mack L. Cheney, MD)

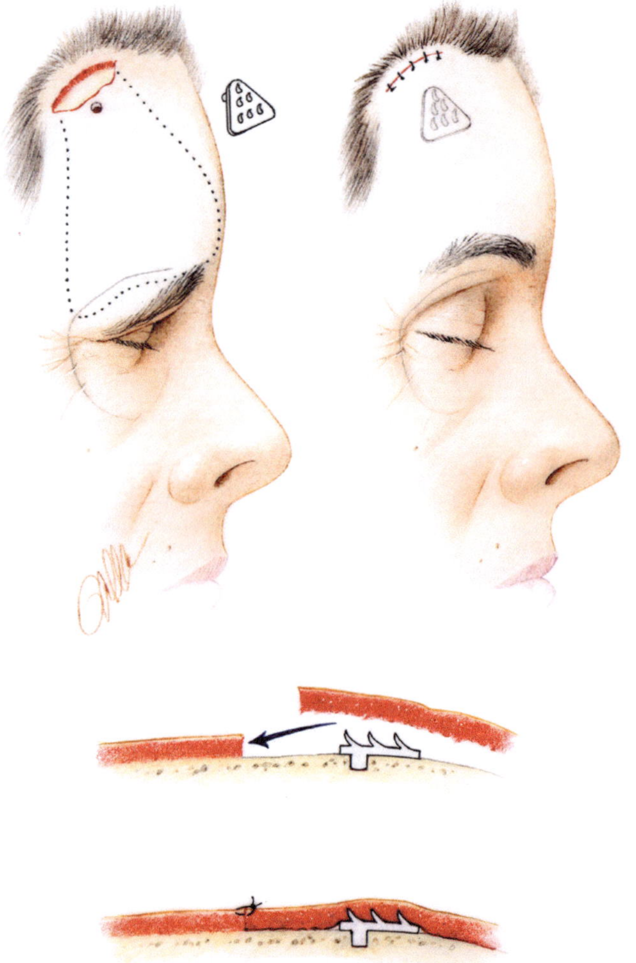

Fig. 16.11 Technique for correction of brow ptosis. Schematic showing lateral views (top) and close-up views of intraoperative (middle) and postoperative (bottom) positions of the tissue with the tine depicted. Note the intradermal position of the tines in the postoperative view. (From Hadlock et al. [33] with permission from Lippincott Williams & Wilkins)

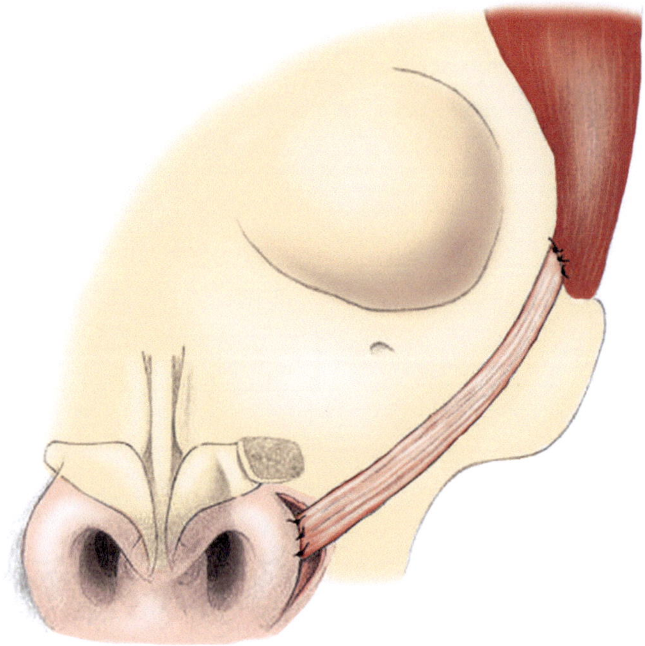

Fig. 16.12 External nasal valve repair via a fascia lata sling from the alar base to the zygoma. (Published with permission © Tessa A. Hadlock, MD and Mack L. Cheney, MD)

Summary

Facial paralysis is a disfiguring and debilitating condition, with its management determined by a large set of clinical variables. A systematic approach to the problem is mandatory. Each facial zone must be evaluated carefully at initial intake as well as longitudinally as the patient's recovery progresses. The complementary roles of reinnervation techniques, muscle transfer, static rehabilitation procedures, adjunctive physical therapy, and chemodenervation must be appreciated. Optimal comprehensive management is most easily accomplished in a multidisciplinary, high-volume setting.

References

1. Orenstein HH, Rohrich RJ, Hand II. Peripheral nerve surgery and tendon transfers. Select Read Plast Surg. 1990;5:1–38.
2. Bremond G, Magnan J. The anatomical and histological features of the facial nerve and their physio-pathological consequences. In: Portmann M, editor. Facial nerve. New York: Masson; 1985. p. 8–11.
3. Anderson RG. Facial nerve disorders. Select Read Plast Surg. 1991;6:1–34.
4. Sunderland S. Nerves and nerve injuries. New York: Churchill Livingstone; 1978.
5. Mackinnon SE, Dellon AL. Surgery of the peripheral nerve. New York: Thieme; 1988.
6. Anderson RG. Facial nerve disorders and surgery. Select Read Plast Surg. 1994;7:4.
7. Millesi H. Nerve suture and grafting to restore the extratemporal facial nerve. Clin Plast Surg. 1979;6:333–41.
8. Yarbrough WG, Brownlee RE, Pillsbury HC. Primary anastomosis of extensive facial nerve defects: an anatomic study. Am J Otol. 1993;14:238–46.
9. Spector JG, Lee P, Peterein J, Roufa D. Facial nerve regeneration through autologous nerve grafts: a clinical and experimental study. Laryngoscope. 1991;101:537–54.
10. Gavron JP, Clemis JD. Hypoglossal-facial nerve anastomosis: a review of forty cases caused by facial nerve injuries in the posterior fossa. Laryngoscope. 1984;94:1447–50.
11. Conley J. Hypoglossal crossover—122 cases. Trans Sect Otolaryngol Am Acad Ophthalmol Otolaryngol. 1977;84:763–8.
12. Kunihiro T, Kanzaki J, Yoshihara S, et al. Hypoglossal-facial nerve anastomosis after acoustic neuroma resection: influence of the time of anastomosis on recovery of facial movement. ORL J Otorhinolaryngol Relat Spec. 1996;58:32–5.
13. Stennert EI. Hypoglossal facial anastomosis: its significance for modern facial surgery. II. Combined approach in extratemporal facial nerve reconstruction. Clin Plast Surg. 1979;6:471–86.
14. Conley J, Baker DC. Hypoglossal-facial nerve anastomosis for reinnervation of the paralyzed face. Plast Reconstr Surg. 1979;63:63–72.
15. May M. Nerve substitution techniques. In: May M, Schaitkin BM, editors. The facial nerve. New York: Thieme; 2000. p. 611–33.
16. Atlas MD, Lowinger DS. A new technique for hypoglossal-facial nerve repair. Laryngoscope. 1997;107:984–91.
17. Klebuc MJ. Facial reanimation using the masseter-to-facial nerve transfer. Plast Reconstr Surg. 2011;127(5):1909–15.
18. Scaramella LF. Cross-face facial nerve anastomosis: historical notes. Ear Nose Throat J. 1996;75:343, 347–52, 354.
19. Glickman LT, Simpson R. Cross-facial nerve grafting for facial reanimation: effect on normal hemiface motion. J Reconstr Microsurg. 1996;12:201–2.
20. Rubin LR, Rubin JP, Simpson RL, Rubin TR. The search for the neurocranial pathways to the fifth nerve nucleus in the reanimation of the paralyzed face. Plast Reconstr Surg. 1999;103:1725–8.
21. Cheney ML, McKenna MJ, Megerian CA, Ojemann RG. Early temporalis muscle transposition for the management of facial paralysis. Laryngoscope. 1995;105:993–1000.
22. Cheney ML, Megerian C, McKenna M. Rehabilitation of the paralyzed face. In: Cheney ML, editor. Facial surgery: plastic and reconstructive. Baltimore: Williams & Wilkins; 1997. p. 655–94.
23. Rubin LR. Reanimation of the paralyzed face, new approaches: contributions by international researchers and surgeons. St. Louis: Mosby; 1977. p. 11–5.
24. Baker DC, Conley J. Regional muscle transposition for rehabilitation of the paralyzed face. Clin Plast Surg. 1979;6:317–31.
25. Aszmann OC, Ebmer JM, Dellon AL. The anatomic basis for the innervated mylohyoid/digastric flap in facial reanimation. Plast Reconstr Surg. 1998;102:369–72.
26. Terzis JK, Kalantarian B. Microsurgical strategies in 74 patients for restoration of dynamic depressor muscle mechanism: a neglected target in facial reanimation. Plast Reconstr Surg. 2000;105:1917–31.
27. Fine NA, Pribaz JJ, Orgill DP. Use of the innervated platysma flap in facial reanimation. Ann Plast Surg. 1995;34:326–30.
28. Harii K, Ohmori K, Torii S. Free gracilis muscle transplantation, with microneurovascular anastomoses for the treatment of facial paralysis. A preliminary report. Plast Reconstr Surg. 1976;57:133–43.
29. Manktelow RT, Zuker RM. Muscle transplantation by fascicular territory. Plast Reconstr Surg. 1984;73:751–7.
30. Zuker RM, Manktelow RT. A smile for the Mobius' syndrome patient. Ann Plast Surg. 1989;22:188–94.
31. Urken ML, Cheney ML, Sullivan ML, Biller HF. Atlas of regional and free flaps for head and neck reconstruction. New York: Raven Press; 1995. p. 139–48.
32. Nadol JB Jr. Schwannomas of the facial nerve. In: Nadol JB, Schuhknecht HF, editors. Surgery of the ear and temporal bone. Philadelphia: Raven Press; 1993.
33. Hadlock TA, Greenfield LJ, Wernick-Robinson M, Cheny ML. Multimodality approach to management of the paralyzed face. Laryngoscope. 2006;116:1388.

Hearing and Surgical Considerations in Neurofibromatosis Type 2

17

Kevin A. Peng, Gregory P. Lekovic, and Derald E. Brackmann

Neurofibromatosis type 2 (NF2) is a genetic disorder characterized by benign tumors of the central nervous system. The hallmark of the disease is the presence of bilateral vestibular schwannomas, although additional tumors, such as meningiomas, are commonly seen. The spinal cord and visual tracts are also often affected. Diagnosis is typically made in the third decade of life, and males and females are equally affected. The disorder can be inherited in autosomal dominant fashion, but roughly half of patients represent *de novo* mutations. This chapter describes the management strategy for patients with bilateral vestibular schwannomas.

Diagnosis

The most common presentation of NF2 is the presence of bilateral vestibular schwannomas as noted on cross-sectional imaging. However, diagnostic criteria for NF2 have been expanded, and a diagnosis can be made in the following presentations [1]:

- A first-degree relative with a diagnosis of NF2 with either of the following:
  - A unilateral vestibular schwannoma
  - Any two of the following: meningioma, schwannoma, glioma, neurofibroma, posterior subcapsular lenticular opacities
- A unilateral vestibular schwannoma and any two of the following: meningioma, schwannoma, glioma, neurofibroma, posterior subcapsular lenticular opacities
- Multiple meningiomas and either of the following:
  - A unilateral vestibular schwannoma
  - Any two of the following: schwannoma, glioma, neurofibroma, posterior subcapsular lenticular opacities

The age of diagnosis of NF2 is variable. Tumors manifest as early as the first decade of life and as late as the seventh decade of life. There is a large breadth of symptom severity, ranging from slow-growing bilateral schwannomas to early-onset, aggressive intracranial and spinal tumors [2] (Table 17.1).

NF2 must be distinguished from neurofibromatosis 1 (NF1), which is caused by a mutation in neurofibromin, located on chromosome 17. NF1 is characterized by multiple pigmented lesions termed café-au-lait spots; while NF2 patients may also exhibit these lesions, they typically have far fewer than NF1 patients. NF1 patients also typically possess numerous neurofibromas, which manifest as cutaneous nodules. Other characteristics specific to NF1 include optic nerve gliomas, benign eye tumors termed Lisch nodules, and axillary freckling [1].

Table 17.1 Characteristics of NF2

Autosomal dominant
Incidence 1:33,000–40,000 live births
merlin gene, chromosome 22
Age of onset variable; diagnosis made most commonly in the third decade of life
Bilateral eighth cranial nerve tumors
Presence of spinal tumors, including ependymomas
Neurofibromas
Meningiomas
Schwannomas of another cranial nerve
Gliomas
Juvenile posterior subcapsular lenticular opacities

K. A. Peng
House Clinic Foundation, Los Angeles, CA, USA

G. P. Lekovic
Division of Neurosurgery, House Clinic, House Ear Institute, Los Angeles, CA, USA

D. E. Brackmann (✉)
Neurotology and Otolaryngology, House Clinic, Inc., Los Angeles, CA, USA
e-mail: dbrackmann@houseclinic.com

N. C. Bambakidis et al. (eds.), *Surgery of the Cerebellopontine Angle*, https://doi.org/10.1007/978-3-031-12507-2_17

Genetics

NF2 is caused by a mutation in merlin, also termed schwannomin or neurofibromin 2, a cytoskeletal tumor suppressor protein encoded by the gene *NF2* located on chromosome 22q12.2. The incidence of NF2 has been estimated at around 1 in every 30,000–40,000 live births. It is inherited in autosomal dominant fashion, although half of cases represent *de novo* mutations in the gene.

NF2 has classically been divided into Wishart and Gardner phenotypes, representing more severe and less severe patterns of disease, respectively. More recent research has demonstrated correlations between genetic alterations and disease phenotype, with truncation mutations associated with a more severe phenotype and missense mutations associated with a less severe phenotype. The most salient predictor of disease severity is the age at diagnosis, with patients diagnosed at younger ages demonstrating more severe phenotypes [3].

A majority of patients with NF2 demonstrate the classic form, with germline mutations in the NF2 gene dictating the clinical phenotype. Recent research in the genetic characteristics of NF2 has revealed that mosaicism, or the presence of the NF2 mutation in some, but not all, of an affected individual's cells, occurs in about 30–35% of NF2 patients. Mosaicism occurs when the NF2 mutation occurs after embryogenesis and cell division, resulting in the pathological mutation in only a fraction of a patient's cells. Patients with mosaic NF2 typically have a milder disease phenotype than those with germline NF2.

Tumors in NF2 are thought to develop via the two-hit hypothesis. The first hit occurs when one copy of the NF2 gene is mutated, either in germline or mosaic fashion. The second hit occurs when the additional copy of the NF2 gene is mutated, termed a somatic mutation [4]. A three-hit hypothesis has also been postulated. When both copies of the NF2 gene are mutated in Schwann cells, there is a loss of tumor suppression, and tumor formation commences. NF2 has been implicated in other neoplasms and malignancies, including mesothelioma and thyroid cancers.

Vestibular Schwannomas

Bilateral vestibular schwannomas are the hallmark of NF2. Vestibular schwannomas are benign tumors of the superior and/or inferior vestibular nerves. Due to the proximity of the vestibular and cochlear nerve fibers, vestibular schwannomas compress and invade the cochlear nerve, causing hearing loss and tinnitus. Vestibular symptoms occur less frequently, likely owing to the capacity for central compensation in the setting of a gradual vestibular loss. As a result, hearing loss is the most common presenting symptom of NF2.

The facial nerve, which runs in close proximity to the vestibulocochlear nerve, may also be affected. Facial nerve schwannomas are encountered much more commonly in NF2 patients and can cause symptoms such as facial twitching and paralysis. Facial nerve compression from a large vestibular schwannoma may also cause similar symptoms.

Schwannomas Involving Other Cranial Nerves

Schwannomas along other cranial nerves are often seen in NF2. Lower cranial nerve schwannomas can lead to dysphagia, which is a leading cause of morbidity and eventual mortality in NF2 patients. Upper cranial nerve schwannomas can involve the oculomotor nerves; trigeminal nerve schwannomas are also commonly seen.

Meningiomas

In addition to schwannomas, intracranial meningiomas are often seen in NF2 patients. Meningiomas are benign proliferations of the cerebral meninges and occur at various locations along the inner table of the calvarium. When they are located near the internal auditory canal (IAC) and cerebellopontine angle (CPA), they may mimic the presentation of a vestibular schwannoma. As in sporadic cases, meningiomas are most commonly World Health Organization (WHO) grade I, although an increased incidence of WHO grade II (atypical) meningiomas has been reported in NF2 patients.

Collision Tumors

NF2 patients may sometimes present with complex tumors in the CPA comprising multiple adjacent tumors growing in close proximity (Fig. 17.1) [5]. Such collision tumors most commonly consist of confluent vestibular, cochlear, facial, trigeminal, and/or lower cranial nerve schwannomas; combined schwannomas and meningiomas are also commonly seen. Importantly, the presence of collision tumors is not always appreciable based on preoperative imaging and, when unrecognized, may complicate the prognosis for hearing preservation and facial nerve function. Schwannomas of the lower cranial nerves are typically not resected, even partially, when contributing to CPA collision tumors in order to preserve lower cranial nerve function. For giant collision tumors, translabyrinthine or combined petrosal approaches are sometimes necessary to obtain sufficient exposure for safe tumor removal.

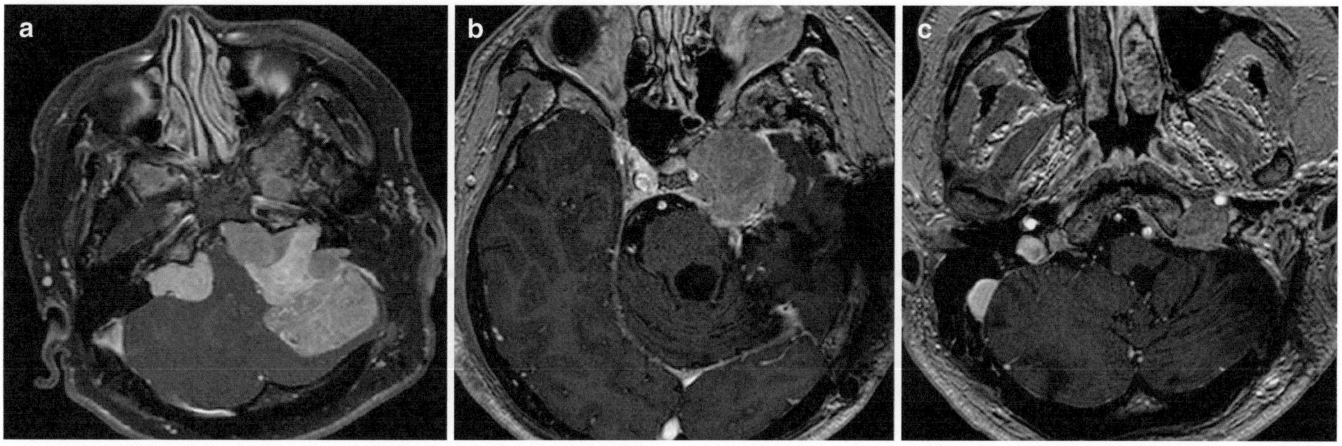

Fig. 17.1 Large collision tumor involving the left cerebellopontine angle and multiple cranial nerves in a patient with neurofibromatosis type 2. The patient was blind in the contralateral eye, and the decision was made preoperatively not to resect the trigeminal nerve tumor to preserve corneal sensation. In addition, to minimize risk of dysphagia, the glossopharyngeal nerve tumor was not resected. (**a**) Preoperative magnetic resonance imaging (MRI), axial view, following administration of intravenous contrast. (**b**) Postoperative MRI demonstrating fifth cranial nerve tumor, which was not resected. (**c**) Postoperative MRI demonstrating ninth cranial nerve tumor, which was not resected

Ependymomas

The most common spinal tumors encountered in NF2 patients are spinal ependymomas, which are intramedullary lesions that may cause symptoms due to cord compression and invasion. The cervical spine is most commonly affected, followed by the lumbar and thoracic spine. Ependymomas may also be encountered in the brainstem in this population. Unlike sporadic ependymomas, ependymomas in NF2 generally do not metastasize and do not demonstrate leptomeningeal spread [6].

Ocular Findings

NF2 patients have a predisposition toward lens opacities and specifically for posterior subcapsular lens opacities. Additional ocular findings include wedge cortical cataracts, retinal hamartomas, hyperplastic primary vitreous, and epiretinal membranes [7]. Even less commonly, Lisch nodules, which are commonly seen in NF1, may be encountered in NF2. Vision can be further compromised as a sequela of corneal scarring resulting from neuropathies of cranial nerves V and VII, even in the absence of primary ocular pathology.

Surgical Management of Vestibular Schwannomas and Hearing Rehabilitation in NF2

As with many treatment decisions in NF2, decisions involving vestibular schwannoma resection and hearing preservation and rehabilitation are highly individualized. The surgical management options to be considered, which are not mutually exclusive and may be performed in sequential fashion, include (1) observation without surgical intervention, (2) middle fossa craniotomy with decompression of the IAC without tumor removal, (3) hearing preservation surgery with total tumor removal, (4) retrosigmoid craniotomy with partial tumor removal, (5) nonhearing preservation surgery with total tumor removal, and (6) hearing rehabilitation via an auditory brainstem implant (ABI) or cochlear implant (CI).

Observation Without Surgical Intervention

A common principle in the management of NF2 patients is to preserve any residual hearing in the absence of contraindications to doing so. Previous research has suggested that tumor cells in vestibular schwannomas in NF2 invade the cochlear nerve to a much greater degree than in sporadic vestibular schwannomas, thus making hearing preservation difficult [8]. Clinically, this encourages close monitoring of slowly growing tumors rather than more aggressive surgical resection.

Observation without surgical intervention is recommended when a small tumor is present in an only-hearing ear or when hearing is present bilaterally but the tumors are too large to attempt hearing preservation surgery (roughly exceeding 2.5 cm in greatest diameter). Observation may be preferable when brainstem compression and hydrocephalus are absent. Regular follow-up (initially at 6 months and then annually) is essential, with trending of tumor size and evaluation for hydrocephalus or mass effect.

A standardized approach to magnetic resonance imaging (MRI) evaluation is recommended for accuracy. If volumetric analysis is possible, tumor volume should be followed; barring this, dimensions in three planes should be noted. Clinical examination and audiometric testing are performed regularly to document hearing level and to identify additional cranial neuropathies or signs of increased intracranial pressure. Hearing fluctuation is reported to the clinician, and sudden hearing loss is typically treated with corticosteroid therapy. Surgical intervention is considered if hearing is no longer serviceable or if tumor factors or additional symptomatology mandate resection.

Middle Fossa Craniotomy with Decompression of the IAC

Decompression of the tumor within the IAC is recommended if hearing impairment progresses or fluctuates in a patient under observation. In this approach, cranial nerve monitoring via auditory brainstem response (ABR) and facial nerve electromyography are employed. A middle fossa craniotomy is first performed, and the IAC is then decompressed widely along its superior, anterior, and posterior aspects. The tumor is generally not debulked as prior studies have suggested that intracapsular debulking is associated with rapid regrowth. The goal of this approach is hearing stabilization, although hearing loss remains a prominent risk of the surgery. In a very small number of patients, middle fossa decompression can lead to hearing improvement [9].

Hearing Preservation Surgery with Total Tumor Removal

In select NF2 patients, hearing preservation is a reasonable goal. In general, though, hearing preservation in NF2 patients is often more difficult than in patients with sporadic tumors, likely because of invasion into the cochlear nerve. Because any preserved hearing is important in NF2 patients, the audiological criteria for attempting hearing preservation are relatively more lenient than in patients with sporadic, unilateral vestibular schwannomas.

The choice of surgical approach—middle fossa or retrosigmoid—is determined by tumor location and size. The middle fossa craniotomy is ideal for small intracanalicular tumors and those extending 0.5–1 cm beyond the porus acusticus into the CPA, and it allows for exposure of the entire IAC (Fig. 17.2). The retrosigmoid approach allows greater access to the CPA than the middle fossa craniotomy, but the posterior semicircular canal and vestibule limit access to the fundus of the IAC. Therefore, the retrosigmoid approach is ideally suited for more medial tumors with 1–2 cm of extension into the CPA but without involvement of the fundus.

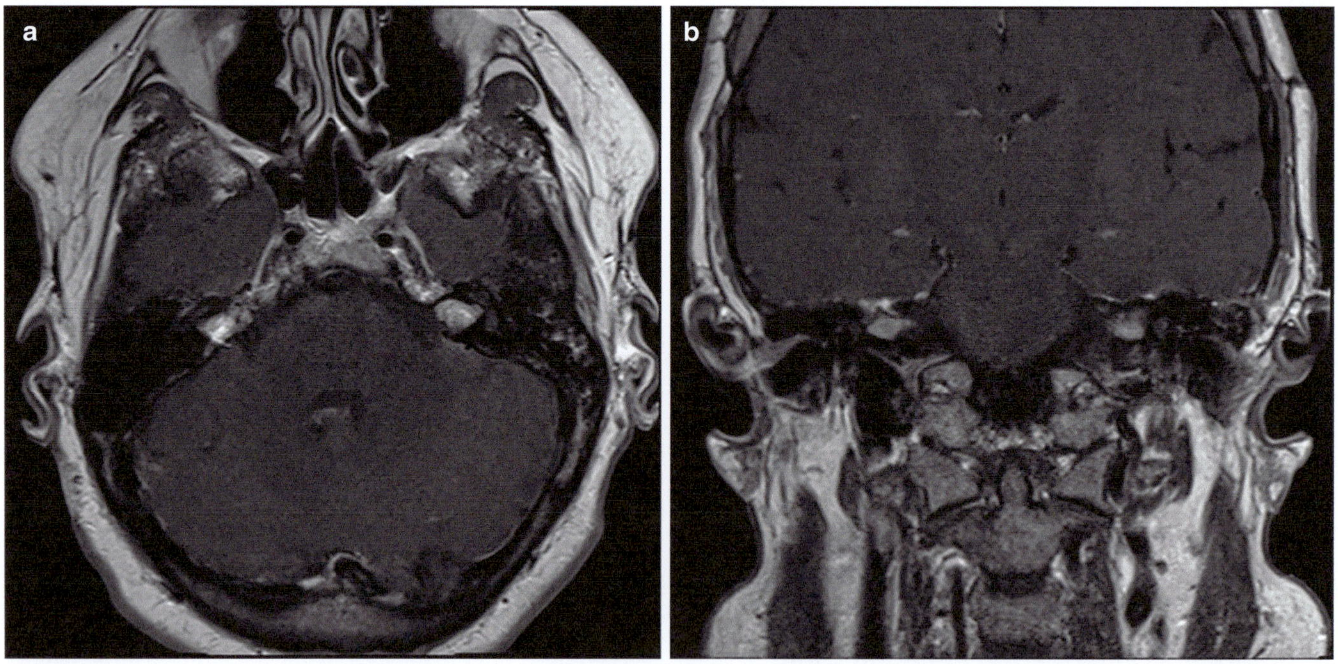

Fig. 17.2 Follow-up magnetic resonance imaging 17 and 20 years following middle fossa craniotomy for resection of bilateral vestibular schwannomas, respectively, demonstrating recurrent vestibular schwannomas bilaterally. Notwithstanding this recurrence, on most recent audiological testing, the patient has serviceable hearing bilaterally (right ear pure-tone average [PTA] 15 dB, word recognition score 100%; left ear PTA 40 dB, word recognition score 92%). (**a**) Axial view, following administration of intravenous contrast. (**b**) Coronal view, postcontrast

Among patients with NF2, few tumors fall into this category. Unless diagnosed early, tumors often reach a large size before hearing is impaired and the diagnosis is made.

The potential for hearing preservation after tumor removal is limited by many factors. It is generally preferred that contralateral hearing be serviceable if tumor removal with hearing preservation is attempted. In addition, tumors should ideally be less than 2.5 cm in greatest diameter for the retrosigmoid approach or 1.5 cm in greatest diameter for the middle fossa approach, although Brackmann and colleagues did not find this to be a significant factor in preserving hearing [10]. Finally, gross total resection should be the surgical objective; regrowth of residual tumors often results in hearing loss with or without further surgery.

In patients with small, bilateral tumors, total tumor removal with attempted hearing preservation on the side with the larger tumor, the greater hearing impairment, or both is recommended. If hearing is preserved at a serviceable level in the first ear, contralateral tumor surgery may be performed after 6 months, which allows for confirmation of stable hearing in the first ear. If hearing preservation is not successful in the first ear, hearing preservation surgery is not attempted in the contralateral ear, and the contralateral tumor is observed.

Some surgeons advocate the removal of the smaller tumor or the tumor on the side with better hearing, with the rationale that hearing preservation is more likely to be achieved. Yet others recommend observation of small- or medium-sized bilateral tumors until deterioration of hearing, mass effect, or both. As with many other decisions in NF2, it is ideal to discuss any treatment philosophy with the patient and arrive together at a management strategy.

Retrosigmoid Craniotomy with Partial Tumor Removal

Partial tumor removal is seldom recommended because even partial tumor removal in patients with NF2 may result in hearing loss and/or tumor regrowth. Still, some surgeons advocate partial tumor removal when patients have good unilateral hearing and a large tumor with mass effect. In this situation, the tumor may be debulked via a retrosigmoid craniotomy. A generous cuff of tumor capsule is left in an attempt to protect the facial and cochlear nerves and the cochlear blood supply.

Nonhearing Preservation Surgery with Total Tumor Removal

When hearing preservation is no longer a consideration, either in the setting of profound hearing loss preoperatively or a large tumor with brainstem compression, even in the presence of useful hearing, total tumor removal with preservation of the facial nerve is the primary goal. The translabyrinthine approach is our preferred approach. It allows for safe tumor removal with minimal cerebellar retraction and maximal exposure of the facial nerve. Furthermore, it allows for direct access to the lateral recess of the fourth ventricle for placement of an ABI as discussed below.

Hearing Rehabilitation Via an ABI or CI

The retrosigmoid and translabyrinthine approaches expose the brainstem, thus allowing placement of an ABI. The ABI, which was conceived by William F. House, MD, and developed at the House Ear Institute in Los Angeles, California in the late 1970s and early 1980s, stimulates the cochlear nucleus of the brainstem directly. It is currently approved by the United States Food and Drug Administration for hearing rehabilitation in NF2 patients aged 12 years and older, either at the time of tumor removal or at a second stage. The electrode array is placed in the lateral recess of the fourth ventricle (Figs. 17.3 and 17.4), and the subcutaneous receiver is located under the scalp [11].

Because the patient population generally requires lifelong surveillance with MRI, the internal magnet is removed intraoperatively following implant testing (typically electrically evoked ABR) for the purposes of both MRI compatibility and to eliminate magnetic shadow. The implant is typically activated several weeks postoperatively. For everyday use, magnetic coupling between the internal receiver–stimulator

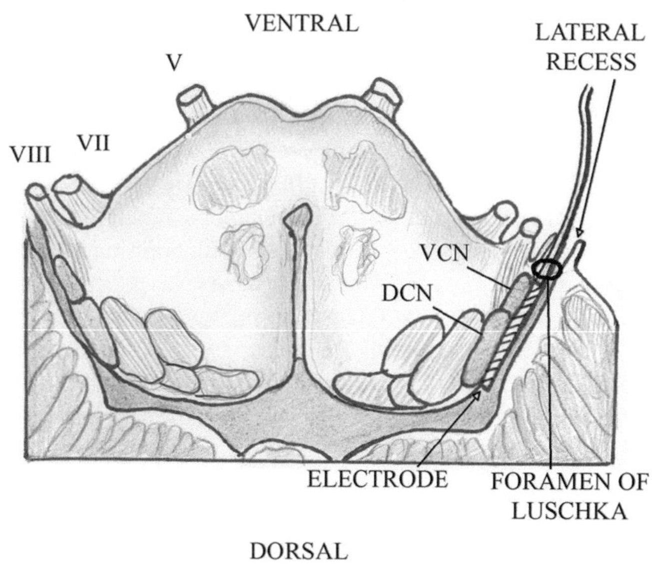

Fig. 17.3 A drawing of an axial cut at the level of the lateral recess of the fourth ventricle. The ABI electrode is placed over the area of the cochlear nucleus, within the lateral recess of the fourth ventricle. (Permission granted to use by the House Ear Institute)

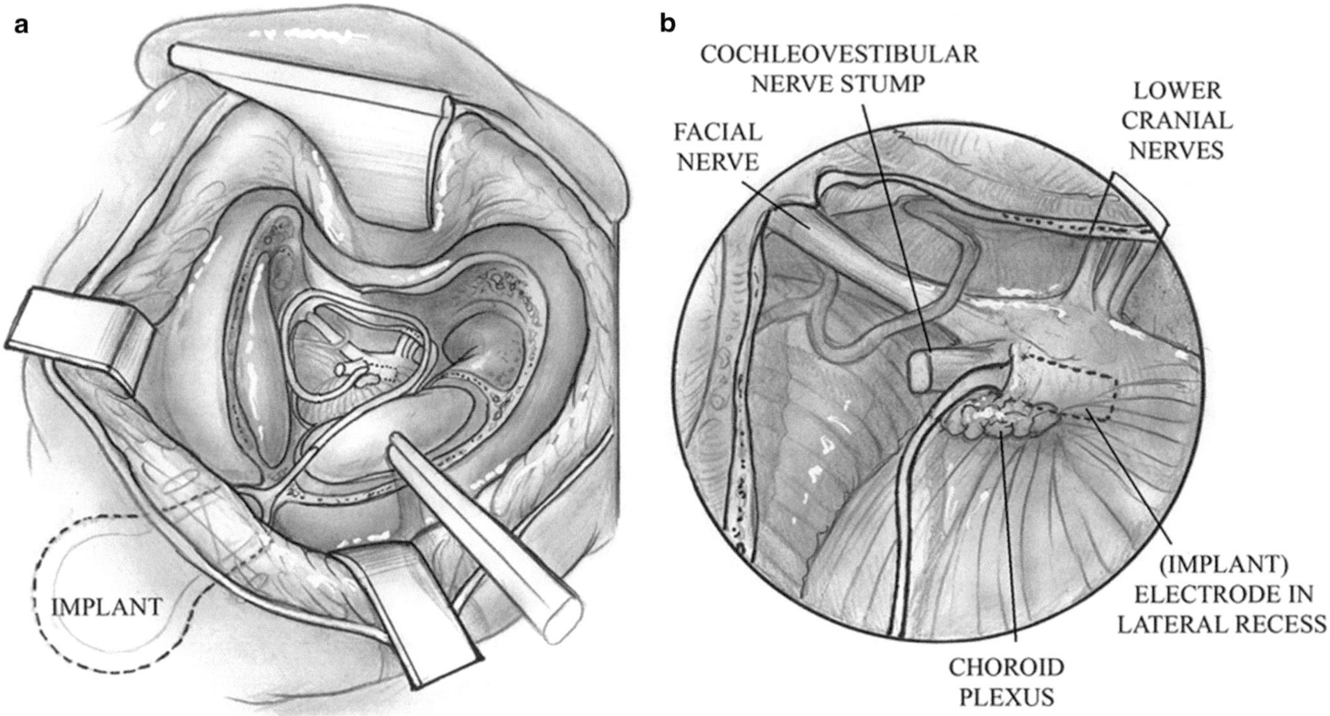

Fig. 17.4 (**a**) An overview of the ABI electrode through a translabyrinthine approach to the cerebellopontine angle and the area of the lateral recess of the fourth ventricle is drawn. The internal receiver and the magnet part of the device are tucked under the periosteum posteriorly. (**b**) The ABI is placed over the area of the cochlear nucleus. The choroid plexus, the stump of the cochleovestibular nerve, the taenia, and the glossopharyngeal nerve are all used as landmarks to position the electrode within the lateral recess of the fourth ventricle. (Permission granted to use by the House Ear Institute)

and the external device is facilitated with the use of an external retainer disc, which is applied to an area of shaved scalp with adhesive. Patients may undergo MRI up to a field strength of 1.5 T, with the external device and retainer disc removed.

Most NF2 patients who rely solely on ABI for auditory perception cannot achieve open-set speech discrimination, though some do. Instead, ABIs provide environmental awareness of sound and augment lip-reading [12]. Some patients with ABIs do not derive meaningful auditory stimulation, but it is difficult to predict performance preoperatively or intraoperatively, even for very large tumors with brainstem deformation or compression, where a subset of patients still performs acceptably with ABIs.

In a select cohort of NF2 patients, a CI may be considered. CIs rely on the presence of an anatomically intact cochlear nerve. While CIs may offer improved speech recognition compared to ABIs, CI function in NF2 patients has been noted almost invariably to decrease over time [13]. This may be secondary to tumor progression in the vicinity of the cochlear nerve or devascularization of the cochlear nerve if surgical resection and/or radiation are performed.

Radiation Therapy for NF2

Control of vestibular schwannoma growth by stereotactic radiosurgery (SRS) is not often recommended for patients with NF2, in part due to the remote risk of malignant transformation and also secondary to the disadvantages of performing radiation therapy on younger patients. Although data on SRS in NF2 are sparse, NF2 vestibular schwannomas respond less well to SRS than sporadic tumors in terms of long-term tumor control as well as hearing preservation. Several case reports suggest that SRS for meningiomas associated with NF2 is more effective than SRS for non-NF2 meningiomas.

As in sporadic cases, radiation to large tumors can lead to significant radiation side effects in the adjacent brainstem and cerebellum, including edema, ventricular obstruction, and resultant hydrocephalus. If salvage surgery is necessary following radiation, the surgical field is significantly more challenging and can occasionally prevent successful placement of an ABI. Because of these considerations, radiation is generally considered only for patients who are poor surgical candidates or for those who refuse surgery. Still, when performed, radiation remains an effective treatment for vestibular schwannomas in NF2 [14].

Surgical Management of Other Tumors in NF2

The management of spinal ependymomas and spinal schwannomas in NF2 is dictated by symptomatology. Growing, symptomatic tumors may warrant surgical intervention, particularly if cord compression is present. Slow-growing or stable tumors may be imaged serially. Similarly, intracranial meningiomas in NF2 are resected if large and/or symptomatic.

Medical Management of NF2

Medical management is considered for growing tumors in NF2 not amenable to surgical resection, including residual and recurrent tumors. Bevacizumab, a monoclonal antibody directed against the vascular endothelial growth factor receptor, has been shown to slow and even reverse tumor growth in select patients. Its use has even been associated with hearing improvement in certain patients. Long-term side effects include proteinuria and hypertension [15]. Additional agents currently under investigation include everolimus and lapatinib among others.

Conclusion

NF2 is an autosomal dominant syndrome characterized by bilateral vestibular schwannomas in addition to schwannomas, meningiomas, ependymomas, and other tumors in the central and peripheral nervous system. Surgical management is performed for small tumors if hearing preservation is attempted; otherwise, it is reserved for large or growing tumors or tumors with nonserviceable hearing. Auditory brainstem implantation remains the mainstay of surgical hearing rehabilitation in carefully selected patients. Emerging medical therapies include the use of bevacizumab, with additional agents under investigation.

References

1. Gutmann DH, Aylsworth A, Carey JC, et al. The diagnostic evaluation and multidisciplinary management of neurofibromatosis 1 and neurofibromatosis 2. J Am Med. 1997;278:51–7.
2. Slattery WH. Neurofibromatosis type 2. Otol Clin N Am. 2015;48:443–60.
3. Asthagiri AR, Parry DM, Butman JA, et al. Neurofibromatosis type 2. Lancet. 2009;373:1974–86.
4. Sainz J, Huynh DP, Figueroa K, Ragge NK, Baser ME, Pulst S-M. Mutations of the neurofibromatosis type 2 gene and lack of the gene product in vestibular schwannomas. Hum Mol Gen. 1994;3:885–91.
5. Pallini R, Tancredi A, Casalbore P, et al. Neurofibromatosis type 2: growth stimulation of mixed acoustic schwannoma by concurrent adjacent meningioma: possible role of growth factors: case report. J Neurosurg. 1998;89:149–54.
6. Mautner V-F, Tatagiba M, Lindenau M, et al. Spinal tumors in patients with neurofibromatosis type 2: MR imaging study of frequency, multiplicity, and variety. Am J Roentgenol. 1995;165:951–5.
7. Bosch MM, Boltshauser E, Harpes P, Landau K. Ophthalmologic findings and long-term course in patients with neurofibromatosis type 2. Am J Ophth. 2006;141:1068–77.
8. Linthicum FH Jr. Unusual audiometric and histologic findings in bilateral acoustic neurinomas. Ann Otol Rhinol Laryngol. 1972;81:433–7.
9. Slattery WH, Hoa M, Bonne N, et al. Middle fossa decompression for hearing preservation: a review of institutional results and indications. Otol Neurotol. 2011;32:1017–24.
10. Brackmann DE, Fayad JN, Slattery WH III, et al. Early proactive management of vestibular schwannomas in neurofibromatosis type 2. Neurosurgery. 2001;49:274–83.
11. Brackmann DE, Hitselberger WE, Nelson RA, et al. Auditory brainstem implant: I. Issues in surgical implantation. Otolaryngol Head Neck Surg. 1993;108:624–33.
12. Otto SR, Brackmann DE, Hitselberger WE, et al. Multichannel auditory brainstem implant: update on performance in 61 patients. J Neurosurg. 2002;96:1063–71.
13. Peng KA, Lorenz MB, Otto SR, et al. Cochlear implantation and auditory brainstem implantation in neurofibromatosis type 2. Laryngoscope. 2018;128(9):2163–9. https://doi.org/10.1002/lary.27181. Epub 2018 Mar 24.
14. Subach BR, Kondziolka D, Lunsford LD, Bissonette DJ, Flickinger JC, Maitz AH. Stereotactic radiosurgery in the management of acoustic neuromas associated with neurofibromatosis type 2. J Neurosurg. 1999;90:815–22.
15. Plotkin SR, Stemmer-Rachamimov AO, Barker FG, et al. Hearing improvement after bevacizumab in patients with neurofibromatosis type 2. N Engl J Med. 2009;361:358–67.

18 Prevention and Management of CSF Leakage Postoperatively

Jacob B. Hunter and George B. Wanna

Introduction

All skull-base surgeons are well aware of the risk of postoperative cerebrospinal fluid (CSF) leaks. It is understood that incising the dura to access the cerebellopontine angle (CPA) will provide a path for CSF to flow from the high intracranial pressure (ICP) region to the low-pressure regions of the temporal bone. Complicating this pressure differential is evidence that suggests CSF pressure significantly increases following vestibular schwannoma (VS) surgery, normalizing within 48 h of surgery [1]. Furthermore, with the presence of a CSF leak, patients risk developing an intracranial infection. Allen and colleagues identified that 3.1% of all their lateral skull-base surgery patients developed postoperative meningitis, calculating that a CSF leak increases a patient's risk of developing meningitis by a factor of 10.2 [2]. Other groups have reported that untreated CSF leaks develop meningitis between 8% and 35% [3].

To avoid developing a postoperative CSF leak and its associated complications, many surgeons suggest taking the time and paying attention to detail throughout the entire procedure, including the surgical approach, tumor exposure, and resection. Nonetheless, a plethora of surgical techniques has been described and outcomes analyzed to best determine which method is best. While many factors contribute to the surgical approach—and no technique is without risk—these studies help surgeons to assess their own outcomes, manage complications, and provide appropriate counsel to patients regarding the risks of surgery.

J. B. Hunter (✉)
Department of Otolaryngology—Head and Neck Surgery, University of Texas Southwestern Medical Center, Dallas, TX, USA
e-mail: Jacob.Hunter@UTSouthwestern.edu

G. B. Wanna
Department of Otolaryngology—Head and Neck Surgery, Icahn School of Medicine of Mount Sinai, New York, NY, USA

Neurology, Icahn School of Medicine of Mount Sinai, New York, NY, USA

Department of Otolaryngology, New York Eye and Ear Infirmary of Mount Sinai and Mount Sinai Beth Israel, New York, NY, USA

Audiology, Hearing and Balance Center, Mount Sinai Health System, New York, NY, USA

Overall Rates

Many studies have compared the rates of CSF leak among the three workhorse surgical approaches to the CPA: translabyrinthine (TL), retrosigmoid (RS), and middle fossa (MF). In one of the largest literature reviews to date exploring CSF leaks following VS surgery, Selesnick and colleagues identified close to 6000 patients among 37 studies (excluding those studies or patients that described combined approaches) and found a CSF leak rate of 9.5%, 10.6%, and 10.6%, in TL, RS, and MF approaches, respectively, which were not significantly different [4]. In a more recent literature review, Ansari and colleagues looked at a number of additional factors and identified 35 studies, accounting for more than 5000 patients, and found that the RS approach led to CSF leaks significantly more frequently compared with the TL or MF approaches, 10.3%, 7.1%, and 5.3%, respectively [5].

In a single institutional review that accounted for 300 total surgeries (100 TL, RS, and MF approaches each), Becker and colleagues found no significant difference between approaches and CSF leaks, with rates of 13%, 10%, and 10%, respectively [6]. Crowson and colleagues reviewed 282 patients who received surgery for VS, 13 of which had previously received radiation, and 12 of which had neurofibromatosis type 2 (NF2), noting that TL approaches had the highest leak rate (12.4%) followed by RS approaches (9.2%) and MF approaches (6.5%), which were not significantly different [7]. Likewise, many other individual center studies, some reviewing as many as 1922 patients, found no significant difference in CSF leak rates between surgical approaches [8–11].

N. C. Bambakidis et al. (eds.), *Surgery of the Cerebellopontine Angle*, https://doi.org/10.1007/978-3-031-12507-2_18

In 624 VS cases, Brennan and colleagues observed a CSF leak rate of 10.7% [12]. While they found that wound leaks occurred more frequently after TL approaches and otorrhea occurred more regularly after RS approaches, the leak rate was not different between approaches [12]. However, in another study, Fishman and colleagues compared their CSF leak rate over a 5-year period with a previous historical control data from their same institution [13]. Identifying 196 VS surgeries, the TL leak rate (5%) was significantly lower compared to RS approaches (8.5%) and MF approaches (8.3%) [13]. Nonetheless, with innumerable variables that play a role in the development of CSF leaks—while universally we cannot state one technique leads to lower CSF leaks as compared to others—one cannot ignore the results of single institutions or surgeons.

Preoperative Issues

Many studies have looked at a multitude of preoperative factors in hopes of determining which patients might be at greater risk of developing postoperative CSF leaks. No consensus exists as to the degree to which patient gender, age, extent of resection, laterality, or tumor size influences the development of CSF leaks.

While Copeland and colleagues found no association between gender and CSF leaks, Russel and colleagues found that men and younger patients were more likely to develop a CSF leak [14, 15]. They speculate that increased physical activities in the postoperative period in younger patients and men might hinder the cephalic venous blood to the heart, leading to disturbances in the absorption of CSF [15]. Similarly, Ludemann and colleagues found that men had higher leak rates, but they speculated that it might be due to greater mastoid pneumatization in men [16].

Assessing the role of age, Becker and colleagues found that patients older than 50 years of age were "suggestive of increased odds of CSF leak" [6]. However, Scheich and colleagues found no difference in CSF leak rates between those patients above and below 50 years of age following MF approaches [17]. Similarly, other groups have found that age is not related to CSF leak, in addition to Selesnick and colleagues' large literature review [4, 14, 18, 19].

As for tumor size, many groups have found no association in individual studies [6, 7, 14, 17, 20, 21], and large literature reviews [4]. Other groups have reported conflicting information. Ludemann reported that smaller tumors were more likely to lead to a CSF leak than larger tumors in RS approaches [16]. However, Slattery and colleagues found that larger tumors were at greater risk of developing postoperative CSF leaks [18]. Similarly, Brennan and colleagues found that tumor size mattered in RS approaches, as opposed to TL cases in which larger tumors were more frequently complicated by CSF leaks [12].

Despite the lack of a statistically significant association with laterality, Copeland and colleagues found a trend for right-sided tumors to have an increased risk of CSF leaks, speculating that prolonged retraction of the dominant sigmoid sinus could result in occlusion and thus elevation in intracranial pressure [14].

Few groups have explored the influence of tumor resection, with Copeland and colleagues finding no association with CSF leaks [14]. Without specifying the reasons for reoperation, Stieglitz and colleagues observed that those patients who undergo reoperation have a significantly higher rate of CSF leaks compared with primary surgery, 11% versus 4.5%, respectively [22].

Copeland and colleagues found that body mass index (BMI), operative time, and TL approaches were all significantly associated with developing a CSF leak [14]. Categorizing patients as overweight (BMI 25–29.9), obese (BMI 30–39), or morbidly obese (BMI ≥40), and comparing the group to normal weight patients, they found that those three groups of patients had a 2.5-fold, 3-fold, and 6-fold increased risk of developing a CSF leak, respectively [14]. In attempting to explain the role of BMI with CSF leaks, Russel and colleagues noted that patients with high BMIs may complicate the procedure due to difficulty manipulating the patient's head, CSF outflow disorders, and increased physical effort to conduct their daily activities following surgery, leading to an increase in CSF pressure [14]. However, while other groups have also identified that BMI is a significant predictor in developing CSF leaks as well as developing a brachial plexopathy [23], Diaz Anadon found no relationship between CSF leak and BMI in 163 patients [24].

Copeland highlights that patients with increased BMI have elevated intracranial pressure at baseline, with elevated intraabdominal pressure in obese patients translating "into higher intrathoracic and cardiac filling pressures, thus decreasing venous return from the brain and ultimately increasing intracranial pressure" [14, 25]. Others have suggested that increased estrogen production from adipose tissue may play a role, with identification of high estrogen levels "in the CSF of obese patients with intracranial idiopathic hypertension" [26]. In addition, obstructive sleep apnea, causing hypoxia and hypercapnia, may lead to cerebral vasodilation and ICP elevation [27, 28].

As to the association with operative time, which is supported by Russel and colleagues, groups speculate that longer cases may lead to surgeon fatigue and/or accumulation of blood and proteinaceous debris in the CSF, contributing to poor closure and/or a transient communicating hydrocephalus [14, 15]. However, Arlt and colleagues found no correlation between operative times and rates of CSF leak [20].

Crowson and colleagues included a small number of NF2 patients in their institutional review as well as a few patients who had previously received radiation, observing that patients with NF2 did not have a significantly higher CSF leak rates (8.3%) compared with those without NF2 (10.4%) [7]. Likewise, there was no significant difference in the CSF leak rate between those patients who had preoperative stereotactic radiosurgery and those who didn't (7.7% and 10.4%, respectively) [7].

In those patients requiring combined surgical approaches, data suggest that those patients are more likely to develop CSF leaks compared with TL, RS, or MF approaches alone. In their review of more than 300 patients, Bryce and colleagues found that those patients who underwent a combined TL-MF approach had an overall leak rate of 13.4%, with surgical repair needed in 6.2% of patients and meningitis developing in 5.3% of patients [21].

Some studies have even explored placing a lumbar drain (LD) preoperatively. Nonaka and colleagues reviewed their experience of preoperatively placing an LD in 410 VS patients prior to surgery, reporting a CSF leak rate of 7.6% [29]. Bien and colleagues provided an additional case series of 78 patients who had an LD placed preoperatively in patients undergoing skull-base surgery compared with those patients who had no LD placement, noting a reduction in the CSF leak rate from 35% to 12% when an LD was placed [30]. LDs are not without complications that include CSF over-drainage, meningitis, and pneumocephalus, which will be discussed later [31].

In Crowson and colleagues' review, they sought to assess the role of the preoperative use of an LD prior to surgery [7]. Reviewing 282 patients who had VS resections with all three approaches, 78.0% had a preoperative LD, generally left for 1 day following an RS approach, and never more than 5 days [7]. In total, 29 patients (10.3%) had a CSF leak, 38.0% of which occurred during their operative admission [7]. Of those who had no LD placed, 14.5% developed a CSF leak, compared with 9.1% who had a preoperative LD placed ($p = 0.24$) [7]. They caution that preoperative use of an LD should be avoided if the goal is to prevent a CSF leak [7].

Translabyrinthine Approach

While several studies have demonstrated no significant difference in CSF leak rates among the various approaches, closing TL approaches provides unique challenges with difficulty reapproximating the dura given the angle of approach. As a result, a plethora of techniques can minimize the risk of CSF leak following TL approaches.

While initial techniques used muscle to close TL defects, Glasscock and colleagues found that muscle could be very small in some women, prompting them to use abdominal fat [32]. However, Montgomery and colleagues first introduced the fat graft several years earlier in 1966 to reduce the risk of CSF leaks following CPA surgery [33]. It wasn't until 1982 that House and colleagues described using strips of fat, opposed to one large fat graft [34].

Emphasizing the importance of fat, Wu and colleagues published their outcomes in 277 patients who underwent TL VS resections with the evolution of three different closure techniques [35]. In one method, they used a piece of fascia lata to cover the dural defect along with tissue glue, followed by several pieces of fat on the fascia, and reported a CSF leak rate of 28.2%, 7.7% of which required reoperation [35]. In the second method, they created a large musculoperiosteal flap to compress the fat in addition to their previous method, which did not change the CSF leak rate [35]. However, when they removed the fascia in the last group—placing the fat directly into the operative field and closing with a musculoperiosteal flap as well as not placing any glue—the CSF leak rate was reduced to 7.4%, with a 3.7% reoperation rate [35].

Thinking that counterpressure to the fat may reduce CSF leak rates, researchers and surgeons conducted studies that describe a number of techniques to provide such counterpressure. Bambakidis and colleagues initially reported their experience with their first 15 patients with titanium mesh and hydroxyapatite (HA) cranioplasty following a TL approach, with no reported complications [36]. In a later study from the same center, Manjila and colleagues reported no CSF leaks in 27 more patients, though they didn't report a length of follow-up [37]. In a larger cohort but describing a similar technique in using a titanium mesh, Fayad and colleagues utilized a titanium mesh cranioplasty after TL approach in 389 patients, reporting a leak rate of 3.3%, which was significantly less than two other cohorts from the same center [38].

Nonetheless, published and anecdotal accounts caution against too much fat. Chen and colleagues describe three cases in which their fat graft prolapsed into the CPA, causing brain stem compression and leading to neurological deterioration [39]. These were identified on postoperative days 1, 3, and 1, respectively, with two patients able to follow commands following removal of some fat [39].

With concerns about cost and infection with a titanium mesh, Hillman and Shelton previously described the use of a resorbable plate following a TL approach in 71 patients, reporting a 12.7% leak rate, with no surgical site infections [40]. However, in comparing their sample with 149 consecutive patients who were closed with a fat graft alone, they found no significant differences in CSF leak rates, LD placements, or surgical revisions [40]. In comparing their experience with Fayad and colleagues, they questioned if the resorbable plate was not as effective at creating counterpressure compared with titanium mesh, or whether subtle technical variations between groups account for the differences [40].

However, in a later study also using a resorbable mesh, Hunter and colleagues reported their CSF leak outcomes of 53 patients who underwent TL approaches for VS, packing the middle ear with muscle and Surgicel®, utilizing a dural substitute to reconstruct the posterior fossa and internal auditory canal (IAC) dura, followed by an abdominal fat graft and a resorbable mesh plate, which can be warmed to increase compression, followed by a multilayered closure (Fig. 18.1) [41]. While they reported a CSF leak rate of 1.9%, they compared their technique with 1441 prior TL approaches from their same institution, all closed with a traditional fat graft closure without mesh, and a CSF leak rate of 11.6%, noting that their technique with the resorbable mesh led to a significant reduction in their institution's CSF leak [41]. Looking at subtle technical differences in regard to the case, they also found no difference in CSF leak rates in those patients who had a posterior tympanotomy and those who didn't [41]. In a subsequent study to determine whether the resorbable plate method was cost-effective, Chern and colleagues reported that the technique was indeed, noting that any cranioplasty exceeding approximately $5000 is not cost-effective [42].

In another technique, groups have used HA cement with and without titanium mesh. Arriaga and Chen describe closing patients with a HA cranioplasty, with their first report noting a reduction of their CSF leak rate from 12.5% to 3.7% in 54 patients when compared to a cohort where only autologous fat was used [43]. Interestingly, in the first seven patients of their cohort, they placed HA cement over the dural defect, filling the remaining mastoid cavity with HA cement [43]. With a CSF leak developing in two of these patients, they modified their technique to place an abdominal

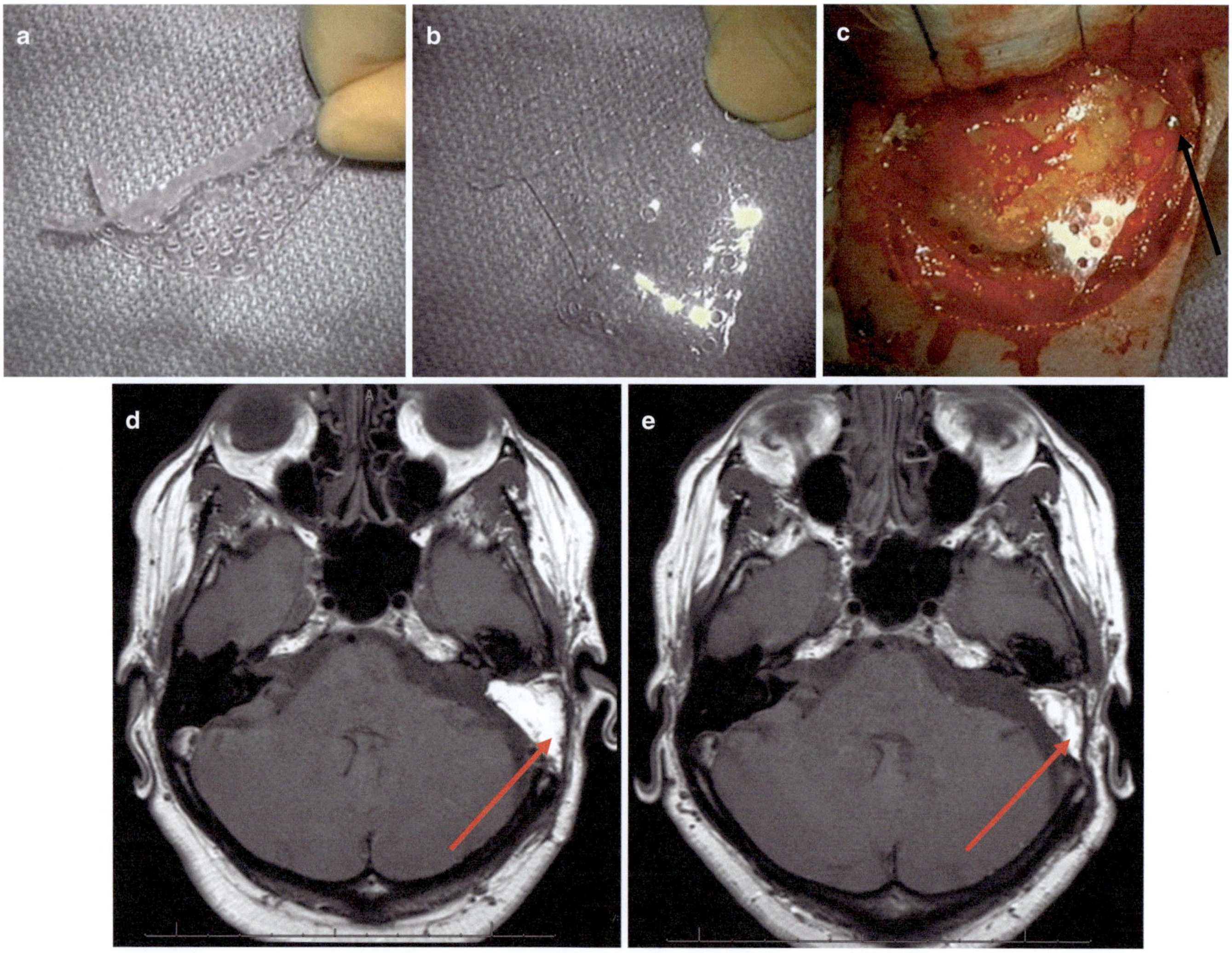

Fig. 18.1 Resorbable mesh cranioplasty. (**a**, **b**) Images demonstrate a trimmed and molded resorbable mesh prior to placement. (**c**) The resorbable mesh is shown in situ, with an arrow pointing to one of several screws used to secure the mesh to the patient. (**d**, **e**) Axial T1 MR images 3 and 12 months postoperatively, respectively, from a left translabyrinthine craniectomy for a vestibular schwannoma. The arrows highlight the resorbable mesh

fat graft through the dural defect, leaving the fat medial to the mastoid antrum and vertical segment of the facial nerve, and filling the remainder of the cavity with HA cement [43]. They then placed a suction drain lateral to the cement, reapproximating the skin, and removing the drain the next day [43]. They noted that one patient developed a delayed wound infection 1 year after surgery, requiring them to remove the cement, but no CSF was encountered. Another patient developed a seroma, which resolved with pressure dressing [43]. They also mention that, at that time, HA cements cost about $80 per gram, with an average need of 25 grams to fill the mastoid cavity [43], but they rationalize that a reduced CSF leak with their technique, reducing the need for further hospitalizations and treatment, justifies their costs [43].

With concerns that HA can lead to infections in skull-base surgery or injure the facial nerve [44–47], the same centers retrospectively reviewed their long-term experience in using the HA cement cranioplasty with an abdominal fat graft to close the surgical defect following a TL approach [48]. The centers summarize the results of three surgeons, none of whom open a posterior tympanotomy, though some pack the antrum and retrofacial air cells with muscle and others pack the eustachian tube (ET) antrum with alternating muscle and Surgicel® [48]. They found an incidence of either CSF leak or infection of 1.9%, or combined 3.8%, among 369 patients [48]. They found that their complication rate is consistent with previously published HA cement cases, with complication rates from 3.4% to 7.7% [45, 47, 49].

While many of these studies have concentrated on using fat and a variety of techniques to provide counter pressure, several other studies have looked at subtle technical differences that may account for differences in CSF leak rates. Glasscock and colleagues describe amputating the head of the malleus and placing it in the ET, filling the entire middle ear with muscle [32]. Cueva and Mastrodimos open a posterior tympanotomy and pack the ET with the incus and small pieces of muscle in the middle ear [50]. In a separate study, Jacob and colleagues assessed their experience at packing the ET with Proplast®, a polymer of polytetrafluoroethylene and carbon filaments, finding that there was no significant difference in CSF leak rates between those patients who had the ET packed and those who did not but found that the Proplast® extruded in 3.3% of patients, leading to delayed purulent otorrhea [10]. In a different study, Saliba and colleagues sought to assess the incidence of CSF rhinorrhea after systematic obliteration of the ET following a TL approach [51]. Opening a posterior tympanotomy and removing the incus, the ET is obliterated with musculoperiosteal fragments, bone wax, fibrin glue, and Surgicel®, followed by placement of "hashed abdominal fat," mixed with fibrin glue, which is injected into the middle ear and surrounding air cells of the IAC [51]. They compared their modified technique with another technique in which the ET is not packed. While there was no significant difference in CSF leaks between groups, the modified technique demonstrated no CSF rhinorrhea [51]. Six cases were seen in the original technique.

Goddard and colleagues reported a 0% CSF leak rate following TL approaches in 61 patients over a mean follow-up period of 31.3 months [52]. They did not open a posterior tympanotomy, left the incus in place, and packed the middle ear with temporalis muscle [52]. Further packing any exposed air cells with more muscle, they placed a larger piece of muscle just lateral to the incus, laying a fascia graft across laterally, followed by an abdominal fat graft [52]. While they did not report one CSF leak, they did note that one patient develop an abdominal graft harvest site infection [52].

Netto and colleagues assessed the role of a biosynthetic dura, performing a retrospective review of 34 patients undergoing VS removal with either the TL approach or the enlarged TL approach [53]. Eighteen of the patients had the dura closed with abdominal fat, while 16 had the dura closed with biosynthetic dura plus abdominal fat [53]. Both techniques obliterated the ET with the incus, and the middle ear was packed through the assistance of a posterior tympanotomy with muscle. While a musculoperiosteal flap was placed over the layered fat strips, which were carefully placed over the posterior fossa in the first procedure, in the second procedure, two layers of a synthetic dural substitute made from porcine small intestinal submucosa were placed under the bone medial to the sigmoid sinus, replacing the posterior fossa dura [53]. Fibrin glue was then used to seal the dural substitute to the bone, with fat placed medial and lateral to the dural substitute, followed by two more strips of dural substitute covering all the abdominal fat [53]. They had one CSF in each group, with an incisional leak in the first group, managed conservatively by oversewing it, while the patient in the second group developed significant drainage on postoperative day 2, with incisional drainage as well as otorrhea; thus, an LD was placed, along with the administration of acetazolamide [53]. The drain was removed after 4 days, the patients were observed for 3 more days, and they were discharged with acetazolamide for 15 more days, with both patients demonstrating no further leakage after 1 year [53]. While the authors found no difference in CSF leak rates between procedures, they emphasize that obliterating the middle ear with small pieces of muscle is key in avoiding CSF leaks [53].

In response to Mangus and colleagues' review, Ben Ammar and colleagues noted that muscle can atrophy and fat can dissolve, so they pack the middle ear with dry periosteum [54]. In one of the larger single institutional studies to date, Merkus and colleagues report a CSF leak rate of 0.8% following 1803 patients who underwent TL approaches for VS, emphasizing that they do not open a posterior tympanotomy. Instead, they obliterate mastoid air cells soon after they are opened as closure becomes more difficult once CSF comes in contact with them. The middle ear and attic are then packed with dried periosteum harvested at the beginning of the case [55]. From the same center, Falcioni and colleagues emphasized closing the attic with periosteum along with conserving the "fascioperiosteal flap," removing "the incus in a correct way," and "fixing the skin flap to the underlying surface"—all keys to reducing CSF leaks [56]. While the topic of temporal bone pneumatization is discussed in RS approaches, Kalamarides and colleagues commented that if the temporal bone was highly pneumatized on a preoperative CT scan, the canal was overclosed (Fig. 18.2) and the ET was obliterated [57].

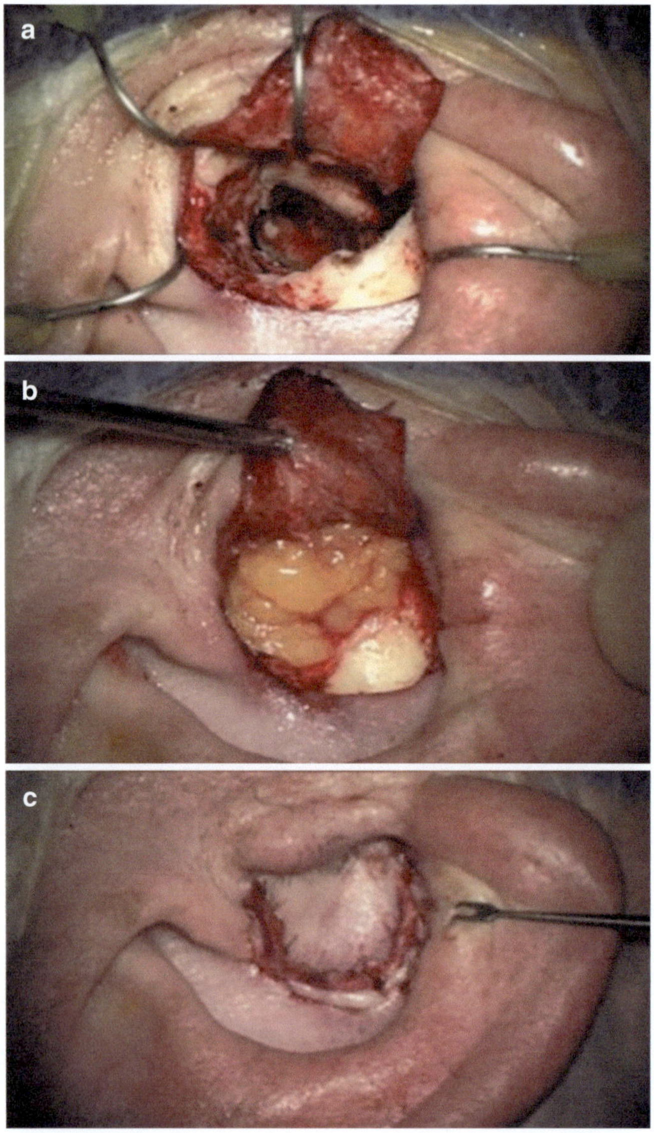

Fig. 18.2 Demonstration of a modified Rambo ear canal overclosure. (**a**) A right ear canal has had all squamous epithelium removed, with lateral elevation of the tragal skin. (**b**) Fat is harvested and placed within the ear canal. (**c**) Tragal skin is sutured to the conchal bowl skin

Retrosigmoid Approaches

In comparison with the TL approach, the RS approach usually provides the opportunity to primarily close the dura. Nonetheless, many practitioners caution that pneumatization of the temporal bone may play a significant role in determining who develops a CSF leak, with opened air cells providing a path for CSF. Rhoton and colleagues even postulated that air cells in the posterior wall of the IAC, which he termed "posteromedial cells," were influential in the development of postoperative CSF rhinorrhea [58]. Despite these issues, many groups report CSF leak rates from 2.2% to 9.2% [12, 13, 16, 38, 50, 59].

In 24 patients, Azad and colleagues describe their IAC closure technique following an RS approach, taking autologous fat graft, placing it over the IAC, covering it with Surgicel® to secure the graft, and then reinforcing with fibrin glue [44]. The dural defect is closed with 4–0 Nurolon sutures, with muscle or fat placed to ensure a watertight seal, followed by waxing of any retromastoid air cells [44]. More autologous fat is placed, followed by a Medpor® titanium implant and multi-layered closure.(Azad) After a mean follow-up time of 20.6 months, they reported no CSF leaks, meningitis, or pseudomeningocele formation [44]. They highlight that "preventing CSF leakage is the most effective method of avoiding and minimizing postoperative complications" [44]. They also mention that fat is an ideal material for the IAC defect, as it is easy to apply, contouring the defect, "and remains insert as a long term implant into the defect" [44]. However, they admit that infections associated with fat have been reported and that revascularization of the fat graft ensures long-term protection [60, 61].

Ludemann and colleagues describe their outcomes in 420 patients who underwent RS approaches, sealing opened air cells with muscle in 238 patients or fat from around the incision in 137 patients [16]. They fixed all plugs with fibrin glue, reporting CSF leak rates of 2.2% and 5.7% with fat and muscle, respectively, which was not statistically significantly different, though men (5.6%) had CSF leaks more frequently than women (3.4%) [16]. They admit that the surgeries using fat were performed after those that utilized muscle, thus the learning curve of the surgeon could account for the difference [16]. Despite the finding that larger tumors tend to have fewer CSF leak rates than smaller tumors, they found that the largest tumors had a higher rate of leaks [16].

With Fishman and colleagues showing that their TL approaches had significantly fewer CSF leaks compared to the other approaches, they postulated that use of a Palva periosteal flap, or "saloon door" flaps, over the petrous bone in retrosigmoid approaches as well as paying attention to air cell tracts led to the decrease in CSF leak rates [13]. They note that the Palva periosteal flap provides counterpressure to the abdominal fat graft in TL approaches and that a temporalis free graft is incorporated into RS dural defects to create a watertight seal [13]. They seal all with fibrin glue to avoid malpositioning [13].

Arlt and colleagues reviewed 81 patients who had multilayered dural closures following RS approaches [20]. With at least 1 year of follow-up, 41 patients were sealed with the "sandwich technique," with TissueFleece® and Spongostan® placed in the subdural space, followed by closure of the dura and placement of Tachosil®, a patch with fibrinogen and thrombin, over the sutured dura [20]. In a comparison group of 40 patients, only the epidural Tachosil® was placed [20]. With the surgeon determining at the time of surgery which technique was to be used, they found no difference between the techniques, with three CSF leaks found in patients receiving the sandwich technique and four in the monolayer technique [20].

Arlt and colleagues emphasize that it is necessary to have a watertight dural closure following RS approaches [20]. Hardy and colleagues obliterated all exposed air cells with fat or bone pate and replaced the dural flap, which was reinforced with fascia lata and fibrin glue [62]. Cueva and Mastrodimos emphasized waxing the mastoid air cells prior to opening the dura while the exposed air cells around the IAC are waxed following tumor removal [50]. Other techniques include using HA bone cement, muscle or fat (with or without fibrin glue), or Tachocomb® [59, 63]. Baird and colleagues describe a technique using HA cement to reconstruct the drilled IAC, reporting an incisional CSF leak rate of 7.7% in 280 patients compared with 6.7% in a control group [63]. Arlt and colleagues also caution that using muscle in the IAC might make it difficult to differentiate remnant or recurrent tumor on follow-up magnetic resonance imaging [20].

Further supporting the role that air cells play in the development of CSF rhinorrhea, Hoffman and colleagues showed that failing to drill the posterior wall of the IAC reduced the incidence of CSF leaks to 0% [19]. Thus, given the role air cells play in CSF leaks following RS approaches, Stieglitz and colleagues looked at how petrosal air cells may influence CSF leaks [22]. In reviewing 22 patients with CSF leaks and comparing them with 78 control patients, they assessed preoperative CT scans and found that smaller tumors showed more pneumatization of the posterior wall of the IAC compared with larger tumors [22]. However, they noted that pneumatization in the posterior wall was present in 26.1% of patients with CSF leaks compared to 28.6% in those without (Fig. 18.3). While temporal bones had pneumatized posterior walls more frequently in smaller tumors compared to larger tumors, 34.9% and 24.1%, respectively, the authors theorized that larger tumors might obliterate air cells by widening the IAC [22]. The pneumatization rates have been supported by other studies, with Lang and Kerr noting that 22% of patients had pneumatized posteromedial air cells in a cadaver study, while Yamakami and colleagues found pneumatization in the posteromedial wall in 17% of 168 patients [64, 65]. However, running counter to their argument, Stieglitz and colleagues admit that their CSF leak cohort and control groups had similar ratios of smaller and larger tumors [22]. They also recognize that smaller tumors tend be located within the IAC, thus requiring more extensive drilling of the posterior wall, which has also been observed by a number of other studies and could contribute to increased CSF leaks [6, 13, 20, 22, 56].

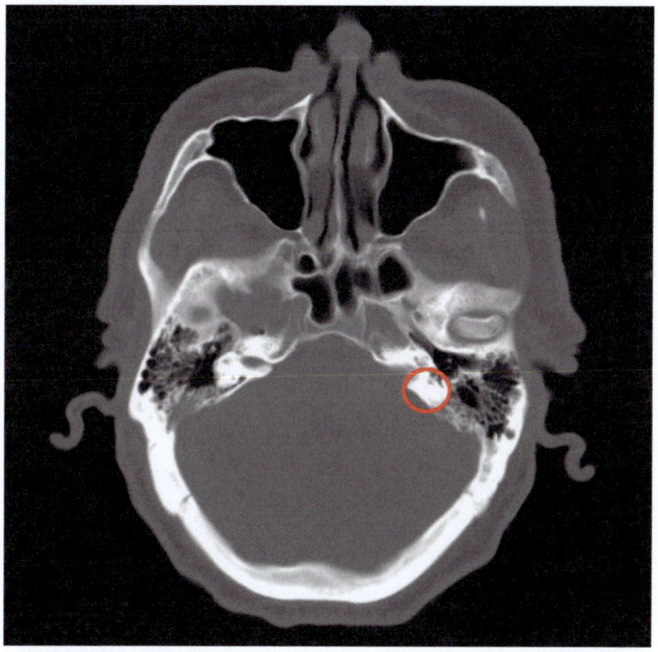

Fig. 18.3 Preoperative axial CT temporal bone image in a patient with a left vestibular schwannoma, with a red circle highlighting the lack of pneumatization of the temporal bone posterior to the left internal auditory canal

Middle Fossa Approach

CSF leaks following the MF approach are the result of either leaking through the fundus of the IAC laterally or opening into air cells in a well pneumatized temporal bone. Various studies report CSF leak rates following MF approaches, ranging from 4% to 19% [4–6, 8, 11, 13, 18, 66, 67].

In another study, Scheich and colleagues report their outcomes of 203 patients who underwent MF approaches with at least 12 months minimum follow-up [68]. After tumor removal, they plug the IAC defect with temporalis muscle, followed by fibrin glue, covering all open air cells with bone wax or fibrin glue, replacing the craniotomy bone plate and muscle flap, and placing a subcutaneous suction drain and soft pressure dressing [68]. Including patients as old as 78 years of age, they reported a CSF leak rate of 12.8%, all but one of which presented as rhinorrhea beginning 1–7 days after surgery [68]. The CSF leaks were self-limiting in 69% of cases after a median of 4 days, though 5 patients required an LD and three required revision surgery [68]. Like the RS approach, Schiech found that the presence of pneumatized mastoid air cells correlated with CSF leakage [17]. Cueva and Mastrodimos, similar to their closure technique following an RS approach, wax all exposed bone on MF approaches and place a fascia graft, if the middle ear is entered, and either fat or absorbable gelatin foam on top of the fascia graft [50]. Weber and Gantz place a temporalis muscle plug and fascia graft, followed by a bone graft [69].

Other Approaches

As mentioned previously, beyond the three workhorse approaches to the IAC and CPA, other approaches are thought to lead to increased CSF leaks. In regard to closure techniques, in presigmoid-retrolabyrinthine approaches (Fig. 18.4), Cueva and colleagues describe using a large, 5-cm areolar temporalis fascia graft, double layering the graft over the antrum and bony ear canal, protecting the middle ear and ossicles, and placing the fat graft into the mastoid cavity [50]. Likewise, in the far lateral transcondylar approach, other authors utilize a large areolar temporalis fascia and a cuff of muscle from the mastoid tip, followed by interrupted woven 4-0 nylon sutures in an attempt to primarily close the dura. They then place fascia over the exposed dura, waxing all exposed mastoid air cells, followed by an abdominal fat graft, buttressed by the posterior belly of the digastric muscle [50].

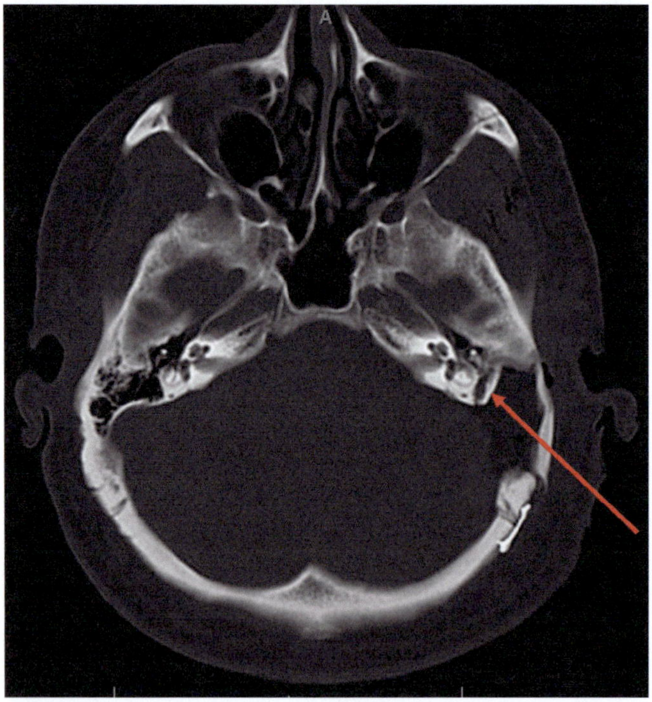

Fig. 18.4 Postoperative axial CT temporal bone image from a patient who underwent a left presigmoid-retrolabyrinthine approach to remove a trochlear schwannoma. The dura was closed primarily, followed by placement of a fat graft within the antrum, and bony plate from the mastoid cortex was harvested (red arrow) and wedged into the antrum, followed by more fat. The patient did well postoperatively, with no evidence of cerebrospinal fluid leak

Management Options

With numerous reports detailing many different techniques in hopes of preventing CSF leaks, they still occur and will continue to occur. With CSF leaks, patients are at risk for meningitis, which is thought to be the second most common complication after VS surgery, occurring in 1–7% of cases [66, 70]. Conservative measures include bed rest, head elevation, fluid restriction, pressure dressings, acetazolamide, and suturing incisional leaks. However, there is no agreement as to how long one should maintain conservative measures, let alone acetazolamide doses and frequency. Becker and colleagues kept patients on acetazolamide for 1 month after resolution of the CSF leak [6]. Several studies have assessed the success rate of conservative measures based on the presenting symptoms or initial approach. Mangus and colleagues found that only 10% of 115 incisional CSF leaks required more than conservative management compared to 59% of those patients who presented with CSF rhinorrhea [11]. Brennan and colleagues found that patients with rhinorrhea following TL approaches required surgery "significantly more often than RS leaks" [12]. In Selesnick and colleagues' large review of the literature for the best management of CSF leaks, they concluded that incisional leaks are best managed with pressure dressings, head of bed elevation, bed rest, and resuturing the surgical incision as well as an LD, with rhinorrhea requiring surgical intervention, with no specific technique superior to another [71].

Some believe that LD placement is a conservative measure, with some studies reporting success rates of an LD in 57–90% of cases [71, 72]. Allen and colleagues retrospectively reviewed 508 transdural lateral skull-base cases, 63 of which required subarachnoid drainage in an attempt to manage CSF leaks [73]. As a protocol, in addition to the LD, patients with CSF rhinorrhea or otorrhea received a pressure dressing, head elevation, and bed rest, with CSF drainage every 4 h, 10–15 mL/h, over 5 days [73]. While the CSF leaks were found an average of 5 days after surgery, ranging from 0 to 24 days, their protocol was successful in 76.2% of patients, significantly more so after TL approaches (90%) compared to RS approaches (50%) [73]. In regard to presenting symptoms, drainage was successful in all patients who had incisional leakage compared to 71.1% in those patients with CSF rhinorrhea and 55.6% in those with CSF otorrhea [73]. Hardy and colleagues performed lumbar punctures daily in all patients postoperatively for 3–5 days with a CSF leak rate of 13% in the first 100 cases, all of which occurred in the first 42 patients [62]. In the subsequent 188 patients following a change in wound closure protocol, which they detail, they reported only two cases of rhinorrhea, both of which required reexploration, and a third patient requiring an LD for an incisional leak, with a CSF leak rate of 1.6% [62].

However, as highlighted earlier, LDs are not without risks. In Allen and colleagues' study, complications included headaches in 28.6% of patients, nausea and vomiting in 22.2%, meningitis in six patients, along with premature catheter dislodgement in three cases, and a retained catheter in the lumbar thecal sac, requiring a lumbar laminectomy [73]. In addition, one patient had the stopcock dislodge, which was noted after the patient was found unconscious, recovering after the LD was closed [73]. Of those with meningitis, half were diagnosed after the LD was placed (diagnosed an average of 18.2 days following surgery) [73]. They also found no difference in the timing of diagnosing the CSF leak and the success of the LD [73]. Other complications have included severe neurologic deterioration, tentorial herniation, and tension pneumocephalus [74].

In Crowson and colleagues' review, they observed that the length of stay was significantly longer when a CSF leak occurred—9.8 versus 5.7 days without a CSF leak [7]. They noted a 5.32% complication rate, with five LDs falling out early, three leaking, two overdrained, and individual cases of a retained tip requiring a laminectomy, a clotted off lumbar drain, and a positive culture [7].

But like acetazolamide dosing, there is no agreed upon protocol for LD management. Following their RS series, Arlt and colleagues would place an LD for 5 days if a CSF was noted, draining 150–250 mL/day, but if leakage continued by day 3, a second operation was performed [20]. Stieglitz report draining between 150 and 200 mL in 24 h [22]. If after 7 days the leak persists, patients underwent surgical revision [22]. Sheich and colleagues drain 10 mL/h, not exceeding 250 mL/day, clamping the day prior to removal [17].

Kalamarides and colleagues treated all patients with CSF leaks with two lumbar punctures, with all opening pressures recorded; thus, 30 mL of CSF was discarded when the CSF pressure was above 15 cm H_2O, while 15 mL was discarded if less, along with daily acetazolamide at 750 mg orally for 7 days [57]. Six patients required a third lumbar puncture if the leak persisted, with surgical revision planned if the conservative treatment failed after 3 days [57]. They found that CSF leaks presented on average 7 days after the procedure, ranging from postoperative day 2 to 21, with patients whose CSF leak resolved having significantly higher mean initial CSF pressures compared to those that failed (18 cm H_2O versus 8 cm H_2O) [57]. While Lazard and colleagues were unable to compare opening CSF pressures, they noted in their twelve CSF leaks that the mean opening CSF pressure was 24 ± 5 cm H_2O, reflective of intracranial hypertension [9]. Nonetheless, Lazard and colleagues report that all their leaks resolved with multiple lumbar punctures, between two and three, along with acetazolamide at 500 mg by mouth daily for 5 days and wound closure reinforcement [9]. All but one patient's CSF leak resolved with this algorithm, with one patient requiring a lumbar peritoneal shunt on postoperative day 13 [9].

Becker and colleagues place a lumboperitoneal drain if an incisional leak does not resolve with an LD, differentiating those patients with CSF rhinorrhea and noting that those with "sniffles" (thought to be low volume leaks) can be treated differently from those patients with copious drainage [6]. In the latter, they placed an LD for 3 days, while in the former, they are conservatively managed with acetazolamide and without an LD [6]. Furthermore, those patients who presented with CSF leaks after postoperative day 4 were treated with immediate LD placement [6].

Russel and colleagues identified 275 patients who underwent TL approaches, reporting a CSF leak rate of 12.0% [15]. They found that resuturing the wound was effective in 15.1% of cases, an LD in 24.2%, and surgical revision to obstruct the petromastoidectomy in 60.6%, with 25% of surgical revision cases requiring at least one more surgical attempt to stop the CSF leak [15]. Mamikolgu and colleagues reported their outcomes of 81 patients with VS larger than 3 cm, all of whom underwent TL approaches, with a 17% CSF leak rate, all of which were managed with pressure dressings and/or lumbar punctures or drains [75]. In regard to MF approaches, revision surgery rates are between 0% and 2% [6, 66, 76, 77].

Recalcitrant Cases

Despite the variety of approaches and techniques to prevent a CSF leak as well as the protocols and practices used to fix such a leak, CSF leaks have still persisted despite multiple attempts at LD and surgical revision (Fig. 18.5). Generally, surgical revision entails overclosing the ear canal and plugging the ET. Some authors have suggested reexploring the closure or placing more abdominal fat. However, several studies have demonstrated that some patients need multiple surgical revisions, with Mangus and colleagues noting that 21% of those treated surgically required a second intervention [11, 13, 19, 21]. One such technique is overclosing the ET from the nose. First described by Kwartler and colleagues in 1996, they scarified the lumen of the ET with a middle ear rasp and packed it with autologous muscle, infolding the mucosal flaps and cauterizing the outer surface, covering it with an absorbable gelatin sponge and leaving posterior nasal packing for 5 days [78].

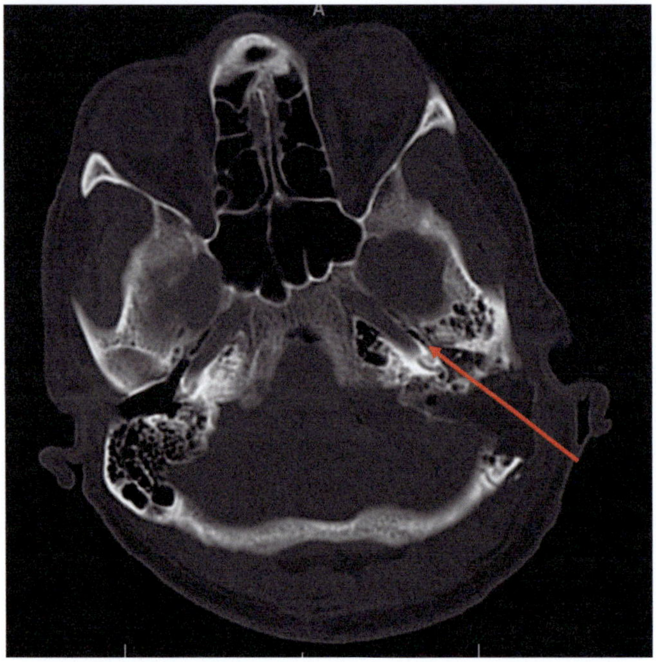

Fig. 18.5 Postoperative axial CT temporal bone image in a patient who had a left translabyrinthine craniectomy for a vestibular schwannoma. Postoperatively, the patient developed rhinorrhea, consistent with cerebrospinal fluid. The images demonstrate a well-aerated petrous apex as well as continued aeration near the eustachian tube. The patient returned to the operating room where the eustachian tube orifice was enlarged to better facilitate packing with muscle. The patient has done well postoperatively, with no evidence of cerebrospinal fluid leak

Orlandi and Shelton describe a modification, cauterizing the inferior 2–3 mm of the ET orifice and closing the orifice with a 4-0 monofilament suture with two passes [79]. In a more recent study, Lemonnier and colleagues summarized their results in nine patients who presented with CSF rhinorrhea following lateral skull-base surgery, managed with endoscopic endonasal closure of the ET [80]. Lemonnier and colleagues describe microdebriding the distal ET circumferentially, followed by circumferentially cauterizing the ET at a depth of 3 mm, obliterating the proximal portion of the ET with an acellular dermal graft, and closing the orifice with a 3-0 Vicryl suture and occasionally as many as three sutures [80]. They reported that seven patients had successful closure, with two requiring revision, both of which underwent a failed revision endoscopic closure; thus, they underwent definitive treatment via either an RS or TL approach [80]. In a variation in these techniques, Sataloff and colleagues describe incising the ET mucosa at a depth of about 1 cm with a Rosen knife with palatal retraction, everting the mucosa, excoriating the inner surface with a rasp, and placing a purse-string suture circumferentially around the ET in five cases [81].

In another recalcitrant CSF leak, Glasscock and colleagues describe removing the osseous portion of the ET down to the isthmus via a MF approach, removing the mucosa and tensor tympani muscle, and placing orthopedic bone glue into the ET [32]. In a similar approach, Grant and colleagues describe a transcochlear approach to repair persistent CSF leaks in four separate cases, drilling out and packing air cell tracts medial to the cochlea with bone wax as well as placing Proplast® into the ET [82]. In two patients with failed endoscopic closure of their ET, Netterville and colleagues have performed a transglenoid approach to the ET in persistent CSF leaks [83], drilling the isthmus and occluding it with Hydroset® (personal communication).

Conclusion

Ultimately, while no substantial conclusions can be made on the surgical approach, patient preoperative factors, or intraoperative techniques, no additional agreement exists as to how they are best managed if they do occur. While it is generally thought meticulous surgical technique, from the incision to the final stitch, minimizes the risk of developing a CSF leak, and surgical techniques will continue to be explored, patients undergoing CPA surgery need to be counseled that the risk of developing a CSF leak remains, along with concomitant complications of meningitis and managing such a leak.

References

1. Laing RJ, Smielewski P, Czosnyka M, Quaranta N, Moffat DA. A study of perioperative lumbar cerebrospinal fluid pressure in patients undergoing acoustic neuroma surgery. Skull Base Surg. 2000;10(4):179–85.
2. Allen KP, Isaacson B, Kutz JW, Purcell PL, Roland PS. The association of meningitis with postoperative cerebrospinal fluid fistula. J Neurol Surg B Skull Base. 2012;73(6):401–4.
3. Daudia A, Biswas D, Jones NS. Risk of meningitis with cerebrospinal fluid rhinorrhea. Ann Otol Rhinol Laryngol. 2007;116(12):902–5.
4. Selesnick SH, Liu JC, Jen A, Newman J. The incidence of cerebrospinal fluid leak after vestibular schwannoma surgery. Otol Neurotol. 2004;25(3):387–93.
5. Ansari SF, Terry C, Cohen-Gadol AA. Surgery for vestibular schwannomas: a systematic review of complications by approach. Neurosurg Focus. 2012;33(3):E14.
6. Becker SS, Jackler RK, Pitts LH. Cerebrospinal fluid leak after acoustic neuroma surgery: a comparison of the translabyrinthine, middle fossa, and retrosigmoid approaches. Otol Neurotol. 2003;24(1):107–12.
7. Crowson MG, Cunningham CD 3rd, Moses H, Zomorodi AR, Kaylie DM. Preoperative lumbar drain use during acoustic neuroma surgery and effect on CSF leak incidence. Ann Otol Rhinol Laryngol. 2016;125(1):63–8.
8. Sameshima T, Fukushima T, McElveen JT Jr, Friedman AH. Critical assessment of operative approaches for hearing preservation in small acoustic neuroma surgery: retrosigmoid vs middle fossa approach. Neurosurgery. 2010;67(3):640–4; discussion 644–5.
9. Lazard DS, Tosello M, Bozorg-Grayeli A, et al. Early complications and symptoms of cerebellopontine angle tumor surgery: a prospective analysis. Eur Arch Otorhinolaryngol. 2011;268(11):1575–82.

10. Jacob A, Bortman JS, Robinson LL Jr, Yu L, Dodson EE, Welling DB. Does packing the eustachian tube impact cerebrospinal fluid rhinorrhea rates in translabyrinthine vestibular schwannoma resections? Otol Neurotol. 2007;28(7):934–8.
11. Mangus BD, Rivas A, Yoo MJ, et al. Management of cerebrospinal fluid leaks after vestibular schwannoma surgery. Otol Neurotol. 2011;32(9):1525–9.
12. Brennan JW, Rowed DW, Nedzelski JM, Chen JM. Cerebrospinal fluid leak after acoustic neuroma surgery: influence of tumor size and surgical approach on incidence and response to treatment. J Neurosurg. 2001;94(2):217–23.
13. Fishman AJ, Marrinan MS, Golfinos JG, Cohen NL, Roland JT Jr. Prevention and management of cerebrospinal fluid leak following vestibular schwannoma surgery. Laryngoscope. 2004;114(3): 501–5.
14. Copeland WR, Mallory GW, Neff BA, Driscoll CL, Link MJ. Are there modifiable risk factors to prevent a cerebrospinal fluid leak following vestibular schwannoma surgery? J Neurosurg. 2015;122(2):312–6.
15. Russel A, Hoffmann CP, Nguyen DT, Beurton R, Parietti-Winkler C. Can the risks of cerebrospinal fluid leak after vestibular schwannoma surgery be predicted? Otol Neurotol. 2017;38(2):248–52.
16. Ludemann WO, Stieglitz LH, Gerganov V, Samii A, Samii M. Fat implant is superior to muscle implant in vestibular schwannoma surgery for the prevention of cerebrospinal fluid fistulae. Neurosurgery. 2008;63(1 Suppl 1):ONS38–42; discussion 42–3.
17. Scheich M, Ginzkey C, Ehrmann-Muller D, Shehata-Dieler W, Hagen R. Management of CSF leakage after microsurgery for vestibular schwannoma via the middle cranial fossa approach. Eur Arch Otorhinolaryngol. 2016;273(10):2975–81.
18. Slattery WH 3rd, Francis S, House KC. Perioperative morbidity of acoustic neuroma surgery. Otol Neurotol. 2001;22(6):895–902.
19. Hoffman RA. Cerebrospinal fluid leak following acoustic neuroma removal. Laryngoscope. 1994;104(1 Pt 1):40–58.
20. Arlt F, Trantakis C, Krupp W, et al. Cerebrospinal fluid leak after microsurgical surgery in vestibular schwannomas via retrosigmoidal craniotomy. Neurol Res. 2011;33(9):947–52.
21. Bryce GE, Nedzelski JM, Rowed DW, Rappaport JM. Cerebrospinal fluid leaks and meningitis in acoustic neuroma surgery. Otolaryngol Head Neck Surg. 1991;104(1):81–7.
22. Stieglitz LH, Giordano M, Gerganov VM, Samii A, Samii M, Ludemann WO. How obliteration of petrosal air cells by vestibular schwannoma influences the risk of postoperative CSF fistula. Clin Neurol Neurosurg. 2011;113(9):746–51.
23. Mantravadi AV, Leonetti JP, Burgette R, Pontikis G, Marzo SJ, Anderson D. Body mass index predicts risk for complications from transtemporal cerebellopontine angle surgery. Otolaryngol Head Neck Surg. 2013;148(3):460–5.
24. Diaz Anadon A, Lassaletta L, Roda JM, Bouzas JG. [CSF fistulae following surgery for cerebellopontine angle tumours and their relationship with the body mass index]. Acta Otorrinolaringol Esp. 2009;60(5):318–24.
25. Sugerman HJ, DeMaria EJ, Felton WL 3rd, Nakatsuka M, Sismanis A. Increased intra-abdominal pressure and cardiac filling pressures in obesity-associated pseudotumor cerebri. Neurology. 1997;49(2):507–11.
26. Toscano V, Sancesario G, Bianchi P, Cicardi C, Casilli D, Giacomini P. Cerebrospinal fluid estrone in pseudotumor cerebri: a change in cerebral steroid hormone metabolism? J Endocrinol Invest. 1991;14(2):81–6.
27. Jennum P, Borgesen SE. Intracranial pressure and obstructive sleep apnea. Chest. 1989;95(2):279–83.
28. Purvin VA, Kawasaki A, Yee RD. Papilledema and obstructive sleep apnea syndrome. Arch Ophthalmol. 2000;118(12):1626–30.
29. Nonaka Y, Fukushima T, Watanabe K, et al. Contemporary surgical management of vestibular schwannomas: analysis of complications and lessons learned over the past decade. Neurosurgery. 2013;72(2 Suppl Operative):ons103–15; discussion ons115.
30. Bien AG, Bowdino B, Moore G, Leibrock L. Utilization of preoperative cerebrospinal fluid drain in skull base surgery. Skull Base. 2007;17(2):133–9.
31. Acikbas SC, Akyuz M, Kazan S, Tuncer R. Complications of closed continuous lumbar drainage of cerebrospinal fluid. Acta Neurochir. 2002;144(5):475–80.
32. Glasscock ME 3rd, Dickins JR. Complications of acoustic tumor surgery. Otolaryngol Clin N Am. 1982;15(4):883–95.
33. Montgomery WW, Ojemann RG, Weiss AD. Suboccipital-translabyrinthine approach for acoustic neuroma. Arch Otolaryngol. 1966;83(6):566–9.
34. House JL, Hitselberger WE, House WF. Wound closure and cerebrospinal fluid leak after translabyrinthine surgery. Am J Otol. 1982;4(2):126–8.
35. Wu H, Kalamarides M, Garem HE, Rey A, Sterkers O. Comparison of different wound closure techniques in translabyrinthine acoustic neuroma surgery. Skull Base Surg. 1999;9(4):239–42.
36. Bambakidis NC, Munyon C, Ko A, Selman WR, Megerian CA. A novel method of translabyrinthine cranioplasty using hydroxyapatite cement and titanium mesh: a technical report. Skull Base. 2010;20(3):157–61.
37. Manjila S, Weidenbecher M, Semaan MT, Megerian CA, Bambakidis NC. Prevention of postoperative cerebrospinal fluid leaks with multilayered reconstruction using titanium mesh-hydroxyapatite cement cranioplasty after translabyrinthine resection of acoustic neuroma. J Neurosurg. 2013;119(1):113–20.
38. Fayad JN, Schwartz MS, Slattery WH, Brackmann DE. Prevention and treatment of cerebrospinal fluid leak after translabyrinthine acoustic tumor removal. Otol Neurotol. 2007;28(3):387–90.
39. Chen TC, Maceri DR, Levy ML, Giannotta SL. Brain stem compression secondary to adipose graft prolapse after translabyrinthine craniotomy: case report. Neurosurgery. 1994;35(3):521–3; discussion 523–4.
40. Hillman TA, Shelton C. Resorbable plate cranioplasty after the translabyrinthine approach. Otol Neurotol. 2011;32(7):1171–4.
41. Hunter JB, Sweeney AD, Carlson ML, et al. Prevention of postoperative cerebrospinal fluid leaks after translabyrinthine tumor resection with resorbable mesh cranioplasty. Otol Neurotol. 2015;36(9):1537–42.
42. Chern A, Hunter JB, Bennett ML. Cost analysis of cerebrospinal fluid leaks and cerebrospinal fluid leak prevention in patients undergoing cerebellopontine angle surgery. Otol Neurotol. 2017;38(1):147–51.
43. Arriaga MA, Chen DA. Hydroxyapatite cement cranioplasty in translabyrinthine acoustic neuroma surgery. Otolaryngol Head Neck Surg. 2002;126(5):512–7.
44. Azad T, Mendelson ZS, Wong A, Jyung RW, Liu JK. Fat graft-assisted internal auditory canal closure after retrosigmoid transmeatal resection of acoustic neuroma: technique for prevention of cerebrospinal fluid leakage. J Clin Neurosci. 2016;24: 124–7.
45. Kveton JF, Coelho DH. Hydroxyapatite cement in temporal bone surgery: a 10 year experience. Laryngoscope. 2004;114(1): 33–7.
46. Matic D, Phillips JH. A contraindication for the use of hydroxyapatite cement in the pediatric population. Plast Reconstr Surg. 2002;110(1):1–5.
47. Poetker DM, Pytynia KB, Meyer GA, Wackym PA. Complication rate of transtemporal hydroxyapatite cement cranioplasties: a case series review of 76 cranioplasties. Otol Neurotol. 2004;25(4): 604–9.
48. Volsky PG, Hillman TA, Stromberg KJ, et al. Hydroxyapatite cement cranioplasty following translabyrinthine approach: long-term study of 369 cases. Laryngoscope. 2017;127(9):2120–5.

49. Kerr RG, Hearst MJ, Samy RN, et al. Delayed extrusion of hydroxyapatite cement after transpetrosal reconstruction. Neurosurgery. 2009;64(3):527–31; discussion 531–2.
50. Cueva RA, Mastrodimos B. Approach design and closure techniques to minimize cerebrospinal fluid leak after cerebellopontine angle tumor surgery. Otol Neurotol. 2005;26(6):1176–81.
51. Saliba I, Shinghal T, Nehme J, Dufour JJ. Eustachian tube obliteration in translabyrinthine vestibular schwannoma excision: cerebrospinal fluid rhinorrhea and middle ear status. J Otolaryngol Head Neck Surg. 2011;40(5):367–75.
52. Goddard JC, Oliver ER, Lambert PR. Prevention of cerebrospinal fluid leak after translabyrinthine resection of vestibular schwannoma. Otol Neurotol. 2010;31(3):473–7.
53. Netto AA, Colafemina JF, Centeno RS. Dural defect repair in translabyrinthine acoustic neuroma surgery and its implications in cerebrospinal fluid leak occurrence. J Neurol Surg B Skull Base. 2012;73(5):327–30.
54. Ben Ammar M, Merkus P, Di Lella F, Sanna M. Management of CSF leak after vestibular schwannoma surgery. Otol Neurotol. 2012;33(3):491–2.
55. Merkus P, Taibah A, Sequino G, Sanna M. Less than 1% cerebrospinal fluid leakage in 1,803 translabyrinthine vestibular schwannoma surgery cases. Otol Neurotol. 2010;31(2):276–83.
56. Falcioni M, Mulder JJ, Taibah A, De Donato G, Sanna M. No cerebrospinal fluid leaks in translabyrinthine vestibular schwannoma removal: reappraisal of 200 consecutive patients. Am J Otol. 1999;20(5):660–6.
57. Kalamarides M, Grayeli AB, Bouccara D, Redondo A, Rey A, Sterkers O. Opening cerebrospinal fluid pressure guides the management of cerebrospinal fluid leakage after acoustic neuroma surgery. Otol Neurotol. 2004;25(5):769–72.
58. Rhoton AL Jr. Microsurgery of the internal acoustic meatus. Surg Neurol. 1974;2(5):311–8.
59. Samii M, Matthies C. Management of 1000 vestibular schwannomas (acoustic neuromas): surgical management and results with an emphasis on complications and how to avoid them. Neurosurgery. 1997;40(1):11–21; discussion 21–3.
60. Black P. Cerebrospinal fluid leaks following spinal or posterior fossa surgery: use of fat grafts for prevention and repair. Neurosurg Focus. 2000;9(1):e4.
61. Yamaguchi M, Matsumoto F, Bujo H, et al. Revascularization determines volume retention and gene expression by fat grafts in mice. Exp Biol Med (Maywood). 2005;230(10):742–8.
62. Hardy DG, Macfarlane R, Moffat DA. Wound closure after acoustic neuroma surgery. Br J Neurosurg. 1993;7(2):171–4.
63. Baird CJ, Hdeib A, Suk I, et al. Reduction of cerebrospinal fluid rhinorrhea after vestibular schwannoma surgery by reconstruction of the drilled porus acusticus with hydroxyapatite bone cement. J Neurosurg. 2007;107(2):347–51.
64. Lang J, Kerr AG. Pneumatization of the posteromedial air-cell tract. Clin Otolaryngol Allied Sci. 1989;14(5):425–7.
65. Yamakami I, Uchino Y, Kobayashi E, Yamaura A. Computed tomography evaluation of air cells in the petrous bone—relationship with postoperative cerebrospinal fluid rhinorrhea. Neurol Med Chir (Tokyo). 2003;43(7):334–8; discussion 339.
66. Arts HA, Telian SA, El-Kashlan H, Thompson BG. Hearing preservation and facial nerve outcomes in vestibular schwannoma surgery: results using the middle cranial fossa approach. Otol Neurotol. 2006;27(2):234–41.
67. Heman-Ackah SE, Golfinos JG, Roland JT Jr. Management of surgical complications and failures in acoustic neuroma surgery. Otolaryngol Clin N Am. 2012;45(2):455–70, x.
68. Scheich M, Ginzkey C, Ehrmann Muller D, Shehata Dieler W, Hagen R. Complications of the middle cranial fossa approach for acoustic neuroma removal. J Int Adv Otol. 2017;13(2):186–90.
69. Weber PC, Gantz BJ. Results and complications from acoustic neuroma excision via middle cranial fossa approach. Am J Otol. 1996;17(4):669–75.
70. Sanna M, Taibah A, Russo A, Falcioni M, Agarwal M. Perioperative complications in acoustic neuroma (vestibular schwannoma) surgery. Otol Neurotol. 2004;25(3):379–86.
71. Selesnick SH, Liu JC, Jen A, Carew JF. Management options for cerebrospinal fluid leak after vestibular schwannoma surgery and introduction of an innovative treatment. Otol Neurotol. 2004;25(4):580–6.
72. Roland PS, Marple BF, Meyerhoff WL, Mickey B. Complications of lumbar spinal fluid drainage. Otolaryngol Head Neck Surg. 1992;107(4):564–9.
73. Allen KP, Isaacson B, Purcell P, Kutz JW Jr, Roland PS. Lumbar subarachnoid drainage in cerebrospinal fluid leaks after lateral skull base surgery. Otol Neurotol. 2011;32(9):1522–4.
74. Basauri LT, Concha-Julio E, Selman JM, Cubillos P, Rufs J. Cerebrospinal fluid spinal lumbar drainage: indications, technical tips, and pitfalls. Crit Rev Neurosurg. 1999;9(1):21–7.
75. Mamikoglu B, Wiet RJ, Esquivel CR. Translabyrinthine approach for the management of large and giant vestibular schwannomas. Otol Neurotol. 2002;23(2):224–7.
76. Shelton C, Brackmann DE, House WF, Hitselberger WE. Middle fossa acoustic tumor surgery: results in 106 cases. Laryngoscope. 1989;99(4):405–8.
77. Rabelo de Freitas M, Russo A, Sequino G, Piccirillo E, Sanna M. Analysis of hearing preservation and facial nerve function for patients undergoing vestibular schwannoma surgery: the middle cranial fossa approach versus the retrosigmoid approach—personal experience and literature review. Audiol Neurootol. 2012;17(2):71–81.
78. Kwartler JA, Schulder M, Baredes S, Chandrasekhar SS. Endoscopic closure of the eustachian tube for repair of cerebrospinal fluid leak. Am J Otol. 1996;17(3):470–2.
79. Orlandi RR, Shelton C. Endoscopic closure of the eustachian tube. Am J Rhinol. 2004;18(6):363–5.
80. Lemonnier LA, Tessema B, Kuperan AB, et al. Managing cerebrospinal fluid rhinorrhea after lateral skull base surgery via endoscopic endonasal eustachian tube closure. Am J Rhinol Allergy. 2015;29(3):207–10.
81. Sataloff RT, Zavod MB, Myers DL. Otogenic cerebrospinal fluid rhinorrhea: a new technique for closure of cerebrospinal fluid leak. Am J Otol. 2000;21(2):240–3.
82. Grant IL, Welling DB, Oehler MC, Baujan MA. Transcochlear repair of persistent cerebrospinal fluid leaks. Laryngoscope. 1999;109(9):1392–6.
83. Langerman A, Naslund TC, Netterville JL. Skull base approach to carotid artery lesions: technique, indications, and outcomes. J Neurol Surg B Skull Base. 2012;73(3):163–7.

Part IV

Nonschwannomatous Lesions of the CPA

Temporal Bone Neoplasms

19

Nauman F. Manzoor, Thomas Ostergard, Maroun T. Semaan, Sarah Mowry, Nicholas C. Bambakidis, and Cliff A. Megerian

Various benign and malignant neoplasms can involve the temporal bone and extend to adjacent areas of the skull base. The rarity of these neoplasms and the unfamiliarity of primary care physicians with both the disease and its manifestations can delay diagnosis. Dealing with lesions that originate in the temporal bone and extend into the cerebellopontine angle (CPA) presents a formidable challenge to surgeons and clinicians in terms of appropriate counseling, prediction of deficits, and choice of a treatment modality to achieve favorable and realistic outcomes. These lesions often present in an advanced stage. As the size of the tumor increases, it compresses, distorts, or infiltrates adjacent nerves and vessels. The onset of symptoms is often gradual, and the time course depends on the location of the lesion. The histological subtype and biological behavior of tumors are also paramount in the choice of a treatment modality and in patient counseling. The treatment of these lesions involves a multidisciplinary team that includes a neurosurgeon, neurotologist, neuroradiologist, radiation oncologist, otolaryngologist/reconstructive surgeon, audiologist, and ancillary team, such as a vestibular and speech therapist.

Differential Diagnosis

The differential diagnosis of lesions of the temporal bone mirrors that for lesions of the CPA in general. In this chapter, we divide the temporal bone into the regions corresponding to the apex and petroclival junction, medial surface, superior surface, inferior surface, and middle and lateral surfaces (Table 19.1, Figs. 19.1, 19.2, 19.3, 19.4, 19.5, and 19.6). The medial surface contains the internal auditory canal, posterior fossa dura, and endolymphatic sac. The superior surface contains the floor of the middle cranial fossa. The inferior surface contains the jugular foramen and its contents. The middle and lateral surfaces contain the middle ear cleft, mastoid portion, and external auditory canal (EAC).

This chapter reviews common lesions that arise within the boundaries of the petrous bone and that extend medially to involve the CPA and its vicinity. Malignant neoplasms arising from more lateral areas of the temporal bone and extending into the CPA tend to be advanced, and their prognosis is usually poor. Benign neoplasms are likewise advanced and extensively involve the contents of the temporal bone. Their surgical resection is laborious and often incomplete, necessitating adjunctive treatment. Only lesions intimately involved with the temporal bone and not covered elsewhere in this book are reviewed.

N. F. Manzoor
Department of Otolaryngology—Head and Neck Surgery and Neurological Surgery, University Hospitals Cleveland Medical Center, Case Western University School of Medicine, Cleveland, OH, USA

T. Ostergard
Carolina Neurosurgery and Spine Associates, Greensboro, NC, USA

M. T. Semaan
Otolaryngology—Otology, University Hospitals Cleveland Medical Center, Cleveland, OH, USA

S. Mowry
Department of Otolaryngology—Head and Neck Surgery, University Hospitals Cleveland Medical Center, Case Western University School of Medicine, Cleveland, OH, USA

N. C. Bambakidis (✉)
Neurological Surgery, The Neurological Institute, University Hospitals of Cleveland, Case Western Reserve University School of Medicine, Cleveland, OH, USA
e-mail: Nicholas.Bambakidis2@UHhospitals.org

C. A. Megerian
University Hospitals Health System, Department of Otolaryngology-Head and Neck Surgery, Department of Neurological Surgery, Case Western Reserve University School of Medicine, Cleveland, OH, USA
e-mail: cliff.megerian@uhhospitals.org

N. C. Bambakidis et al. (eds.), *Surgery of the Cerebellopontine Angle*, https://doi.org/10.1007/978-3-031-12507-2_19

Table 19.1 Differential diagnosis of lesions of the CPA and temporal bone

Petrous apex and petroclival region[a]	Medial temporal surface[b]	Superior temporal surface[c]	Middle and lateral temporal bone[d]	Inferior temporal bone[e]
Petroclival meningiomas	Schwannomas (CN VII and VII)	Middle fossa meningiomas	Paragangliomas (glomus tympanicum)	Paragangliomas (glomus jugulare and vagale)
Schwannomas (CN V)	Meningiomas of the IAC or CPA	Schwannomas of CN VII (geniculate ganglion)	Schwannomas of CN VII (mastoid portion)	Schwannomas of CN IX, X, XI, and XII
Chondrosarcomas	Endolymphatic sac tumors	Geniculate ganglion hemangiomas	Adenomas	Meningiomas of jugular foramen
Rhabdomyosarcomas			Adenocarcinomas	Chondrosarcomas
Osteosarcomas			Ceruminous adenomas	Osteosarcomas
Leukemia, lymphomas, and plasmocytomas			Adenoid cystic carcinomas	
Metastatic disease			Ceruminous adenocarcinomas	
Cholesterol granulomas[f]			Squamous cell carcinomas	
Epidermoids: Primary cholesteatomas of the petrous apex[a]			Carcinoid tumors	

CN cranial nerve, *CPA* cerebellopontine angle, *IAC* internal auditory canal
[a]See Fig. 19.1
[b]See Figs. 19.2 and 19.3
[c]See Fig. 19.4
[d]See Fig. 19.5
[e]See Fig. 19.6
[f]Non-neoplastic disease entities discussed briefly because of their pathological importance in lesions affecting the CPA

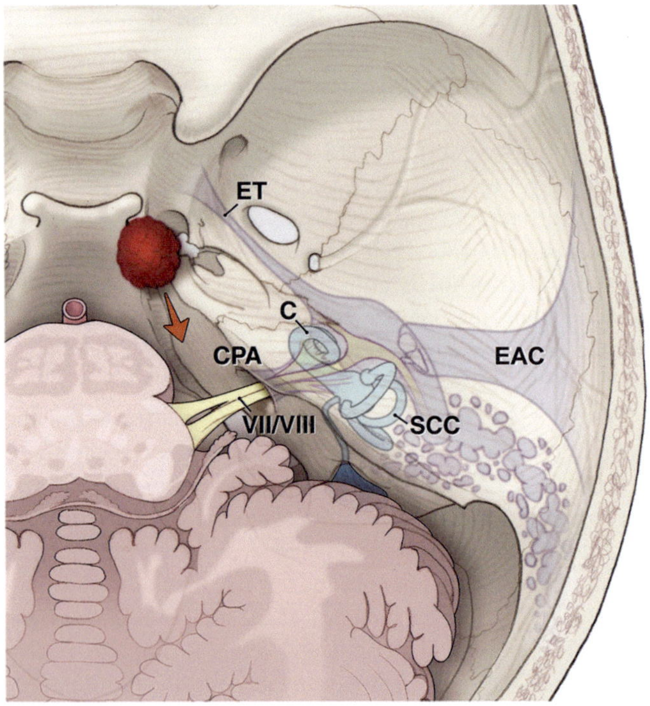

Fig. 19.1 Neoplasm originating in the region of the petroclival junction and petrous apex can involve the CPA by medial and posterior extension. *C* cochlea, *CPA* erebellopontine angle, *EAC* external auditory canal, *ET* eustachian tube, *SCC* semicircular canals, *VII/VIII* cranial nerves VII and VIII complex. Reproduced with permission from Barrow Neurological Institute

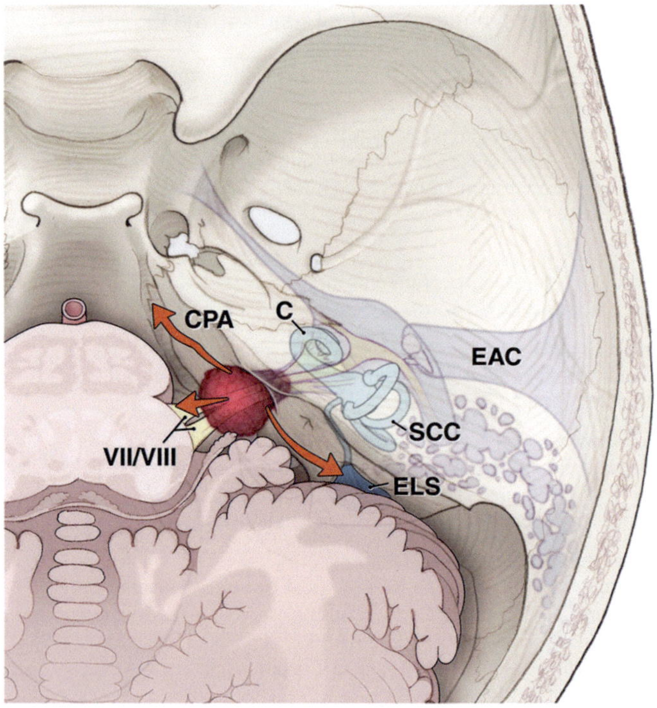

Fig. 19.2 Neoplasms originating from the region of the internal auditory canal can involve the CPA by extending medially and anterosuperiorly. *C* cochlea, *CPA* erebellopontine angle, *EAC* external auditory canal, *ELS* endolymphatic sac, *SCC* semicircular canals, *VII/VIII* cranial nerves VII and VIII complex. Reproduced with permission from Barrow Neurological Institute

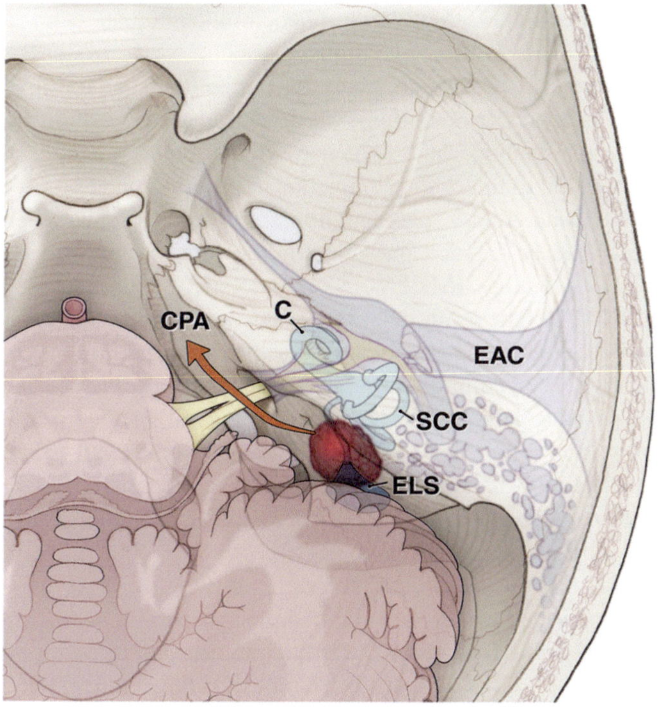

Fig. 19.3 Neoplasms originating from the region of the endolymphatic sac and posterior petrous ridge can involve the CPA by extending anteriorly. *C* cochlea, *CPA* erebellopontine angle, *EAC* external auditory canal, *ELS* endolymphatic sac, *SCC* semicircular canals. Reproduced with permission from Barrow Neurological Institute

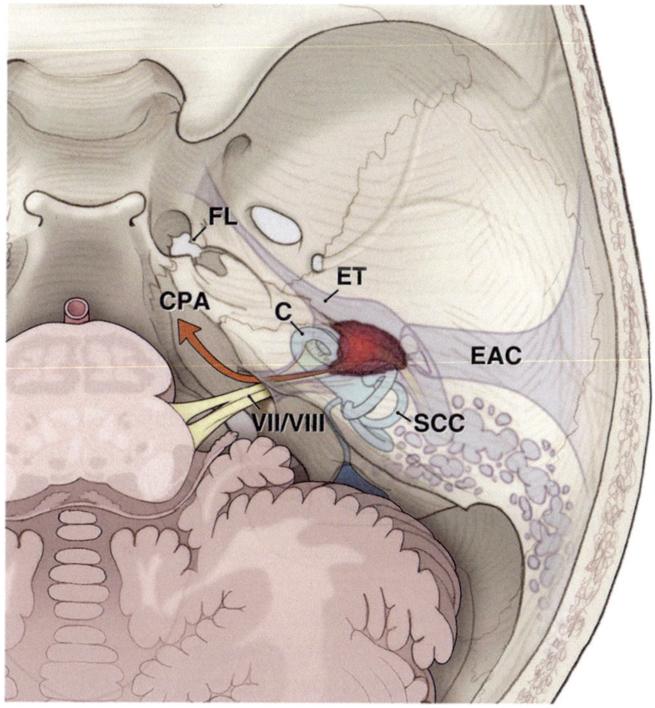

Fig. 19.4 Neoplasms originating from the region of the geniculate ganglion and floor of the middle cranial fossa can spread to the CPA by extending medially and anteriorly. *C* cochlea, *CPA* cerebellopontine angle, *EAC* external auditory canal, *ET* eustachian tube, *FL* foramen lacerum, *SCC* semicircular canals, *VII/VIII* cranial nerves VII and VIII complex. Reproduced with permission from Barrow Neurological Institute

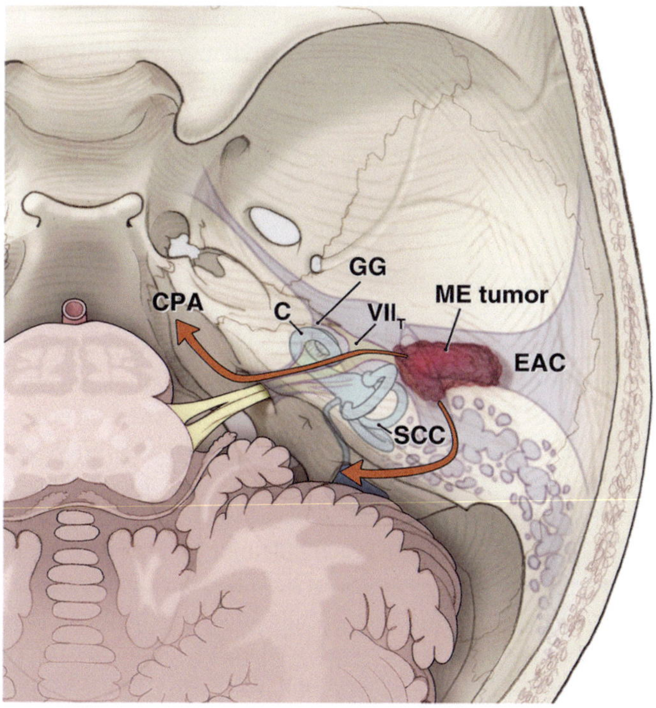

Fig. 19.5 Neoplasms originating from the lateral aspect of the temporal bone, external auditory canal, or middle ear can extend to the CPA by spreading medially, posteromedially (via the mastoid and perilabyrinthine air-cell systems), or anteriorly (via the petrous or infralabyrinthine air-cell systems). *C* cochlea, *CPA* cerebellopontine angle, *EAC* external auditory canal, *ET* eustachian tube, *ME* middle ear, *SCC* semicircular canals; *GG* geniculate ganglion, *VIIT* tympanic portion of CN VII. Reproduced with permission from Barrow Neurological Institute

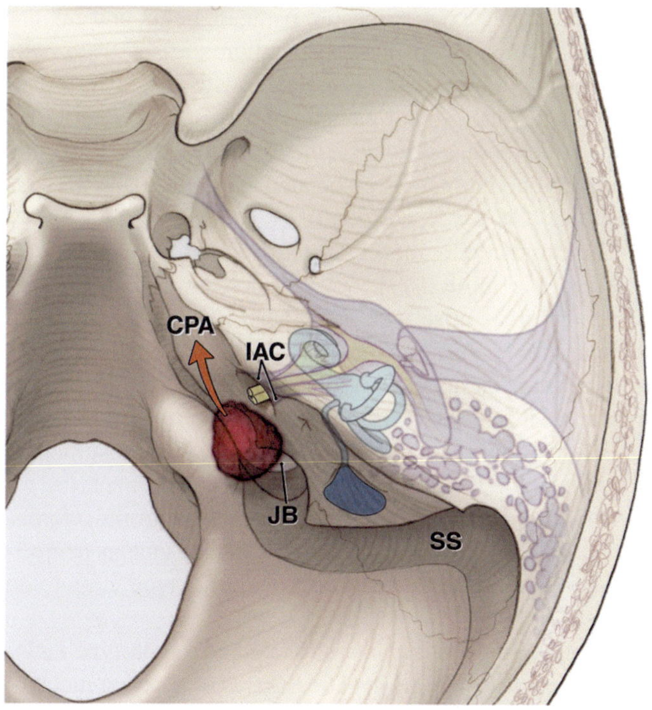

Fig. 19.6 Neoplasms originating from the region of the jugular bulb and lower cranial nerves extend to the CPA by spreading anteriorly and superiorly. *CPA* cerebellopontine angle, *IAC* internal auditory canal, *JB* jugular bulb, *SS* sigmoid sinus. Reproduced with permission from Barrow Neurological Institute

Temporal Bone Paragangliomas

Temporal bone paragangliomas (glomus tumors) are tumors arising from the extraadrenal paraganglionic tissue. They are slow-growing tumors, usually benign and highly vascular. During embryogenesis, paraganglionic tissue is derived from the migration of neural crest cells in close association with the autonomic nervous system. Within the head and neck, these cell rests are predominantly distributed throughout the middle ear in close association with Jacobson's nerve (branch of the glossopharyngeal nerve, cranial nerve [CN IX]) and Arnold's nerve (branch of the vagus nerve, CN X), the jugular foramen, CN X, and the carotid body [1]. In 1941, Guild coined the term glomus-tissue, referring to the vascularized ganglionic tissue along the adventitia of the jugular bulb and promontory. In 1953, he also published an anatomical study detailing formation of glomus tissue along Jacobson's and Arnold's nerves, which forms the basis of origin of tympanic paraganglioma [2]. In 1945, Harry Rosenwasser successfully removed the first temporal bone paraganglioma that he described as a tumor of the middle ear, resembling a carotid body [3].

In the past, various terminology has been used to describe these tumors, including glomus tumors, nonchromaffin paragangliomas, and chemodectomas. Contemporary literature emphasizes the use of the term paraganglioma, which will be used in this text [4, 5].

The most common head and neck paragangliomas are carotid body tumors. Within the temporal bone, two types of paragangliomas exist: tympanic paraganglioma and jugular paraganglioma. Tympanic paraganglioma arises from rests of paraganglionic tissue associated with Jacobson's and Arnold's nerves. Jugular paraganglioma is believed to arise from similar paraganglionic rests within the adventitia of the jugular bulb, intimately associated with the pars nervosa structures (CN IX, X, and XI).

The estimated incidence of extraadrenal paragangliomas is 1 per one million [1]. Seventy percent of extraadrenal paragangliomas arise within the head and neck region and the majority (> 95%) are nonsecretory [1]. No ethnic predilection has been noted, and they commonly manifest in the fourth and fifth decades of life. The only phenotypic modifier of theses tumors is high-altitude living with postulations about hypoxia as a driver of tumor development [6, 7]. Historically, both paraganglioma and pheochromocytomas have been linked with hereditary syndromes such as neurofibromatosis 1, multiple endocrine neoplasia type 2, and von Hippel-Lindau (VHL) disease.

Paraganglioma has evolved to become a prototype endocrine tumor for studying genetics related to aberrant metabolism [8]. The genetic era started with a seminal discovery of mutations in various subunits of succinate dehydrogenase (SDH) [9]. Since then, a plethora of studies have investigated different pathways and key players in tumorigenesis [10–12]. Paragangliomas along with pheochromocytomas carry a (familial) germline mutation in about 40% of cases. Mutations in 12 key genes have been identified, and multiple key pathways (pseudo-hypoxia driven, altered metabolism, kinase signaling, and epigenetic remodeling) have been implicated in tumor development and progression [13]. Five distinct hereditary paraganglioma syndromes have been described so far and harbor germline mutation of various SDH subunits (SDHA, SDHB, SDHC, SDHD, and SDHAF2). These are inherited in autosomal dominant fashion. The genetic screening for various paraganglioma syndromes is becoming more widespread as the phenotypic expression helps guide the workup as well as determines prognosis (e.g., SDHD and SDHAF2 mutations carry high rates of multifocal tumors and are derived from a defective paternal allele, whereas SDHB mutations have about a 50% risk of malignant phenotype [8, 14].

Paragangliomas spread through pathways of least resistance: air cell tracts, vascular channels, naturally occurring fissures, and foramina. Different patterns of intracranial spread, so-called dangerous triangles, have been described [15]. Paragangliomas can travel through the peritubal air cells into the petrous apex, petrous carotid artery, and middle cranial fossa, or through the hypotympanic air-cell tract between the jugular bulb and carotid artery into the posterior fossa; they can involve the CPA structures as well [16, 17].

Malignant paragangliomas are rare and reported in 5% of the cases [18]. The diagnosis of malignancy is based on the confirmed presence of regional (lymphatic) or distant metastasis. Cellular criteria and invasiveness have not been established as prerequisites for the diagnosis of malignant paraganglioma.

Pathology

Paragangliomas contain two cell types: chief cells and sustentacular cells. The chief cells possess secretory granules that contain catecholamines. They are derivatives of neural crest cells and belong to the diffuse neuroendocrine system [1, 19]. Cells that are members of this system are capable of secreting neurotransmitters and have similar cell receptors.

Despite the detection of catecholamine precursors in most paragangliomas, only 1 to 3% of head and neck paragangliomas excrete norepinephrine. Unlike adrenal paragangliomas (pheochromocytomas), extraadrenal paragangliomas rarely produce epinephrine because the rate-converting enzyme phenylethanolamine-N-methyltransferase is absent [20]. On light microscopy, chief cells form clusters (Zellballen) embedded with support cells (sustentacular cells) within an abundant vascular stroma (Fig. 19.7). Mitosis and capsular invasion have been described in benign variants and are not

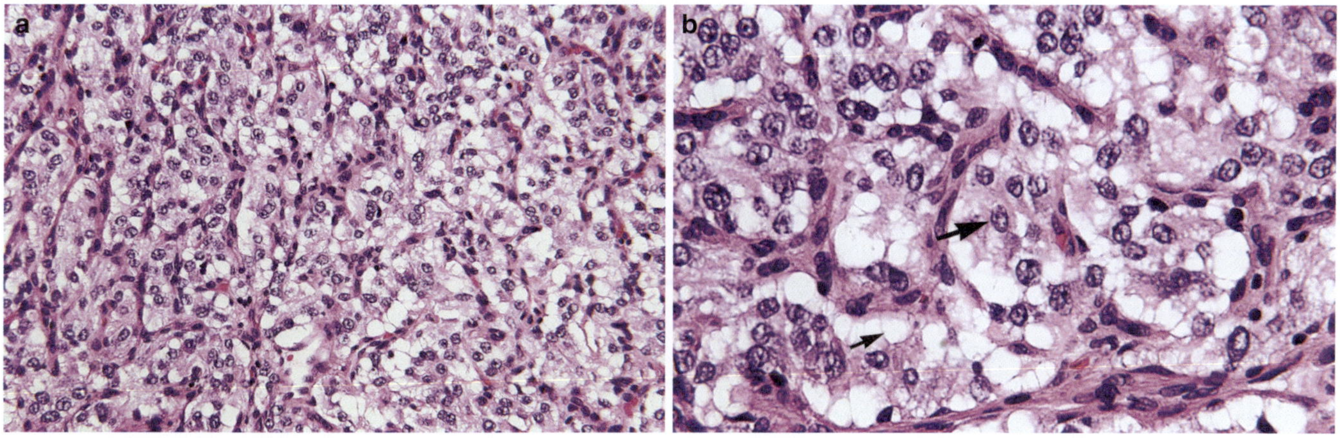

Fig. 19.7 (**a**) Photomicrograph (hematoxylin and eosin stain) of a glomus jugulare. (**b**) Higher magnification photomicrograph (hematoxylin and eosin stain) of a glomus jugulare showing the nest of chief cells (large black arrow). Zellballen are seen with surrounding sustentacular or supportive cells (small black arrow)

considered determinants of malignant behavior. Unmyelinated nerve fibers may be present [1].

Clinical Manifestations

A paraganglioma (PGL) may be sporadic or part of an inherited syndrome (types 1–5) with an autosomal dominant mode of transmission with genetic imprinting and variable penetrance. Certain hereditary forms (PGL1 and PGL2) are characterized by a higher incidence of multicentricity and associated tumors [14, 21]. These paragangliomas exhibit paternal genetic imprinting, such that the offspring of females carrying the mutated gene do not express the phenotype. In contrast, inheriting a mutated copy from the father results in phenotypic expression with high penetrance. In contrast, PGL3 and PGL5 are less common and appear to have less penetrance. PGL4 carries a much higher risk of malignant disease [12, 14].

Early-stage paragangliomas present with symptoms related to involvement of the middle ear cleft. Pulsatile tinnitus and conductive hearing loss are the most common presenting symptoms [4, 22, 23]. A glomus tympanicum tends to spread through pathways of least resistance along the peritubal air cells, intrapetrous carotid artery, and petrous apex. A glomus jugulare manifests with pulsatile tinnitus and cranial neuropathy. Lower cranial neuropathies are present when the tumor erodes the medial wall of the jugular bulb and involves the pars nervosa [4]. These neoplasms tend to spread through the hypotympanic air-cell tract, around the jugular bulb, inferior petrosal sinus, and carotid artery and into the jugular foramen and posterior fossa. Fifty percent of tumors may present with a jugular foramen syndrome [17]. Lower cranial nerve (IX–XII) deficits are variable but common, especially in advanced stage tumors, and present as dysphagia, dysphonia, and aspiration [4, 24]. A glomus tympanicum appears as a retrotympanic red mass on the promontory. When a glomus jugulare erodes into the floor of the hypotympanum, it manifests similarly to a middle ear mass or aural polyp if associated with erosion of the tympanic membrane. Invasion of the middle ear results in conductive hearing loss. Paragangliomas encroach onto the ossicles but do not cause ossicular erosion [25]. Pulsatile tinnitus is an indicator of the tumor's hypervascularity. Brown's sign (tumor blanching with positive pressure using pneumatoscopy) or Aquino's sign (cessation of pulsations with compression of the ipsilateral carotid artery) may be seen [26].

As the tumor invades deeper structures, additional lower cranial neuropathies, sensorineural hearing loss, vertigo, and pain may ensue. Extension of the tumor through the facial recess and retrofacial air cells may result in encasement of the facial nerve. In large tumors, Horner syndrome, facial hypesthesia, and diplopia may follow extension into the carotid artery and intradural or extradural involvement of CN VI [24, 27]. Symptoms of unrelenting headaches, vomiting, and diplopia herald increased intracranial pressure secondary to intracranial involvement and obstruction at the level of fourth ventricle [4]. In one study, the posterior fossa was involved in 50% of the cases with jugular foramen syndrome and in 75% of the cases with CN XII neuropathy [17].

It is prudent not to biopsy a vascular middle ear mass. An aberrant carotid artery or high-riding, dehiscent jugular bulb may appear as a reddish or bluish mass in the hypotympanum and possibly masquerade as a glomus tumor. During a biopsy, proximal control is not possible with either vascular structure. Given the impressive vascularity of paragangliomas, it can be very difficult to obtain hemostasis from the biopsy site.

In cases of multicentricity and in clinical cases of secretory paragangliomas, an appropriate evaluation includes screening for other adrenal and extraadrenal tumors and for familial-type paragangliomas [5]. The incidence of secretory extraadrenal head and neck paraganglioma is low (<4%) [4]. A 24-hour urinary vanillylmandelic acid, plasma catecholamines, and urinary beta-metanephrines and normetanephrines may be obtained as part of the biochemical screening [28]. Patients with an isolated paraganglioma should still be questioned about symptoms of labile hypertension or attacks of headache, anxiety, flushing, and sweating. Given the rarity of functional head and neck paragangliomas, these symptoms are more likely related to an undiagnosed pheochromocytoma, which is important to diagnose preoperatively. Similarly, elevated levels of plasma catecholamines in an isolated head and neck paraganglioma should still prompt a search for a pheochromocytoma. The anesthesia provider should be aware of this diagnosis, and perioperative alpha blockade should be considered to avoid a catecholaminergic crisis. Gadolinium-enhanced magnetic resonance imaging (MRI) of the head and neck is the gold standard for screening for multicentric paragangliomas.

The role of neuroradiology in determining the origin, extent, and nature of the tumor is crucial. Its role is not only limited to characterization of the lesion itself but is also essential in differentiating these lesions from vascular anomalies or temporal bone malignant neoplasms and in screening for other contralateral or ipsilateral lesions in cases of familial paragangliomas [29].

On high-resolution computed tomography (CT) of the temporal bone, a glomus tympanicum in its early phases appears as a well-circumscribed, soft-tissue mass localized on the promontory. The differential diagnosis of a soft-tissue density confined to the promontory includes congenital cholesteatoma, a persistent stapedial artery, and an aberrant carotid artery [30]. Radiographically, glomus jugulare tumors are associated with an irregular erosive enlargement of the jugular plate (floor of the hypotympanum) and the jugulocarotid spine, a pattern described as "moth-eaten" (Fig. 19.8a) [31]. Depending on their origin, these neoplasms can extend through the skull base to involve the jugular foramen in its neural and vascular compartments. Eventually,

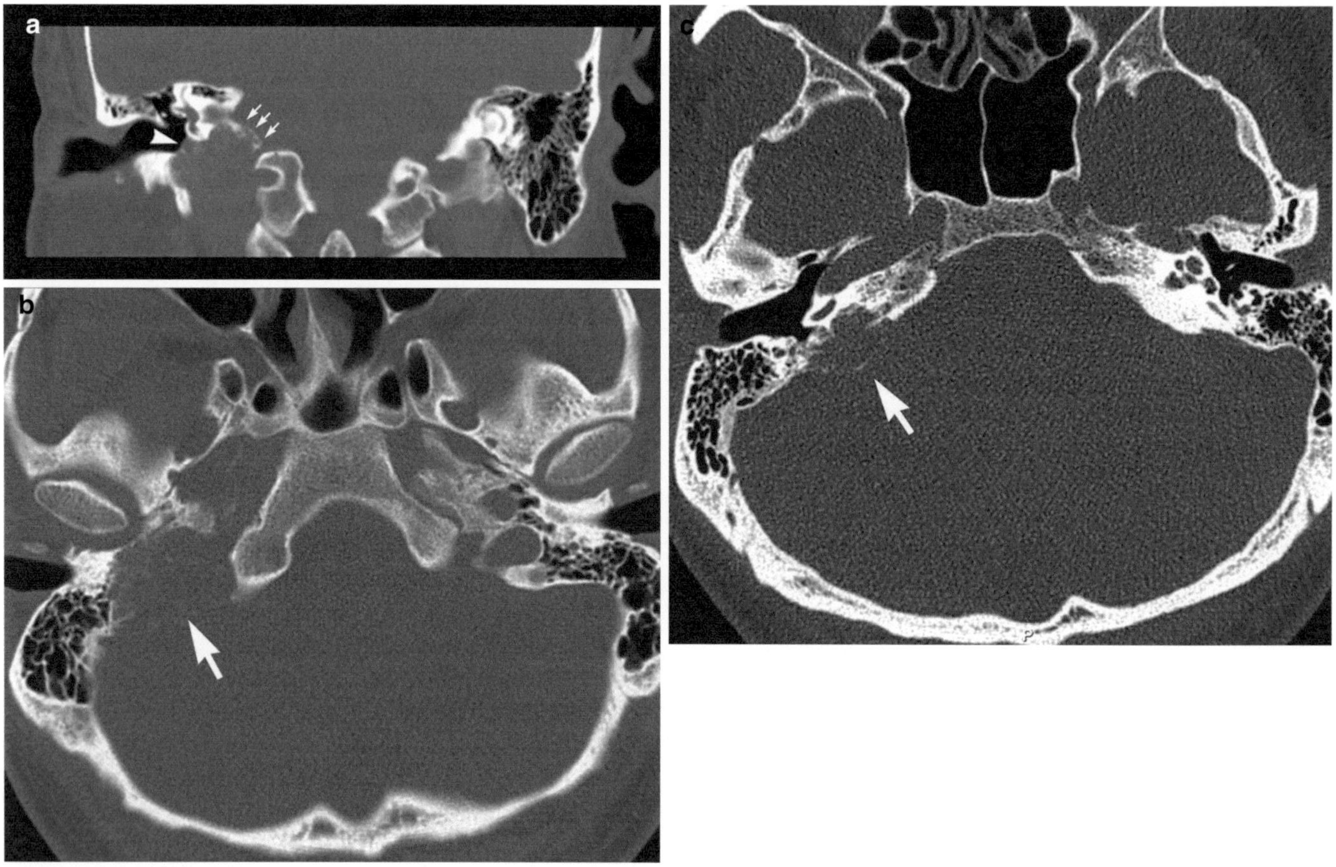

Fig. 19.8 (**a**) High-resolution CT of the temporal bone, coronal view, shows a glomus jugulare extending toward the posterior fossa. Note the irregular borders, moth-eaten appearance (small white arrows), and erosion of the floor of the hypotympanum (arrowhead). (**b**) High-resolution CT of the temporal bone, axial views, shows a lesion extending from the jugular bulb into the posterior fossa consistent with a glomus jugulare. (**c**) Note the moth-eaten appearance and irregular borders

they progress intracranially through intradural or extradural pathways, or extracranially through cervical extension.

Contrast-enhanced MRI is superior for evaluating tumor vascularity, extension along neural foramina, and multicentricity. Magnetic resonance venography is helpful to evaluate patency of the entire venous system and is important to study before making decisions regarding surgical approach [32]. On T1-weighted MRI, paragangliomas appear hypointense and speckled. On gadolinium-enhanced T1-weighted MRI, early and pronounced enhancement reflects the hypervascular nature of the neoplasm. On T2-weighted MRI, paragangliomas are hyperintense. When larger than 2 cm, the serpentine flow void pattern is described as a "salt and pepper" appearance [32, 33].

On catheter angiography, paragangliomas exhibit an intense blush or a "bag of worms" appearance. Magnetic resonance angiography (MRA) may substitute for catheter angiography to evaluate the vascularity of skull-base tumors (Fig. 19.9). However, small vascular anomalies and arterial feeders are best seen on conventional angiography. Catheter angiography also provides the option for preoperative embolization. The latter may decrease intraoperative blood loss and operative time [34]. It is prudent to reassess the cranial nerve function after embolization to ascertain any embolization-related palsy, which is important to document before aggressive surgery is undertaken [4].

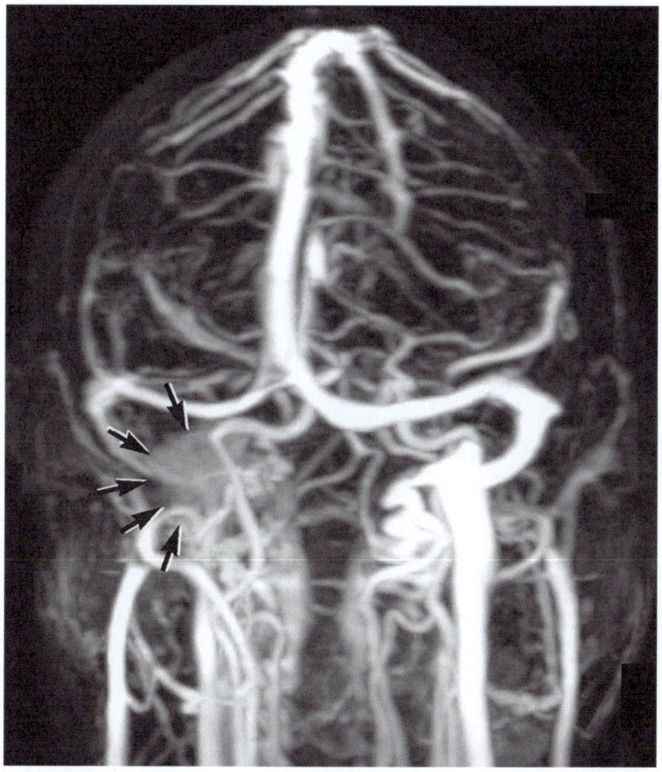

Fig. 19.9 Magnetic resonance venography of a patient with a left glomus jugulare (black arrows). The blush indicates hypervascularity. The magnetic resonance venography is important for assessment of the contralateral venous system. This patient has a patent contralateral jugular system

Classification Schemes

Different classification schemes for paragangliomas have been described to help guide surgeons in the selection of the most appropriate approach to eradicate the disease. The scheme devised by Fisch (Table 19.2) divides these lesions into four categories. Type A tumors are limited to the middle ear. Type B tumors are limited to the tympanomastoid compartment. Type C tumors involve the infralabyrinthine air-cell tract and intrapetrous carotid canal and extend into the petrous apex. Type D tumors have an intracranial extension.

The scheme described by Glasscock and Jackson (Table 19.3) divides jugulotympanic paragangliomas into four types. Type I tumors are small and involve the jugular bulb, middle ear, and mastoid. Type II tumors extend under the internal auditory canal and may have an intracranial extension. Type III tumors extend into the petrous apex with or without an intracranial extension. Type IV tumors extend beyond the petrous apex into the clivus, infratemporal fossa, or both. The House ear group adopted the classification devised by Antonio de la Cruz (Table 19.4). Jugulotympanic paragangliomas are considered tympanic when tumors are entirely confined to the mesotympanum. Tympanomastoid tumors extend beyond the limits of the mesotympanum without eroding the jugular plate. Jugular bulb tumors are confined to the jugular foramen without involvement of the

Table 19.2 Fisch paraganglioma staging system

Tumor type	Location
Type A	Tumor limited to middle ear
Type B	Tumor limited to tympanomastoid area with no infralabyrinthine involvement
Type C	Tumor involves infralabyrinthine compartment of temporal bone and extends into petrous apex
Type D1	Tumors with intracranial extension less than 2 cm
Type D2	Tumors with intracranial extension greater than 2 cm

Table 19.3 Glasscock and Jackson paraganglioma staging system

Tumor type	Location
Type I	Small tumor involving jugular bulb, middle ear, and mastoid
Type II	Tumor extends under internal auditory canal; may have an intracranial extension
Type III	Tumor extends into petrous apex; may have an intracranial extension
Type IV	Tumor extends beyond petrous apex into clivus or infratemporal fossa; may have an intracranial extension

Table 19.4 DE LA CRUZ paraganglioma staging system

Classification	Surgical approach
Tympanic	Transcanal
Tympanomastoid	Mastoid-extended facial recess
Jugular bulb	Mastoid-neck
Carotid artery	Infratemporal fossa
Transdural	Infratemporal fossa/intracranial

carotid artery or an intracranial extension. Carotid artery tumors involve the intrapetrous carotid artery. Transdural tumors extend intracranially.

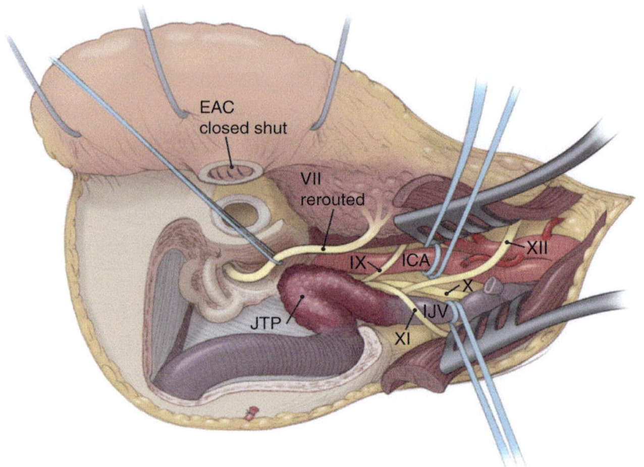

Fig. 19.10 Illustration showing the mastoid neck approach for removal of a large glomus jugulare. The labyrinth is preserved. The external auditory canal has been shut, and the facial nerve is elevated from the fallopian canal and retracted anteriorly. Vascular control is obtained by performing a neck exploration. Many surgeons advocate against rerouting the facial nerve because this maneuver results in a high incidence of facial paralysis. *EAC* external auditory canal, *ICA* internal carotid artery, *IJV* internal jugular vein, *JTP* jugulotympanic paraganglioma. Reproduced with permission from Barrow Neurological Institute

Operative Management

Tympanic paragangliomas may be completely excised via a transcanal approach. To ensure adequate exposure, the tympanic annulus is elevated circumferentially and left attached to the manubrium. The tumor is excised using cup forceps, and hemostasis is performed with hemostatic sealant or absorbable gelatin foam (Gelfoam®). Tympanomastoid tumors are removed via a classic mastoidectomy with an extended facial recess approach. Sometimes this approach can obviate the need to elevate a tympanomeatal flap.

For jugular bulb tumors, the mastoid-neck approach is used (Fig. 19.10). Only after preoperative embolization has been achieved is a mastoidectomy performed. The mastoid tip is removed along with the insertion of the sternocleidomastoid muscle. The posterior belly of the digastric muscle is dissected free and reflected anteriorly to expose the great vessels. The jugular vein is ligated in the neck. The proximal sigmoid sinus is packed extraluminally, and the anterior wall of the segment involved by the tumor is excised while preserving the posterior dural surface of the vein intact. Bleeding from the inferior petrosal sinus is controlled by packing, and the remainder of the tumor is removed. Preoperatively, some centers embolize the inferior petrosal sinus to minimize intraoperative bleeding and to facilitate neural microdissection [35].

Facial nerve rerouting can often be avoided if a fallopian bridge technique is used to access the tumor [36]. This technique involves removal of the retrofacial and infralabyrinthine air-cell tracts. Anatomical factors, such as an anteriorly displaced jugular bulb, may limit exposure.

For carotid artery and intracranial involvement, the infratemporal fossa approaches described by Fisch provide adequate access and corridor for removal of lesions. Detailing the surgical technique is beyond the scope of this discussion. Transdural involvement is addressed by different posterior fossa approaches. Paragangliomas involving the CPA are often extensive, and their treatment involves a combined extradural and intradural approach, which may or may not be a staged procedure [37].

The transpetrosal approaches, with or without facial nerve rerouting, with or without a transcochlear approach with additional craniotomies designed as dictated by tumor extension, may be performed for complete tumor excision [38, 39]. For tumors extending into the CPA without violating the otic capsule, a transsigmoid retrolabyrinthine approach may provide adequate exposure of the upper compartment of the CPA. For lesions with an inferior extension, a retrosigmoid approach, which can be combined with a far-lateral approach, may be needed. Lesions extending to the middle cranial fossa with preserved hearing may be removed using the subtemporal-retrolabyrinthine approach. These extensive operations are often associated with significant morbidity and increased operative time.

For elderly patients or for patients in whom extensive surgery is contraindicated, a limited surgical procedure with adjuvant radiotherapy may be advised. Symptoms have resolved with minimal resultant morbidity [40, 41]. Customized approaches can be used as well to preserve the conductive hearing apparatus, if feasible based on extent of disease [42].

Radiotherapy

Radiotherapy in the form of Gamma Knife radiosurgery (GKRS) or conventional radiotherapy has been used as an adjuvant, salvage, or primary treatment of paragangliomas [43–47]. Traditionally, radiotherapy was favored for poor surgical candidates or patients with bilateral tumors with an increased iatrogenic risk of bilateral vagal nerve dysfunction, or patients that refuse surgery [43]. However, there is an increasing number of publications reporting the use of radiotherapy as a first-line treatment in all patients. Primary radiosurgery for glomus jugulare tumors has been reported in more than 300 patients. A meta-analysis of these data showed 96% tumor control at 36 months.

However, similar to stereotactic radiosurgery for other benign pathologies, rates of long-term tumor control are lacking and provide a consistent concern. These tumors have an estimated growth rate of only 0.8 mm per year, which highlights the need to concentrate on long-term outcomes. Additionally, in long-term follow-up of recurrence following surgical resection, the mean time until recurrence was 82.8 months.

Reports of complications following radiosurgery mainly consist of new cranial nerve palsies. New neurologic deficits occur in 8.5% of patients with 2.1% of these deficits becoming permanent. Importantly, in the literature, these permanent deficits were grade II–IV facial palsies. There were no reported mortalities from radiosurgery. There are unfortunately no randomized control trials that compare radiotherapy and microsurgical treatment of these tumors. Direct comparison of the data, especially with respect to tumor control, is difficult due to the rarity of this tumor, selection bias, and inconsistencies in the data. All of these data also have an important temporal component, as surgeons have improved their technique and use of new technologies both inside and outside the operating room.

Endolymphatic Sac Tumors

Until recently, the entity of endolymphatic sac tumor (ELST) has been widely debated. Primary adenomatous neoplasms of the temporal bone have been reported [48]. In 1988, Gaffey and colleagues [49] referred to low-grade adenocarcinomas of the middle ear as aggressive papillary middle ear tumors. A year later, Heffner [50] described 20 cases of "adenocarcinoma of the endolymphatic sac" (AES). In 1993, Poe and colleagues [51] reported bilateral AES in a patient with VHL disease. Li and colleagues [52] applied the term ELST to the lesion initially described by Heffner.

ELSTs are rare neoplasms of the temporal bone. Their exact prevalence is unknown. They usually occur in sporadic forms but may be hereditary in the context of VHL disease. As of 2002, 43 cases had been reported in the English literature, 13 of which were bilateral [53].

ELSTs originate from the endolymphatic sac epithelium and are centered over the posterior portion of the petrous bone. They invade the posterior petrous ridge and involve the posterior fossa. In advanced stages, the CPA is involved. ELSTs should be considered in the differential diagnosis of a destructive temporal bone lesion involving the posterior fossa and CPA.

Pathology

The origin of ELSTs sparked an active debate. The biological behavior of ELSTs is best described as that of a low-grade neoplasm that is locally aggressive and destructive. Hematogenous metastasis has not been described. However, "drop metastasis" was recently reported in a patient who underwent multiple attempts to excise a large ELST [54]. The initial debate about the cells of origin, which included metaplastic middle ear mucosa, choroid plexus epithelium, and endolymphatic sac epithelium, has been resolved by immunohistochemical analysis of the differential expression of transthyretin [55]. Transthyretin, a known marker of choroid plexus epithelium, was present in five patients with a choroid plexus papilloma and in none of four patients with ELST. Transthyretin is normally detected in choroid plexus epithelium and is absent in epithelial cells of the endolymphatic sac. This differential expression clearly makes a common origin highly unlikely and categorizes these tumors as not originating from the adjacent choroid plexus.

Another interesting histopathological finding was described in the temporal bone of a patient with VHL who succumbed to his disease [56]. The patient harbored a large destructive lesion in his temporal bone thought to be metastatic from papillary thyroid cancer. However, subsequent analysis revealed features consistent with ELST. On the contralateral site, the same patient harbored a small focus of an intraductal in situ papillary tumor confined to the endolymphatic duct. This lesion is believed to be the precursor lesion for ELST and suggested that the endolymphatic duct and sac are the sites of origin of ELST.

A radiographic review of the site of the lesion in 8 patients with ELST suggested that the endolymphatic sac was the epicenter of the lesion [56].

ELSTs are locally aggressive neoplasms that cause bony destruction and infiltration with minimal osteogenesis or sclerosis. Histologically, they contain cystic and papillary components. The epithelium of the papillary component is lined with a single cell layer of cuboidal or low columnar epithelium (Fig. 19.11) [57]. ELST may contain areas of hemosiderin deposits, fibrosis, and cholesterol clefts. The cystic component contains a proteinaceous material reminiscent of thyroid colloid. It stains positively with periodic acid-Schiff stain [50]. Thyroglobulin stains are essential to rule out a metastatic thyroid carcinoma. The hypervascularity of the tumor is reflected by an abundant vascular stroma.

Immunohistochemical analysis shows that ELSTs stain positively with cytokeratin, S-100, and neuron-specific

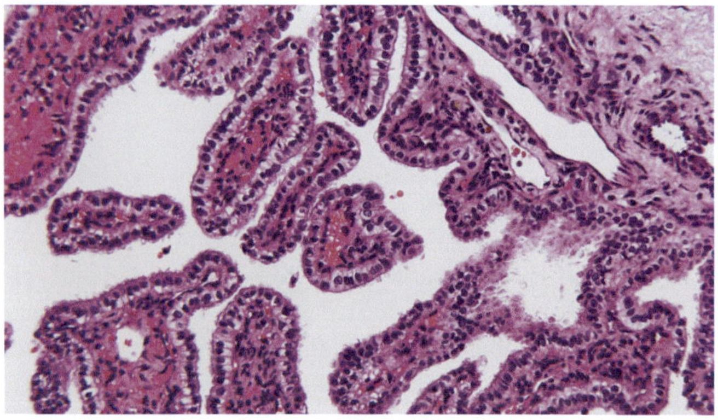

Fig. 19.11 Photomicrograph of an endolymphatic sac tumor showing papillary structures lined with cuboidal cells

enolase, suggesting a neuroectodermal origin [58–60]. However, the absence of reactivity to antibodies directed against glial fibrillary acid protein and transthyretin argues against a glial or choroidal origin [55].

ELST and VHL

VHL is an autosomal dominant disorder due to a germline mutation of the VHL tumor-suppressor gene localized on chromosome 3p25 [61]. The prevalence of the disease is estimated to be 1 in 39,000 [62]. It is characterized by an inherited predisposition to visceral (renal cell carcinomas and cysts, pheochromocytomas, pancreatic neuroendocrine tumors, and reproductive adnexal cystadenomas) and central nervous system (CNS) neoplasms (cerebellar and brainstem hemangioblastomas, retinal angiomas, and ELST) (Fig. 19.12).

In the Online Mendelian Inheritance in Man, an online catalog, ELST has been associated with VHL disease (No. 193300) [63]; it occurs in 11 to 16% of patients with VHL. Bilateral involvement has been described in 30% of the cases of ELST associated with VHL [53].

The phenotypic expression of VHL occurs with loss of both copies of the tumor-suppressor gene. In its hereditary form, a germline mutation results in the absence of one allele. The loss of heterozygosity or "single-hit" mutation of the second allele results in phenotypic expression [64]. In a study of three patients with ELST using fluorescence in situ hybridization analysis, loss of heterozygosity was seen in tumor cells but not in normal adjacent cells [65].

The VHL gene product pVHL regulates the expression of hypoxia-inducible factor-1 (HIF-1) [66–69]. In the absence of hypoxia, pVHL activates the degradation of HIF-1 through the activation of E3 ubiquitin ligase [68, 69]. In hypoxemic conditions and in VHL-deficient cells, the absence of degradation of HIF-1 leads to activation of downstream products: vascular endothelial growth factor, platelet-derived growth factor-B, and transforming-growth factoralpha [68]. The accumulation of these growth factors may play an important role in tumorigenesis.

Clinical Manifestations

ELSTs can occur sporadically or in the context of VHL. If ELSTs occur in the context of VHL, associated tumors may be present at diagnosis. In a study of 121 patients with VHL, 13 (11%) patients showed evidence of 15 ELSTs on MRI [70]. Sensorineural hearing loss; acute, fluctuating, or progressive episodic vertigo; aural fullness; and tinnitus were commonly described [56, 70–72]. These symptoms are reminiscent of Ménière's disease, and their combination occurs in 21% of patients [71]. Auditory and vestibular complaints are present in 59% of VHL patients without evidence of ELST on MRI [70]. Facial weakness is described in 43% of patients [71]. Other cranial neuropathies and headache have been described.

The mechanism of cochleovestibular dysfunction has been postulated [65]. In small ELSTs, obstruction of the endolymphatic duct [73], overproduction of endolymph, intraductal hemorrhage, and neuronal degeneration may be responsible for acute, fluctuating, or progressive hearing loss and vertigo. Evidence of intralabyrinthine hemorrhage may be the first sign of an ELST not detectable on imaging. In large ELST, otic capsule destruction and neuronal degeneration may explain the symptoms described. At this stage, image-detectable ELSTs are diagnosed radiographically.

Diagnosis

A patient diagnosed with VHL should undergo MRI screening for an ELST. A high index of suspicion is needed as early detection may offer the patient the potential benefit of a hearing-preservation surgical approach. Often, these patients are initially diagnosed with Ménière's disease because of their hearing loss and vertigo. Audiologic data can help characterize the type of hearing loss. In most cases, sensorineural hearing loss is present. Conductive loss may be associated with tumors invading the middle ear cleft. Vestibular testing may show caloric weakness but is of limited diagnostic value.

Radiological studies are very useful in the evaluation of suspected ELST. The typical finding on a high-resolution CT of the temporal bone is a destructive lesion confined to the posterior fossa, often centered over the posterior plate of the petrous bone (Fig. 19.13) [56, 74]. The lesion shows stippled, reticular, and speculated areas of calcification [75]. In patients with VHL, evidence of intralabyrinthine hemorrhage on noncontrasted high-resolution CT may be the first sign of a tumor undetectable by imaging [65].

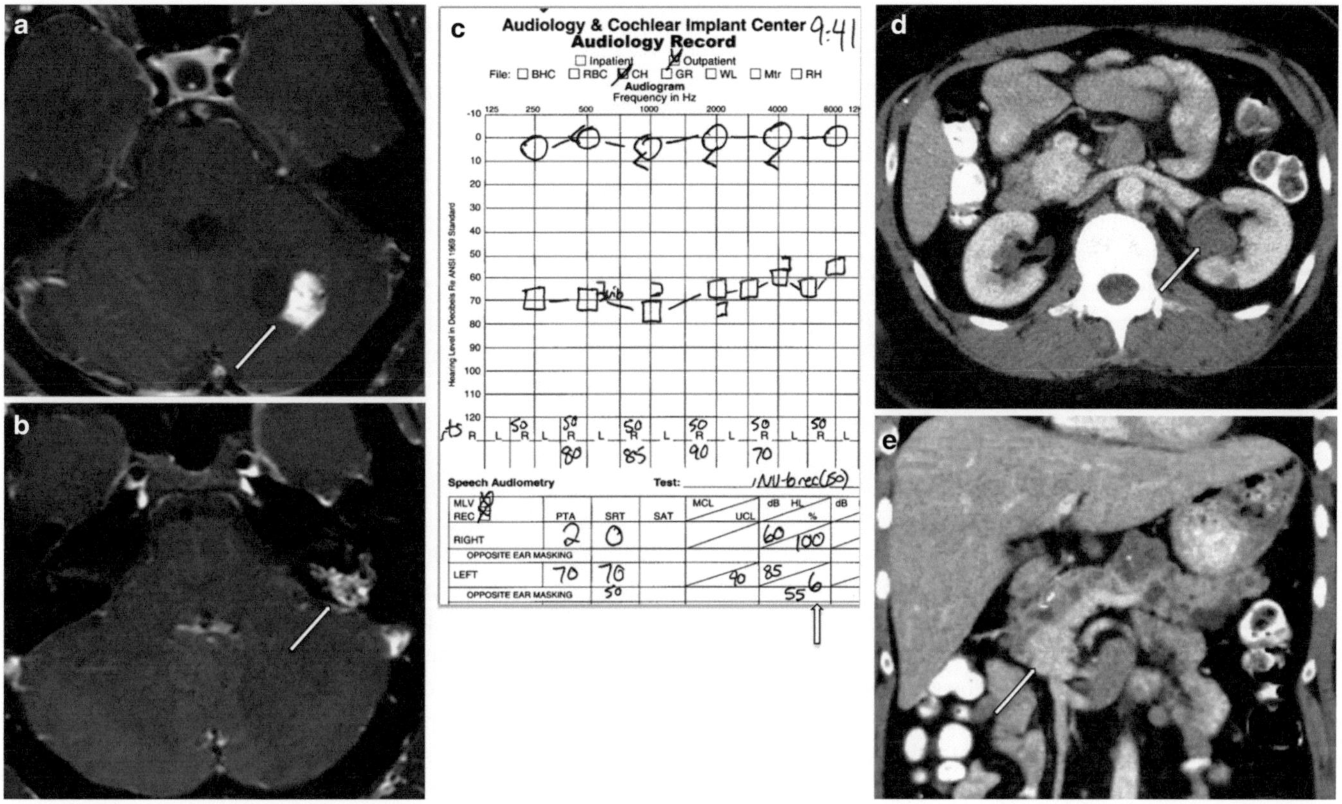

Fig. 19.12 Von Hippel-Lindau (VHL) disease. MRI (axial cuts) revealed (**a**) a cerebellar lesion as well as (**b**) a heterogeneously enhancing lesion centered over the left temporal bone/posterior fossa plate. (**c**) Audiogram revealed left-sided sensorineural hearing loss with poor word discrimination. (**d,** and **e**) Abdominal imaging showed a pancreatic lesion, concerning for neuroendocrine tumor, as well as renal cysts

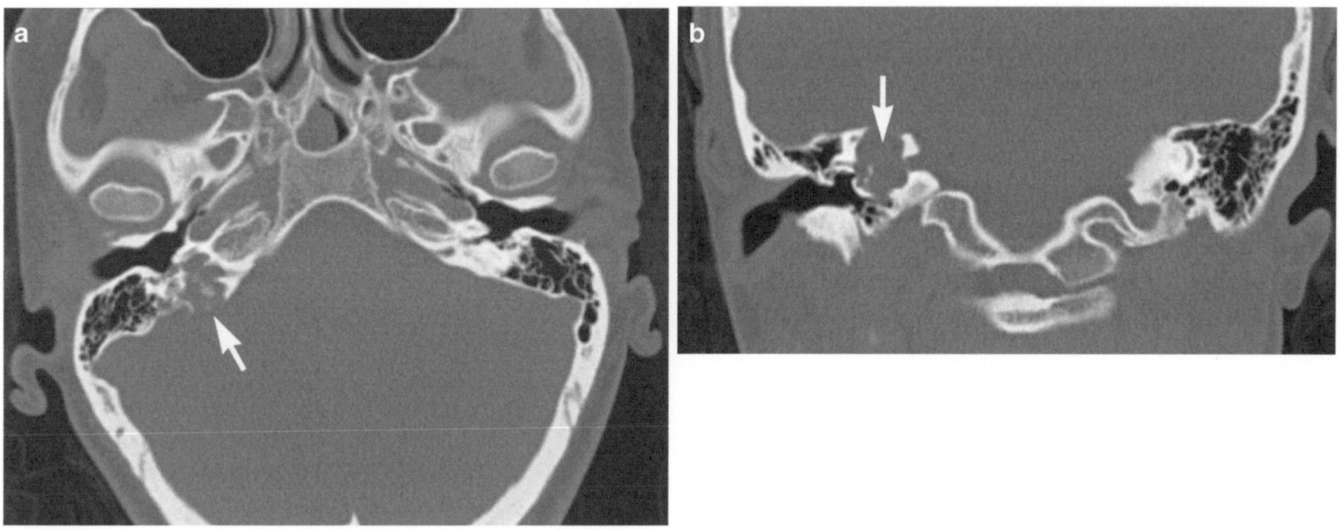

Fig. 19.13 (**a**) High-resolution CT of the temporal bone, axial view, showing endolymphatic sac tumor (white arrow). Note the destructive pattern, the location along the posterior petrous ridge, and the presence of spicules and calcifications. (**b**) Coronal view showing destruction of otic capsule (white arrow)

Follow-up with repeat MRI is recommended. On T1-weighted MRI, intralesional foci of hyperintensity are seen in 79% of tumors larger than 3 cm. Nonenhanced T1-weighted MRIs of tumors less than 3 cm show a circumferential rim of increased intensity [74, 75]. This rim is likely the result of subacute hemorrhage at the periphery of the tumor. ELSTs enhance with gadolinium. On T2-weighted MRI, a heterogenous pattern of intensity is often associated with an internal flow void in tumors larger than 2 cm [74]. The tumor may spread through the posterior fossa dura into more anterior regions, particularly the CPA and jugular foramen.

On catheter angiography, ELSTs are highly vascular. In tumors smaller than 3 cm, the vascular supply is usually only from the external carotid artery. In tumors larger than 3 cm, additional vascular supply is recruited from the posterior circulation [74].

Recently, a staging system with therapeutic implications was described (Table 19.5) [76]. Stage I tumors are confined to the temporal bone and middle ear cleft. Stage II tumors extend to the posterior fossa. Stage III tumors are more advanced, with a middle fossa extension. Stage IV tumors are far-advanced lesions that extend to the clivus and sphenoid.

Treatment

The therapeutic modality depends on the size of the lesion, stage of the tumor, and patient's hearing status (Table 19.5). Several reports of tumor removal showed resolution of vestibular symptoms and stabilization of hearing [71, 72].

In a patient with a stage I ELST and serviceable hearing, the tumor may be completely removed through a retrolabyrinthine transdural approach. This approach allows hearing preservation and tumor removal by excision of the dural base and lip of tumor extending into the endolymphatic duct [53, 72]. However, this approach offers limited access to anteriorly located lesions and a decreased angle of exposure in patients with an anteriorly displaced sigmoid sinus.

Table 19.5 Grading and treatment system for endolymphatic sac tumors [74]

Grade	Tumor extent	Surgical options
I	Confined to temporal bone, middle ear cavity, and/or external auditory canal	Hearing preservation with RLT approach
II	Extension into posterior fossa	Extended RLT approach with labyrinthectomy if hearing poor
III	Extension in posterior fossa and middle cranial fossa	Subtemporal craniotomy with petrosectomy[a]
IV	Extension to clivus and/or sphenoid wing	Staged anterior and posterior fossa techniques[a]

Modified with permission from Lippincott Williams and Wilkins [74]
[a]Preoperative embolization for grades II-IV and postoperative stereotactic radiosurgery for postoperative residual disease may be adjunctive. *RLT* retrolabyrinthine

Hearing preservation surgery is particularly important in patients with VHL, in whom the incidence of bilateral involvement is 30%. Hearing preservation is a desirable goal to avoid the social consequences of profound bilateral hearing impairment.

For larger lesions that extend into the posterior fossa (stage II), hearing may be affected and tumors are removed using an extended retrolabyrinthine transdural approach or translabyrinthine approach. The posterior fossa dura is resected and reconstructed. Failure to remove the dural attachment of the posterior fossa at the site of the endolymphatic sac and the intraductal portion of the tumor may lead to a recurrence [53, 72]. In lesions with a significant posterior fossa or middle fossa extension (stage III) and serviceable hearing, a combined approach involving a subtemporal craniotomy with petrosectomy provides good access without violating the hearing end-organ. In extensive lesions involving the petrous apex and CPA (stage IV), a transcochlear approach can be performed with complete exenteration of the otic capsule and exposure of the carotid canal. However, given the high rate of facial weakness following facial nerve mobilization, many authors have argued that staged anterior and posterior fossa approaches provide a less morbid strategy.

When tumors are excised completely, recurrence is rare. In a small published series [53, 71, 72], complete resolution of vestibular symptoms and stabilization of hearing was achieved when a hearing-preservation procedure was performed.

Hemangiomas of the Geniculate Ganglion and Internal Auditory Canal

Hemangiomas are benign neoplasms of blood vessels. They are the most common neoplasms of infancy. They frequently affect the skin and soft tissue, but bone involvement is also well described. Hemangiomas are not apparent at birth but develop soon thereafter. Their typical progression is characterized by an initial proliferative phase that lasts about 18 months, followed by an involution phase. Regression occurs over 2–9 years, and hemangiomas are gradually replaced by fibrofatty tissues.

Hemangiomas of the skull-base and temporal bone are rare lesions. In 1984, a review of the literature found 21 reported cases of skull-base hemangiomas [77]. In the temporal bone, lesions appear to have a predilection for the internal carotid artery, middle ear, and geniculate ganglion. Pulec is credited for the first description of a geniculate ganglion hemangioma in 1969 [78]. These hemangiomas differ from their pediatric counterparts in that they are often seen in middle-aged individuals and show no clear pattern of involution.

Recent work has confirmed the monoclonal nature of endothelial cell proliferation, which is modulated by a dysregulation in the mediation of endothelial cell growth [79]. Hemangiomas appear as rubbery red or purple masses. Histologically, they are characterized by a proliferation of small- or medium-sized vessels lined by endothelial cells that often appear as cystic spaces filled with blood. In osseous hemangiomas, these proliferating endothelial cells are interspersed within bony trabeculae. The adjacent bone appears "moth-eaten," and bony spicules are occasionally seen [80]. This appearance is not of an invasive nature; rather, it represents a reactive bony change.

Hemangiomas of the geniculate ganglion and internal auditory canal are extraneural tumors that likely originate from the perineural capillary network of the corresponding nerve [81]. Despite their extraneural origin, neural invasion is often seen on histological specimens. This infiltration can be extensive, rendering preservation of the nerve impossible and resulting in nerve transection and subsequent graft placement [82].

Compressive symptoms occur at an early phase even with small tumors involving the internal auditory canal or geniculate ganglion [80]. The floor of the middle fossa is almost always dehiscent over the tumor. Geniculate ganglion hemangiomas may involve the distal part of the facial nerve but do not extend beyond the cochleariform process. Medial growth beyond the labyrinthine portion of the facial nerve toward the internal auditory canal is not seen. However, hemangiomas that arise in the internal auditory canal may extend more medially toward the CPA but not laterally toward the geniculate ganglion [83].

In contrast to the majority of temporal bone neoplasms, the most common presenting symptom associated with geniculate ganglion hemangiomas is progressive facial palsy. Facial nerve paresis may develop even when lesions are small. The facial palsy may mimic idiopathic facial nerve paralysis or Bell's palsy. Responsiveness to steroid therapy does not exclude the diagnosis because discontinuation of steroids is often followed by recurrence of the facial weakness. Less frequently, the onset of facial paralysis is acute [84]. Facial twitching and hemifacial spasms may be the presenting symptoms. These symptoms are indicative of nerve compression or irritation. Involvement of the greater superficial petrosal nerve may result in epiphora or dry eyes.

Extension into the middle ear causes conductive hearing loss by disturbing the ossicular chain. Hemangiomas eroding the otic capsule, creating a cochlear fistula, may cause sensorineural hearing loss. Sensorineural hearing loss may be the presenting symptom associated with hemangiomas of the internal auditory canal [80, 85]. Similar to other symptoms from hemangiomas, hearing loss may occur at very early stages. Tinnitus is also common [80, 85].

Audiometry helps delineate the type of hearing loss. In geniculate ganglion hemangiomas, hearing loss is conductive. The acoustic reflex is usually absent because the site of the lesion is proximal to the exit of the stapedial branch of the facial nerve [82]. Internal auditory canal hemangiomas cause sensorineural hearing loss, even when a lesion is small [80, 85]. A cochlear fistula causes sensorineural hearing loss. However, a fistula may be found at surgery despite a normal preoperative audiogram [82].

Given the overlap in clinical presentation, it is important to distinguish these lesions from facial nerve schwannomas. On MRI, hemangiomas classically are hyperintense on T1-weighted and T2-weighted images. In contrast, schwannomas are typically isointense or hypointense on T1-weighted images. Both lesions homogenously enhance with contrast administration. The notable exception is cavernous hemangiomas, which can be isointense on T1-weighted images. Heterogeneous signal intensity on T2-weighted MRIs is also suggestive of a geniculate hemangioma [83].

On high-resolution temporal bone CT, schwannomas usually are larger masses with sharp bony margins. Roughly half of hemangiomas will produce a "honeycomb" appearance on CT, with hyperdense intratumoral spicules and irregular bony margins. The presence of calcifications in an expansile-appearing, soft-tissue density, "ossifying hemangioma" in the region of the geniculate ganglion is usually diagnostic [83, 84, 86]. The lesion often extends into the labyrinthine portion of the nerve and into the distal tympanic segment. The absence of bony coverage of the middle fossa also suggests a hemangioma. Contrasted MRI is superior for the evaluation of lesions confined to the internal auditory canal, but high-resolution CT may be superior in visualizing a geniculate ganglion lesion [80, 85]. When differentiating these lesions, it is important to remember that the presence of facial paralysis in the context of a small lesion (less than 10 mm) is more suggestive of a hemangioma [80].

Similar to other neoplasms that involve the facial nerve, treatment should be individualized with consideration of anatomic location, preoperative facial nerve function, preoperative hearing function, and the potential need for nerve reconstruction. Surgical resection is the mainstay of therapy for hemangiomas involving the geniculate ganglion and internal auditory canal. For lesions localized to the geniculate ganglion in patients with poor hearing, a transmastoid approach provides exposure to remove the lesion and graft the resected nerve. In the more common situation of patients with preserved hearing, the middle fossa approach provides better access that allows tumor resection and nerve grafting. The approach is typically extradural. The dura is easily elevated from the underlying tumor [80, 84].

Although the neoplasm is essentially extraneural, excision while preserving continuity of the nerve is not always the expected outcome. Neural invasion is frequently noted at surgery [80, 82, 84]. Therefore, preservation of the continuity of the nerve and complete excision of the tumor are not always possible, even when lesions are small. The surgeon should be prepared to graft the nerve with a greater auricular or sural nerve cable graft. Patients should be counseled that there is a high likelihood of severe facial nerve dysfunction following surgery. A cochlear fistula also may be seen intraoperatively in patients with normal preoperative hearing. The postoperative occurrence of significant sensorineural hearing loss is a real risk and patients should be counseled appropriately.

The timing of intervention is a matter of debate. Some advocate early intervention, especially in patients with small lesions, to optimize the chances of facial nerve preservation [80]. Advocates for this approach suggest that smaller lesions have less perineural reaction, increasing the chances of safely freeing the lesion from the nerve. Others believe that neural invasion can be seen at any stage and can be difficult to predict preoperatively. They therefore recommend waiting until facial nerve function is compromised by the tumor, then performing resection and nerve reconstruction. Because the best expected facial nerve outcome after a cable graft is House-Brackmann 3, patients are observed until facial nerve function deteriorates to a House-Brackmann 3 or worse [82]. There is also the concern that this delayed approach leads to poorer facial musculature function after reconstruction, due to facial muscle atrophy and fibrosis. Due to the rarity of these lesions and the need for individualized treatment, no prospective data exist to guide surgeons in choosing an optimal treatment strategy.

Carcinomas of the Temporal Bone

Squamous cell carcinomas are the most frequent primary malignancy of the temporal bone [87]. The neoplasms arise from the skin of the EAC or the middle ear cleft. In the EAC, squamous cell carcinomas are more common than basal cell carcinomas. Their prevalence is 0.8–1.0 per million [88]. Squamous cell carcinomas involving the CPA are often very advanced at the time of presentation and treatment is often palliative. Other types of carcinomatous neoplasms also can affect the temporal bone: adenocarcinomas that arise from salivary glandular tissue or apocrine and eccrine glandular elements in the EAC. Two malignant subtypes have been described: adenoid cystic carcinomas and ceruminous adenocarcinomas (ceruminomas). Their benign counterparts, pleomorphic adenomas and ceruminous adenomas, also may involve the EAC. They typically present as localized submucosal lesions, without extensive infiltration of surrounding soft tissue and neurovascular structures. Owing to their extreme rarity, a detailed discussion of these lesions is beyond the scope of this chapter.

Squamous cell carcinomas are locally invasive. For early-stage lesions, regional metastasis is uncommon [89]. The patterns of extension have been studied [89, 90]. Once the neoplasm becomes invasive, it spreads via pathways of least resistance along neurovascular structures, fissures, and foramina present within the confines of the temporal bone. Anteriorly, tumor cells transverse Santorini's fissures to extend into adjacent soft tissues. This anterior spread results in invasion of the temporomandibular joint capsule, zygomatic root, and infratemporal fossa. Typically, patients become symptomatic with trismus. Inferior spread may involve the stylomastoid foramen, extratemporal facial nerve, ramus of the mandible, and infratemporal fossa. Initially, medial growth of the neoplasm is limited by the presence of the tympanic membrane. However, tumor cells may extend into the middle ear around the tympanic annulus and eventually through the tympanic membrane. Erosion into the posterior wall can result in involvement of the mastoid portion of the temporal bone. Through the posterior and medial routes, tumor growth can progress to involve the ossicular chain, tympanic and mastoid portions of the facial nerve, sigmoid sinus, and intrapetrous portion of the carotid artery. Through involvement of the vestibule via the round and oval windows, the tumor may extend to the internal auditory canal and CPA. Spread along the sigmoid sinus, jugular bulb, and jugular foramen causes lower cranial nerve neuropathies. Involvement of the otic capsule is uncommon, but advanced lesions invade the labyrinth. Further extension and invasion of the posterior fossa dura ultimately result in the tumor entering the posterior fossa and CPA. Superiorly, the tumor can erode into the tegmen and invade the middle fossa and temporal lobe [91].

The histological subtypes differ in their degree of cellular differentiation. In the well-differentiated subtype, a more typical squamous architecture is recognized along with the presence of intercellular bridges and pearls of keratin. As cellular differentiation is lost, these findings disappear. The cellular appearance then becomes more disorganized and atypical. Poorly differentiated squamous cell carcinomas are characterized by numerous mitotic figures with irregular nests of atypical cells. Another rare subtype, spindle cell squamous cell carcinomas, demonstrates spindle-shaped cells with minimal resemblance to normal epithelial cells. This subtype may be difficult to differentiate from certain soft tissue sarcomas.

No clear etiological factor has been identified. Chronic suppurative otitis media has been suggested as a potential cause of middle ear squamous cell carcinomas [92]. Often, squamous cell carcinomas arise in a chronically draining ear. The chronic inflammation results in metaplasia of the middle ear mucosa, with possible progression to carcinoma.

Squamous cell carcinomas can mimic all the signs and symptoms associated with a chronically draining ear. Otorrhea, conductive hearing loss, and bloody ear drainage are common [92]. Severe otalgia, headache, and progressive cranial neuropathy in a draining ear should alert clinicians to the possibility of carcinoma. Examination of the EAC reveals a red, exophytic lesion or a raised ulcerated plaque. If a vascular lesion has been excluded, any suspicious aural polyp should be biopsied [93]. In advanced-stage carcinoma, palpable cervical lymphadenopathy may be present. A palpable parotid mass can represent a primary parotid gland neoplasm with an extension toward the EAC or a sign of involvement of the deep and superficial lobes of the parotid gland by a squamous cell carcinoma originating in the EAC. Squamous cell carcinomas of the temporal bone involving the CPA are advanced lesions that usually destroy the inner ear structures and somewhat involve critical neurovascular structures.

Table 19.6 University of Pittsburgh staging system for temporal bone SCC [92]

Tumor type	Feature
T1	Tumor limited to EAC without bony erosion or evidence of soft tissue extension
T2	Tumor with limited EAC erosion or limited soft tissue involvement (< 0.5 cm)
T3	Tumor eroding osseous EAC with limited soft tissue involvement. Involves middle ear and mastoid
T4	Tumor eroding the cochlea, petrous apex, medial wall of middle ear, carotid canal, jugular foramen, or dura, associated with extensive soft tissue involvement (> 0.5 cm) or causes facial paralysis

SCC squamous cell carcinoma, *EAC* external auditory canal

Audiometry is helpful in delineating the type of hearing loss. Squamous cell carcinomas limited to the middle ear cleft usually cause conductive hearing loss. In a chronically draining ear, the status of the ossicular chain may be affected by the inflammatory process that might have preceded the neoplasm. In lesions extending into the CPA, sensorineural hearing loss is expected.

Imaging is the mainstay of the diagnostic workup. In addition to unraveling the extent of the lesion, imaging is crucial in determining the stage of the neoplasm (Table 19.6). Destruction of the bony architecture and involvement of the otic capsule are best seen on high-resolution CT [94]. Contrasted CT of the temporal bone may show the extent of the tumor in the surrounding soft tissue (Fig. 19.14). A neck CT with contrast shows the presence of cervical metastasis. However, if an intracranial extension is suspected or involve-

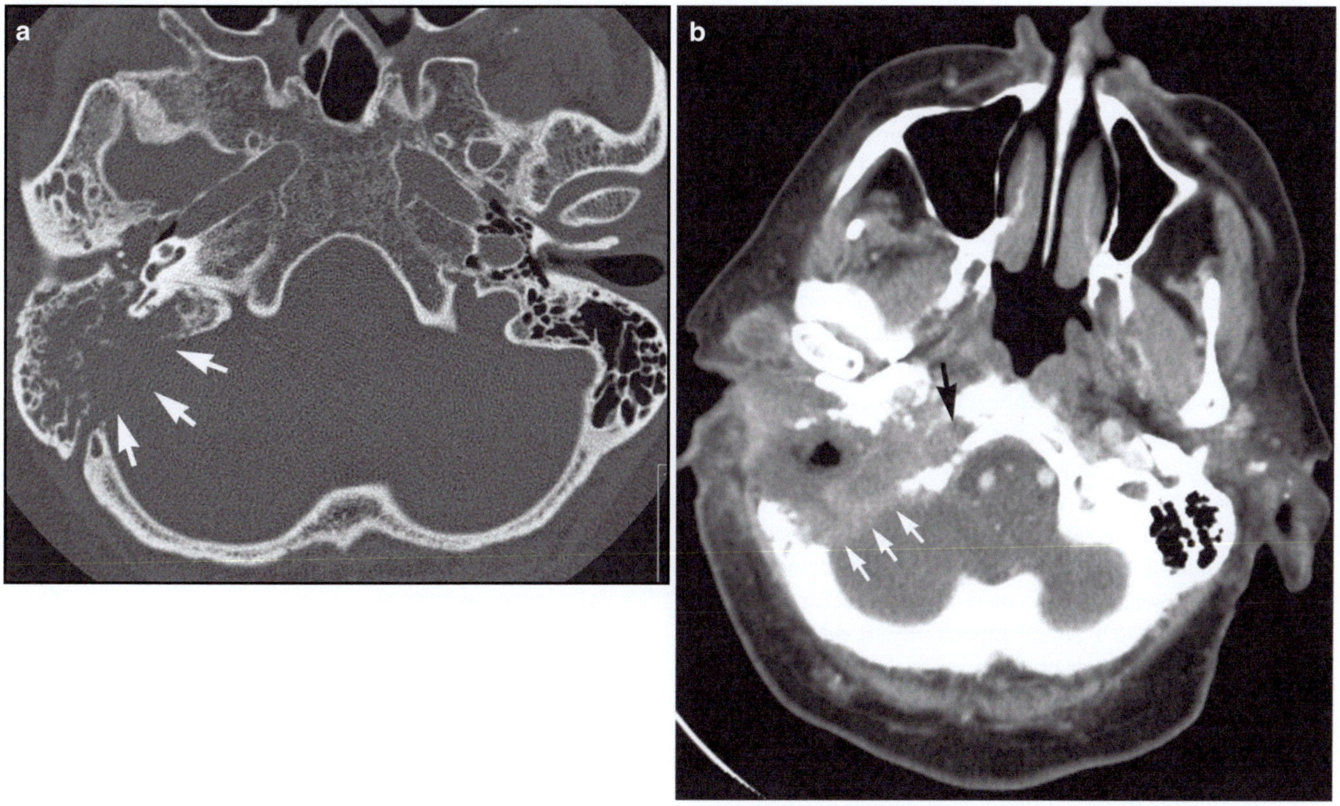

Fig. 19.14 (**a**) CT of the brain shows a destructive process involving the right temporal bone (white arrows). The process extends from the external auditory canal into the posterior fossa and is associated with destruction of the posterior fossa ridge, otic capsule, and mastoid air-cell system. The patient had a squamous cell carcinoma originating from the external auditory canal. (**b**) Note the anterior extension toward the petrous apex (black arrow)

ment of the soft tissue is not clearly evident, MRI with contrast is superior to high-resolution CT. Angiography helps evaluate the patency and integrity of the carotid artery, adequacy of the collateral circulation, and venous drainage. Carotid artery involvement or encasement requires a balloon occlusion test to determine the adequacy of the collateral circulation.

Before a therapeutic modality is selected, accurate knowledge of the tumor's extent, and thus of the T-stage, is essential. Surgical treatment of temporal bone neoplasms with the intent to cure is often a colossal task that requires the integrated efforts of multiple disciplines. The best treatment modality is still debated. En bloc resection of temporal bone neoplasms with adequate margins is not always possible [92, 94–96]. The commonly used alternative of a radical mastoidectomy with postoperative radiotherapy has been associated with poor survival rates at 5 years [93]. Results for advanced temporal bone lesions treated with an extended temporal bone resection, dural excision and grafting, partial resection of the temporal lobe, and postoperative radiotherapy have been encouraging [91]. Aggressive surgical treatment is associated with increased morbidity and mortality rates. Furthermore, postoperative defects often require major reconstruction using a free or regional flap. Obliteration of the resultant cavity and postradiotherapy tissue changes make it difficult to detect a recurrence.

The widely used staging system devised by the University of Pittsburgh has therapeutic implications [95]. A T1 lesion is managed with sleeve resection of the EAC, with preservation of the tympanic membrane and middle ear contents. Such localized lesions are uncommon. For T2 lesions, a lateral temporal bone resection with en bloc removal of the EAC, malleus, incus, and tympanic membrane is usually recommended. An extended facial recess approach is performed, and the bone anterior to the vertical portion of the facial nerve is removed. The tympanic annulus is removed along with the specimen. The facial nerve is followed into the stylomastoid foramen. Anteriorly, the dissection continues toward the zygomatic root superiorly and toward the temporomandibular joint inferiorly. The incudostapedial joint is dislocated, and the tensor tympani tendon is sectioned. Negative margins are confirmed with frozen-section analysis. A lateral temporal bone resection may be performed in conjunction with a partial or total auriculectomy, parotidectomy, and cervical lymphadenectomy. If the auricle has been removed, a fasciocutaneous free-tissue transfer or a regional musculocutaneous flap can be used for reconstruction.

A T3 lesion is treated with subtotal temporal bone resection. All contents of the temporal bone lateral to the internal auditory canal and carotid artery are removed. If resection of the sigmoid sinus or jugular bulb is anticipated, patency of the contralateral venous system should be ascertained. Such a defect is reconstructed using a trapezius flap or a rectus abdominis free-tissue transfer. Total temporal bone resection, with or without sacrifice of the carotid artery, with or without dural excision, and with or without partial resection of the temporal lobe, is recommended for T4 lesions. Adjuvant radiotherapy is advised for both T3 and T4 lesions.

Extensive brain involvement, invasion into the cavernous sinus, infratemporal fossa, and paraspinal muscles are associated with a grim prognosis [97]. Other negative prognostic factors are the presence of nodal metastasis, salvage surgery, and poorly differentiated subtype [98]. With the advent of contemporary skull-base microsurgical techniques and the use of more aggressive treatment, the cure rate for T1 and T2 lesions approximates 100%. In contrast, the cure rates for T3 and T4 lesions are 50 and 38%, respectively [98]. According to the staging system described by Arriaga and colleagues [95], temporal bone squamous cell carcinomas involving the CPA are considered T4 lesions. Treatment of advanced-stage squamous cell carcinomas with a significant extension into the CPA is, at best, palliative.

In summary, the original reports of aggressive surgical resection yielded poor overall survival rates at 5 years [96, 97, 99]. Multiple studies have highlighted the importance of aggressive, extensive surgical resection of lesions followed by postoperative radiotherapy to improve local control [98, 99]. Surgical treatment that sacrifices important neurovascular structures is met with some resistance. Most available data are limited to retrospective reviews of small series. Well-designed studies are needed to help elucidate this approach and to define outcomes better.

Soft Tissue Sarcomas

Soft tissue sarcomas are rare neoplasms derived from cells of mesenchymal origin. Depending on the cell type of origin, different histological variants exist. In the temporal bone, two types are of particular interest: chondrosarcomas and rhabdomyosarcomas. These two entities differ pathologically, clinically, and therapeutically and merit separate discussion.

Rhabdomyosarcomas

Rhabdomyosarcomas account for 5–15% of all childhood neoplasms and for 30% of temporal bone sarcomas [100, 101]. They are the most common malignant neoplasms of the temporal bone in childhood. Forty percent of rhabdomyosarcomas occur in the head and neck [102]. Commonly affected locations in the head and neck are the orbit, middle ear, oral cavity, nasopharynx, and infratemporal fossa [103]. Most occur before the age of 15 years; the mean age at presentation is between 4- and 5-years-old. In the head and neck, rhabdomyosarcomas are divided into three categories: orbital (23%), parameningeal (56%), and nonparameningeal (21%) [102]. Parameningeal denotes tumors that develop near the skull base and adjacent meninges.

Rhabdomyosarcomas are highly aggressive, locally destructive, malignant neoplasms of the soft tissue. Distant metastasis is present in 14% of patients at diagnosis and associated with the possibility of distal spread to the lungs, bone, liver, and brain [104]. In the temporal bone, it is hypothesized that rhabdomyosarcomas originate from the malignant transformation of myocytes residing in the stapedial or tensor tympani muscles. Four histological subtypes have been described: embryonal, alveolar, pleomorphic, and botryoid [105]. In the head and neck, embryonal rhabdomyosarcomas are the most frequently encountered histological subtype (85%) followed by alveolar rhabdomyosarcomas (15%) [102]. Histologically, embryonal rhabdomyosarcomas are characterized by the presence of elongated malignant cells with bipolar processes reminiscent of immature rhabdomyoblasts. A single central nucleus is typically present along with a relatively abundant eosinophilic cytoplasm. Alternating areas of hypercellularity and hypocellularity may be seen. In the hypercellular areas, dense small round blue cells can predominate, thereby including these neoplasms in the differential diagnosis of tumors with small round blue cells. Numerous mitotic figures are present. In hypocellular areas, a myxoid-appearing stroma is present [106].

The alveolar subtype shows clusters of cells resembling epithelial cells reminiscent of the pulmonary alveolus with intervening sheets of connective tissue. Striations can be present along with giant and multinucleated cells [105, 106]. The primitive appearance of some rhabdomyosarcomas makes their recognition difficult. The addition of immunohistochemical analysis is helpful in differentiating some of these cases. Antibodies directed against actin, sarcomeric actin, desmin, myogenin, and myoD1 can be useful [105].

Rhabdomyosarcomas of the middle ear grow and spread by destroying adjacent structures. Medial spread by early involvement and invasion of the fallopian canal is seen [103, 107]. Extension toward the mastoid bone is common. Involvement of the otic capsule and vestibule results in further medial spread toward the internal auditory canal and posterior fossa meninges. Superior extension through the tegmen results in involvement of the middle cranial fossa. Lateral and inferior extension of the neoplasm results in involvement of the EAC and area of the jugular foramen with further extension toward the infratemporal fossa and nasopharynx. Meningeal and CNS involvement portends a poor prognosis and warrants more aggressive therapy.

Diagnosis

In children, rhabdomyosarcomas mimic all the signs and symptoms of chronic suppurative otitis media [87, 101, 108–110]. The prevalence of infectious disease may delay diagnosis. Clinical suspicion should be heightened when patients have a middle ear or EAC mass or polyp, an unrelenting course despite aggressive antibiotic treatment, and pain associated with cranial neuropathy. Early diagnosis and institution of appropriate multimodality therapy are key elements to successful outcomes. Clinically, rhabdomyosarcomas can become symptomatic with earache, a middle ear and EAC mass or polyp, and intermittent bloody otorrhea. As the tumor invades surrounding structures, additional signs and symptoms develop: facial weakness, hearing loss, vertigo, trismus, and headache.

On temporal bone imaging, rhabdomyosarcomas exhibit the characteristics of locally aggressive neoplasms. On high-resolution CT [111], these lesions appear as a soft tissue density associated with infiltrative bony destruction and irregular erosion. The middle ear is commonly affected, and different parts of the petrous bone and adjacent areas are involved depending on the extent of the tumor. The administration of contrast material causes heterogenous enhancement.

MRI is helpful in the evaluation of meningeal and CNS involvement [112, 113]. On T1-weighted MRI, rhabdomyosarcomas typically have a homogenous appearance isointense to muscle. When gadolinium is administered, enhancement helps delineate the soft tissue component. On T2-weighted MRI, rhabdomyosarcomas show a hyperintense signal.

Ultimately, the rhabdomyosarcoma is diagnosed by histological confirmation. Biopsy material may be obtained from an aural polyp or by a myringotomy performed to access the middle ear. Tissue also can be obtained during a planned mastoidectomy.

Treatment

It became evident that treatment of temporal bone rhabdomyosarcomas requires a multimodality approach with surgery, radiation, and multiagent chemotherapy. Before multimodality therapy was available, middle ear and mastoid rhabdomyosarcomas were associated with a grim prognosis. Through the collaborative work of multiple study groups designed to classify and treat patients with rhabdomyosarcomas, the outcome of what was once considered a uniformly fatal disease has been transformed. The cure rate for these chemosensitive tumors now approaches 70% when multimodality therapy is used [114]. This dramatic improvement contrasts with the initial poor results obtained with single modality treatment (overall 5-year survival rate, 28%) [115].

The site, histological subtype, IRS stage, patient's age, and type of treatment are important prognostic factors [102, 116–118]. Parameningeal rhabdomyosarcomas have a worse prognosis than orbital and nonparameningeal rhabdomyosarcoma. Embryonal rhabdomyosarcomas have a better outcome than the alveolar type. Age greater than 10 years or less than 1 year is associated with the poorest outcome.

The current clinical classification used to predict tumor behavior and response to treatment in a given individual is the intergroup rhabdomyosarcoma study (IRS) classification system introduced in 1975 [104]. Group I refers to localized disease; group II refers to microscopic residual or regional disease; group III refers to individuals with incomplete resection or biopsy with gross residual disease; and group IV includes patients with metastatic disease at presentation.

The results of the studies performed by the IRS I through IV have increased understanding of the disease, ultimately reducing mortality rates and increasing the disease-free survival and overall survival rates [104, 119–121]. Before the institution of multimodality therapy, the survival rates for IRS clinical groups I, II, III, and IV were 0, 14, 0, and 0%, respectively [122]. To evaluate and compare the results of multimodality treatment, the IRS conducted a series of studies, IRS I to IV.

The IRS-I study [104] included 686 patients with a rhabdomyosarcoma or an undifferentiated sarcoma followed from 1972 to 1978. The results showed no additional benefit of radiotherapy to combination chemotherapy (vincristine and dactinomycin or vincristine alone) for clinical group I (localized disease completely resected). No benefit was associated with adding a daily low dose of oral cyclophosphamide to the combination of radiation and chemotherapy (vincristine and dactinomycin or vincristine alone) or with adding Adriamycin to the combination of radiation and chemotherapy (vincristine, dactinomycin, and cyclophosphamide). The 5-year survival rates for the entire group and for those with parameningeal rhabdomyosarcomas were 55 and 47%, respectively.

The IRS-II study [121] was conducted between 1978 and 1984 and included 999 patients with rhabdomyosarcoma. All patients were included after surgical treatment. In IRS clinical group III, the use of radiation and intrathecal chemotherapy increased the 5-year survival rate from 47 to 59%.

The IRS-III study [119] was conducted from 1984 to 1991 and included 1062 patients with rhabdomyosarcomas. The major difference in the intervention in the clinical group III was a reduction in the radiation fields for parameningeal rhabdomyosarcomas without intracranial extension and intensification of the chemotherapy regimen. In the clinical group III, the 5-year survival rate increased from 59 to 65%.

The IRS-IV study [120] was conducted from 1991 to 1997 and included 883 patients. For clinical group III, the study compared the efficacy of hyperfractionated radiotherapy with conventional radiotherapy and found no difference.

Currently, for parameningeal rhabdomyosarcomas, which include middle ear rhabdomyosarcomas, the recommended treatment is surgery for biopsy, followed by radiotherapy and chemotherapy. Although complete resection is the mainstay of treatment for trunk and extremity rhabdomyosarcomas, radical resection of parameningeal rhabdomyosarcoma results in high morbidity and is disfiguring. The timing of treatment is important. For parameningeal rhabdomyosarcomas with evidence of intracranial extension, radiotherapy should be given concurrently with chemotherapy [103].

Both chemotherapy and radiotherapy have been associated with complications. Ifosfamide is associated with renal tubular dysfunction. High-dose cyclophosphamide is associated with veno-occlusive disease, and multidrug regimens are associated with acute myelogenous leukemia [120, 123, 124].

The long-term side effects of radiotherapy led to the development of trials in Europe, where radiotherapy has been excluded from the initial management of low-risk groups and reinstituted in the event of recurrence. This rationale is based on the fact that the "salvage gap" can be restored with retreatment. Patients with no relapse who did not receive radiotherapy enjoyed a long-term disease-free survival without late sequelae [101]. Late sequelae include hormonal dysfunction, cognitive dysfunction, facial growth retardation, hearing loss, and dental and visual problems [124]. The application of this rationale to parameningeal rhabdomyosarcomas is not accepted because these patients are considered to be a high-risk group.

Hematologic Malignancies

Rarely the temporal bone may be involved by different hematopoietic malignancies. Most commonly, tumor cells infiltrate the temporal bone and its marrow spaces as part of a systemic disease process. Rarely, isolated involvement may be seen. Leukemia, lymphoma, and plasmacytoma can affect the petrous bone [125–127]. Although all parts of the petrous bone can be affected, the middle ear and mastoid are typically involved.

Leukemia is a neoplastic disorder that affects white blood cells and results in the proliferation and accumulation of a large number of immature lymphohematopoietic cells. By the time of diagnosis, leukemic cells have already infiltrated the bone marrow and spread to some extramedullary sites. The loss of differentiation and lack of apoptosis cause neoplastic cells to accumulate. Based on the particular morphologic and immunophenotypic characteristics of these tumors, different classification schemes have been described.

Detailing each subtype is beyond the scope of this chapter. In the temporal bone, symptoms are caused by infiltration and hemorrhage. Rarely, the hyperviscosity caused by the large number of leukocytes in the circulation can manifest with the acute onset of bilateral hearing loss [128]. Leukemic patients may become symptomatic with middle ear effusions, facial nerve palsy, vertigo, tinnitus, and sensorineural hearing loss [125, 127, 129, 130]. Histopathological studies of human temporal bones show infiltration of the cochleovestibular nerve and facial nerve [125, 131]. Inner ear involvement is uncommon [132]. In rare instances, the CPA is involved by the accumulation of neoplastic granulocytic cells, chloromas, usually seen in patients with acute myelogenous leukemia [133]. The treatment of acute or chronic leukemia involving the temporal bone is medical, and the role of surgery is limited to biopsy.

Lymphomas are neoplastic processes that affect the lymphoid system. Histologically, Hodgkin's lymphoma (HL) is characterized by the presence of Reed-Sternberg cells in a background of inflammatory stroma. HL is classified into different subsets based on morphologic and immunophenotypic criteria. The more common non-Hodgkin's lymphoma (NHL) is a heterogenous group of neoplastic disorders of the lymphoid system that lacks the characteristic cell type seen in HL. Both types of lymphomas infiltrate the bone marrow, middle ear, and eustachian tube mucosa [125, 134, 135]. Patients may present with middle ear effusion, hearing loss, and facial paralysis [136, 137]. Involvement of the temporal bone is less common with HL [138]. If no other extranodal sites are present, surgery is limited to biopsy. Medical management is the mainstay of treatment.

Plasmacytomas, monoclonal proliferation of plasma, or plasmacytoid cells are variants of multiple myeloma and comprise less than 10% of plasma cell dyscrasias [139, 140]. Two clinical forms have been described: solitary plasmacytomas of bone and extramedullary plasmacytomas. Solitary plasmacytomas of bone manifest with isolated bone involvement that usually affects the axial skeleton and extremities without clinical, radiographic, and immunoelectrophoretic evidence of multiple myeloma. Conversion to multiple myeloma usually occurs in more than half of the patients over 4–5 years. Extramedullary plasmacytomas present with a space-occupying lesion that consists of neoplastic proliferation of plasma cells outside the bone marrow—usually the upper aerodigestive tract and paranasal sinuses [126, 139]. Temporal bone involvement is rare. High-resolution CT shows a lytic process occasionally associated with a soft tissue mass [141, 142]. Plasmacytomas usually infiltrate the middle ear and mastoid; however, involvement of the otic capsule has been described [126, 142]. The diagnosis is based on the presence of extramedullary proliferation of monoclonal plasma cells without evidence of multiple myeloma on bone marrow biopsy. Treatment is usually radiotherapy and 25% of plasmacytomas recur. Progression to multiple myeloma is uncommon [143].

Regardless of their pathological type, low-grade and high-grade lymphohematopoietic neoplasms that originate from B or T cells or from plasma cells rarely affect the temporal bone. Clinically, these lesions can mimic any acute or chronic middle ear and mastoid pathology. Neural involvement in the form of hearing loss, tinnitus, vertigo, and facial paralysis is common. A high index of suspicion, mainly in patients with systemic disease, is necessary for timely diagnosis. The CPA is rarely involved, and most reported cases are limited to small series. A list of adjunctive laboratory tests is often necessary for appropriate diagnosis, and treatment is often nonsurgical. Different chemotherapeutic agents are used with or without radiotherapy. Radiotherapy alone is used to treat extramedullary plasmacytomas and isolated lymphomas. The role of the medical oncologist is essential for the care of these patients.

Metastasis of the Temporal Bone

Uncommonly, the temporal bone may harbor a metastasis from various carcinomatous neoplasms. The most common sites of origin are breast, lung, kidney, stomach, prostate, and melanoma [144–146]. In the temporal bone, metastatic disease commonly affects the petrous apex followed by the internal auditory canal [146]. In a study of 1354 CPA lesions, the incidence of metastatic disease was 0.2% [147]. Most published series are small and spaced over many years. The most important mechanism of spread is hematogenous seeding of the marrow-rich portion of the temporal bone. If neoplastic cells gain access to the cerebrospinal fluid-containing spaces, the internal auditory canal and CPA may be involved bilaterally [146].

Clinically, patients may become symptomatic during the course of a known malignancy. Or rarely, the temporal bone may be the revealing site. Hearing loss, facial palsy, and vertigo occur in 60, 50, and 30% of the patients, respectively [145]. The temporal bone may be involved in multiple sites in 20% of patients [146].

Radiographically, metastasis demonstrates a lytic process on high-resolution CT. MRI shows an infiltrative and destructive soft tissue mass with low signal intensity on T1-weighted images and high signal intensity on T2-weighted images. Enhancement is usually present (Fig. 19.15) [113]. The petrous apex is commonly involved, but other sites may be affected. The destructive process on radiologic studies often exceeds the clinical findings [144]. Prognosis is guarded, and treatment is palliative. If clinically indicated, surgery is limited to tissue confirmation. Palliative treatment includes chemotherapy, with or without radiotherapy, as dictated by the nature of the primary lesion.

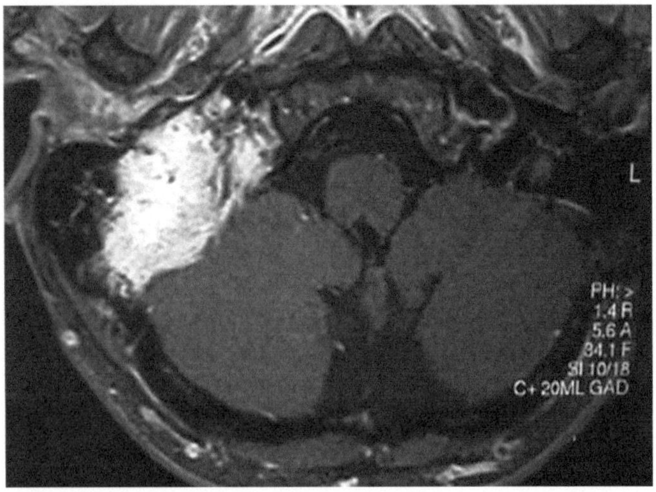

Fig. 19.15 Gadolinium-enhanced MRI of the temporal bone shows an enhancing metastasis from a renal cell carcinoma associated with destruction of the posterior dural plate and invasion of the CPA

Cholesterol Granulomas

Cholesterol granulomas arise in the pneumatized spaces of the temporal bone. Their pathogenesis remains unclear. However, it is believed that cholesterol granulomas result from occlusion of the temporal bone air-cell system. The resultant negative pressure causes hemorrhage into the air-cell system and subsequently a foreign-body reaction and formation of an inflammatory granuloma. The formed granuloma expands to involve adjacent areas, including the CPA [148, 149].

As the disease process enlarges, CN VI, VII, VIII, and IV may be compressed. Hearing loss, tinnitus, vertigo, and headache are common. Imaging is the mainstay of diagnosis. On high-resolution CT, cholesterol granulomas appear as nonenhancing punched-out lesions isodense to the brain. The borders are typically smooth, and rim enhancement is occasionally seen [113]. On T1-and T2-weighted MRIs, cholesterol granulomas show a distinct increased intensity that is unique to these lesions [113, 148]. No enhancement to gadolinium occurs.

Unlike primary cholesteatomas of the petrous apex, cholesterol granulomas require a drainage procedure. The petrous apex can be accessed for drainage by a transmastoid infralabyrinthine approach or a transcanal intracochlear approach [150–152]. Symptoms are controlled, and preoperative cranial nerve function recovers in more than 80% of treated cases [150].

Conclusion

A variety of benign and malignant neoplasms can affect the temporal bone and its vicinity. The anatomic proximity of the CPA explains its frequent involvement by lesions originating from the temporal bone. The signs and symptoms reflect the extent and site of involvement. Radiographic studies are essential when evaluating patients suspected of having CPA pathology. Different factors may alter the choice of treatment. These factors may depend on the patient, lesion, and surgeon.

Dealing with lesions of the temporal bone and CPA can overwhelm even the most astute physician. The patient should be at the center of the discussion and should be offered unbiased treatment alternatives. Informed consent is a key portion of the process, and appropriate counseling often requires repetitive office visits with different specialists. A multidisciplinary approach incorporating the talents of different physicians gives patients the best chance of achieving a favorable outcome.

References

1. Williams MD, Rich TA. Paragangliomas arising in the head and neck: a morphologic review and genetic update. Surg Pathol Clin. 2014;7:543–57.
2. Guild SR. The glomus jugulare, a nonchromaffin paraganglion, in man. Ann Otol Rhinol Laryngol. 1953;62:1045–71.
3. Rosenwasser H. Glomus jugulare tumors: I. historical background. Arch Otolaryngol. 1968;88:3–5.
4. Wanna GB, Sweeney AD, Haynes DS, Carlson ML. Contemporary management of jugular paragangliomas. Otolaryngol Clin N Am. 2015;48:331–41.
5. Moore MG, Netterville JL, Mendenhall WM, Isaacson B, Nussenbaum B. Head and neck paragangliomas: an update on evaluation and management. Otolaryngol Head Neck Surg. 2016;154:597–605.
6. Astrom K, Cohen JE, Willett-Brozick JE, Aston CE, Baysal BE. Altitude is a phenotypic modifier in hereditary paraganglioma type 1: evidence for an oxygen-sensing defect. Hum Genet. 2003;113:228–37.
7. Cerecer-Gil NY, Figuera LE, Llamas FJ, et al. Mutation of SDHB is a cause of hypoxia-related high-altitude paraganglioma. Clin Cancer Res. 2010;16:4148–54.
8. Favier J, Amar L, Gimenez-Roqueplo AP. Paraganglioma and phaeochromocytoma: from genetics to personalized medicine. Nat Rev Endocrinol. 2015;11:101–11.
9. Baysal BE, Ferrell RE, Willett-Brozick JE, et al. Mutations in SDHD, a mitochondrial complex II gene, in hereditary paraganglioma. Science. 2000;287:848–51.
10. Astuti D, Hart-Holden N, Latif F, et al. Genetic analysis of mitochondrial complex II subunits SDHD, SDHB and SDHC in paraganglioma and phaeochromocytoma susceptibility. Clin Endocrinol. 2003;59:728–33.
11. Mhatre AN, Li Y, Feng L, Gasperin A, Lalwani AK. SDHB, SDHC, and SDHD mutation screen in sporadic and familial head and neck paragangliomas. Clin Genet. 2004;66:461–6.
12. Fishbein L. Pheochromocytoma and paraganglioma: genetics, diagnosis, and treatment. Hematol Oncol Clin North Am. 2016;30:135–50.
13. Dahia PL. Pheochromocytoma and paraganglioma pathogenesis: learning from genetic heterogeneity. Nat Rev Cancer. 2014;14:108–19.
14. Benn DE, Robinson BG, Clifton-Bligh RJ. 15 years of paraganglioma: clinical manifestations of paraganglioma syndromes types 1-5. Endocr Relat Cancer. 2015;22(4):T91–103.
15. Spector GJ, Sobol S, Thawley SE, Maisel RH, Ogura JH. Panel discussion: glomus jugulare tumors of the temporal bone. Patterns of invasion in the temporal bone. Laryngoscope. 1979;89:1628–39.

16. Kinney SE. Glomus jugulare tumor surgery with intracranial extension. Otolaryngol Head Neck Surg. 1980;88:531–5.
17. Spector GJ, Ciralsky RH, Ogura JH. Glomus tumors in the head and neck: III. Analysis of clinical manifestations. Ann Otol Rhinol Laryngol. 1975;84:73–9.
18. Manolidis S, Shohet JA, Jackson CG, Glasscock ME. Malignant glomus tumors. Laryngoscope. 1999;109:30–4.
19. Gulya AJ. The glomus tumor and its biology. Laryngoscope. 1993;103:7–15.
20. Myssiorek D. Head and neck paragangliomas: an overview. Otolaryngol Clin N Am. 2001;34:829–36.
21. McCaffrey TV, Meyer FB, Michels VV, Piepgras DG, Marion MS. Familial paragangliomas of the head and neck. Arch Otolaryngol Head Neck Surg. 1994;120:1211–6.
22. Green JD, Brackmann DE, Nguyen CD, Arriaga MA, Telischi FF, De la Cruz A. Surgical management of previously untreated glomus jugulare tumors. Laryngoscope. 1994;104:917–21.
23. Fayad JN, Keles B, Brackmann DE. Jugular foramen tumors: clinical characteristics and treatment outcomes. Otol Neurotol. 2010;31:299–305.
24. Spector GJ, Gado M, Ciralsky R, Ogura JH, Maisel RH. Neurologic implications of glomus tumors in the head and neck. Laryngoscope. 1975;85:1387–95.
25. Brown LA. Glomus jugulare tumor of the middle ear; clinical aspects. Laryngoscope. 1953;63:281–92.
26. Sweeney AD, Carlson ML, Wanna GB, Bennett ML. Glomus tympanicum tumors. Otolaryngol Clin N Am. 2015;48:293–304.
27. Jackson CG, Harris PF, Glasscock ME, et al. Diagnosis and management of paragangliomas of the skull base. Am J Surg. 1990;159:389–93.
28. Schwaber MK, Glasscock ME, Nissen AJ, Jackson CG, Smith PG. Diagnosis and management of catecholamine secreting glomus tumors. Laryngoscope. 1984;94:1008–15.
29. Ong CK, Fook-Hin CV. Imaging of jugular foramen. Neuroimaging Clin N Am. 2009;19:469–82.
30. Lo WW, Solti-Bohman LG, Lambert PR. High-resolution CT in the evaluation of glomus tumors of the temporal bone. Radiology. 1984;150:737–42.
31. Lo WW, Solti-Bohman LG. High-resolution CT of the jugular foramen: anatomy and vascular variants and anomalies. Radiology. 1984;150:743–7.
32. Weber AL, McKenna MJ. Radiologic evaluation of the jugular foramen. Anatomy, vascular variants, anomalies, and tumors. Neuroimaging Clin N Am. 1994;4:579–98.
33. Woolen S, Gemmete JJ. Paragangliomas of the head and neck. Neuroimaging Clin N Am. 2016;26:259–78.
34. Murphy TP, Brackmann DE. Effects of preoperative embolization on glomus jugulare tumors. Laryngoscope. 1989;99(12):1244–7.
35. Lustig LR, Jackler RK. The variable relationship between the lower cranial nerves and jugular foramen tumors: implications for neural preservation. Am J Otol. 1996;17(4):658–68.
36. Odat H, Shin SH, Odat MA, Alzoubi F. Facial nerve management in jugular paraganglioma surgery: a literature review. J Laryngol Otol. 2016;130(3):219–24.
37. Bacciu A, Medina M, Ait Mimoune H, et al. Lower cranial nerves function after surgical treatment of Fisch class C and D tympanojugular paragangliomas. Eur Arch Otorhinolaryngol. 2015;272(2):311–9.
38. Blevins NH, Jackler RK, Kaplan MJ, Gutin PH. Combined transpetrosal-subtemporal craniotomy for clival tumors with extension into the posterior fossa. Laryngoscope. 1995;105(9 Pt 1):975–82.
39. Carlson ML, Driscoll CL, Garcia JJ, Janus JR, Link MJ. Surgical management of giant transdural glomus jugulare tumors with cerebellar and brainstem compression. J Neurol Surg B Skull Base. 2012;73(3):197–207.
40. Miller JP, Semaan M, Einstein D, Megerian CA, Maciunas RJ. Staged gamma knife radiosurgery after tailored surgical resection: a novel treatment paradigm for glomus jugulare tumors. Stereotact Funct Neurosurg. 2009;87(1):31–6.
41. Maniglia AJ, Sprecher RC, Megerian CA, Lanzieri C. Inferior mastoidectomy-hypotympanic approach for surgical removal of glomus jugulare tumors: an anatomical and radiologic study emphasizing distances between critical structures. Laryngoscope. 1992;102(4):407–14.
42. Papaspyrou K, Mewes T, Tóth M, Schmidtmann I, Amedee RG, Mann WJ. Hearing results after hypotympanotomy for glomus tympanicum tumors. Otol Neurotol. 2011;32(2):291–6.
43. Willen SN, Einstein DB, Maciunas RJ, Megerian CA. Treatment of glomus jugulare tumors in patients with advanced age: planned limited surgical resection followed by staged gamma knife radiosurgery: a preliminary report. Otol Neurotol. 2005;26(6):1229–34.
44. Krych AJ, Foote RL, Brown PD, Garces YI, Link MJ. Long-term results of irradiation for paraganglioma. Int J Radiat Oncol Biol Phys. 2006;65(4):1063–6.
45. Pemberton LS, Swindell R, Sykes AJ. Radical radiotherapy alone for glomus jugulare and tympanicum tumours. Oncol Rep. 2005;14(6):1631–3.
46. Pollock BE. Stereotactic radiosurgery in patients with glomus jugulare tumors. Neurosurg Focus. 2004;17(2):E10.
47. Sheehan J, Kondziolka D, Flickinger J, Lunsford LD. Gamma knife surgery for glomus jugulare tumors: an intermediate report on efficacy and safety. J Neurosurg. 2005;102(Suppl):241–6.
48. Hyams VJ, Michaels L. Benign adenomatous neoplasm (adenoma) of the middle ear. Clin Otolaryngol Allied Sci. 1976;1(1):17–26.
49. Gaffey MJ, Mills SE, Fechner RE, Intemann SR, Wick MR. Aggressive papillary middle-ear tumor. A clinicopathologic entity distinct from middle-ear adenoma. Am J Surg Pathol. 1988;12(10):790–7.
50. Heffner DK. Low-grade adenocarcinoma of probable endolymphatic sac origin a clinicopathologic study of 20 cases. Cancer. 1989;64(11):2292–302.
51. Poe DS, Tarlov EC, Thomas CB, Kveton JF. Aggressive papillary tumors of temporal bone. Otolaryngol Head Neck Surg. 1993;108(1):80–6.
52. Li JC, Brackmann DE, Lo WW, Carberry JN, House JW. Reclassification of aggressive adenomatous mastoid neoplasms as endolymphatic sac tumors. Laryngoscope. 1993;103(12):1342–8.
53. Megerian CA, Haynes DS, Poe DS, Choo DI, Keriakas TJ, Glasscock ME 3rd. Hearing preservation surgery for small endolymphatic sac tumors in patients with von Hippel-Lindau syndrome. Otol Neurotol. 2002;23(3):378–87.
54. Bambakidis NC, Rodrigue T, Megerian CA, Ratcheson RA. Endolymphatic sac tumor metastatic to the spine: case report. J Neurosurg Spine. 2005;3(1):68–70.
55. Megerian CA, Pilch BZ, Bhan AK, McKenna MJ. Differential expression of transthyretin in papillary tumors of the endolymphatic sac and choroid plexus. Laryngoscope. 1997;107(2):216–21.
56. Megerian CA, McKenna MJ, Nuss RC, et al. Endolymphatic sac tumors: histopathologic confirmation, clinical characterization, and implication in von Hippel-Lindau disease. Laryngoscope. 1995;105(8 Pt 1):801–8.
57. Schindler RA. The ultrastructure of the endolymphatic sac in man. Laryngoscope. 1980;90(6 Pt 2):1–39.
58. Levin RJ, Feghali JG, Morganstern N, Llena J, Bradley MK. Aggressive papillary tumors of the temporal bone: an immunohistochemical analysis in tissue culture. Laryngoscope. 1996;106(2 Pt 1):144–7.
59. Feghali JG, Levin RJ, Llena J, Bradley MK, Kantrowitz AB. Aggressive papillary tumors of the endolymphatic sac: clinical and tissue culture characteristics. Am J Otol. 1995;16(6):778–82.

60. Batsakis JG, El-Naggar AK. Papillary neoplasms (Heffner's tumors) of the endolymphatic sac. Ann Otol Rhinol Laryngol. 1993;102(8 Pt 1):648–51.
61. Latif F, Tory K, Gnarra J, et al. Identification of the von Hippel-Lindau disease tumor suppressor gene. Science. 1993;260(5112):1317–20.
62. Neumann HP, Wiestler OD. Clustering of features and genetics of von Hippel-Lindau syndrome. Lancet. 1991;338(8761):258.
63. Sgambati MT, Stolle C, Choyke PL, et al. Mosaicism in von Hippel-Lindau disease: lessons from kindreds with germline mutations identified in offspring with mosaic parents. Am J Hum Genet. 2000;66(1):84–91.
64. Knudson AG Jr. Genetics of human cancer. J Cell Physiol Suppl. 1986;4:7–11.
65. Lonser RR, Kim HJ, Butman JA, Vortmeyer AO, Choo DI, Oldfield EH. Tumors of the endolymphatic sac in von Hippel-Lindau disease. N Engl J Med. 2004;350(24):2481–6.
66. Glasker S, Lonser RR, Tran MG, et al. Effects of VHL deficiency on endolymphatic duct and sac. Cancer Res. 2005;65(23):10847–53.
67. Qi H, Gervais ML, Li W, DeCaprio JA, Challis JR, Ohh M. Molecular cloning and characterization of the von Hippel-Lindau-like protein. Mol Cancer Res. 2004;2(1):43–52.
68. Kaelin WG Jr. The von Hippel-Lindau tumor suppressor gene and kidney cancer. Clin Cancer Res. 2004;10(18 Pt 2):6290S–5S.
69. Maher ER, Kaelin WG Jr. von Hippel-Lindau disease. Medicine (Baltimore). 1997;76(6):381–91.
70. Manski TJ, Heffner DK, Glenn GM, et al. Endolymphatic sac tumors. A source of morbid hearing loss in von Hippel-Lindau disease. JAMA. 1997;277(18):1461–6.
71. Hansen MR, Luxford WM. Surgical outcomes in patients with endolymphatic sac tumors. Laryngoscope. 2004;114(8):1470–4.
72. Kim HJ, Butman JA, Brewer C, et al. Tumors of the endolymphatic sac in patients with von Hippel-Lindau disease: implications for their natural history, diagnosis, and treatment. J Neurosurg. 2005;102(3):503–12.
73. Hassard AD. Identification of endolymphatic sac tumors. Otolaryngol Head Neck Surg. 1985;93(3):445.
74. Mukherji SK, Albernaz VS, Lo WW, et al. Papillary endolymphatic sac tumors: CT, MR imaging, and angiographic findings in 20 patients. Radiology. 1997;202(3):801–8.
75. Ho VT, Rao VM, Doan HT, Mikaelian DO. Low-grade adenocarcinoma of probable endolymphatic sac origin: CT and MR appearance. AJNR Am J Neuroradiol. 1996;17(1):168–70.
76. Bambakidis NC, Megerian CA, Ratcheson RA. Differential grading of endolymphatic sac tumor extension by virtue of von Hippel-Lindau disease status. Otol Neurotol. 2004;25(5):773–81.
77. Glasscock ME 3rd, Smith PG, Schwaber MK, Nissen AJ. Clinical aspects of osseous hemangiomas of the skull base. Laryngoscope. 1984;94(7):869–73.
78. Pulec JL. Facial nerve tumors. Ann Otol Rhinol Laryngol. 1969;78(5):962–82.
79. Boye E, Yu Y, Paranya G, Mulliken JB, Olsen BR, Bischoff J. Clonality and altered behavior of endothelial cells from hemangiomas. J Clin Invest. 2001;107(6):745–52.
80. Shelton C, Brackmann DE, Lo WW, Carberry JN. Intratemporal facial nerve hemangiomas. Otolaryngol Head Neck Surg. 1991;104(1):116–21.
81. Gjuric M, Koester M, Paulus W. Cavernous hemangioma of the internal auditory canal arising from the inferior vestibular nerve: case report and review of the literature. Am J Otol. 2000;21(1):110–4.
82. Isaacson B, Telian SA, PE MK, Arts HA. Hemangiomas of the geniculate ganglion. Otol Neurotol. 2005;26(4):796–802.
83. Lo WW, Horn KL, Carberry JN, et al. Intratemporal vascular tumors: evaluation with CT. Radiology. 1986;159(1):181–5.
84. Eby TL, Fisch U, Makek MS. Facial nerve management in temporal bone hemangiomas. Am J Otol. 1992;13(3):223–32.
85. Lo WW, Shelton C, Waluch V, et al. Intratemporal vascular tumors: detection with CT and MR imaging. Radiology. 1989;171(2):445–8.
86. Curtin HD, Jensen JE, Barnes L Jr, May M. "Ossifying" hemangiomas of the temporal bone: evaluation with CT. Radiology. 1987;164(3):831–5.
87. Devaney KO, Boschman CR, Willard SC, Ferlito A, Rinaldo A. Tumours of the external ear and temporal bone. Lancet Oncol. 2005;6(6):411–20.
88. Morton RP, Stell PM, Derrick PP. Epidemiology of cancer of the middle ear cleft. Cancer. 1984;53(7):1612–7.
89. Michaels L, Wells M. Squamous cell carcinoma of the middle ear. Clin Otolaryngol Allied Sci. 1980;5(4):235–48.
90. Leonetti JP, Smith PG, Kletzker GR, Izquierdo R. Invasion patterns of advanced temporal bone malignancies. Am J Otol. 1996;17(3):438–42.
91. Moffat DA, Grey P, Ballagh RH, Hardy DG. Extended temporal bone resection for squamous cell carcinoma. Otolaryngol Head Neck Surg. 1997;116(6 Pt 1):617–23.
92. Kinney SE. Squamous cell carcinoma of the external auditory canal. Am J Otol. 1989;10(2):111–6.
93. Conley J, Schuller DE. Malignancies of the ear. Laryngoscope. 1976;86(8):1147–63.
94. Arriaga M, Curtin HD, Takahashi H, Kamerer DB. The role of preoperative CT scans in staging external auditory meatus carcinoma: radiologic-pathologic correlation study. Otolaryngol Head Neck Surg. 1991;105(1):6–11.
95. Arriaga M, Curtin H, Takahashi H, Hirsch BE, Kamerer DB. Staging proposal for external auditory meatus carcinoma based on preoperative clinical examination and computed tomography findings. Ann Otol Rhinol Laryngol. 1990;99(9 Pt 1):714–21.
96. Lesser RW, Spector GJ, Devineni VR. Malignant tumors of the middle ear and external auditory canal: a 20-year review. Otolaryngol Head Neck Surg. 1987;96(1):43–7.
97. Kinney SE, Wood BG. Malignancies of the external ear canal and temporal bone: surgical techniques and results. Laryngoscope. 1987;97(2):158–64.
98. Moffat DA, Wagstaff SA, Hardy DG. The outcome of radical surgery and postoperative radiotherapy for squamous carcinoma of the temporal bone. Laryngoscope. 2005;115(2):341–7.
99. Spector JG. Management of temporal bone carcinomas: a therapeutic analysis of two groups of patients and long-term followup. Otolaryngol Head Neck Surg. 1991;104(1):58–66.
100. Kraus DH, Saenz NC, Gollamudi S, et al. Pediatric rhabdomyosarcoma of the head and neck. Am J Surg. 1997;174(5):556–60.
101. Jaffe BF, Fox JE, Batsakis JG. Rhabdomyosarcoma of the middle ear and mastoid. Cancer. 1971;27(1):29–37.
102. Stevens MC. Treatment for childhood rhabdomyosarcoma: the cost of cure. Lancet Oncol. 2005;6(2):77–84.
103. Wharam MD Jr. Rhabdomyosarcoma of Parameningeal sites. Semin Radiat Oncol. 1997;7(3):212–6.
104. Maurer HM, Beltangady M, Gehan EA, et al. The intergroup rhabdomyosarcoma study-I. a final report. Cancer. 1988;61(2):209–20.
105. Nakhleh RE, Swanson PE, Dehner LP. Juvenile (embryonal and alveolar) rhabdomyosarcoma of the head and neck in adults. A clinical, pathologic, and immunohistochemical study of 12 cases. Cancer. 1991;67(4):1019–24.
106. Newton WA Jr, Soule EH, Hamoudi AB, et al. Histopathology of childhood sarcomas, intergroup rhabdomyosarcoma studies I and II: clinicopathologic correlation. J Clin Oncol. 1988;6(1):67–75.
107. Jan MM. Facial paralysis: a presenting feature of rhabdomyosarcoma. Int J Pediatr Otorhinolaryngol. 1998;46(3):221–4.

108. Potter GD. Embryonal rhabdomyosarcoma of the middle ear in children. Cancer. 1966;19(2):221–6.
109. Ruymann FB. Rhabdomyosarcoma in children and adolescents. A review. Hematol Oncol Clin North Am. 1987;1(4):621–54.
110. Verma PL, Marwaha AR. Embryonal rhabdomyosarcoma of the middle ear and mastoid. J Laryngol Otol. 1972;86(1):67–71.
111. Latack JT, Hutchinson RJ, Heyn RM. Imaging of rhabdomyosarcomas of the head and neck. AJNR Am J Neuroradiol. 1987;8(2):353–9.
112. Maroldi R, Farina D, Palvarini L, et al. Computed tomography and magnetic resonance imaging of pathologic conditions of the middle ear. Eur J Radiol. 2001;40(2):78–93.
113. Jackler RK, Parker DA. Radiographic differential diagnosis of petrous apex lesions. Am J Otol. 1992;13(6):561–74.
114. Raney RB, Anderson JR, Barr FG, et al. Rhabdomyosarcoma and undifferentiated sarcoma in the first two decades of life: a selective review of intergroup rhabdomyosarcoma study group experience and rationale for intergroup rhabdomyosarcoma study V. J Pediatr Hematol Oncol. 2001;23(4):215–20.
115. Sutow WW, Lindberg RD, Gehan EA, et al. Three-year relapse-free survival rates in childhood rhabdomyosarcoma of the head and neck: report from the intergroup rhabdomyosarcoma study. Cancer. 1982;49(11):2217–21.
116. Breneman JC, Lyden E, Pappo AS, et al. Prognostic factors and clinical outcomes in children and adolescents with metastatic rhabdomyosarcoma–a report from the intergroup rhabdomyosarcoma study IV. J Clin Oncol. 2003;21(1):78–84.
117. Joshi D, Anderson JR, Paidas C, et al. Age is an independent prognostic factor in rhabdomyosarcoma: a report from the soft tissue sarcoma Committee of the Children's oncology group. Pediatr Blood Cancer. 2004;42(1):64–73.
118. Meza JL, Anderson J, Pappo AS, Meyer WH, Children's OG. Analysis of prognostic factors in patients with nonmetastatic rhabdomyosarcoma treated on intergroup rhabdomyosarcoma studies III and IV: the Children's oncology group. J Clin Oncol. 2006;24(24):3844–51.
119. Crist W, Gehan EA, Ragab AH, et al. The third intergroup rhabdomyosarcoma study. J Clin Oncol. 1995;13(3):610–30.
120. Crist WM, Anderson JR, Meza JL, et al. Intergroup rhabdomyosarcoma study-IV: results for patients with nonmetastatic disease. J Clin Oncol. 2001;19(12):3091–102.
121. Maurer HM, Gehan EA, Beltangady M, et al. The intergroup rhabdomyosarcoma study-II. Cancer. 1993;71(5):1904–22.
122. Schuller DE, Lawrence TL, Newton WA Jr. Childhood rhabdomyosarcomas of the head and neck. Arch Otolaryngol. 1979;105(12):689–94.
123. Sung L, Anderson JR, Donaldson SS, et al. Late events occurring five years or more after successful therapy for childhood rhabdomyosarcoma: a report from the soft tissue sarcoma Committee of the Children's oncology group. Eur J Cancer. 2004;40(12):1878–85.
124. Paulino AC, Simon JH, Zhen W, Wen BC. Long-term effects in children treated with radiotherapy for head and neck rhabdomyosarcoma. Int J Radiat Oncol Biol Phys. 2000;48(5):1489–95.
125. Okura SI, Kaga K. Temporal bone pathology of leukemia and malignant lymphoma with middle ear effusion. Auris Nasus Larynx. 1994;21(1):1–7.
126. Panosian MS, Roberts JK. Plasmacytoma of the middle ear and mastoid. Am J Otol. 1994;15(2):264–7.
127. Paparella MM, Berlinger NT, Oda M, El-Fiky F. Otological manifestations of leukemia. Laryngoscope. 1973;83(9):1510–26.
128. Harada T, Namiki S, Kawabata I. Acute profound sensorineural hearing loss as the initial manifestation of acute leukemia–report of a case. Auris Nasus Larynx. 2000;27(4):359–62.
129. Zappia JJ, Bunge FA, Koopmann CF Jr, McClatchey KD. Facial nerve paresis as the presenting symptom of leukemia. Int J Pediatr Otorhinolaryngol. 1990;19(3):259–64.
130. Kurtz JE, Andres E, Veillon F, et al. Hearing loss due to acute leukemia. Am J Med. 2000;109(6):509–10.
131. Zechner G, Altmann F. The temporal bone in leukemia. Histological studies. Ann Otol Rhinol Laryngol. 1969;78(2):375–87.
132. Berlinger NT, Koutroupas S, Adams G, Maisel R. Patterns of involvement of the temporal bone in metastatic and systemic malignancy. Laryngoscope. 1980;90(4):619–27.
133. Gokcan MK, Batikhan H, Calguner M, Tataragasi AI. Unilateral hearing loss as a presenting manifestation of granulocytic sarcoma (chloroma). Otol Neurotol. 2006;27(1):106–9.
134. Takahara T, Sando I, Bluestone CD, Myers EN. Lymphoma invading the anterior eustachian tube. Temporal bone histopathology of functional tubal obstruction. Ann Otol Rhinol Laryngol. 1986;95(1 Pt 1):101–5.
135. Nicolaides A, McFerran DJ, Croxson G. Non-Hodgkins lymphoma of the temporal bone. J Laryngol Otol. 1988;102(10):928–31.
136. Lang EE, Walsh RM, Leader M. Primary middle-ear lymphoma in a child. J Laryngol Otol. 2003;117(3):205–7.
137. Merkus P, Copper MP, Van Oers MH, Schouwenburg PF. Lymphoma in the ear. ORL J Otorhinolaryngol Relat Spec. 2000;62(5):274–7.
138. Paparella MM, El-Fiky FM. Ear involvement in malignant lymphoma. Ann Otol Rhinol Laryngol. 1972;81(3):352–63.
139. Wax MK, Yun KJ, Omar RA. Extramedullary plasmacytomas of the head and neck. Otolaryngol Head Neck Surg. 1993;109(5):877–85.
140. Abemayor E, Canalis RF, Greenberg P, Wortham DG, Rowland JP, Sun NC. Plasma cell tumors of the head and neck. J Otolaryngol. 1988;17(7):376–81.
141. Ruenes R, Palacios E. Plasmacytoma of the petrous temporal bone. Ear Nose Throat J. 2003;82(9):672.
142. George JC, Caldemeyer KS, Kreipke DL, Chalian AA, Moran CC. Solitary plasmacytoma of the mastoid bone presenting as coalescent mastoiditis. Arch Otolaryngol Head Neck Surg. 1994;120(12):1393–4.
143. Yetiser S, Talas D, Akkaya A, Deveci S. Plasmacytoma of the temporal bone: management with a combination of surgery and radiotherapy. Acta Otolaryngol. 2001;121(8):915–8.
144. Adams GL, Paparella MM, el-Fiky FM. Primary and metastatic tumors of the temporal bone. Laryngoscope. 1971;81(8):1273–85.
145. Schuknecht HF, Allam AF, Murakami Y. Pathology of secondary malignant tumors of the temporal bone. Ann Otol Rhinol Laryngol. 1968;77(1):5–22.
146. Streitmann MJ, Sismanis A. Metastatic carcinoma of the temporal bone. Am J Otol. 1996;17(5):780–3.
147. Brackmann DE, Bartels LJ. Rare tumors of the cerebellopontine angle. Otolaryngol Head Neck Surg (1979). 1980;88(5):555–9.
148. Arriaga MA, Brackmann DE. Differential diagnosis of primary petrous apex lesions. Am J Otol. 1991;12(6):470–4.
149. Jackler RK, Cho M. A new theory to explain the genesis of petrous apex cholesterol granuloma. Otol Neurotol. 2003;24(1):96–106. discussion 106
150. Brackmann DE, Toh EH. Surgical management of petrous apex cholesterol granulomas. Otol Neurotol. 2002;23(4):529–33.
151. Fong BP, Brackmann DE, Telischi FF. The long-term follow-up of drainage procedures for petrous apex cholesterol granulomas. Arch Otolaryngol Head Neck Surg. 1995;121(4):426–30.
152. Giddings NA, Brackmann DE, Kwartler JA. Transcanal infracochlear approach to the petrous apex. Otolaryngol Head Neck Surg. 1991;104(1):29–36.

Congenital Rest Lesions and Rare Tumors

20

Madjid Samii, Sam Safavi-Abbasi, Christian Herold, and Amir Samii

In 1902, Henneberg and Koch first used the term cerebellopontine angle (CPA) in their report of two patients with bilateral vestibular schwannomas in the location that they described as *Kleinhirnbrüeckenwinkels* [1], a term still used in German. The CPA contains a variety of neurovascular structures. It is outlined by the meninges of the CPA cistern and the bony structures of the posterior fossa. Overall, lesions of the CPA account for 6–10% of all intracranial tumors [2, 3]. With a prevalence of 80–90%, vestibular schwannomas represent the majority of these lesions, followed by meningiomas and epidermoids [2–4]. The remaining lesions are encountered less frequently. Embryologic remnants and metastasis account for many CPA tumors. Thus, neurosurgeons encounter a variety of rare lesions in this location.

This chapter focuses on the less common, "unusual" CPA lesions. This group includes embryologic remnants and maldevelopmental masses such as epidermoid, dermoid, and arachnoid cysts; lipomas, nonvestibular schwannomas, and CPA metastases; exophytic and skull-base tumors; and other rare lesions. In treating many of these lesions since 1968, it is the senior author's (M. Samii) personal experience that, regardless of the size and origin of a lesion, the lateral suboccipital retrosigmoid retromastoid approach offers an exquisite route to the different pathologies that can involve this location.

M. Samii (✉) · A. Samii
International Neuroscience Institute—Hannover, Hannover, Germany
e-mail: samii@ini-hannover.de

S. Safavi-Abbasi
Flagstaff Neurosurgery, Flagstaff, AZ, USA

C. Herold
Department of Biomedical Imaging and Image-guided Therapy Medical, Medical University of Vienna, Vienna General Hospital, Vienna, Austria

Department of Radiology, Johns Hopkins Medical Institutions, Baltimore, MD, USA

General Principles of the Lateral Suboccipital Retrosigmoid Approach

Although the retrosigmoid approach is described elsewhere in this text, the authors' technique is reviewed briefly. The procedure may be performed with the patient in a semisitting (lounging) or supine position (with the head turned 60° toward the contralateral side) [2, 3]. For the semisitting position, the back of the operating table is elevated to 30°. The head is turned 30° to the side of the craniotomy, placed in a head-fixation device, and flexed slightly. The head and neck are in a natural anatomical position, without strain or compromise of the cervical venous drainage. The patient is padded appropriately. Arterial blood pressure is monitored, and a central venous catheter is placed in the right atrium. Precordial Doppler ultrasonography is used to monitor for signs of air embolism. The risk of air embolism is decreased by elevating the legs to the level of the right atrium of the heart.

Preoperative bone window computerized tomography (CT) and magnetic resonance imaging (MRI) show individual anatomic variations in the location of the posterior fossa, emissary veins, and jugular bulb, as well as in the relationship of the tumor to the internal auditory canal (IAC) and other bony structures [5]. Preoperative X-rays of the cervical spine are obtained routinely to detect possible spinal abnormalities and to prevent medullary compression. Somatosensory evoked potentials (SSEPs) are monitored throughout the case.

Before the skin is incised, the mastoid eminence, digastric groove, and inion should be palpated and identified. A curvilinear skin incision is then placed behind the ear, 1.5–2 cm medial to the mastoid process. The incision reaches from just above the superior nuchal line to the level of C1. The trapezius and splenius capitis muscles are detached from the superior nuchal line. The occipital artery and the greater occipital nerve are preserved. Great care should be taken to avoid injury to the vertebral artery.

N. C. Bambakidis et al. (eds.), *Surgery of the Cerebellopontine Angle*, https://doi.org/10.1007/978-3-031-12507-2_20

A suboccipital craniectomy is executed. Important landmarks are the external occipital protuberance that overlies the sinus confluence and the superior nuchal line overlying the transverse sinus. A single bur hole is placed below the Frankfurt horizontal line, 3 cm behind the external auditory canal [2, 3, 6]. Frameless stereotactic guidance is not used routinely when planning the craniectomy; use of the anatomic landmarks is preferred.

The dura is separated carefully, and the bone is removed with rongeurs until the craniectomy is 3–4 cm in diameter. The transverse sinus and its junction with the sigmoid sinus should be exposed. Emissary veins are exposed cautiously with a diamond drill and then coagulated to avoid air embolism.

After the tumor is removed, hemostasis is carefully attained. The mastoid air cells are sealed with autologous muscle or with fat and fibrin glue, and the wound is closed in multiple layers.

Anatomical Considerations

The complex anatomy of the CPA is discussed elsewhere. However, an understanding of the anatomy of the posterior fossa cisterns is crucial for surgery involving the CPA. Any approach to this region is directed through the subarachnoid cisterns. These cisterns create a natural corridor through which the major intracranial vessels and cranial nerves can be approached. We emphasize complete knowledge of their location and relationship to critical neurovascular structures, including the interpeduncular cistern, prepontine cistern, premedullary cistern, quadrigeminal cistern, cisterna magna, cerebellopontine cistern, and cerebellomedullary cistern (Fig. 20.1) [7, 8]. Of major importance for the lateral suboccipital retrosigmoid approach are the paired cerebellopontine and cerebellomedullary cisterns and the unpaired premedullary cistern.

As its name implies, the cerebellopontine cistern is located between the anterolateral surface of the pons and cerebellum. The lateral border is formed by the petrous temporal bone. When viewed on axial images, this cistern forms a triangular space. At the level of the tentorium, this cistern is separated from the superiorly situated ambient, or perimesencephalic cistern, by the lateral pontomesencephalic membrane. The anterior pontine membrane separates the cerebellopontine cistern from the more medially located unpaired prepontine cistern. The trigeminal, abducens, facial, and vestibulocochlear nerves pass through the cerebellopontine cistern. Its outer arachnoidal membrane extends into the IAC around the facial and vestibulocochlear nerves. The superior cerebellar and anterior inferior cerebellar arteries (AICA) also course through the cerebellopontine cistern. The veins in this cistern join near the trigeminal nerve, where they form the superior petrosal veins, which usually drain into the superior petrosal sinus [9].

The premedullary cistern is located between the lower part of the clivus and the anterior surface of the medulla. It is separated from the prepontine cistern by the medial ponto-

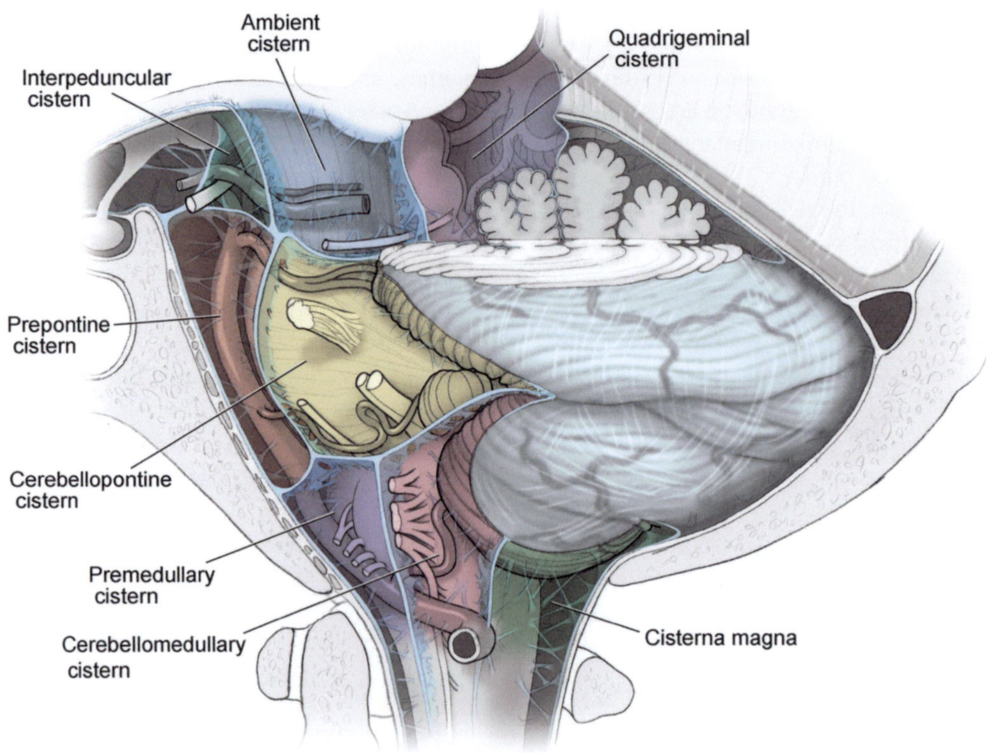

Fig. 20.1 Anatomical representation of the basilar cisterns in a sagittal view. These cisterns create a natural corridor through which the major intracranial vessels and cranial nerves can be approached. Pictured are the interpeduncular cistern, prepontine cistern, premedullary cistern, quadrigeminal cistern, cisterna magna, cerebellopontine cistern, and cerebellomedullary cistern. Reproduced with permission from Barrow Neurological Institute

medullary membrane. The rootlets of the hypoglossal nerve join and pass through the posterior aspect of this cistern. Inferiorly, the premedullary cistern is continuous with the anterior spinal cistern. After ascending through the foramen magnum, the vertebral arteries enter the anterior spinal cistern inferiorly. The major veins in this cistern are the transverse medullary veins, the median anterior medullary vein, and the vein of the pontomedullary sulcus [8, 9].

The cerebellomedullary cistern is the more lateral aspect of the premedullary cistern and the more inferior aspect of the cerebellopontine cistern. It is separated from the latter by the lateral pontomedullary membrane and from the former by the trabeculae anterior to the lower cranial nerves [7, 8]. The inferior border of the cerebellomedullary cistern is at the level of the foramen magnum. The vertebral artery enters the dura at the lower border of this cistern and exits to enter the premedullary cistern. The glossopharyngeal and vagus nerves and the medullary portion of the accessory nerve arise within and course through the cerebellomedullary cistern into the jugular foramen. The posterior inferior cerebellar artery (PICA) enters the cerebellomedullary cistern, reaching the anterior aspect of the rootlets of the glossopharyngeal, vagus, and accessory nerves. The artery passes dorsally between the rootlets near the medulla to enter the cisterna magna. The major veins in the cerebellomedullary cistern are the vein of the pontomedullary sulcus, the lateral medullary vein, the retro-olivary vein, and the lateral part of the transverse medullary veins [9]. The fourth ventricle communicates with this cistern through the foramen of Luschka [7, 8].

Once the arachnoid membrane forming the posterior wall of the cerebellopontine, cerebellomedullary, and premedullary cisterns is exposed and opened, the structures within these three cisterns are in the center of the lateral suboccipital retrosigmoid approach. The surgeon then has an excellent view of their configurations.

General Techniques of Surgical Resection

After the dura is opened, the remainder of the entire procedure is performed using the operating micro-scope. The dura is usually opened along the sigmoid and transverse sinuses. To provide extra space, to avoid compression of the cerebellum, and to improve the surgical exposure, the lateral cerebellomedullary cistern is opened and cerebrospinal fluid (CSF) is withdrawn. The lower cranial nerves are identified and protected with a wet cottonoid. The cerebellum is also covered with a moist cottonoid, and a brain retractor is placed to offer support and to provide exposure [2, 3].

Large tumors may fill the entire CPA and usually must be debulked before the cranial nerves can be identified. In the case of medium-sized tumors, the vestibulocochlear and facial nerves are typically easily identified medially at the brainstem. Small intracanalicular lesions, however, may not be visible in the CPA. In such cases, the IAC must be opened as a first step to identify the lateral tumoral extension. First, a circle of dura is excised from the petrous bone posterior to the IAC. Next, the posterior wall of the meatus is drilled with a high-speed diamond bur under continuous irrigation. Early drilling is performed with a 4–5 mm bur. As the fundus is approached, smaller diamond burs are used.

Review of preoperative CT scans to determine the position of the jugular bulb is essential before the porus is drilled. In case of a highly positioned jugular bulb, drilling proceeds cautiously to avoid violating the bulb. Drilling of the posterior wall of the IAC skeletonizes the jugular bulb so that it can be pressed down. Thereafter, the remaining bone of the posterior wall of the IAC can be drilled away.

Care must be taken to avoid opening or injuring the semicircular canals and vestibule, especially if the tumor has an extreme lateral extension. The remaining distance to the fundus must be evaluated constantly by making use of an angulated micro-instrument. If the semicircular canals are opened inadvertently, suctioning of the perilymph and endolymph must be avoided. The fenestration should be closed with fascia and sealed with fibrin glue immediately.

As the fundus is approached, the drilling continues in a medial-to-lateral direction. In this way, the bone plate between the IAC, ampulla of the semicircular canal, and jugular bulb can be thinned in 0.1 mm increments with the diamond bur without injuring the peripheral vestibular apparatus or jugular bulb. To avoid entering the labyrinth, at least 2 mm of bone should remain from the fundus of the IAC. A small autologous muscle or fat graft is applied to the opened portion of the IAC to prevent formation of a CSF fistula.

Using the retrosigmoid approach to the CPA and petroclival region, we distinguish different surgical "floors," which are determined by the arrangement of the cranial nerves within the CPA [3]. These floors create the surgical opening to the tumor. One aperture is between the caudal cranial nerves and the seventh and eighth cranial nerves. Another opening is between the facial, vestibulocochlear, and trigeminal nerves. For the supratentorial portion of a tumor, the opening is between the trigeminal and trochlear nerves and tentorial edges. To avoid mechanical or thermal injury to these structures, moist cottonoids should be used for protection. It is crucial to recognize that vascular structures can be encased by tumor. The AICA is of special anatomical interest because its disturbance can result in infarction of the lateral brainstem with catastrophic consequences [2, 3].

Tumor invasion into the cranial nerve foramina can make visualization of the cranial nerves difficult. In such cases, tumor should be resected piecemeal rather than en bloc. Great attention must be paid to prevent injury to the sixth cranial nerve. Especially with large tumors, this nerve is not visible until late in the procedure. Therefore, coagulation of tumor tissue must be avoided in the vicinity of the abducens nerve. Once the tumor is debulked, the abducens nerve should be identified at the brainstem and followed to its entry point in Dorello's canal.

The operative field is irrigated continuously with saline solution to maintain good visualization. As in vestibular schwannoma surgery, the auditory and facial nerves should be monitored routinely. If the amplitude of the waveforms changes, the surgeon must stop the procedure and change the strategy for resection. The suboccipital route offers the best opportunities for preservation and for reconstruction of the facial nerve. To avoid additional surgeries, reconstructive procedures may be performed during the same operative setting [2, 3].

Epidermoids and Dermoids

Epidermoids and dermoids are both ectoderm-lined inclusion cysts, but their complexity differs. Enclosed ectodermal cysts may arise when the surface ectoderm fails to separate entirely from the underlying neural tube [10, 11]. They also may result from abnormal sequestration or invagination of surface ectoderm along the embryologic sites of dermal fusion that form the eyes, ears, and face [10, 12]. Implantation of epidermoids can also be iatrogenic after lumbar puncture and has been reported in all age groups. Stab and puncture wounds can also cause a traumatic implantation.

Epidermoid tumors represent 0.2–1.8% of intracranial tumors. Their most common location in the central nervous system is the CPA. Epidermoids represent 4.6–6.3% of all CPA lesions and are the third most common lesion of the CPA after vestibular schwannomas and meningiomas [2, 13]. Thus, epidermoids are much more common than dermoids. Dermoids are midline lesions that rarely invade the CPA laterally. They contain elements from all layers of skin. Thus, fat, hair, and sebaceous glands can be found in addition to squamous epithelium. Dermoids may be associated with dermal sinuses to the skin surface and may cause focal changes in skin pigmentation, tufts of external hair, and, in the spinal cord, spina bifida [12].

In both lesions, rupture of the cyst can cause aseptic meningitis. Repeated episodes of such granulomatous meningitis may then lead to hydrocephalus in patients with dermoids and epidermoids. Dermoid cysts usually contain a mucoid, brown, oily fluid. Epidermoids usually contain a pearly, flaky material. In 1829, the French pathologist Jean Cruveilhier described these tumors as "pearly tumors" (tumeur perlée) [13]. Malignant change of dermoids and epidermoids to squamous cell carcinoma is extremely rare but fatal [14, 15].

On CT scans, epidermoid cysts usually appear as low-density cystic masses with irregular margins. In contrast to arachnoid cysts, which constitute the main differential diagnosis, epidermoid cysts produce no adjacent bony reaction on CT [10, 16]. On T1-and T2-weighted MRIs, the signal intensity of epidermoids is usually higher than that of CSF, with heterogeneous and marbled features (Fig. 20.2). On conventional MRIs, however, the signal intensity is often similar to that of CSF [11]. Diffusion-weighted images and fluid-attenuated inversion recovery sequences (FLAIR) are newer imaging modalities that allow differentiation of epidermoid and arachnoid cysts and also confirmation of the presence of residual tumor [17]. Due to their fatty content, dermoid cysts have negative attenuation values on CT scans and high signal intensity on T1-weighted MRIs [11, 16]. They may have calcifications [16].

Intracranial epidermoid and dermoid cysts usually grow slowly [10, 11, 13, 18]. Their clinical presentation is thus delayed, and symptoms depend on the close adhesions of the cystic capsule and compression of neurovascular structures. Facial nerve involvement and unilateral hearing loss are the most common presenting symptoms. However, facial nerve symptoms occur earlier than with vestibular schwannomas [2, 13]. Some patients may present with a classic trigeminal neuralgia or constant neuralgic pain [2, 18]. Rarely, malignant transformation has been described [19–21]. These cysts have also been associated with abnormalities of the craniovertebral junction and Klippel-Feil cervical fusion defects [22].

Even large tumors that extend beyond the CPA can usually be managed through the retrosigmoid approach [10, 11, 13]. Since 1984, most cases have been managed through this approach (Table 20.1). Goel and colleagues described 96 cases, 85 of which were managed with the suboccipital approach; their resection rate was 48% [36]. Because hearing can improve or recover, a translabyrinthine approach should not be used to treat patients with a dermoid or epidermoid of the CPA, if possible [38]. However, the surgical approach must be tailored to the location and extent of an individual lesion to ensure optimal exposure.

Bilateral lesions that involve the cranial nerves on both sides constitute a surgical challenge. Resection of these masses in a stepwise manner is emphasized. Significant time should be allowed between the two procedures to allow the recovery of possible deficits, especially of the lower cranial nerves.

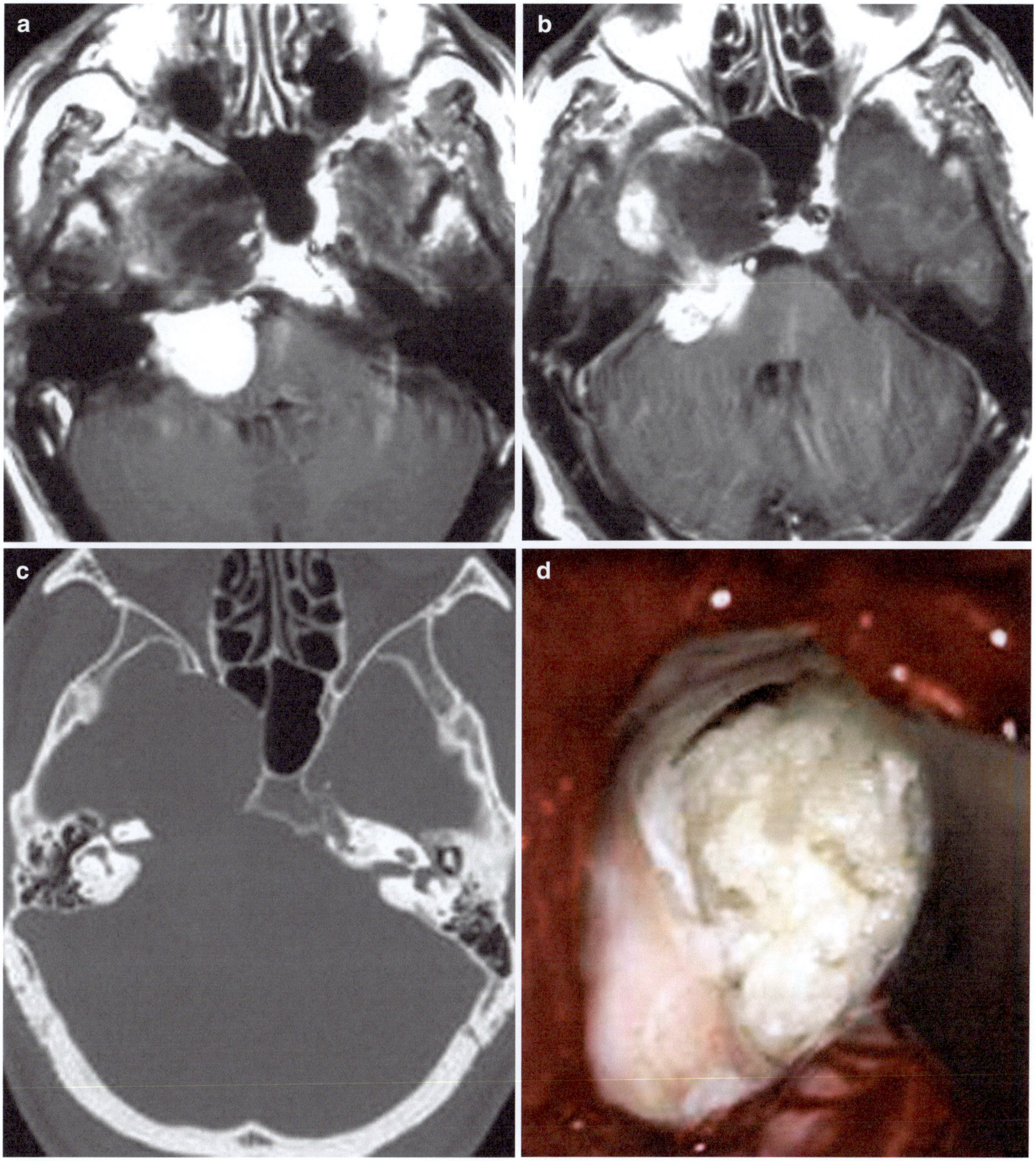

Fig. 20.2 Axial MRIs with contrast enhancement show a cerebellopontine angle epidermoid cyst (**a**) with an extension in the middle fossa (**b**). CT scan shows extension and widening of the internal auditory meatus (**c**). Intraoperative view shows the typical pearly appearance of an epidermoid tumor (**d**)

Table 20.1 Summary of approaches and surgical resection rates in treatment of epidermoid tumors in a review of major surgical series over 22 years

Reference	Suboccipital (No.)	Subtemporal (No.)	Combination (No.)	Removal rate (%)
Fischer et al. [23]	6	–	–	na
Berger and Wilson [10]	11	–	1 (suboccipital and frontotemporal)	0
Sabin et al. [24]	10	3	7 (supra- and infratentorial)	5
Salazar et al. [25]	10	2	4 (suboccipital and subtemporal)	0
Morard and De Tribolet [26]	5	–	–	na
deSouza et al. [27]	23	–	4 (suboccipital and middle fossa)	18
Yasargil et al. [11]	22	–	–	97
Altschuler et al. [28]	10	–	1 (retromastoid and frontotemporal)	na
Lunardi et al. [29]	16	1	–	35
Vinchon et al. [30]	5	–	4 (suboccipital and subtemporal)	55
Samii et al. [13]	40	–	–	75
Mohanty et al. [31]	23	1	1 (suboccipital and subtemporal)	48
Talacchi et al. [32]	17	3	–	55
Mallucci et al. [33]	6	–	–	62
Kobata et al. [18]	30	–	–	56
Lakhdar et al. [34]	9	1	–	40
Schroeder et al. [35]	5	–	–	37
Goel et al. [36]	85	9	2 (suboccipital and subtemporal)	48
Safavi-Abbasi et al. [37]	11	1	–	75

na not available

The capsule is thin and adherent to the arachnoid at numerous sites. Once the capsule is observed, the cyst can be entered and its soft contents removed first to debulk the tumor. Afterward, the matrix can be separated from the neurovascular structures under optimal visualization. The strategy is then to remove the tumor completely in one region before moving to the next region. In this way, no small tumor remnants are overlooked and the risk of regrowth is lowered. As a final step, all the corners of the CPA should be inspected with an endoscope, and the surgical field should be irrigated to ensure removal of remnants.

In the senior author's experience with the surgical resection of more than 100 CPA epidermoids through the suboccipital retromastoid approach, total removal was achieved safely in more than 75% of cases. Postoperative deficits are primarily related to the degree that the cystic capsule of dermoids and epidermoids adheres to the neurovascular structures. Consequently, it is advisable to leave small portions of the capsule rather than risk a surgical catastrophe [10, 13].

Arachnoid Cysts

Arachnoid cysts are pouch-like intraarachnoid masses that supposedly form by splitting of the arachnoid membrane [39]. Typically, these cysts are considered to be congenital lesions. Examples in the literature, however, suggest that a subgroup may be acquired [40].

The neuroimaging characteristics of arachnoid cysts almost exactly match those of CSF (Fig. 20.3) [16]. The lesions have smooth, rounded edges. They displace neurovascular structures and may erode adjacent bone structures. In the CPA, arachnoid cysts essentially behave as locally expanding masses and may become quite large [41]. They can manifest with various "posterior fossa symptoms" such as hearing loss, vertigo, tinnitus, cranial nerve weakness, or other unusual symptoms [42–47]. Often, however, the presentation is associated with vague, nonspecific complaints such as headaches and dizziness [39].

Various surgical techniques such as stereotactic puncture, shunting, cyst fenestration, radical open resection, and endoscopic management have been used to treat these lesions [39, 48–50]. Conservative management of asymptomatic cases with clinical and radiological follow-up will identify cases that may require surgical intervention. Surgical therapy and technique should be based on the following criteria: cystic growth; compression of neurovascular structures; and, most importantly, the patient's signs and symptoms, especially progressive clinical worsening. Patients with compression of cranial nerve, or brainstem and related symptoms usually profit from surgical treatment. The best way to prevent a recurrence is to resect the entire cyst wall. The suboccipital route permits safe exposure of the cyst and surrounding neurovascular structures [39]. Regardless of the procedure used for treatment, outcomes tend to be excellent with appropriate selection of surgical indications and techniques [51–53].

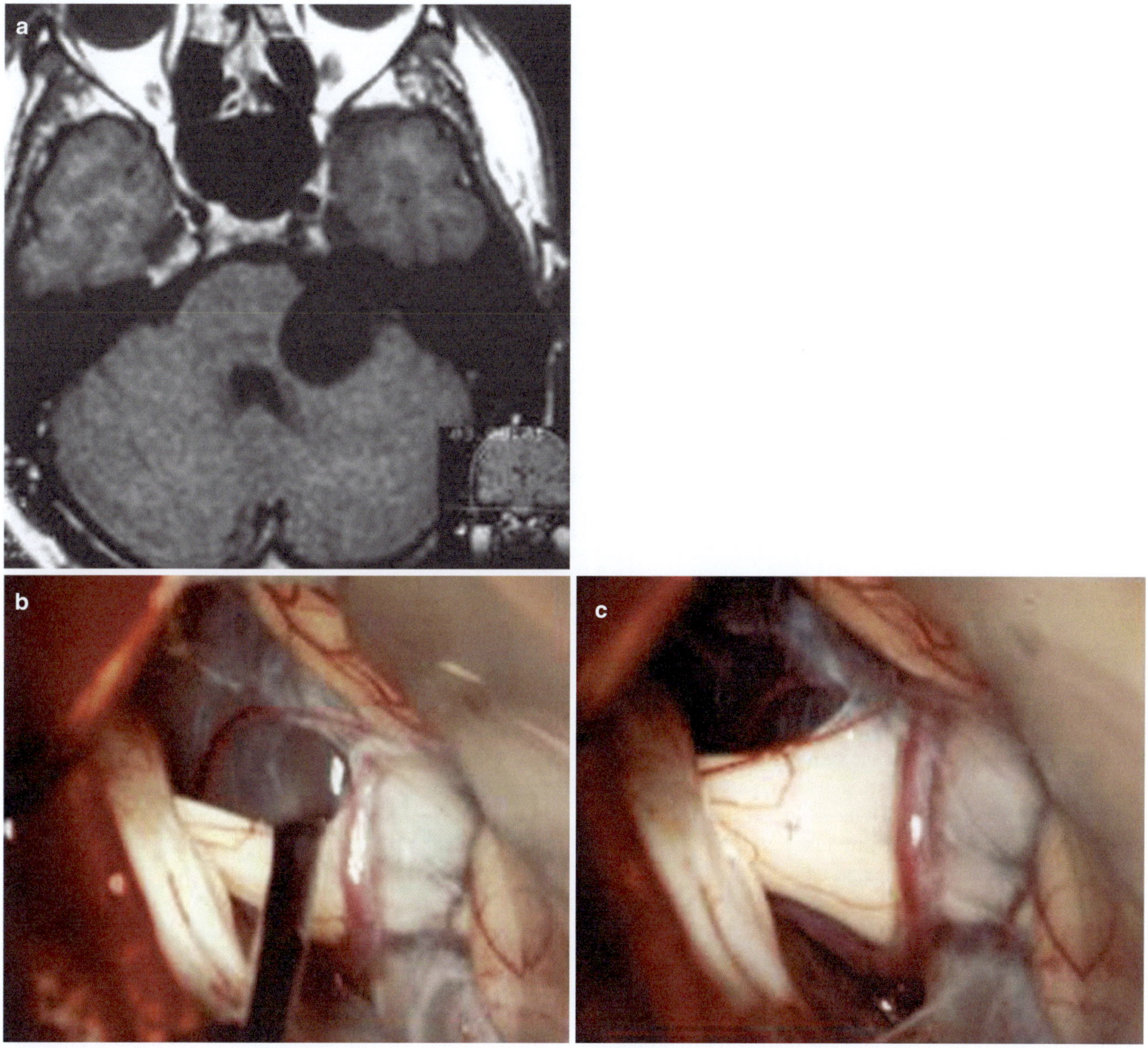

Fig. 20.3 Preoperative MRI (**a**) and intraoperative images (**b** and **c**) of a cerebellopontine angle arachnoid cyst

Nonvestibular Schwannomas

Intracranial schwannomas compose about 8% of all primary brain tumors [2, 3]. All cranial nerve schwannomas may occur as posterior fossa masses because of the location of the cranial nerves within the posterior fossa cisterns. The trigeminal nerve is the second most commonly involved cranial nerve, and trigeminal neurinomas account for 0.8–8% of intracranial schwannomas [54, 55]. Other cranial nerve schwannomas are uncommon, and preoperative radiological investigation is essential to establish their precise location (Fig. 20.4). Schwannomas also can manifest as intracranial or extracranial skull-base tumors. MR imaging has revolutionized their preoperative diagnosis, but CT and plain X-rays are still useful in defining bony architecture and skull-base anatomy for preoperative planning.

On plain X-rays, trigeminal neurinomas of the middle fossa and dumbbell-shaped lesions usually produce a sharp-edged bone defect in the floor of the middle fossa involving the foramen ovale, foramen spinosum, and petrous apex. The lateral aspect and dorsum of the sella, anterior clinoid process, and superior orbital fissure may be involved with some trigeminal schwannomas. In the case of jugular foramen schwannomas, plain X-ray and bone window CT scans show enlargement of the jugular foramen and bony destruction. On MRI the jugular bulb may not be patent [54, 56]. Clinically,

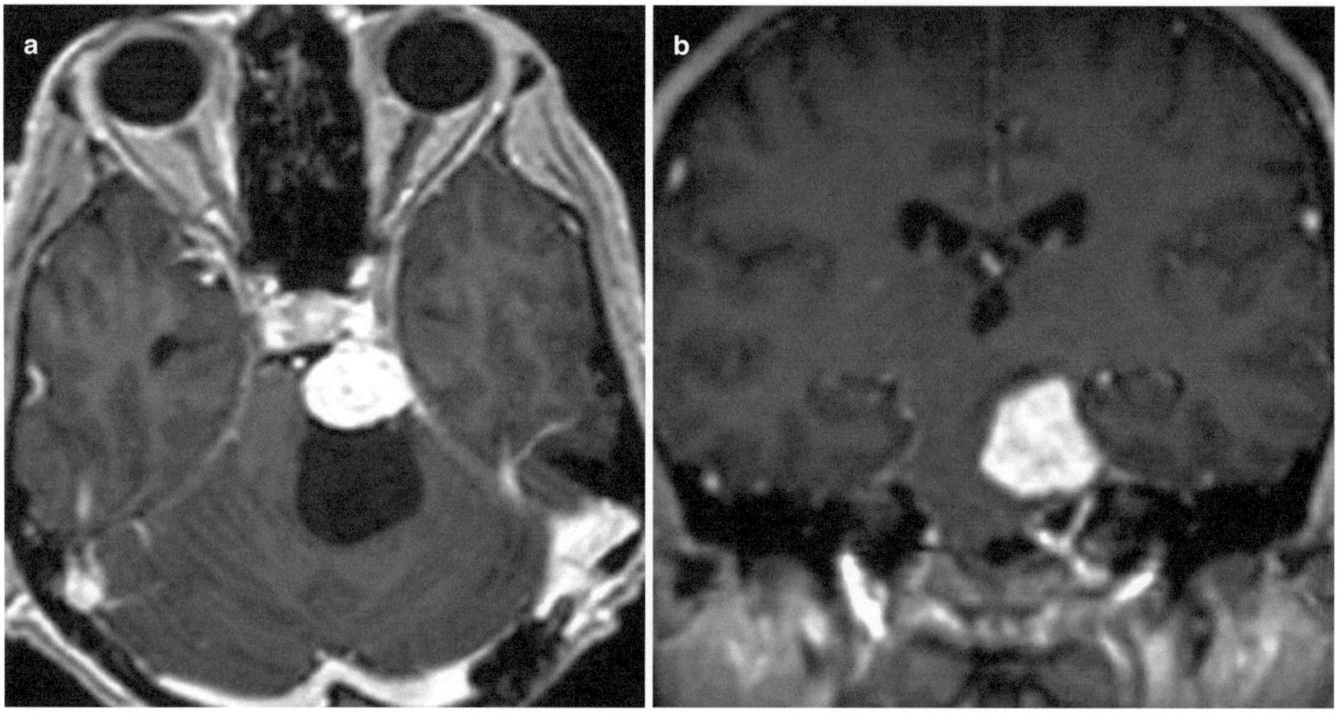

Fig. 20.4 Axial (**a**) and coronal (**b**) MRIs of a trochlear schwannoma in the posterior fossa associated with a cyst

sensation may be decreased in all three branches of the nerve. Facial pain may occur but is not a consistent feature of trigeminal schwannomas. Other symptoms associated with compression of other neurovascular structures also occur.

In 1955 Jefferson classified these tumors into three types: type 1 tumors, mainly in the middle fossa; type 2 tumors, mainly in the posterior fossa; and type 3 tumors with extension into both cranial fossae (Fig. 20.5) [56]. We have classified these tumors, depending on their radiological features, into four subtypes. Type A tumors are predominantly located in the middle cranial fossa. Type B tumors are located in the posterior fossa. Type C tumor are dumbbell-shaped and extend into both cranial fossae. Type D tumors are primarily extracranial tumors with some degree of intracranial extension.

Finally, we usually use a frontotemporal craniotomy and an epidural or transsylvian approach for type A tumors. A low temporal craniotomy and zygomatic osteotomy may be necessary to avoid excessive retraction. A retrosigmoid craniectomy is the favored approach for type B tumors. Dumbbell-shaped tumors with extension into two cranial fossae are the most difficult to excise completely. In the past, we usually used a combined or staged modification of retromastoid and subtemporal approaches. For meningiomas of the petroclival region with an extension to Meckel's cave, we developed and used a modification of the retrosigmoid approach (retrosigmoidal suprameatal transpetrosal apex approach) in 1982 to open Meckel's cave [57]. This approach is also ideal for removing dumbbell-shaped trigeminal schwannomas. Type D tumors usually originate from the mandibular or maxillary divisions of the trigeminal nerve and reach into the infratemporal fossa through the foramen ovale or foramen rotundum. An extradural subtemporal-infratemporal approach through a preauricular-infratemporal skin incision is typically selected. If an intradural extension is present, this approach can be combined with a temporal craniotomy. Great care must be taken to avoid injury of the facial nerve within parotid tissue and the petrous section of the carotid artery.

Schwannomas arising from the ninth, tenth, and eleventh cranial nerves compose only about 2.9% of all cranial schwannomas [54, 56]. These tumors are usually reviewed collectively as *jugular foramen schwannomas* because the actual nerve of origin often cannot be determined (Fig. 20.6). Symptoms may not manifest before the tumor becomes large. These tumors are rare in the first decade of life. Their occurrence in young patients should raise the suspicion of neurofibromatosis 2.

Size and origin of the tumor define the clinical presentation and also the appropriate surgical approach. Tumors that arise proximally mainly extend intracranially and manifest as masses involving the posterior fossa or CPA. Tumors arising in the midsection of the nerve expand the temporal bone. Distal lesions usually present as extracranial, skull-base, or cervical tumors.

We have classified these tumors into four types [56]. Type A tumors are primarily CPA masses with minimal extension into the jugular foramen. Type B tumors are primarily in the

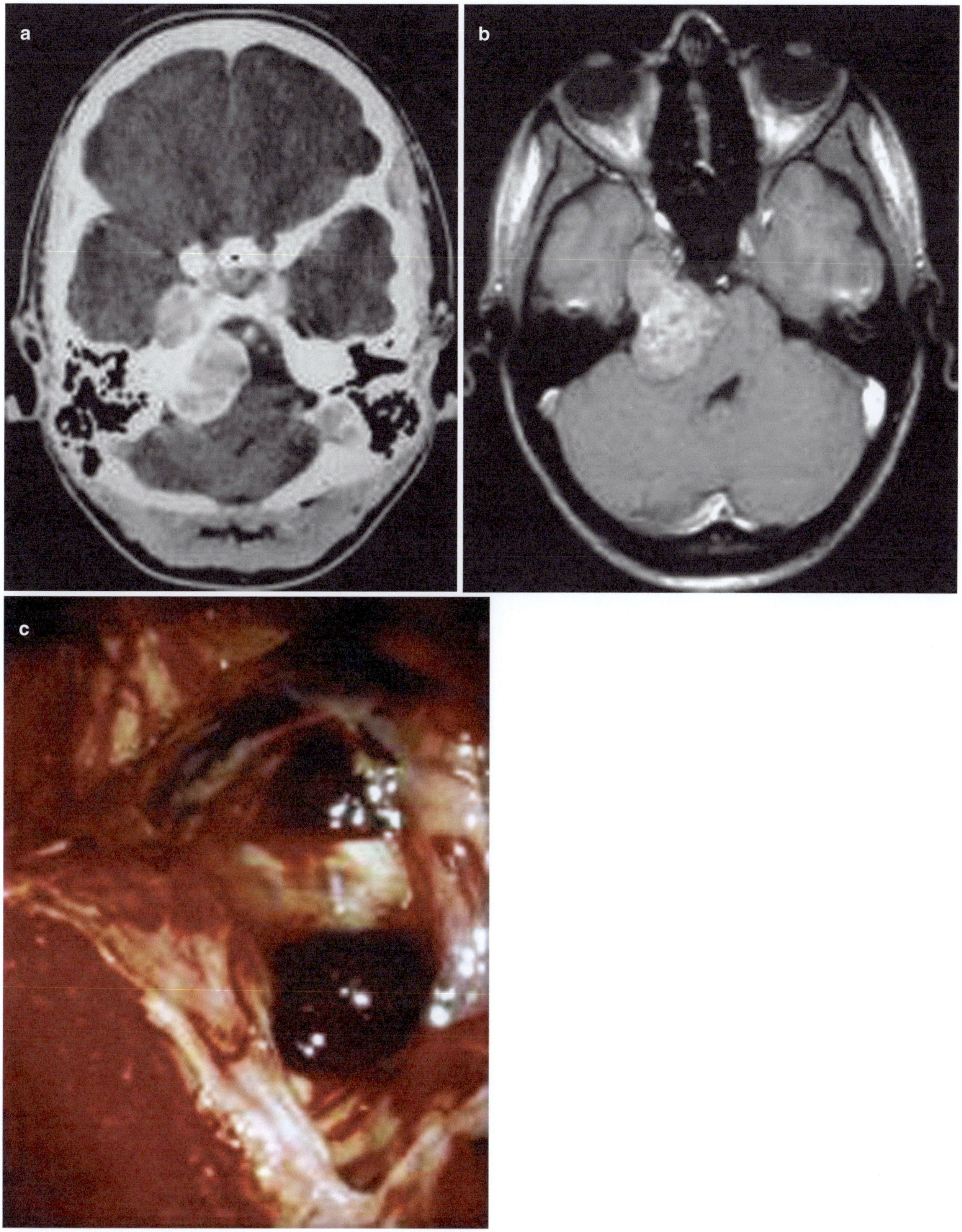

Fig. 20.5 CT scan (**a**) and MRI (**b**) of a large melanotic trigeminal neurinoma with an extension into multiple cranial fossae. Intraoperative view (**c**) after complete resection and preservation of the fifth cranial nerve

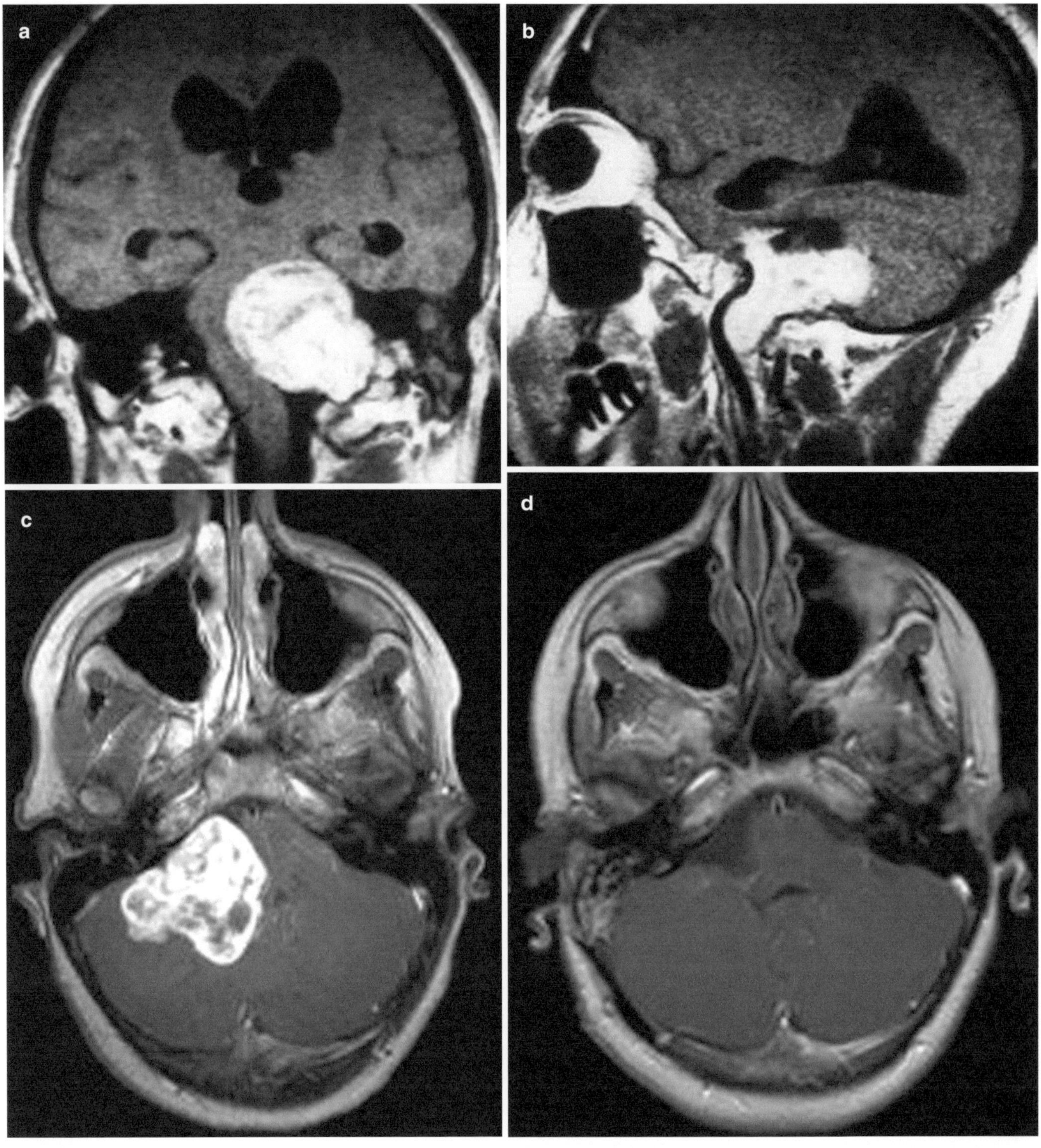

Fig. 20.6 Coronal (**a**) and sagittal (**b**) contrast-enhanced MRIs of a large jugular foramen schwannoma displacing the brainstem. Axial images contrasted MRI of another patient with a very large schwannoma of the jugular foramen before (**c**) and after (**d**) operative management

jugular foramen with some intracranial extension. Type C tumors are primarily extracranial, and type D tumors are dumbbell-shaped lesions with intra-and extracranial components. By virtue of the proximity of the jugular foramen to the IAC, patients with type A and B tumors often become symptomatic with symptoms referable to the seventh and eighth cranial nerves. The lateral suboccipital craniectomy provides good exposure for type A tumors. A single-stage combined cervical-transmastoid approach usually provides sufficient exposure for all other types of tumor [56, 57].

Metastatic and Exophytic Lesions

Although rare, metastasis to the CPA complicates the differential diagnosis of space-occupying lesions in this region (Fig. 20.7). Carcinoma of the lung and adenocarcinoma of the breast are most commonly encountered, probably related to their overall high rates of occurrence. However, gastrointestinal and genitourinary carcinomas as well as various other metastatic tumors, such as squamous cell carcinomas of the oropharynx, malignant lymphomas, malignant fibrous mesotheliomas, thyroid cancers, and malignant melanomas, may involve the CPA. Metastatic melanomas have a special predilection for hematogenous seeding of the IAC [16]. Tissue in the central nervous system is a common site of metastasis. Primary CPA melanoma is extremely rare; however, bilateral IAC involvement may occur with both metastatic and primary CPA melanomas.

Metastatic lesions are usually associated with an acute onset of uni or bilateral hearing loss or other cranial neuropathies. Symptoms may include nonspecific symptoms such as headache, ataxia, or nausea. Facial palsy is common and occurs more suddenly as compared with schwannomas, meningiomas, or other benign slow-growing tumors. Facial palsy may therefore be misdiagnosed as Bell's palsy.

Because of their hypervascularity, metastatic tumors usually enhance with intravenous contrast administration. Peritumoral edema disproportionate to the size of the mass can occur and is best detected on T2-weighted MRIs. Unlike benign tumors of the CPA, metastatic tumors seldom become large before they are diagnosed. Rather, they manifest early with fulminant and rapidly progressive symptoms. Their radiographic appearance, however, is variable and may resemble more common lesions in this location. Thus, the rapid onset of symptoms and a history of malignancy should prompt consideration of the diagnosis.

Yet, a history of previous malignancy and the subsequent appearance of a lesion in the CPA does not necessarily imply metastasis because second tumors can occur. Cases that arouse suspicion preoperatively require a thorough systemic evaluation. CSF cytology and serum tumor antigen examination are helpful. Frequently, a diagnosis cannot be obtained before surgery, and a neuropathologic examination of the tissue is needed to obtain the final diagnosis.

Complete tumor removal is usually the goal of surgical therapy. Often, the choice between therapeutic and palliative resection and tissue biopsy must be decided during surgical resection. Thus, the risk of injury to cranial nerves and quality of life must be weighed against the goal of oncologic intervention, especially considering the radio- and chemosensitivity of some lesions. However, local excision of solitary lesions can be remarkably beneficial [2, 3].

Parenchymal tumors that grow exophytically, such as medulloblastomas and gliomas, may extend into the CPA and mimic other lesions in this location [58]. At the lateral foramen of Luschka, the ependymal lining of the ventricle becomes everted and turns into the subarachnoid space of the cistern. Ependymomas and papillomas of the choroids plexus may grow through outlets of the fourth ventricle. Thus, a fourth ventricular component may be visible on MRI. The clinical and radiological presentation of intraaxial tumors, however, may be similar to that of the more common extraaxial lesions.

When patients become symptomatic with symptoms of short duration, rapid progression to brainstem dysfunction, hydrocephalus, and surrounding parenchymal edema associated with a relatively small mass, an intraaxial origin should be suspected. Extraaxial masses are uncommon in childhood. Therefore, a CPA mass in a child should raise the suspicion for an exophytically growing parenchymal mass [58]. As for other CPA masses, a retrosigmoid craniotomy usually provides good access to the tumor. Again, pathologic examination of the tissue is often needed to obtain the final diagnosis.

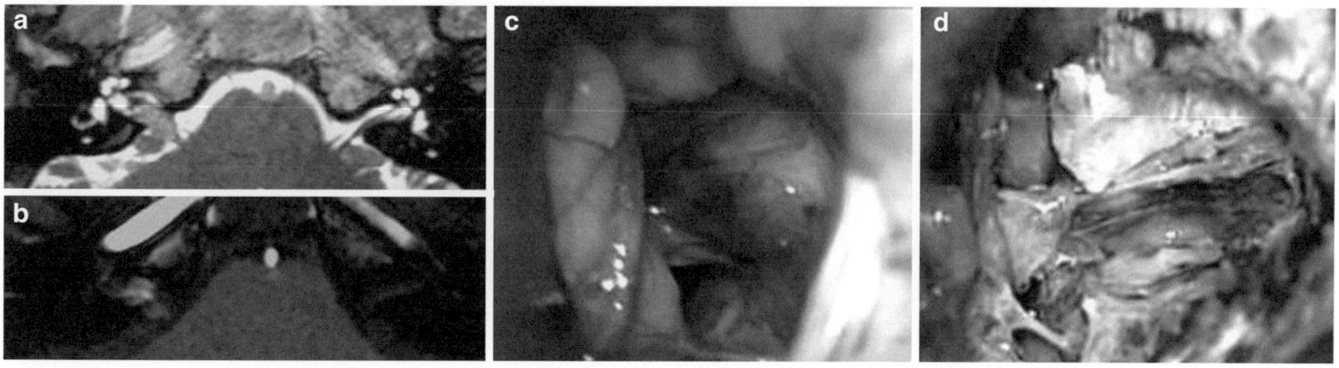

Fig. 20.7 Axial MRI (**a** and **b**) after contrast enhancement (**a**) of an intracanalicular vascular malformation. Intraoperative view shows the typical appearance of a cavernous malformation (**c**). Complete removal of the lesion and hematoma was associated with preservation of the facial and vestibulocochlear nerve complexes (**d**)

Lipomas

Clinically, lipomas can manifest like vestibular schwannomas and be associated with widening of the IAC on CT and MRI. A completely intracanalicular appearance is also possible. As cited by Samii and colleagues [2], in 1859, Klob found the first CPA lipoma at autopsy of a patient with hearing loss. Like other fatty tissues, lipomas are usually isointense or hypointense on T2-weighted MRIs. Typically, they appear bright on T1-weighted MRI [16]. This appearance is unique. However, some dermoids and epidermoids with a high fat content may appear fairly similar on MRI. On CT scans, lipomas usually appear as homogeneous, hypodense, and nonenhancing lesions [2]. These tumors are characterized by a high degree of neurovascular infiltration. Our experience has shown that surgery should be avoided because the natural history of these lesions is associated with far fewer complications than neurosurgical interventions.

Conclusions

Congenital rest lesions and other rare tumors of the CPA compose a subgroup of unusual disease entities that pose unique treatment challenges. Sound surgical judgment and experience in their management are critical in achieving excellent outcomes and long periods of disease-free survival.

References

1. Henneberg R, Koch M. Über "centrale" Neurofibromatose und die geschwüelste des Kleinhirnbrüeckenwinkels (Acusticusneurinome). Arch F Psychiatry. 1902;36:251–304.
2. Samii M, Draf W, Lang J. Surgery of the skull base: an interdisciplinary approach. Berlin: Springer; 1989.
3. Samii M, Cheatham ML, Becker DP. Atlas of cranial base surgery. Berlin: Springer; 1994.
4. Brackmann DE, Bartels LJ. Rare tumors of the cerebellopontine angle. Otolaryngol Head Neck Surg. 1980;88:555–9.
5. Matthies C, Samii M, Krebs S. Management of vestibular schwannomas (acoustic neuromas): radiological features in 202 cases—their value for diagnosis and their predictive importance. Neurosurgery. 1997;40:469–81.
6. Lang J Jr, Samii A. Retrosigmoidal approach to the posterior cranial fossa. An anatomical study. Acta Neurochir. 1991;111:147–53.
7. Matsuno H, Rhoton AL Jr, Peace D. Microsurgical anatomy of the posterior fossa cisterns. Neurosurgery. 1988;23:58–80.
8. Rhoton AL Jr. The posterior fossa cisterns. Neurosurgery. 2000;47:S287–97.
9. Matsushima T, Rhoton AL Jr, de Oliveira E, Peace D. Microsurgical anatomy of the veins of the posterior fossa. J Neurosurg. 1983;59:63–105.
10. Berger MS, Wilson CB. Epidermoid cysts of the posterior fossa. J Neurosurg. 1985;62:214–9.
11. Yasargil MG, Abernathey CD, Sarioglu AC. Microneurosurgical treatment of intracranial dermoid and epidermoid tumors. Neurosurgery. 1989;24:561–7.
12. Smirniotopoulos JG, Chiechi MV. Teratomas, dermoids, and epidermoids of the head and neck. Radiographics. 1995;15:1437–55.
13. Samii M, Tatagiba M, Piquer J, Carvalho GA. Surgical treatment of epidermoid cysts of the cerebellopontine angle. J Neurosurg. 1996;84:14–9.
14. Link MJ, Cohen PL, Breneman JC, Tew JM Jr. Malignant squamous degeneration of a cerebellopontine angle epidermoid tumor. Case report. J Neurosurg. 2002;97:1237–43.
15. Tamura K, Aoyagi M, Wakimoto H, et al. Malignant transformation eight years after removal of a benign epidermoid cyst: a case report. J Neuro-Oncol. 2006;79:67–72.
16. Bonneville F, Sarrazin JL, Marsot-Dupuch K, et al. Unusual lesions of the cerebellopontine angle: a segmental approach. Radiographics. 2001;21:419–38.
17. Sirin S, Gonul E, Kahraman S, Timurkaynak E. Imaging of posterior fossa epidermoid tumors. Clin Neurol Neurosurg. 2005;107:461–7.
18. Kobata H, Kondo A, Iwasaki K. Cerebellopontine angle epidermoids presenting with cranial nerve hyperactive dysfunction: pathogenesis and long-term surgical results in 30 patients. Neurosurgery. 2002;50:276–85.
19. Abramson RC, Morawetz RB, Schlitt M. Multiple complications from an intracranial epidermoid cyst: case report and literature review. Neurosurgery. 1989;24:574–8.
20. Michael LM, Moss T, Madhu T, Coakham HB. Malignant transformation of posterior fossa epidermoid cyst. Br J Neurosurg. 2005;19:505–10.
21. Mohanty A, Kolluri VR, Santosh V. Squamous cell carcinomatous change in a posterior fossa epidermoid: case report with a review of the literature. Br J Neurosurg. 1996;10:493–5.
22. Chandra PS, Gupta A, Mishra NK, Mehta VS. Association of craniovertebral and upper cervical anomalies with dermoid and epidermoid cysts: report of four cases. Neurosurgery. 2005;56:E1155.
23. Fischer G, Bret P, Hor F, et al. Epidermoid cysts of the cerebellopontile angle. 6 cases. Neurochirurgie. 1984;30:365–72.
24. Sabin HI, Bordi LT, Symon L. Epidermoid cysts and cholesterol granulomas centered on the posterior fossa: twenty years of diagnosis and management. Neurosurgery. 1987;21:798–805.
25. Salazar J, Vaquero J, Saucedo G, Bravo G. Posterior fossa epidermoid cysts. Acta Neurochir. 1987;85:34–9.
26. Morard M, De Tribolet N. Epidermal cysts of the cerebellopontile angle. Neurochirurgie. 1988;34:253–7.
27. deSouza CE, deSouza R, da Costa S, et al. Cerebellopontine angle epidermoid cysts: a report on 30 cases. J Neurol Neurosurg Psychiatry. 1989;52:986–90.
28. Altschuler EM, Jungreis CA, Sekhar LN, et al. Operative treatment of intracranial epidermoid cysts and cholesterol granulomas: report of 21 cases. Neurosurgery. 1990;26:606–13.
29. Lunardi P, Missori P, Innocenzi G, et al. Long-term results of surgical treatment of cerebello-pontine angle epidermoids. Acta Neurochir. 1990;103:105–8.
30. Vinchon M, Pertuzon B, Lejeune JP, et al. Intradural epidermoid cysts of the cerebellopontine angle: diagnosis and surgery. Neurosurgery. 1995;36:52–6.
31. Mohanty A, Venkatrama SK, Rao BR, et al. Experience with cerebellopontine angle epidermoids. Neurosurgery. 1997;40:24–9.
32. Talacchi A, Sala F, Alessandrini F, et al. Assessment and surgical management of posterior fossa epidermoid tumors: report of 28 cases. Neurosurgery. 1998;42:242–51.
33. Mallucci CL, Ward V, Carney AS, et al. Clinical features and outcomes in patients with non-acoustic cerebellopontine angle tumours. J Neurol Neurosurg Psychiatry. 1999;66:768–71.

34. Lakhdar A, Sami A, Naja A, et al. Epidermoid cyst of the cerebellopontine angle. A surgical series of 10 cases and review of the literature. Neurochirurgie. 2003;49:13–24.
35. Schroeder HW, Oertel J, Gaab MR. Endoscope-assisted microsurgical resection of epidermoid tumors of the cerebellopontine angle. J Neurosurg. 2004;101:227–32.
36. Goel A, Muzumdar D, Desai K. Anterior tentorium-based epidermoid tumours: results of radical surgical treatment in 96 cases. Br J Neurosurg. 2006;20:139–45.
37. Safavi-Abbasi S, Di Rocco F, Bambakidis N, et al. Has management of epidermoid tumors of the cerebellopontine angle improved? A surgical synopsis of the past and present. Skull Base. 2008;18(2):85–98.
38. Chu CK, Tseng HM, Young YH. Clinical presentation of posterior fossa epidermoid cysts. Eur Arch Otorhinolaryngol. 2006;263:548–51.
39. Samii M, Carvalho GA, Schuhmann MU, Matthies C. Arachnoid cysts of the posterior fossa. Surg Neurol. 1999;51:376–82.
40. Krisht AF, O'Brien MS. Acquired mirror-image cerebellopontine angle arachnoid cysts: case report. Neurosurgery. 1992;30:798–800.
41. Lancon JA, Ellis AL. Giant posterior fossa arachnoid cyst. Pediatr Neurosurg. 2004;40:151–2.
42. Cartwright MJ, Eisenberg MB, Page LK. Posterior fossa arachnoid cyst presenting with an isolated twelfth nerve paresis. Case report and review of the literature. Clin Neurol Neurosurg. 1991;93:69–72.
43. Haberkamp TJ, Monsell EM, House WF, et al. Diagnosis and treatment of arachnoid cysts of the posterior fossa. Otolaryngol Head Neck Surg. 1990;103:610–4.
44. Hadley MN, Grahm TW, Daspit CP, Spetzler RF. Otolaryngologic manifestations of posterior fossa arachnoid cysts. Laryngoscope. 1985;95:678–81.
45. O'Reilly RC, Hallinan EK. Posterior fossa arachnoid cysts can mimic Ménière's disease. Am J Otolaryngol. 2003;24:420–5.
46. Pirotte B, Morelli D, Alessi G, et al. Facial nerve palsy in posterior fossa arachnoid cysts: report of two cases. Childs Nerv Syst. 2005;21:587–90.
47. Yousaf I, Flynn P, McKinstry CS, Choudhari KA. Posterior fossa arachnoid cyst presenting with unilateral tremor. Br J Neurosurg. 2005;19:191–2.
48. Choi JU, Kim DS, Huh R. Endoscopic approach to arachnoid cyst. Childs Nerv Syst. 1999;15:285–91.
49. Dwarakanath S, Suri A, Mahapatra AK, et al. Endoscopic assisted excision of a retroclival arachnoid cyst presenting as hysterical breathlessness. Childs Nerv Syst. 2006;22:424–7.
50. Schroeder HW, Gaab MR, Niendorf WR. Neuroendoscopic approach to arachnoid cysts. J Neurosurg. 1996;85:293–8.
51. Daneyemez M, Gezen F, Akboru M, et al. Presentation and management of supratentorial and infratentorial arachnoid cysts. Review of 25 cases. J Neurosurg Sci. 1999;43:115–21.
52. Erdincler P, Kaynar MY, Bozkus H, Ciplak N. Posterior fossa arachnoid cysts. Br J Neurosurg. 1999;13:10–7.
53. Galassi E, Tognetti F, Frank F, et al. Infratentorial arachnoid cysts. J Neurosurg. 1985;63:210–7.
54. Al Mefty O, Ayoubi S, Gaber E. Trigeminal schwannomas: removal of dumbbell-shaped tumors through the expanded Meckel cave and outcomes of cranial nerve function. J Neurosurg. 2002;96:453–63.
55. Samii M, Migliori MM, Tatagiba M, Babu R. Surgical treatment of trigeminal schwannomas. J Neurosurg. 1995;82:711–8.
56. Samii M, Babu RP, Tatagiba M, Sepehrnia A. Surgical treatment of jugular foramen schwannomas. J Neurosurg. 1995;82:924–32.
57. Samii M, Tatagiba M, Carvalho GA. Retrosigmoid intradural suprameatal approach to Meckel's cave and the middle fossa: surgical technique and outcome. J Neurosurg. 2000;92:235–41.
58. Ahn MS, Jackler RK. Exophytic brain tumors mimicking primary lesions of the cerebellopontine angle. Laryngoscope. 1997;107:466–71.

21 Vascular Lesions of the Cerebellopontine Angle

Simone E. Dekker, Robert W. Tarr, Warren R. Selman, and Shakeel A. Chowdhry

Lesions of the cerebellopontine angle (CPA) offer a unique challenge to neurosurgeons because of their close proximity to the brainstem and cranial nerves. Although not as common as schwannomas and meningiomas, a number of vascular disorders can also arise in this region. Diagnostic and therapeutic advances have dramatically improved outcomes for patients affected by these lesions. The purpose of this chapter is to provide a systematic and comprehensive review of the most common vascular lesions that occur in the region of the CPA, including vascular compression syndromes, aneurysms, cavernous malformations, and hemangioblastomas. The principal diagnostic and therapeutic considerations for each lesion are discussed.

Vascular Loop Compression

Cranial nerve compression by vascular loops in the CPA is a well-recognized phenomenon. The most common vascular compression syndrome is trigeminal neuralgia, which involves compression of the trigeminal nerve by the superior cerebellar artery (SCA), posterior inferior cerebellar artery (PICA), or more rarely, an ectatic basilar artery [1, 2]. The transverse pontine veins are frequently involved in compression of the trigeminal nerve. These veins pass close to the trigeminal nerve to reach the bridging veins that enter the superior petrosal sinus. Hemifacial spasm is caused by compression at the facial nerve root entry zone by the anterior inferior cerebellar artery (AICA), PICA, or vertebral artery, in decreasing order of frequency (Fig. 21.1) [3]. Because the relationship of the vessels to the cranial nerves must be assessed, digital subtraction angiography is not very useful when vascular loop compression is suspected. Thin-section high-resolution T2-weighted magnetic resonance imaging (MRI) (e.g., FIESTA sequence) of the CPA with a 3-Tesla magnet can sometimes clarify the diagnosis (Fig. 21.2) [1, 4, 5]. However, a negative MRI does not necessarily rule out compression. The differential diagnosis for vascular loop compression includes a PICA or vertebral artery aneurysm, and arteriovenous malformation (AVM) involving the CPA, and vertebrobasilar dolichoectasia [1].

The treatment of choice for vascular loop compression syndromes is microvascular decompression via a variation in the lateral suboccipital/retrosigmoid approach. The trigeminal nerve is exposed through an infratentorial lateral supracerebellar approach, which allows the nerve to be decompressed in the lateral portion of the cerebellar tentorial surface. Facial nerve decompression is best performed through a lateral suboccipital infrafloccular approach, which exposes the inferior portion of the petrosal surface [6]. These approaches offer excellent visualization of the compressed nerve root entry zone while minimizing cerebellar retraction, which is associated with injury to the eighth cranial nerve [6–8]. Most series report a long-term success rate of more than 90% [9–14]. Endoscopic visualization in these

S. E. Dekker (✉) · W. R. Selman
Department of Neurological Surgery, The Neurological Institute, University Hospitals Cleveland Medical Center, Case Western Reserve University, Cleveland, OH, USA

R. W. Tarr
Radiology, Neurology, Neurological Surgery, University Hospitals Cleveland Medical Center, Case Western Reserve University School of Medicine, Cleveland, OH, USA

S. A. Chowdhry
NorthShore Neurological Institute, Evanston, IL, USA

N. C. Bambakidis et al. (eds.), *Surgery of the Cerebellopontine Angle*, https://doi.org/10.1007/978-3-031-12507-2_21

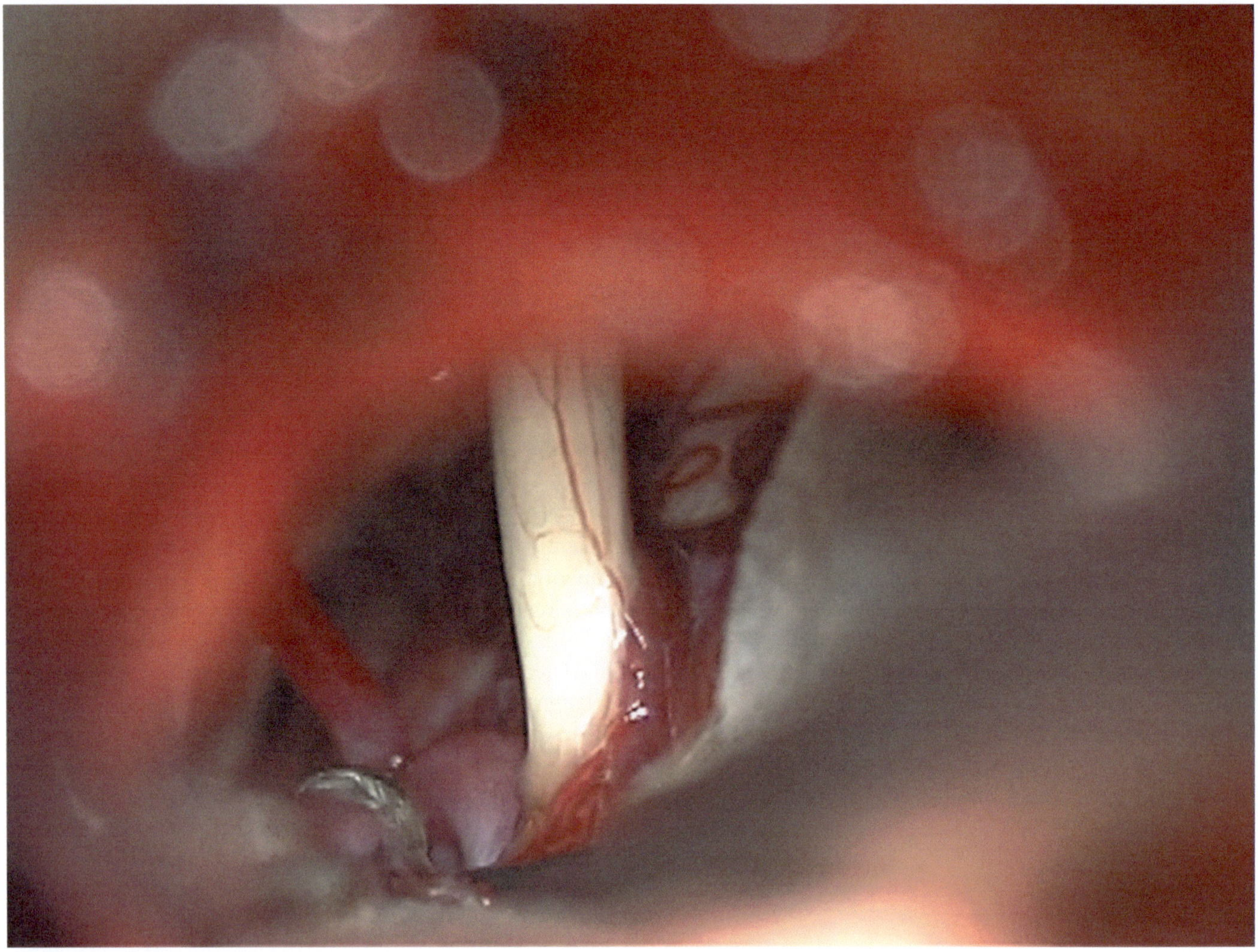

Fig. 21.1 Patient with left-sided hemifacial spasm. The intraoperative view demonstrates compression of the left facial nerve at root entry zone by a loop of the anterior inferior cerebellar artery (arrow)

approaches can be utilized as well to allow for improved visualization when smaller craniotomies are made [15].

Other less invasive options for treatment of cranial neurovascular compression syndromes include stereotactic radiosurgery (SRS), percutaneous balloon compression, percutaneous glycerol rhizotomy, and percutaneous radiofrequency thermal rhizotomy. SRS carries the lowest rate of long-term success and may be a good option for patients with multiple sclerosis and those unable to undergo other treatment options. Rhizotomies are effective but often with less long-term durability than microvascular decompression and often with limited ability to treat V1 symptoms. Microvascular decompression offers the highest long-term success rate with lower risk of facial numbness than the other treatment options.

In vertebrobasilar dolichoectasia, the offending vessel is an ectatic elongated vertebrobasilar system. Vertebrobasilar dolichoectasia most often manifests with symptoms of thromboembolic ischemia in the posterior circulation territory or with hemorrhage. Rarely, it causes symptoms from direct compression of cranial nerves or the brainstem (Fig. 21.3). Zaidi and colleagues reviewed the surgical strategies and clinical outcomes of microvascular decompression for hemifacial spasm secondary to vertebrobasilar dolichoectasia [16]. Employing Teflon pledgets alone provided good symptom relief with acceptable morbidity. Sling transposition can be used to augment decompression in patients with long segment compression [16].

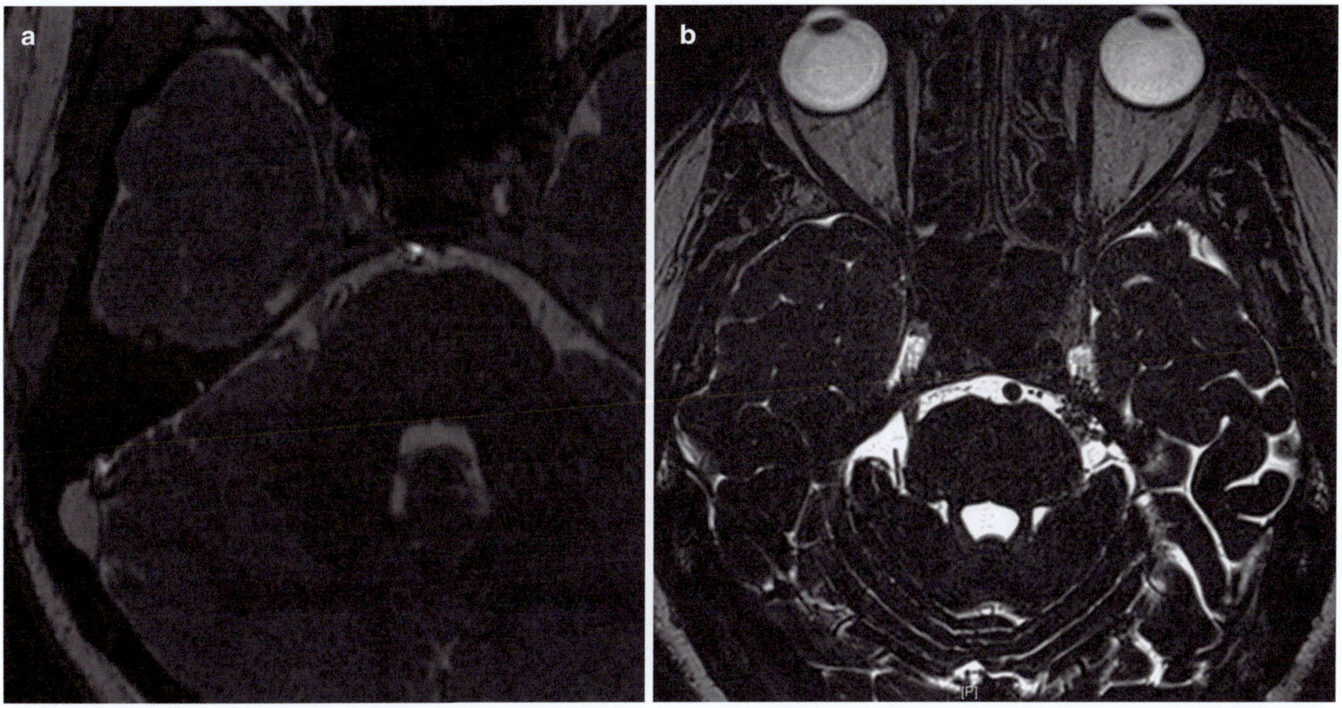

Fig. 21.2 (**a**) The FIESTA sequence can reveal the site of arterial compression as in this patient with right-sided trigeminal neuralgia. (**b**) The FIESTA sequence depicts a small arteriovenous malformation (AVM) causing left-sided trigeminal neuralgia (arrow). Treatment of the AVM with stereotactic radiosurgery resulted in resolution of symptoms

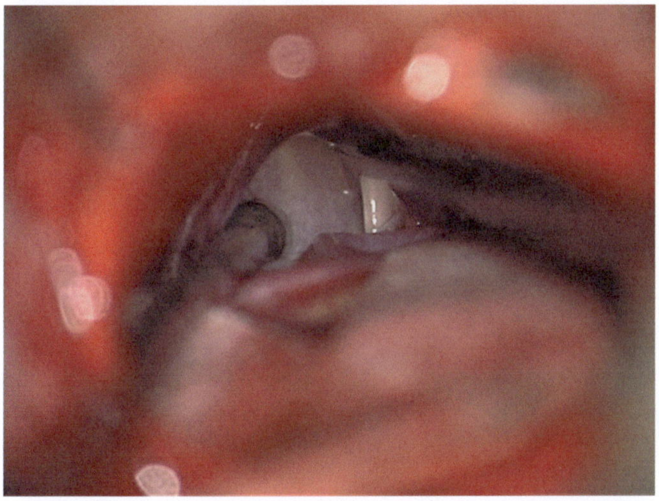

Fig. 21.3 Left retrosigmoid approach. A dolichoectactic basilar artery (directly under suction) causes direct compression of the trigeminal nerve (elevated by dissector)

Aneurysms

Fusiform Aneurysms

Atherosclerotic fusiform aneurysmal dilatation of the vertebrobasilar system is especially challenging for neurosurgeons to treat. This condition often manifests with posterior circulation thromboembolic disease and is associated with a poor prognosis. Occasionally, fusiform aneurysmal dilation of a tortuous vertebrobasilar system can cause CPA syndrome. Treatment of fusiform aneurysms can include deconstructive measures (e.g., unilateral/bilateral vertebral sacrifice or basilar artery occlusion after confirmation of adequate collateral circulation), stent-assisted coil embolization, and flow diversion [17]. If collateral circulation is inadequate, external carotid artery-to-posterior circulation bypass grafting should be performed before endovascular therapy or surgical trapping (Fig. 21.4) [18]. Staged endovascular occlusion of the vertebral arteries can also lead to aneurysmal thrombosis by altering flow dynamics [19]. The elimination of pulsatile blood flow in the thrombosed aneurysm usually improves symptoms of mass effect; although in the case of dissecting fusiform atherosclerotic aneurysms, there is an ongoing dynamic process of clot lysis and formation. For these aneurysms, complete occlusion of flow into the aneurysm is necessary for the thrombosed portion of the aneurysm to decrease in size.

Saccular Aneurysms

Aneurysms occur commonly in the posterior circulation at the basilar apex, PICA origin, SCA origin, and vertebrobasilar junction. SCA aneurysms and vertebral/PICA aneurysms

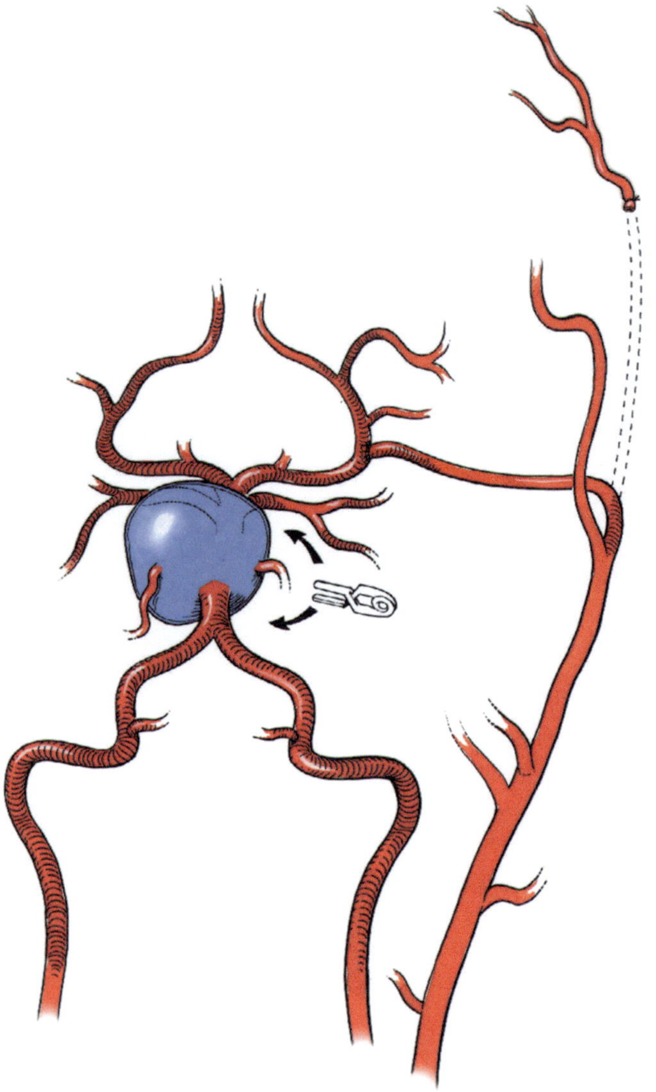

Fig. 21.4 The involvement of this giant midbasilar aneurysm with perforators makes it unsuitable for clipping. The flow to the aneurysm is reversed with an aneurysm clip, placed either proximally or distally, and it is revascularized with an STA-to-PCA bypass. The distal circulation must be bypassed with an anastomosis from the STA or occipital artery into the PCA or superior cerebellar artery. Reproduced with permission from Barrow Neurological Institute

are covered elsewhere in this book. Here we will focus on the more uncommonly encountered AICA aneurysm. The AICA arises from the mid to lower third of the basilar artery (Fig. 21.5) and is divided into three segments. The premeatal segment extends from the exit of the AICA from the basilar artery to the seventh and eighth cranial nerve complex and provides perforators to the brainstem. The meatal segment is related to the internal auditory canal and may also give off small perforating branches. Finally, the postmeatal segment, which is distal to the seventh and eighth cranial nerve complex, subsequently divides into rostral and caudal branches. The internal auditory (labyrinthine) artery is a branch of the rostral division of the postmeatal segment. The distal AICA then joins branches of the PICA and the SCA to supply the cerebellum.

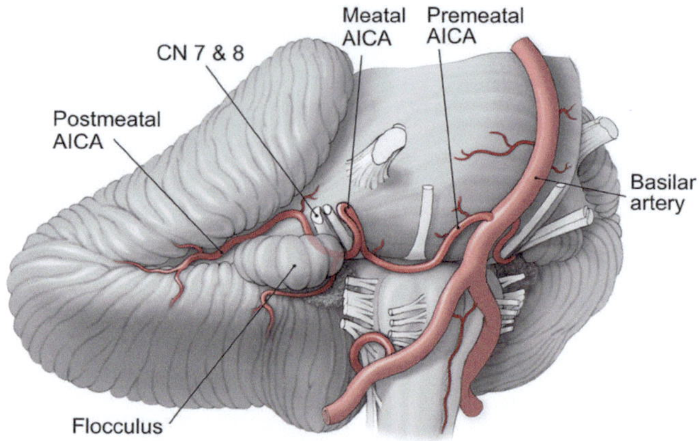

Fig. 21.5 Illustration shows the exit of the anterior inferior cerebellar artery from the basilar artery and its course. Reproduced with permission from Barrow Neurological Institute

Patients with saccular AICA aneurysms typically become symptomatic with subarachnoid hemorrhage (SAH). Because of its proximity to many vital structures, an unruptured AICA aneurysm may also cause neurological deficits related to local mass effect, including cranial nerve deficits (particularly facial palsy and hearing loss from compression of the seventh and eighth cranial nerves), long-tract signs from brainstem compression, and occipital or retromastoid headache.

Diagnosis of SAH associated with an aneurysm is straightforward or when a flow-void on MRI or magnetic resonance angiography (MRA) demonstrates a signal consistent with an aneurysm. However, diagnosis of aneurysms causing symptoms of mass effect can be more challenging. Occasionally, heterogeneous MRI signal loss occurs, depending on the particular flow dynamics within the aneurysm [20]. The signal characteristics of partially thrombosed aneurysms are even more variable. Such aneurysms can masquerade as CPA tumors such as acoustic neuromas or meningiomas [20]. A high degree of suspicion and factors such as sudden presentation of symptoms can help attain the correct preoperative diagnosis of AICA aneurysms. Digital subtraction angiography remains the gold standard for the evaluation of these aneurysms (Fig. 21.6). In some centers, computed tomography angiography (CTA) has replaced conventional angiography as the initial diagnostic study in patients suspected of harboring aneurysms.

AICA aneurysms can be categorized into proximal and distal types. Proximal aneurysms arise from the basilar–AICA junction or at the premeatal segment. Distal aneurysms usually arise from the rostral postmeatal branch. Suzuki and colleagues proposed that the AICA can be sacrificed distal to the internal auditory branch because of anasto-

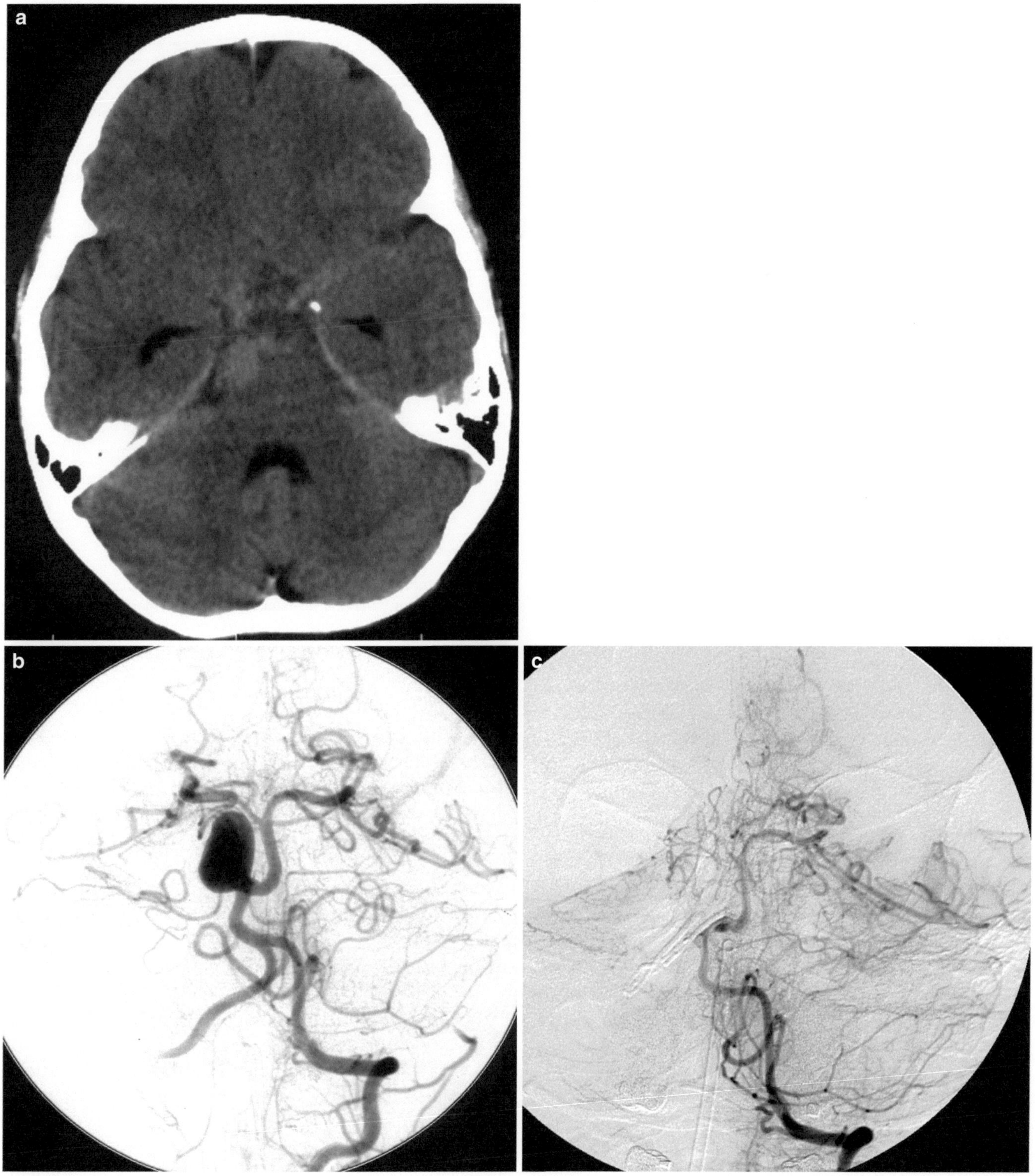

Fig. 21.6 (**a**) On noncontrasted computed tomography, a giant anterior inferior cerebellar artery (AICA) aneurysm appears as a hyperdense mass in the cerebellopontine angle. (**b**) Cerebral angiogram shows the giant AICA aneurysm. (**c**) Postoperative angiogram confirms successful clipping of the aneurysm with preservation of the parent vessel. From Gonzalez LF et al. [21], reproduced with permission from Lippincott Williams & Wilkins

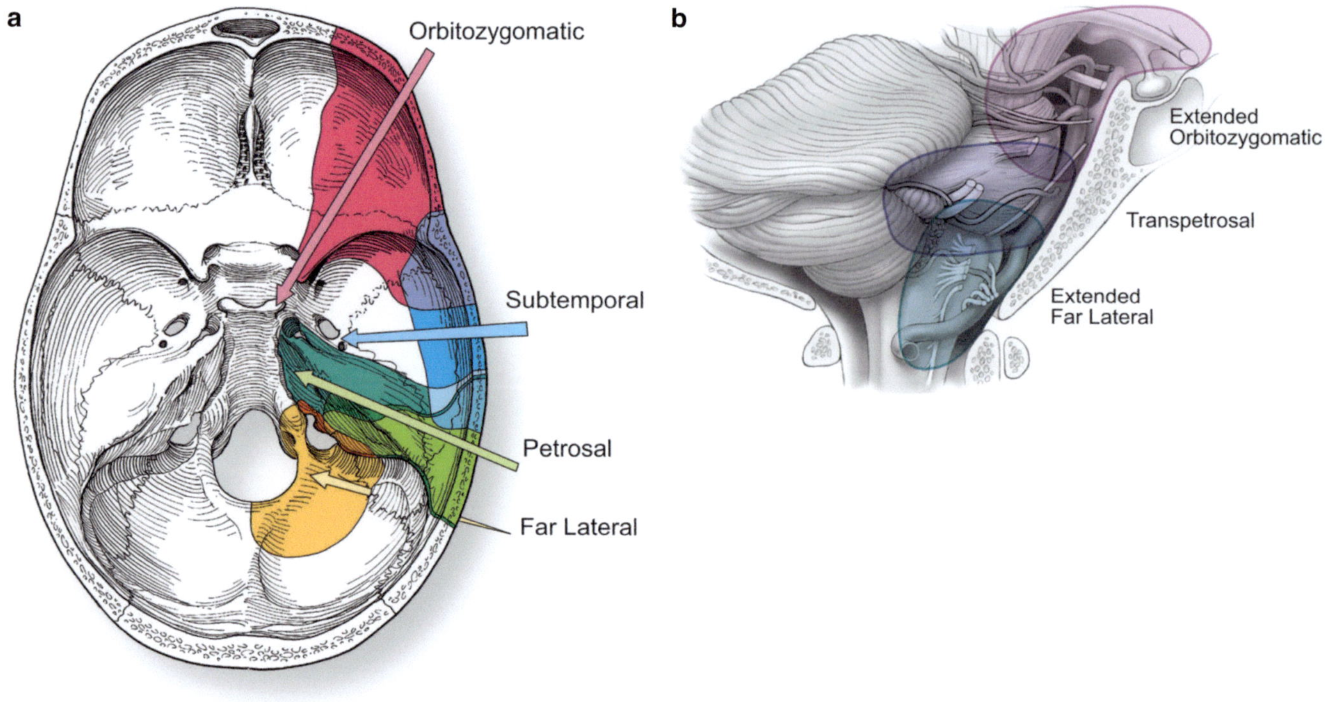

Fig. 21.7 Illustrations showing (**a**) axial and (**b**) sagittal views of surgical approaches for clipping complex aneurysms involving the cerebellopontine angle. The approach must be tailored to the size, configuration, and precise location of the aneurysm. A significant amount of bone may need to be removed to obtain adequate exposure of large or complex lesions. In such cases, the extended orbitozygomatic, transpetrosal, or extended far-lateral approaches may be considered as surgical options. Reproduced with permission from Barrow Neurological Institute

motic connections with branches of PICA and SCA [22]. However, the adequacy of these anastomotic vessels is extremely difficult to assess intraoperatively and during cerebral angiography [21].

Aneurysms of the AICA are exceedingly rare. In the series reported by Gonzalez and colleagues of more than 3500 saccular aneurysms treated surgically during a 16-year period, a mere 34 (1.7%) arose from the AICA [23]. Of these, 21 became symptomatic with SAH. Of the 13 unruptured aneurysms, seven manifested with brainstem compression. Eight aneurysms were giant (> 2.5 cm). Depending on the anatomic features of the aneurysm, various surgical approaches, including the retrosigmoid, far-lateral, transcochlear, translabyrinthine, and orbitozygomatic (Fig. 21.7), were used. Important considerations in choosing a surgical approach include the height of the aneurysm relative to the clivus and the position of the aneurysm along the course of the AICA. Among the 19 patients in this series for whom long-term follow-up information was available, 56% developed neurologic complications, including cranial nerve palsy (68%), cerebrospinal fluid (CSF) leakage (18%), hemiparesis (13%), and orbital hematoma (5%). Cranial nerve injury included palsy of the sixth (68%), seventh (23%), and eighth (17%) cranial nerves. At discharge, the mean Glasgow Coma Scale score for these patients was not significantly different than at admission. The high complication rate in such experienced hands underscores the difficulty involved with the surgical management of AICA aneurysms.

Treatment of Aneurysms

Choice of Surgical Approach

Treatment of AICA aneurysms requires expertise in vascular, endovascular, and skull-base surgical techniques. The unique difficulty associated with clipping these aneurysms partially reflects their location near the skull base and their proximity to multiple cranial nerves. The two most important factors in choosing a surgical approach are the craniocaudal location of the aneurysm in relation to the clivus and its mediolateral location along the course of the artery.

To visualize AICA aneurysms effectively, a corridor must be developed between the temporal bone and the CPA. Because of its anteroposterior oblique trajectory, the orbitozygomatic approach provides the best visualization of high-riding aneurysms. When using this approach, the posterior clinoid process must be drilled to expose the basilar artery. Drilling must proceed judiciously because it increases the risk of cranial nerve palsies, particularly of the third cranial nerve (Fig. 21.8).

Historically, the subtemporal corridor has been used to approach basilar trunk aneurysms. Drake and colleagues exposed 32 of 41 AICA aneurysms through a subtemporal-transtentorial approach [24–26]. More recently, however, Spetzler's team used the subtemporal and subtemporal-transtentorial approach only once in the surgical treatment of 41 AICA aneurysms. They attributed the scarcity of its use to the high rate of associated morbidity [23]. Today this approach is used mainly for visualizing midclival aneurysms (Fig. 21.9). Besides enabling drilling of the petrous apex, use of the subtemporal-transtentorial approach allows the tentorial edge to be opened to increase the extent of exposure. However, doing so significantly increases the risk of injury to the fourth cranial nerve. Significant morbidity can also follow retraction of the temporal lobe, especially the dominant side.

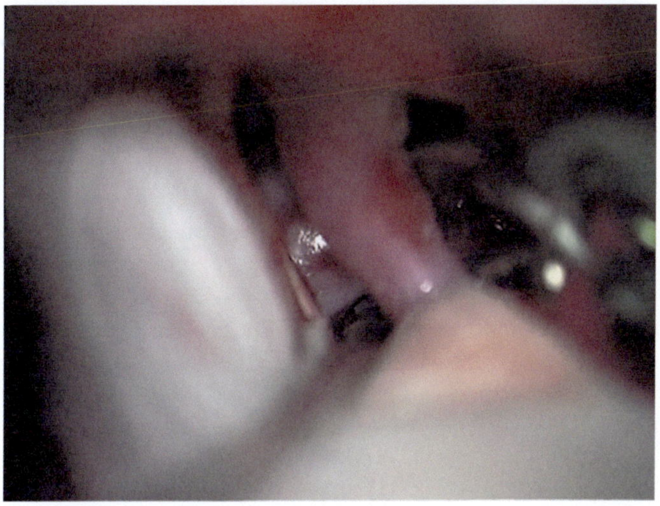

Fig. 21.8 Intraoperative view of left orbitozygomatic approach for basilar apex aneurysm clipping. Note the visualization of the medial anterior inferior cerebellar artery between clip blades

Because of its versatility and relatively low risk of complications, the retrosigmoid approach is the most common avenue for AICA aneurysm surgery. Skeletonization and lateral retraction of the transverse-sigmoid junction allow minimal retraction on the cerebellum. The premeatal AICA can then be seen between the fifth and seventh cranial nerves. During subsequent dissection, care must be exercised as it is easy to injure the sixth cranial nerve. The retrosigmoid approach offers good access to distal AICA aneurysms off the meatal and postmeatal segments. Alone or in combination with the retrosigmoid approach, the far-lateral approach can be used to expose low-lying aneurysms near the vertebrobasilar junction. This combination approach is especially useful for giant AICA aneurysms [23].

Transpetrosal approaches (transcochlear and translabyrinthine) provide the most direct route to the brainstem [27–32]. However, these approaches are associated with significant morbidity, such as deafness, facial nerve palsy, and CSF leakage. Spetzler's group advocates the use of the

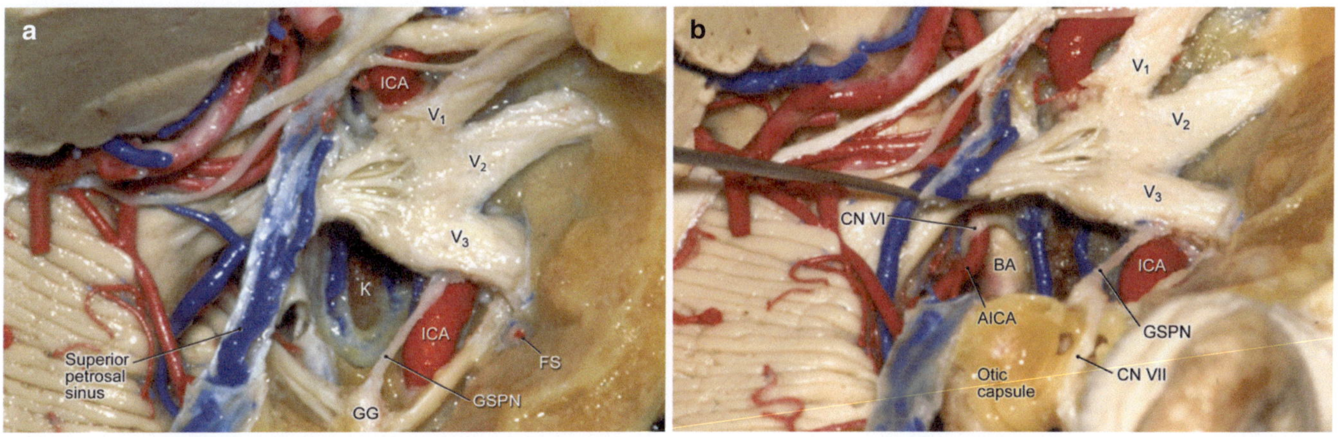

Fig. 21.9 Photographs of a cadaveric dissection show the right middle fossa. (**a**) The petrous apex has been drilled in Kawase's area, the "door" to the posterior fossa from the middle fossa. (**b**) The superior petrosal sinus has been sectioned, and the dura of the posterior fossa has been removed to expose the basilar artery and anterior inferior cerebellar artery (AICA). *BA* basilar artery, *CN VI* sixth cranial nerve, *FS* foramen spinosum, *GG* geniculate ganglion, *GSPN* greater superficial petrosal nerve, *ICA* internal carotid artery, *K* Kawase's area, V_1 ophthalmic branch of the trigeminal nerve, V_2 maxillary branch of the trigeminal nerve, and V_3 mandibular branch of the trigeminal nerve. From Gonzales LF, Amin-Hanjani S, Bambakidis NC, Spetzler RF: Skull base approaches to the basilar artery. Neurosurg Focus 19(2):E3, 2005. With permission from *Journal of Neurosurgery*

transpetrosal approach for select patients with giant aneurysms [23]. In their series, bilateral AICA aneurysms were clipped successfully through the transpetrosal approach, using the wide corridor made possible through a transcochlear approach. Transoral-transfacial approaches to AICA aneurysms have also been reported, although they are associated with exceedingly high rates of morbidity [27, 33–36].

Hypothermic cardiac arrest with barbiturate cerebral protection is historically an important adjunct for surgery of basilar and AICA aneurysms [37]. This technique allows deflation of the aneurysm, permitting manipulation and dissection of its dome from the pons and brainstem perforators with decreased risk of intraoperative hemorrhage. This technique is especially helpful for giant aneurysms that invaginate into the pons. More recently, adenosine has been utilized to reduce blood flow for a brief period of time in cases where proximal control cannot be readily obtained or when intraoperative rupture is encountered.

Rarely, dissecting AICA aneurysms also involve the CPA. Hancock and Millar reported a spontaneous AICA dissection in a patient with brainstem ischemic symptoms [38]. The patient's initial MRI showed a lesion of the CPA consistent with hematoma, but delayed high-resolution MRI demonstrated a decrease in size and evolution of signal characteristics consistent with signal void and serpentine contrast enhancement. Cerebral angiography showed a fusiform dilatation of the left AICA with an unusual corkscrew lumen. The diagnosis of spontaneous AICA dissection is suggested by evolution of signal characteristics on MRI, shrinkage of the lesion over time, and a clinical presentation consistent with occlusion of the vestibular and perforating branches of the AICA.

Endovascular Options for Aneurysms

The rapidly evolving field of endovascular surgery has revolutionized the treatment of aneurysms. Because of the high morbidity and mortality rates associated with vertebrobasilar aneurysm surgery, most experts now consider detachable coil embolization as the first line of treatment. Successful coil embolization requires an adequate dome-to-neck ratio and the ability to maneuver a microcatheter into the aneurysm dome to deliver the detachable coils. Most AICA aneurysms arise from the proximal portion of the artery. Therefore, the microcatheter can usually be manipulated into the aneurysm dome. If complete packing of the aneurysm is determined to carry a risk of parent vessel occlusion due to protruding loops of coil, it may be wise to leave a small remnant uncoiled. After clipping or endovascular treatment, any neck remnant can be observed with serial angiograms, and repeat coil embolization can be performed if growth is observed. Flow diversion has also proven to be an effective treatment option for posterior circulation aneurysms.

Deconstructive therapy with endovascular vertebral or basilar artery occlusion may be used if direct coiling of the aneurysm is infeasible or if a giant aneurysm indents the pons, or as an adjunct to flow diversion or surgical bypass. The parent vessel is occluded by altering local blood flow dynamics, thereby aiding in thrombosis of the aneurysm. Balloon test occlusion should be performed first to identify patients who can tolerate permanent vessel occlusion. Distal extracranial-intracranial bypass may be required before endovascular occlusion of the parent vessel in patients who fail balloon test occlusion. Before the procedure, all patients with unruptured aneurysms begin antiplatelet therapy to reduce the risk of antegrade parent vessel thrombosis, which can have devastating results. When not contraindicated, the patient is heparinized during the procedure to an activated clotting time of two times the baseline value.

Giant AICA aneurysms often invaginate into and compress the pons. Traditionally, coiling such aneurysms was considered contraindicated because of fear that the coil mass would increase compression on the brainstem. Recently, however, it has been shown that coiling of giant aneurysms can actually decrease mass effect and local parenchymal inflammation [39–41]. Balloon-assisted techniques and the placement of flexible Neuroform™ stents across the neck of an aneurysm are valuable when the aneurysmal dome-to-neck ratio is unfavorable. More recently, flow diversion provides a technically more straightforward option for these complex lesions (Fig. 21.10).

Although technically more difficult, distal AICA aneurysms can also be treated with endovascular means (Fig. 21.11). However, because there is usually adequate collateral supply to the brainstem and cerebellum from the ipsilateral PICA and SCA, distal AICA aneurysms may be treated with parent vessel occlusion distal to the internal auditory branch [22].

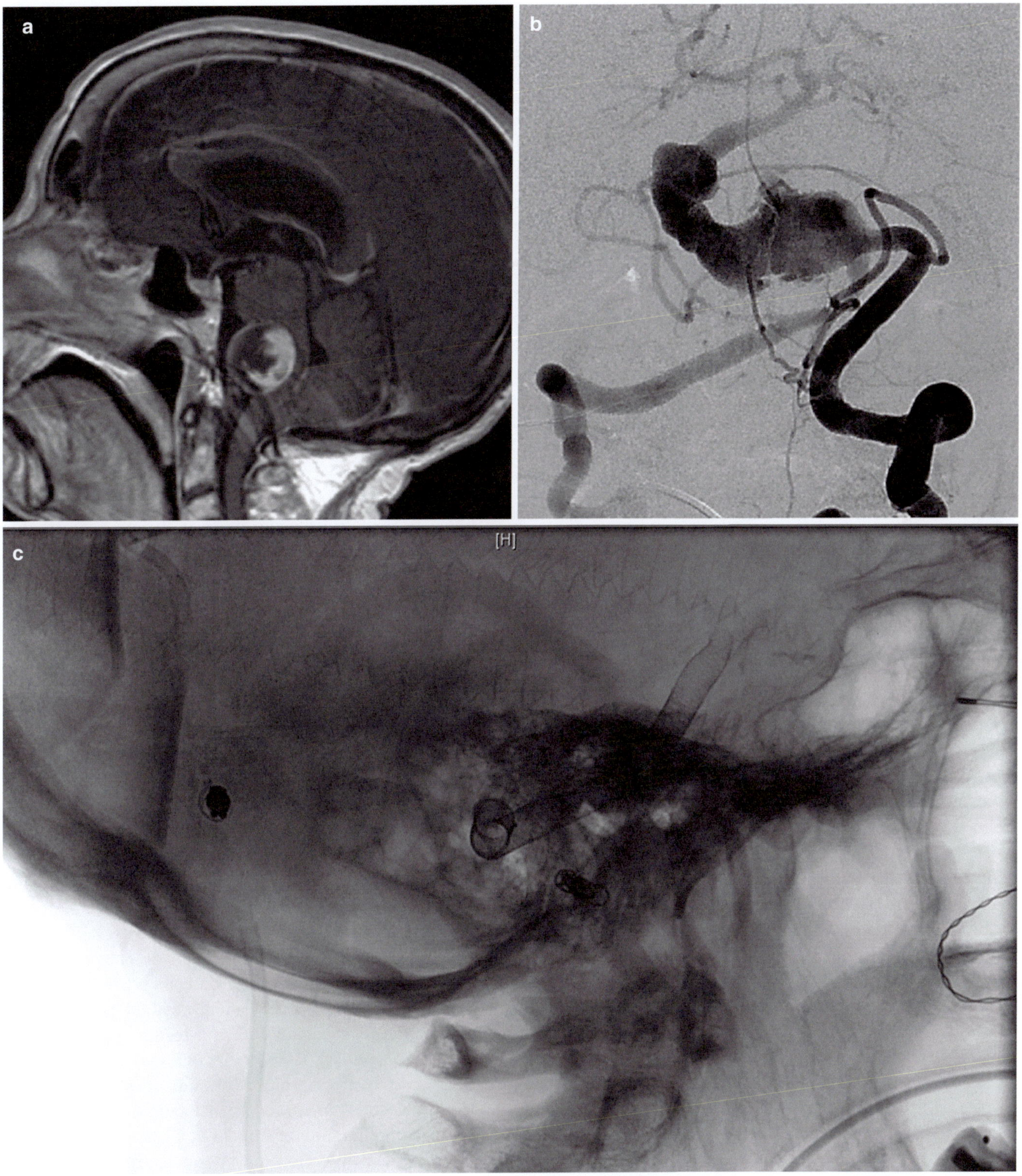

Fig. 21.10 A giant midbasilar aneurysm seen on (**a**) sagittal T1-weighted magnetic resonance imaging and (**b**) anteroposterior angiography following left vertebral artery injection. This aneurysm was treated with (**c**) deconstruction of the right vertebral artery distal to the posterior inferior cerebellar artery and flow diversion with pipeline flow diverting stents 2 weeks after a ventriculoperitoneal shunt had been placed.

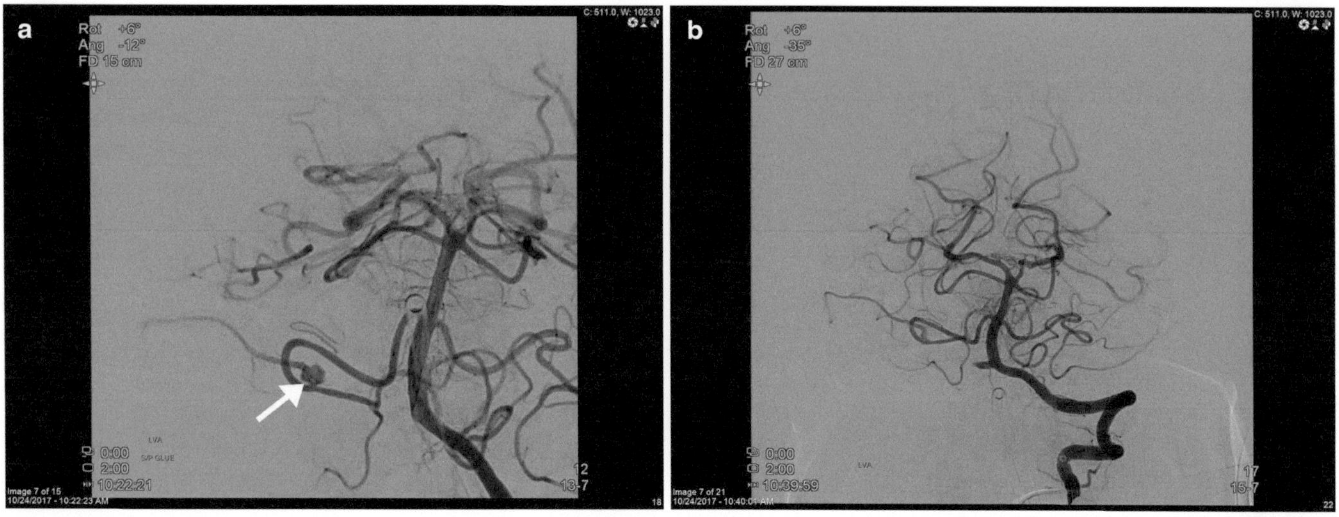

Fig. 21.11 (**a**) A ruptured 5-mm right anterior inferior cerebellar artery dissecting aneurysm arising from the postmeatal segment seen on Townes view following left vertebral artery injection (arrow). (**b**) The aneurysm was treated with embolization with no residual filling

Arteriovenous Malformations

AVMs, which consist of arteriovenous shunting without an intervening capillary bed, are the most common symptomatic intracranial vascular malformations. Seven to 25% of AVMs occur in the posterior fossa [42–49], cerebellum, brainstem, and CPA, in decreasing order of frequency [50, 51].

AVMs constitute fewer than 1% of all CPA lesions [52–54]. They are located at the pial surface of the brainstem or cerebellum and do not invade the parenchyma [44, 54]. They usually receive their arterial supply from dilated branches of the AICA or SCA [55] and drain into the prepontine and petrosal sinuses. Unlike AVMs in the cerebellum and brainstem, which often become symptomatic with hemorrhage, AVMs of the CPA most frequently cause symptoms related to mass effect. Patients often have symptoms of cranial nerve dysfunction, usually hearing loss or facial weakness [44, 54]. Trigeminal neuralgia or hemifacial spasm can also occur [56–59]. From a series of 1257 microvascular decompressions, Tsubaki and colleagues reported three AVMs of the CPA causing trigeminal neuralgia [56]. Most of these lesions can be identified preoperatively with high-resolution MRI of the CPA. Rarely, a vascular malformation mimics a purely intracanalicular acoustic neuroma [50, 52], appearing as an enhancing lesion on MRI. In the setting of hearing loss and facial palsy disproportionate to the size of the tumor, it is prudent to obtain a cerebral angiogram to rule out an intracanalicular AVM.

There are two main options for definitive treatment of AVMs involving the CPA: surgery and stereotactic radiosurgery. Because the morbidity rate associated with surgery is high [60], radiosurgery has been advocated as first-line treatment for brainstem AVMs, especially for very old patients or those with major medical problems. More aggressive treatment is necessary for CPA AVMs with hemorrhagic presentation versus those with non-hemorrhagic presentation. Yet, the ideal treatment for hemorrhagic cases remains unclear [61].

Gamma Knife radiosurgery (GKS) is an effective and safe treatment option for patients who do not require urgent relief of facial pain (Fig. 21.2). In a series of 80 parenchymal and 7 subpial AVMs, Massager and colleagues reported that 73% of the brainstem AVMs were totally obliterated 3 years after GKS; 74% of these patients had presented with hemorrhage before GKS [60]. The mean treatment volume was 1.3 mL, and the median prescription dose was 21.3 Gray. One disadvantage of GKS is the risk of bleeding for 2–3 years after therapy before the AVM is obliterated. In Massager's series, 3 of 87 patients had repeat hemorrhage after GKS and one patient died [60]. In this series, 19 patients with angiographic evidence of incomplete obliteration underwent repeat GKS. Nishiro and colleagues described the use of GKS for six patients presenting with hemorrhagic onset of symptoms. All cases resulted in favorable outcomes except for one patient who experienced rebleeding after GKS, which was caused by the repeated rupture of a feeder aneurysm [61]. Treatment of cerebral AVMs with GKS may fail for several reasons: inadequate definition of nidus, large volume of nidus, low dose of radiation, recanalization, and radioresistance related to intranidal fistula [62].

Microsurgical resection may be indicated in cases with moderate-to-severe neurological deficits due to the initial hemorrhage. Moreover, surgery may be considered for AVMs with perinidal aneurysms unsuitable for embolization (Fig. 21.12) [61]. Because of the superficial location and venous drainage of AVMs involving the CPA, these lesions usually are more amenable to surgical resection than those deeper in the parenchyma. Standard microsurgical technique

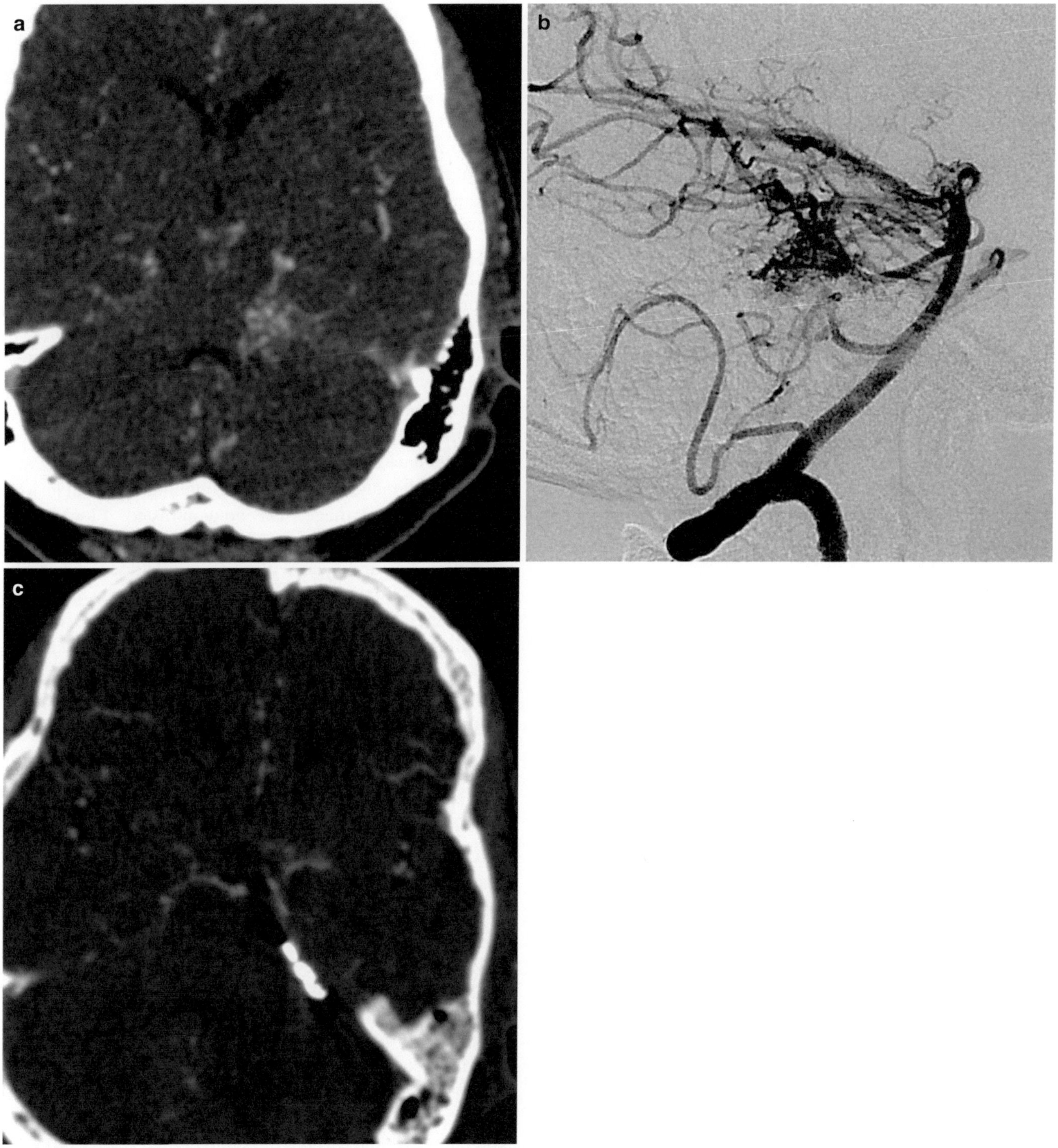

Fig. 21.12 A ruptured left-sided arteriovenous malformation seen on (**a**) axial computed tomography angiography (CTA) and (**b**) lateral angiogram with left vertebral artery injection. (**c**) Postoperative CTA following resection.

through the retrosigmoid craniotomy described earlier provides excellent access to the CPA. The main advantage of surgery is complete resection of the AVM, without the risk of rebleeding that is present for 2–3 years after radiosurgery. Han and colleagues described a series of microsurgical resections of brainstem AVMs. In all seven patients with a lateral pontine-type AVM, the nidi were completely resected without any neurological deterioration, even though four of the seven patients had preoperative neurological deficits with a modified Rankin Scale score > 3 [63]. Nozaki and colleagues investigated surgical results for eight CPA AVMs [64]. All eight patients had hemorrhage on initial presentation with preoperative neurological deficits, such as cranial nerve palsy and ataxia. Total microsurgical resection was performed in all patients, but three patients experienced a worsening of preexisting deficits [64]. Preoperative MRI, including time-of-flight and constructive interference in steady state imaging, can provide useful information for determining the nidus-nerve relationship, thus limiting intraoperative nerve root injury [61].

The association between intracranial AVMs and aneurysms is well documented [65–70]. Redekop and colleagues reported a 15% incidence of aneurysms among 632 patients with AVMs (5.5% intranidal and 11% flow related) [71]. The presence of an AVM-associated aneurysm is associated with a significantly higher risk of hemorrhage [72, 73]. Occasionally, these aneurysms rapidly expand, causing rapidly progressive cranial nerve palsy [74]. If an AVM involving the CPA is treated surgically, the associated aneurysm can be clipped intraoperatively. In patients undergoing radiosurgery, optimal treatment may involve endovascular coiling, depending on the type of aneurysm [75]. Because aneurysms arising from distal feeding arteries near the nidus have a high rate of regression after AVM obliteration (80% in Redekop's series [71]), radiosurgery alone may be adequate for distal flow-related aneurysms. Alternatively, embolization can be useful to obliterate aneurysms on distal feeding arteries before radiosurgery. In contrast, aneurysms on the proximal feeding arteries thrombose only 4% of the time after AVM obliteration [71]. Therefore, they require endovascular coiling before radiosurgery.

Glue embolization of large intracranial AVMs is reported to improve outcome by reducing operative blood loss and decreasing the incidence of normal perfusion pressure breakthrough [76, 77]. However, more recent data indicate that complete obliteration of cerebral AVMs with glue embolization is successful in only 15–20% of cases [78]. As described, embolization is most useful for the obliteration of aneurysms associated with AVMs involving the CPA.

Cavernous Malformations

Cavernous malformations (cavernous angiomas, cavernomas) are benign vascular hamartomas that consist of endothelial-lined vascular channels without intervening normal brain tissue. They are filled with blood products of different ages. They can occur throughout the central nervous system but are rarely seen at the CPA. In their series of 426 consecutive operative cases of lesions of the CPA or internal auditory canal, Kohan and colleagues reported only one cavernous malformation [79]. Overall, only a few cases have been reported [80–82]. Engh and colleagues performed a systematic literature review on cavernous malformations of the CPA and included 15 cases relevant to this disease. They found that hearing loss (86.7%) and facial paresis (53.8%) are the most common clinical signs associated with this tumor. The largest series of brainstem cavernous malformations consists of 100 patients [83]. In this series, 15 lesions were at the pontomesencephalic junction and 10 were in the pontomedullary junction. The number at the CPA was not identified. Brainstem cavernous malformations are always associated with venous anomalies.

CT can be negative in 30–50% of patients with cavernous malformations. When visible, these lesions appear as rounded hyperdense lesions with or without calcium. On T2-weighted MRI, the classic "mulberry" appearance is surrounded by a hypointense rim of hemosiderin. T2-weighted gradient echo MRI shows a prominent susceptibility effect (blooming) and is the most sensitive diagnostic sequence. Fluid-attenuated inversion recovery (FLAIR) and T2-weighted images may show surrounding edema in lesions with acute hemorrhage. On noncontrasted T1-weighted images, cavernous malformations range from isointense to hyperintense to brain, and often have loculated regions of increased signal consistent with blood products. Angiographically, these lesions are occult, but associated anomalies such as venous angiomas may be visualized.

The natural history of a cavernous malformation involves repeated hemorrhages that gradually increase its size and number of vascular channels. As a result, cavernous malformations in the CPA usually manifest with progressive hearing loss, facial weakness secondary to mass effect, or both [80, 81]. Because of their location at the pial surface and the lack of surrounding brain parenchyma to contain hemorrhages, they can also present with devastating SAH or with intraparenchymal hemorrhage into the brainstem.

Because they tend to enlarge over time, cavernous malformations of the CPA are usually resected surgically. Their peripheral location facilitates a surgical approach. Intraparenchymal brainstem cavernous malformations are associated with a relatively high rate of operative morbidity. Nonetheless, they are usually recommended for surgical resection because of their tendency to enlarge progressively from repeated hemorrhage [83]. Although complete resection is curative, it may be infeasible if the lesion is intimately associated with the seventh or eighth cranial nerves [80, 81]. Any associated venous malformation should be preserved to avoid venous infarction (Fig. 21.13).

Amin-Hanjani and colleagues reported their experience with proton-beam radiosurgery in the treatment of 98 cases of "surgically inaccessible" cavernous malformations [84]. After a latency of 2 years, they reported a reduction in annual hemorrhage rate from 17.3 to 4.5% per lesion. The associated incidence of permanent neurological deficit was 16%, and the mortality rate was 3%. Kondziolka and colleagues

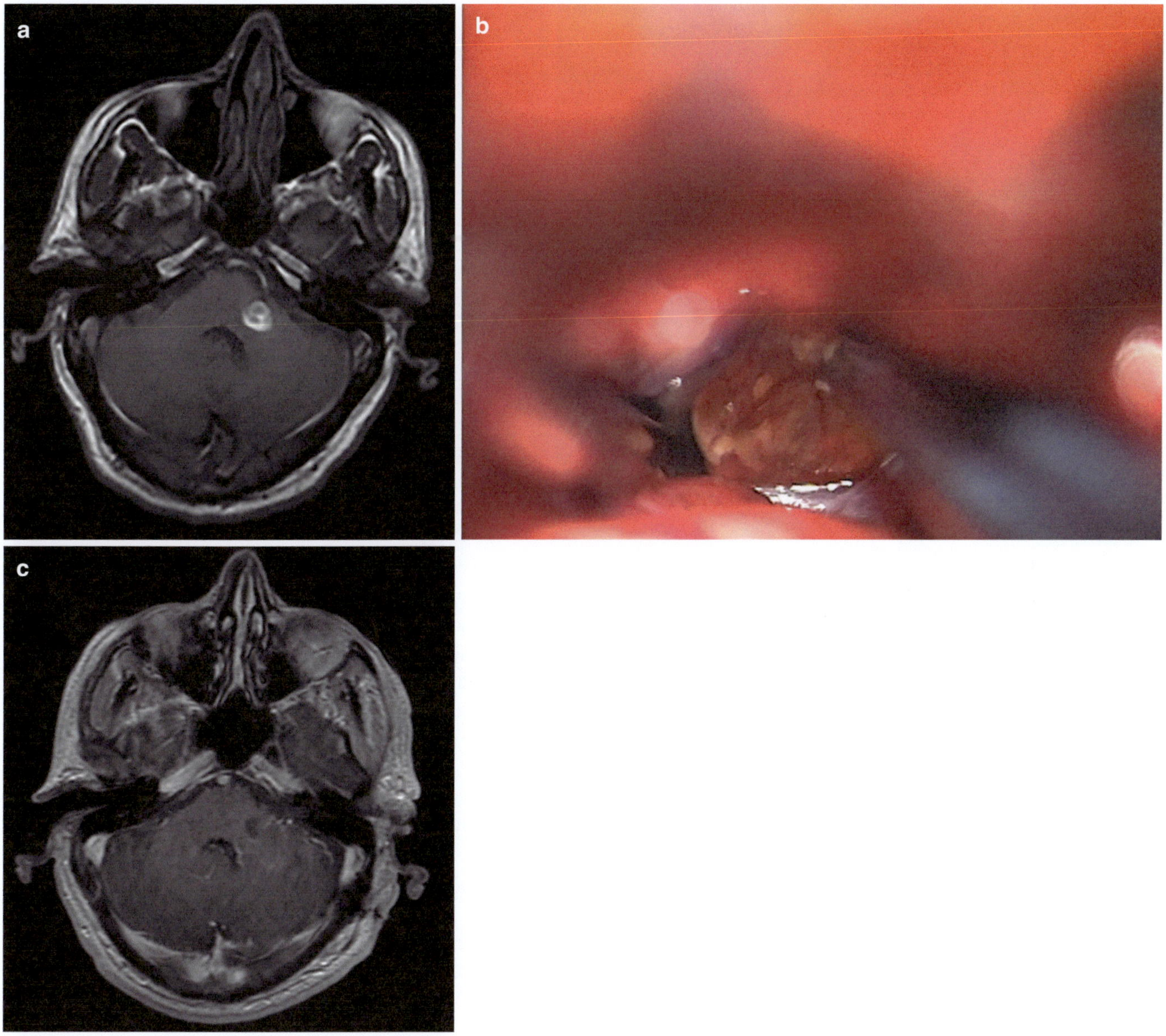

Fig. 21.13 A left-sided cavernous malformation situated in the cerebellar peduncle. (**a**) Preoperative T1-weighted axial magnetic resonance imaging (MRI) following gadolinium administration. (**b**) The cerebellopontine fissure is opened to allow a more direct route to the tumor, which can be seen during resection. (**c**) Postoperative T1-weighted gadolinium-enhanced axial MRI

used GKS to treat 47 patients with cavernous malformations in critical areas, 27 of which were in the brainstem [85]. The annual hemorrhage rate decreased from 56 to 8.8% per lesion after a latency of 2 years. After radiosurgery, 26% of the patients in this series experienced neurological deterioration. The main criticism of the above studies is that their pretreatment hemorrhage rate was much higher than previously reported, which may overstate the efficacy of treatment [86–97]. Additionally, given the natural history of cavernous malformations to have periods of quiescence between hemorrhages, the short-term follow-up is a significant limitation in the data. In any case, surgery is indicated for accessible cavernous malformations in the CPA as for any other lesion associated with a significant risk of hemorrhage.

Hemangioblastomas

Hemangioblastomas are benign vascular tumors of unclear origin associated with von Hippel-Lindau disease (VHL) in 25–40% of cases. They usually manifest in adults as a cystic intraaxial posterior fossa mass with an enhancing nodule. As many as 40% of hemangioblastomas lack a cystic component; when present, the cyst wall seldom enhances.

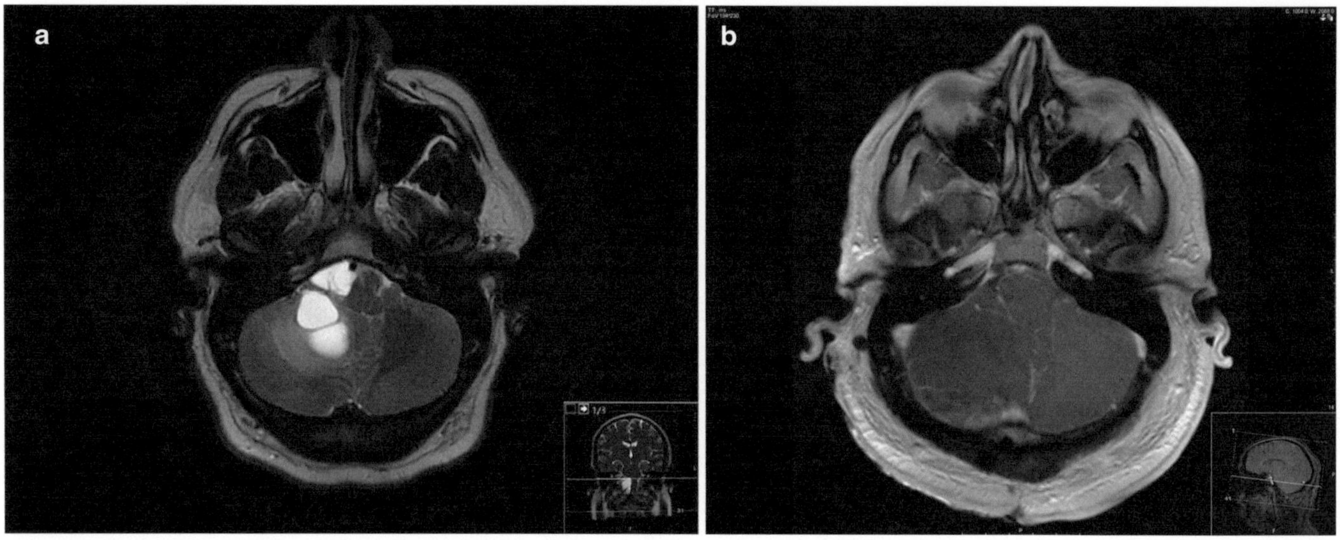

Fig. 21.14 (**a**) Cystic hemangioblastoma seen on preoperative axial T2-weighted imaging. A mural nodule was seen on gadolinium-enhanced imaging. (**b**) Gadolinium-enhanced axial T1-weighted imaging following resection via a far-lateral approach

Hemangioblastomas rarely reach the cerebellar surface and extend into the CPA. The differential diagnosis includes cystic astrocytoma, metastasis, cavernous malformation, and clear cell ependymoma. Angiography shows a highly vascular nodule with a prolonged blush and the occasional presence of an early-draining vein. The diagnosis is usually made with MRI, and angiography is rarely required. Surgical resection is the standard therapy for hemangioblastomas (Fig. 21.14). Depending on the relationship of the feeding artery and vascular nodule, preoperative embolization may be a useful adjunct.

Cheng and colleagues described 23 patients with CPA hemangioblastomas who underwent surgical resection [98]. Gross total resection was achieved in 96% of the cases. After surgery, the symptoms improved in 78%, remained unchanged in 13%, and in 9% of the cases the symptoms were aggravated. Patients with cystic hemangioblastomas exhibited better neurologic improvement versus patients with solid tumors. Moreover, a higher incidence of postoperative complications was found in patients with maximal tumor diameter of >3 cm or solid tumors. Patients with VHL disease are more likely to have a local recurrence [98].

Patrice and colleagues reported 38 hemangioblastomas treated with stereotactic radiosurgery [99]. Eight patients were treated for multiple hemangioblastomas (24 tumors) with a median tumor dose of 15.5 Gray. The 2-year actuarial rate of freedom from progression was 86%, and 78% of the surviving patients remained neurologically stable or improved. No significant permanent neurological complications were observed. A higher radiation dose and smaller tumor volume were significantly associated with better tumor control.

In summary, surgery is recommended in cases of uncertain diagnosis and for accessible hemangioblastomas exhibiting significant mass effect associated with symptoms. Small tumors or multifocal hemangioblastomas associated with VHL disease may be effectively treated with stereotactic radiosurgery [100].

Other Hypervascular Lesions

Hemangiopericytomas and paragangliomas are other hypervascular lesions that can occur in the CPA. Hemangiopericytomas and paragangliomas are discussed in Chap. 20 Congenital Rest Lesions and Rare Tumors.

Conclusion

A variety of vascular lesions occur at the CPA and can become symptomatic from thromboembolism, hemorrhage, or direct mass effect on the brainstem or cranial nerves. Vascular loop compression syndromes are the most common and can be treated surgically or with radiosurgery. Aneurysms in this location can also be treated effectively as can vascular malformations (AVMs and cavernous malformations) and tumors (hemangioblastomas). Advances in endovascular surgery, microneurosurgical techniques, and stereotactic radiosurgery have resulted in better outcomes for patients affected by these lesions.

References

1. Hearnsberger HR. Vascular loop compression, CPA-IAC. In: Osborn AG, Blaser SI, Salzman KL, et al., editors. Diagnostic imaging: brain. 2nd ed. Salt Lake City: Amirsys; 2004. p. 24–7.
2. Zakrzewska JM. Diagnosis and differential diagnosis of trigeminal neuralgia. Clin J Pain. 2002;18:14–21.
3. Tan NC, Chan LL, Tan EK. Hemifacial spasm and involuntary facial movements. QJM. 2002;95:493–500.
4. Majoie CB, Verbeeten B Jr, Dol JA, Peeters FL. Trigeminal neuropathy: evaluation with MR imaging. Radiographics. 1995;15:795–811.
5. Kazawa N, Togashi K, Ito J. The anatomical classification of AICA/PICA branching and configurations in the cerebellopontine angle area on 3D-drive thin slice T2WI MRI. Clin Imaging. 2013;37:865–70.
6. Hitotsumatsu T, Matsushima T, Inoue T. Microvascular decompression for treatment of trigeminal neuralgia, hemifacial spasm, and glossopharyngeal neuralgia: three surgical approach variations: technical note. Neurosurgery. 2003;53:1436–41.
7. Jannetta PJ, McLaughlin MR, Casey KF. Technique of microvascular decompression. Technical note. Neurosurg Focus. 2005;18:E5.
8. Jannetta PJ. Selection criteria for the treatment of cranial rhizopathies by microvascular decompression (honored guest lecture). Clin Neurosurg. 1997;44:69–77.
9. Chong YJ, Zhu GT, Duan DY, et al. Clinical analysis of 2643 cases of trigeminal neuralgia treated by microvascular decompression. Zhonghua Wai Ke Za Zhi. 2005;43:1407–9.
10. Kondo A. Microvascular decompression surgery for trigeminal neuralgia. Stereotact Funct Neurosurg. 2001;77:187–9.
11. Chung SS, Chang JH, Choi JY, et al. Microvascular decompression for hemifacial spasm: a long-term follow-up of 1,169 consecutive cases. Stereotact Funct Neurosurg. 2001;77:190–3.
12. Moffat DA, Durvasula VS, Stevens King A, et al. Outcome following retrosigmoid microvascular decompression of the facial nerve for hemifacial spasm. J Laryngol Otol. 2005;119:779–83.
13. Goto Y, Matsushima T, Natori Y, et al. Delayed effects of the microvascular decompression on hemifacial spasm: a retrospective study of 131 consecutive operated cases. Neurol Res. 2002;24:296–300.
14. Zhao W, Shen J, Pu C. Microvascular decompression for hemifacial spasm: experience of 215 cases. Zhonghua Yi Xue Za Zhi. 2001;81:1121–3.
15. Kabil MS, Eby JB, Shahinian HK. Endoscopic vascular decompression versus microvascular decompression of the trigeminal nerve. Minim Invasive Neurosurg. 2005;48:207–12.
16. Zaidi HA, Awad AW, Chowdhry SA, Fusco D, Nakaji P, Spetzler RF. Microvascular decompression for hemifacial spasm secondary to vertebrobasilar dolichoectasia: surgical strategies, technical nuances and clinical outcomes. J Clin Neurosci. 2015;22(1):62–8.
17. Hassan T, Ezura M, Takahashi A. Treatment of giant fusiform aneurysms of the basilar trunk with intra-aneurysmal and basilar artery coil embolization. Surg Neurol. 2004;62:455–62.
18. Terasaka S, Itamoto K, Houkin K. Basilar trunk aneurysm surgically treated with anterior petrosectomy and external carotid artery-to-posterior cerebral artery bypass: technical note. Neurosurgery. 2002;51:1083–7.
19. Omahen DA, Findlay JM. A giant fusiform basilar aneurysm treated by bilateral vertebral artery occlusion. J Clin Neurosci. 2004;11:324–8.
20. Sarkar A, Link MJ. Distal anterior inferior cerebellar artery aneurysm masquerading as a cerebellopontine angle tumor: case report and review of literature. Skull Base. 2004;14:101–6.
21. Nishimoto A, Fujimoto S, Tsuchimoto S, et al. Anterior inferior cerebellar artery aneurysm. Report of three cases. J Neurosurg. 1983;59:697–702.
22. Suzuki K, Meguro K, Wada M, et al. Embolization of a ruptured aneurysm of the distal anterior inferior cerebellar artery: case report and review of the literature. Surg Neurol. 1999;51:509–12.
23. Gonzalez LF, Alexander MJ, McDougall CG, Spetzler RF. Anteroinferior cerebellar artery aneurysms: surgical approaches and outcomes—a review of 34 cases. Neurosurgery. 2004;55:1025–35.
24. Drake CG. Surgical treatment of ruptured aneurysms of the basilar artery. Experience with 14 cases. J Neurosurg. 1965;23:457–73.
25. Drake CG. The surgical treatment of aneurysms of the basilar artery. J Neurosurg. 1968;29:436–46.
26. Drake CG, Peerless SG, Hernesniemi JA. Surgery of vertebrobasilar aneurysms: London, Ontario experience on 1767 patients. New York: Springer; 1995.
27. Seifert V, Stolke D. Posterior transpetrosal approach to aneurysms of the basilar trunk and vertebrobasilar junction. J Neurosurg. 1996;85:373–9.
28. Lawton MT, Daspit CP, Spetzler RF. Transpetrosal and combination approaches to skull base lesions. Clin Neurosurg. 1996;43:91–112.
29. Kawase T, Toya S, Shiobara R, Mine T. Transpetrosal approach for aneurysms of the lower basilar artery. J Neurosurg. 1985;63:857–61.
30. Steward DL, Pensak ML. Transpetrosal surgery techniques. Otolaryngol Clin N Am. 2002;35:367–91.
31. Tummala RP, Coscarella E, Morcos JJ. Transpetrosal approaches to the posterior fossa. Neurosurg Focus. 2005;19:E6.
32. Seifert V. Direct surgery of basilar trunk and vertebrobasilar junction aneurysms via the combined transpetrosal approach. Neurol Med Chir (Tokyo). 1998;38(Suppl):86–92. https://doi.org/10.2176/nmc.38.suppl_86.
33. Crockard HA, Koksel T, Watkin N. Transoral transclival clipping of anterior inferior cerebellar artery aneurysm using new rotating applier. Technical note. J Neurosurg. 1991;75:483–5.
34. de los Reyes RA, Kantrowitz AB, Detwiler PW, et al. Transoral-transclival clipping of a giant lower basilar artery aneurysm. Surg Neurol. 1992;38:379–82.
35. Hitchcock E, Cowie R. Transoral-transclival clipping of a midline vertebral artery aneurysm. J Neurol Neurosurg Psychiatry. 1983;46:446–8.
36. Saito I, Takahashi H, Joshita H, et al. Clipping of vertebrobasilar aneurysms by the transoral transclival approach. Neurol Med Chir (Tokyo). 1980;20:753–8.
37. Spetzler RF, Hadley MN, Rigamonti D, et al. Aneurysms of the basilar artery treated with circulatory arrest, hypothermia, and barbiturate cerebral protection. J Neurosurg. 1988;68:868–79.
38. Hancock JH, Millar JS. Spontaneous dissection of the anterior inferior cerebellar artery. Neuroradiology. 2000;42:535–8.
39. Gruber A, Killer M, Bavinzski G, Richling B. Clinical and angiographic results of endosaccular coiling treatment of giant and very large intracranial aneurysms: a 7-year, single-center experience. Neurosurgery. 1999;45:793–803.
40. Sluzewski M, Menovsky T, van Rooij WJ, Wijnalda D. Coiling of very large or giant cerebral aneurysms: long-term clinical and serial angiographic results. AJNR Am J Neuroradiol. 2003;24:257–62.
41. Ross IB, Weill A, Piotin M, Moret J. Endovascular treatment of distally located giant aneurysms. Neurosurgery. 2000;47:1147–52.
42. Apfelbaum RI. Surgery for tic douloureux. Clin Neurosurg. 1983;31:351–68.
43. Chou SN, Erickson DL, Oritiz-Suarez HJ. Surgical treatment of vascular lesions in the brain stem. J Neurosurg. 1975;42:23–31.

44. Drake CG. Surgical removal at arteriovenous malformations from the brain stem and cerebellopontine angle. J Neurosurg. 1975;43:661–70.
45. Drake CG, Friedman AH, Peerless SJ. Posterior fossa arteriovenous malformations. J Neurosurg. 1986;64:1–10.
46. Jellinger K. Vascular malformations of the central nervous system: a morphological overview. Neurosurg Rev. 1986;9:177–216.
47. Lessell S, Ferris EJ, Feldman RG, Hoyt WF. Brain stem arteriovenous malformations. Arch Ophthalmol. 1971;86:255–9.
48. Perret G, Nishioka H. Report on the cooperative study of intracranial aneurysms and subarachnoid hemorrhage. Section VI. Arteriovenous malformations. An analysis of 545 cases of cranio-cerebral arteriovenous malformations and fistulae reported to the cooperative study. J Neurosurg. 1966;25:467–90.
49. Solomon RA, Stein BM. Management of arteriovenous malformations of the brain stem. J Neurosurg. 1986;64:857–64.
50. Linskey ME, Jannetta PJ, Martinez AJ. A vascular malformation mimicking an intracanalicular acoustic neurilemoma. Case report. J Neurosurg. 1991;74:516–9.
51. McCormick WF, Hardman JM, Boulter TR. Vascular malformations ("angiomas") of the brain, with special reference to those occurring in the posterior fossa. J Neurosurg. 1968;28:241–51.
52. Brackmann DE, Bartels LJ. Rare tumors of the cerebellopontine angle. Otolaryngol Head Neck Surg. 1980;88:555–9.
53. Martuza RL, Parker SW, Nadol JB Jr, et al. Diagnosis of cerebellopontine angle tumors. Clin Neurosurg. 1985;32:177–213.
54. Viale GL, Pau A, Viale ES, Turtas S. Angiomas of the cerebellopontine angle. J Neurol. 1981;225:259–67.
55. O'Shaughnessy BA, Getch CC, Bendok BR, Batjer HH. Microsurgical resection of infratentorial arteriovenous malformations. Neurosurg Focus. 2005;19:E5.
56. Tsubaki S, Fukushima T, Tamagawa T, et al. Parapontine trigeminal cryptic angiomas presenting as trigeminal neuralgia. J Neurosurg. 1989;71:368–74.
57. Maher CO, Atkinson JL, Lane JI. Arteriovenous malformation in the trigeminal nerve. Case report. J Neurosurg. 2003;98:908–12.
58. Nagata S, Fujii K, Nomura T, et al. Hemifacial spasm caused by CP angle AVM associated with ruptured aneurysm in the feeding artery—case report. Neurol Med Chir (Tokyo). 1991;31:406–9.
59. Kim Y, Tanaka A, Kimura M, et al. Arteriovenous malformation in the cerebellopontine angle presenting as hemifacial spasm—case report. Neurol Med Chir (Tokyo). 1991;31:109–12.
60. Massager N, Regis J, Kondziolka D, et al. Gamma knife radiosurgery for brainstem arteriovenous malformations: preliminary results. J Neurosurg. 2000;93(Suppl 3):102–3.
61. Nishino K, Hasegawa H, Morita K, Fukuda M, Ito Y, Fujii Y, Sato M. Clinical characteristics of arteriovenous malformations in the cerebellopontine angle cistern. J Neurosurg. 2017;126:60–8.
62. Kwon Y, Jeon SR, Kim JH, et al. Analysis of the causes of treatment failure in gamma knife radiosurgery for intracranial arteriovenous malformations. J Neurosurg. 2000;93(Suppl 3):104–6.
63. Han SJ, Englot DJ, Kim H, Lawton MT. Brainstem arteriovenous malformations: anatomical subtypes, assessment of "occlusion in situ" technique, and microsurgical results. J Neurosurg. 2015;122:107–17.
64. Nozaki K, Hashimoto N, Kikuta K, Takagi Y, Kikuchi H. Surgical applications to arteriovenous malformations involving the brainstem. Neurosurgery. 2006;58(4 Suppl 2):ONS-270–9.
65. Boucquey JP. Arteriovenous angiomas (arteriovenous aneurysms) of the posterior fossa. Acta Neurol Psychiatr Belg. 1965;65:335–48.
66. Verbiest H. Arteral and arteriovenous aneurysms of the posterior fossa. Psychiatr Neurol Neurochir. 1962;65:329–69.
67. Vitale A, Terracciano S. Arteriovenous aneurysms of the posterior cranial fossa. Rass Int Clin Ter. 1961;41:304–19.
68. Gibson RM, Melo AN. Angiographic finding of an aneurysm and arteriovenous malformation in the posterior cranial fossa in a case of subarachnoid haemorrhage. J Neurol Neurosurg Psychiatry. 1960;23:237–8.
69. Kondziolka D, Nixon BJ, Lasjaunias P, et al. Cerebral arteriovenous malformations with associated arterial aneurysms: hemodynamic and therapeutic considerations. Can J Neurol Sci. 1988;15:130–4.
70. Lasjaunias P, Piske R, Terbrugge K, Willinsky R. Cerebral arteriovenous malformations (C. AVM) and associated arterial aneurysms (AA). Analysis of 101 C. AVM cases, with 37 AA in 23 patients. Acta Neurochir. 1988;91:29–36.
71. Redekop G, TerBrugge K, Montanera W, Willinsky R. Arterial aneurysms associated with cerebral arteriovenous malformations: classification, incidence, and risk of hemorrhage. J Neurosurg. 1998;89:539–46.
72. Brown RD Jr, Wiebers DO, Forbes GS. Unruptured intracranial aneurysms and arteriovenous malformations: frequency of intracranial hemorrhage and relationship of lesions. J Neurosurg. 1990;73:859–63.
73. Perata HJ, Tomsick TA, Tew JM Jr. Feeding artery pedicle aneurysms: association with parenchymal hemorrhage and arteriovenous malformation in the brain. J Neurosurg. 1994;80:631–4.
74. Neimat JS, Hoh BL, McKenna MJ, et al. Aneurysmal expansion presenting as facial weakness: case report and review of the literature. Neurosurgery. 2005;56:190.
75. Matsumaru Y, Hyodo A, Tsuboi K, et al. Brainstem arteriovenous malformation with a pedicle aneurysm treated by endovascular surgery and proton-beam radiosurgery—case report. Neurol Med Chir (Tokyo). 1996;36:716–20.
76. Zhao J, Wang C, Wang S, et al. Combination of intraoperative embolization with surgical resection for treatment of giant cerebral arteriovenous malformation. Chin Med J. 1999;112: 273–7.
77. Endo H, Osawa SI, Matsumoto Y, Endo T, Sato K, Niizuma K, Fujimura M, Tominaga T. Embolization of ruptured arteriovenous malformations in the cerebellopontine angle cistern. Neurosurg Rev. 2018;41(1):173–82.
78. Yu SC, Chan MS, Lam JM, et al. Complete obliteration of intracranial arteriovenous malformation with endovascular cyanoacrylate embolization: initial success and rate of permanent cure. AJNR Am J Neuroradiol. 2004;25:1139–43.
79. Kohan D, Downey LL, Lim J, et al. Uncommon lesions presenting as tumors of the internal auditory canal and cerebellopontine angle. Am J Otol. 1997;18:386–92.
80. Ohkuma A, Sugimoto S, Ando H, et al. Cavernous angioma in the cerebellopontine angle: a case report. No Shinkei Geka. 1993;21:367–71.
81. Bordi L, Pires M, Symon L, Cheesman AD. Cavernous angioma of the cerebello-pontine angle: a case report. Br J Neurosurg. 1991;5:83–6.
82. Engh JA, Kostov D, St Martin MB, Yeaney G, Rothfus W, Hirsch B, Kassam AB. Cavernous malformation tumors: a case study and review of the literature. Otol Neurotol. 2010 Feb;31(2):294–8. https://doi.org/10.1097/MAO.0b013e3181c34bf2.
83. Porter RW, Detwiler PW, Spetzler RF, et al. Cavernous malformations of the brainstem: experience with 100 patients. J Neurosurg. 1999;90:50–8.
84. Amin-Hanjani S, Ogilvy CS, Candia GJ, et al. Stereotactic radiosurgery for cavernous malformations: Kjellberg's experience with proton beam therapy in 98 cases at the Harvard cyclotron. Neurosurgery. 1998;42:1229–36.
85. Kondziolka D, Lunsford LD, Flickinger JC, Kestle JR. Reduction of hemorrhage risk after stereotactic radiosurgery for cavernous malformations. J Neurosurg. 1995;83:825–31.

86. Zabramski JM, Wascher TM, Spetzler RF, et al. The natural history of familial cavernous malformations: results of an ongoing study. J Neurosurg. 1994;80:422–32.
87. Del Curling O, Kelly DL Jr, Elster AD, Craven TE. An analysis of the natural history of cavernous angiomas. J Neurosurg. 1991;75:702–8.
88. Moynahan EJ. Natural history of cavernous haemangiomata. Lancet. 1960;1:227.
89. Aiba T, Tanaka R, Koike T, et al. Natural history of intracranial cavernous malformations. J Neurosurg. 1995;83:56–9.
90. Robinson JR, Awad IA, Little JR. Natural history of the cavernous angioma. J Neurosurg. 1991;75:709–14.
91. Kondziolka D, Lunsford LD, Kestle JR. The natural history of cerebral cavernous malformations. J Neurosurg. 1995;83:820–4.
92. Ziyal IM, Ozgen T. Natural history of brainstem cavernous malformations. Neurosurgery. 2001;49:1023–4.
93. Kupersmith MJ, Kalish H, Epstein F, et al. Natural history of brainstem cavernous malformations. Neurosurgery. 2001;48:47–53.
94. Moriarity JL, Clatterbuck RE, Rigamonti D. The natural history of cavernous malformations. Neurosurg Clin N Am. 1999;10:411–7.
95. Moriarity JL, Wetzel M, Clatterbuck RE, et al. The natural history of cavernous malformations: a prospective study of 68 patients. Neurosurgery. 1999;44:1166–71.
96. Dorsch NWC, McMahon JHA. Intracranial cavernous malformations—natural history and management. Crit Rev Neurosurg. 1998;8:154–68.
97. Porter PJ, Willinsky RA, Harper W, Wallace MC. Cerebral cavernous malformations: natural history and prognosis after clinical deterioration with or without hemorrhage. J Neurosurg. 1997;87:190–7.
98. Cheng J, Liu W, Zhang S, Lei D, Hui X. Clinical features and surgical outcomes in patients with cerebellopontine angle Hemangioblastomas: retrospective series of 23 cases. World Neurosurg. 2017 Jul;103:248–56.
99. Patrice SJ, Sneed PK, Flickinger JC, et al. Radiosurgery for hemangioblastoma: results of a multiinstitutional experience. Int J Radiat Oncol Biol Phys. 1996;35:493–9.
100. Park YS, Chang JH, Chang JW, Chung SS, Park YG. Gamma knife surgery for multiple hemangioblastomas. J Neurosurg. 2005;102 Suppl:97–101. https://doi.org/10.3171/jns.2005.102.s_supplement.0097.

Part V

Cases and Approaches (Animations and Videos)

Case 1: Retrosigmoid Approach for Vestibular Schwannoma

22

Simone E. Dekker and Nicholas C. Bambakidis

Summary

A 45-year-old woman was treated with a retrosigmoid approach to a vestibular schwannoma.

Case Presentation

A 45-year-old woman presented with progressive hearing loss and dizziness. Figure 22.1 shows preoperative images of this patient.

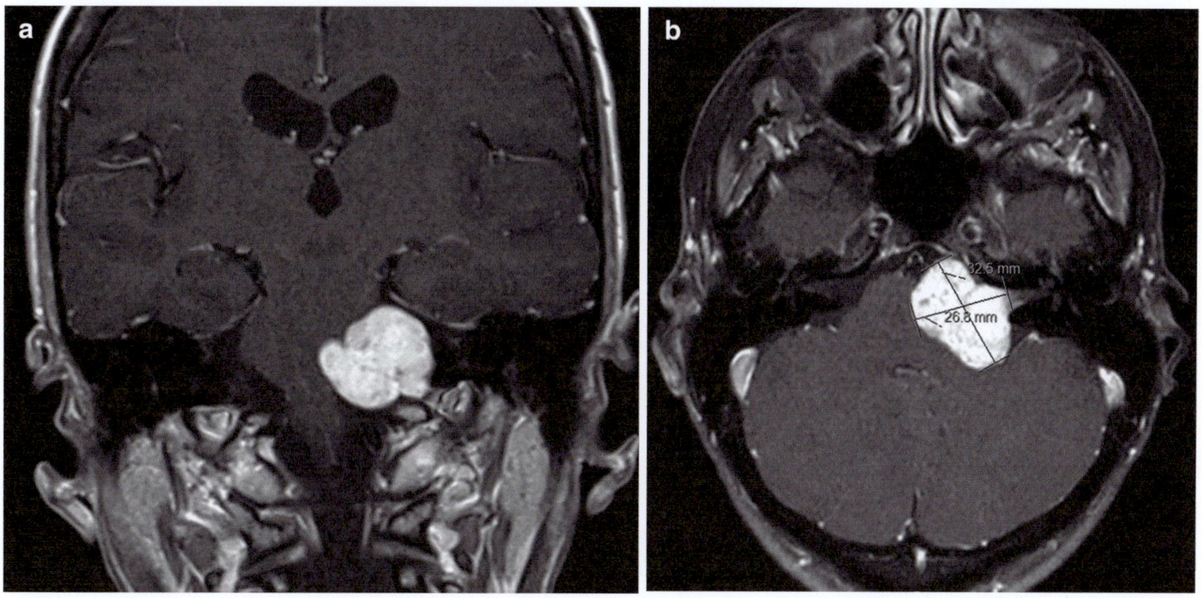

Fig. 22.1 Preoperative imaging: (**a**) coronal and (**b**) axial

Supplementary Information The online version contains supplementary material available at [https://doi.org/10.1007/978-3-031-12507-2_22].

S. E. Dekker
Department of Neurological Surgery, The Neurological Institute, University Hospitals Cleveland Medical Center, Case Western Reserve University, Cleveland, OH, USA

N. C. Bambakidis (✉)
Neurological Surgery, The Neurological Institute, University Hospitals of Cleveland, Case Western Reserve University School of Medicine, Cleveland, OH, USA
e-mail: Nicholas.Bambakidis2@UHhospitals.org

N. C. Bambakidis et al. (eds.), *Surgery of the Cerebellopontine Angle*, https://doi.org/10.1007/978-3-031-12507-2_22

Approach

We used a retrosigmoid approach (Fig. 22.2), beginning with a burr hole near the asterion. We continued with a suboccipital craniotomy, with high-speed drill, exposing the borders of the transverse and sigmoid sinuses. The borders of the transverse and sigmoid sinuses are exposed with care to preserve the emissary vein. The dura is carefully incised, flapped anteriorly, and the cerebellopontine contents are exposed.

Alternatives

Conservative medical management with serial observation is an alternative.

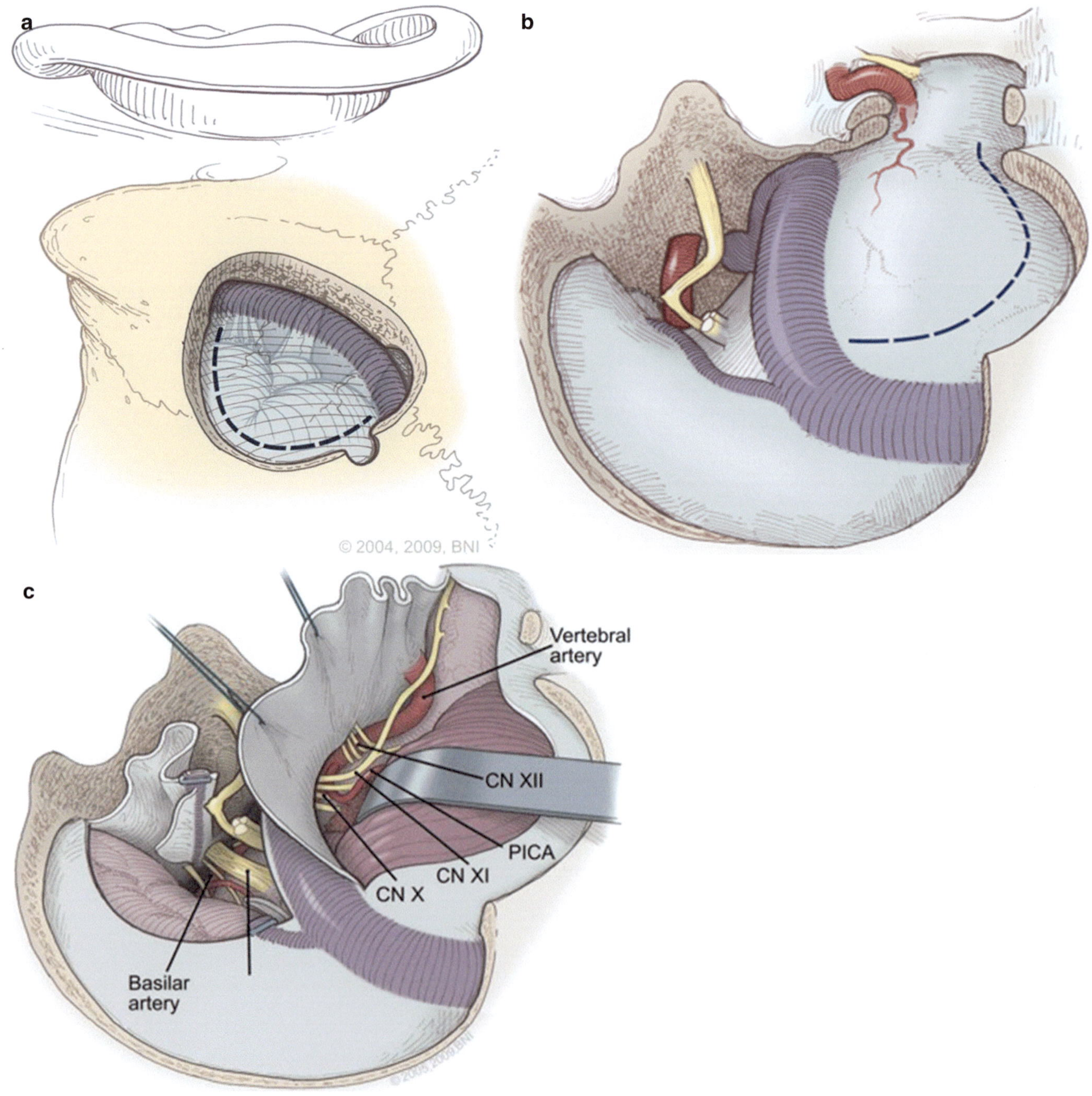

Fig. 22.2 Illustration of a retrosigmoid approach. (**a**) Illustration shows the semicircular opening of the dura with a wide base toward the sigmoid sinus. Note the underlying anatomic structures. (**b**) After the transverse and sigmoid sinuses have been skeletonized, the dura can be opened by cutting the retrosigmoid dura (green dashed lined). (**c**) Exposure of the contents of the posterior fossa. Sequential movement of the operating microscope and judicious retraction of the sigmoid sinus affords a view almost as complete as that afforded by its division. This strategy minimizes the risk of venous injury or infarction. *CN* cranial nerve, *PICA* posterior inferior cerebellar artery

Positioning

The patient was positioned in a supine position with the head turned to the right.

Incision

A curvilinear skin incision was made 1–2 cm behind the pinna through the asterion to the mastoid tip.

Operation

The operative video shows tumor resection using a retrosigmoid approach (See Video 22.1).

Post-op

Postoperative course was initially uneventful, and the patient was discharged on postoperative day (POD) 3 (Fig. 22.3).

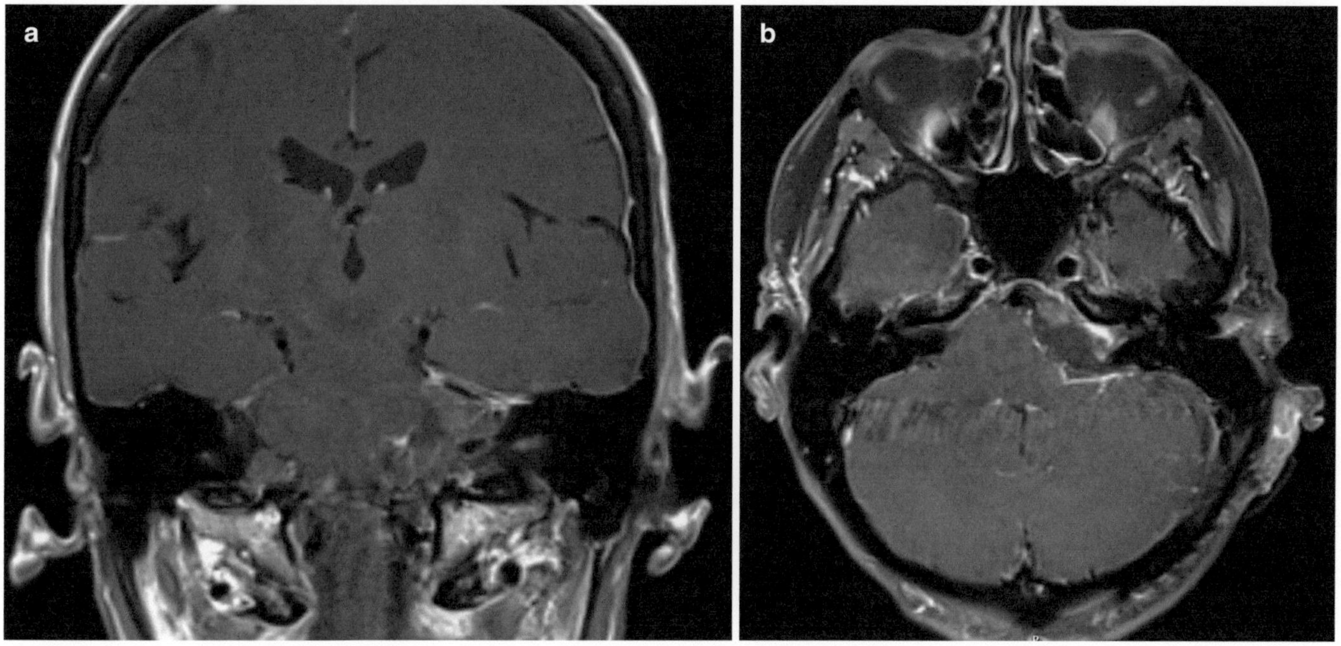

Fig. 22.3 Postoperative imaging: (**a**) coronal and (**b**) axial

Outcome

On POD 5, the patient developed delayed facial weakness (House-Brackmann grade 3), which resolved slowly over 6 weeks to normal facial function.

Pearls and Pitfalls

- If possible, the course of the facial nerve should be recognized early in the case to aid in anatomic preservation.
- Once the facial nerve course is identified, internal debulking can usually be performed rapidly.
- Intradural drilling of the internal carotid artery allows for distal facial nerve identification.
- Delayed facial weakness is not uncommon but may take several weeks to resolve [1].

Discussion

In retrosigmoid approaches to vestibular schwannomas with significant intracanalicular extension, it is important to drill off the posterior aspect of the internal carotid artery. Care must be taken to avoid injury to adjacent otologic structures. Delayed facial palsy is not an uncommon occurrence after vestibular schwannoma resection, with a reported rate of 16% in a single institution study. Development of facial palsy occurs at a mean of POD 12 but typically resolves by POD 33. Patients with a gross total tumor resection or undergoing a retrosigmoid approach may be at higher risk of delayed facial palsy, but they recover normal or near-normal function.

Reference

1. Carlstrom LP, Copeland WR III, Neff BA, Castner ML, Driscoll CL, Link MJ. Incidence and risk factors of delayed facial palsy after vestibular schwannoma resection. Neurosurgery. 2016;78(2):251–5.

Case 2: Combined Transpetrosal Approach with Hearing Preservation for Resection of a Meningioma

23

Simone E. Dekker and Nicholas C. Bambakidis

Summary

This case illustrates a combined transpetrosal approach with hearing preservation.

Case Presentation

A 50-year-old female presented with facial pain and numbness. Her hearing was normal (Fig. 23.1).

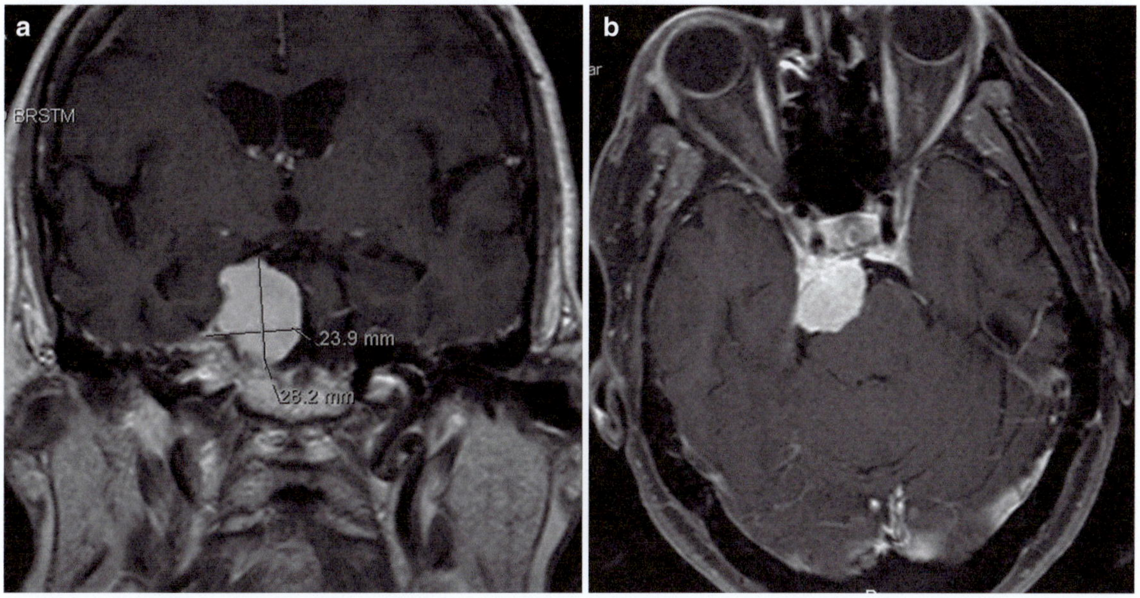

Fig. 23.1 Preoperative imaging: (**a**) coronal and (**b**) axial

Supplementary Information The online version contains supplementary material available at [https://doi.org/10.1007/978-3-031-12507-2_23].

S. E. Dekker
Department of Neurological Surgery, The Neurological Institute, University Hospitals Cleveland Medical Center, Case Western Reserve University, Cleveland, OH, USA

N. C. Bambakidis (✉)
Neurological Surgery, The Neurological Institute, University Hospitals of Cleveland, Case Western Reserve University School of Medicine, Cleveland, OH, USA
e-mail: Nicholas.Bambakidis2@UHhospitals.org

N. C. Bambakidis et al. (eds.), *Surgery of the Cerebellopontine Angle*, https://doi.org/10.1007/978-3-031-12507-2_23

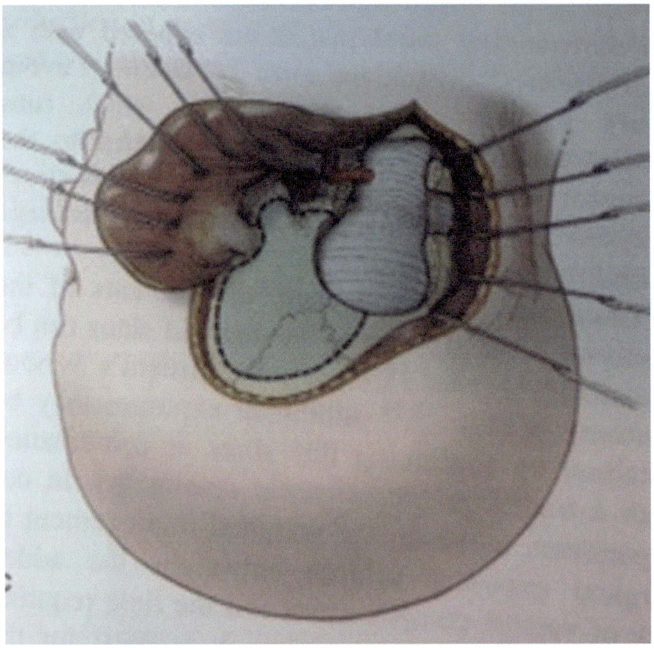

Fig. 23.2 Illustration of a combined subtemporal with transpetrosal approach

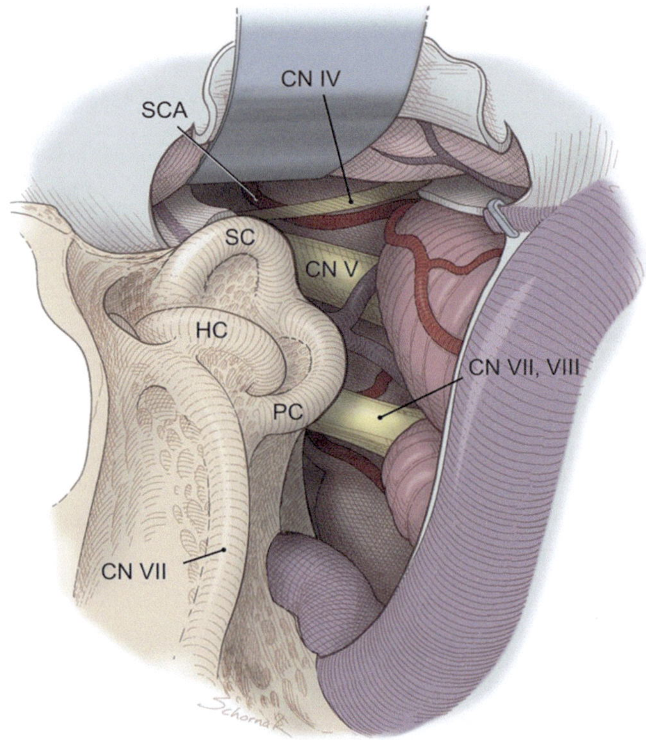

Fig. 23.3 Representation of the surgical view. APC ampulla of posterior canal, ASC ampulla of superior canal, CC crus commune, CN cranial nerve, HC horizontal canal, SC superior canal, SCA superior cerebellar artery

Approach

We used a combined subtemporal with transpetrosal approach (Fig. 23.2).

Alternatives

This tumor has a large supratentorial component, so a retrosigmoid approach is inadequate. If the patient was older, an orbitozygomatic approach from above or retrosigmoid approach from below might be considered to debulk only.

Anatomy

A representation of the surgical view is shown in Fig. 23.3.

Positioning

The patient was positioned in a supine position with the head turned left in 30°.

Incision

The skin incision may extend below the foramen magnum along a paramedian course for the far-lateral exposure (dashed line in Fig. 23.4). Extension superiorly in a curvilinear fashion over the pinna to the root of the zygoma allows a subtemporal craniotomy to be incorporated (dotted line).

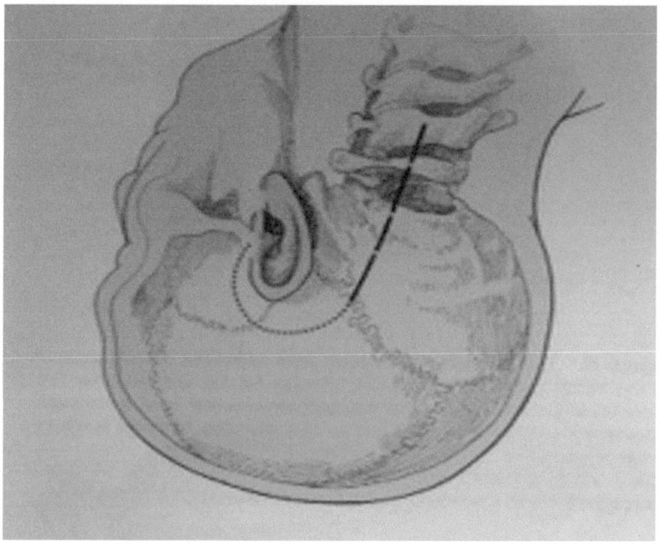

Fig. 23.4 Representation of surgical incision

Operation

A combined transpetrosal approach with hearing preservation is shown in the narrated operative video (see Video 23.1).

Post-op

The patient had a transient CN IV deficit postoperatively (Fig. 23.5).

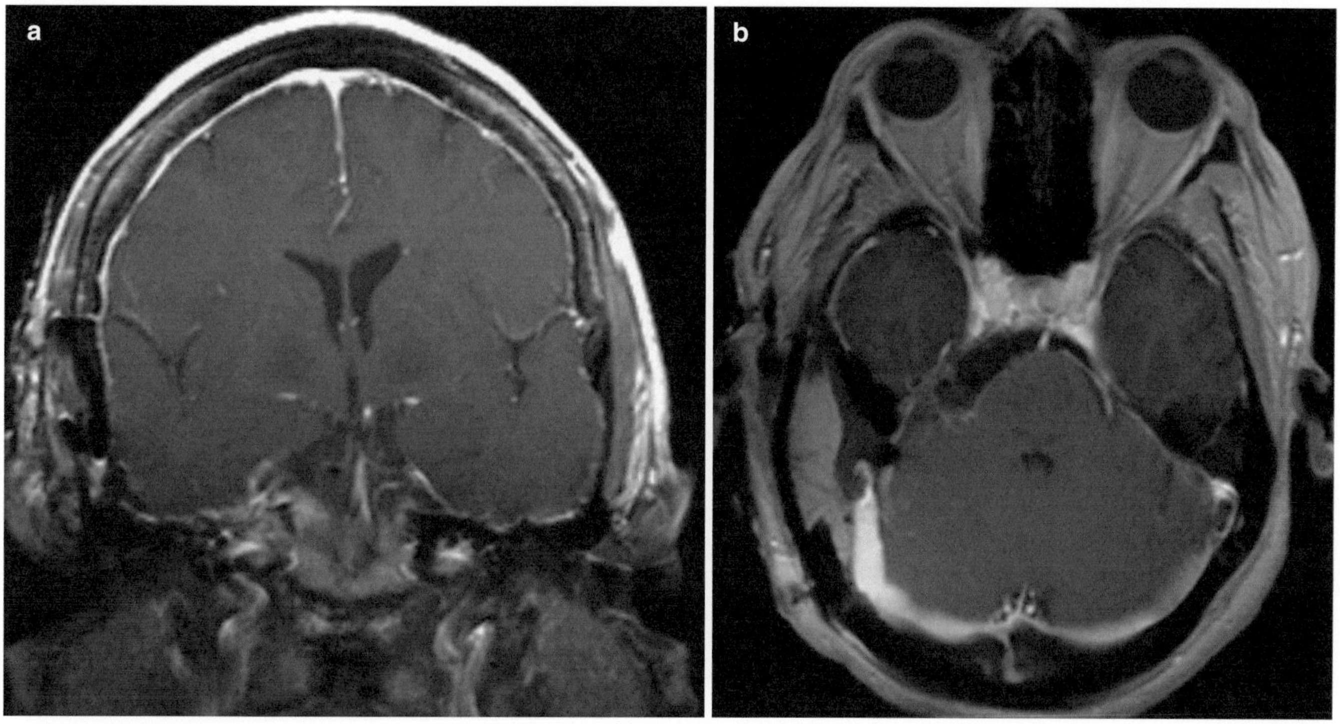

Fig. 23.5 Postoperative imaging: (a) coronal and (b) axial

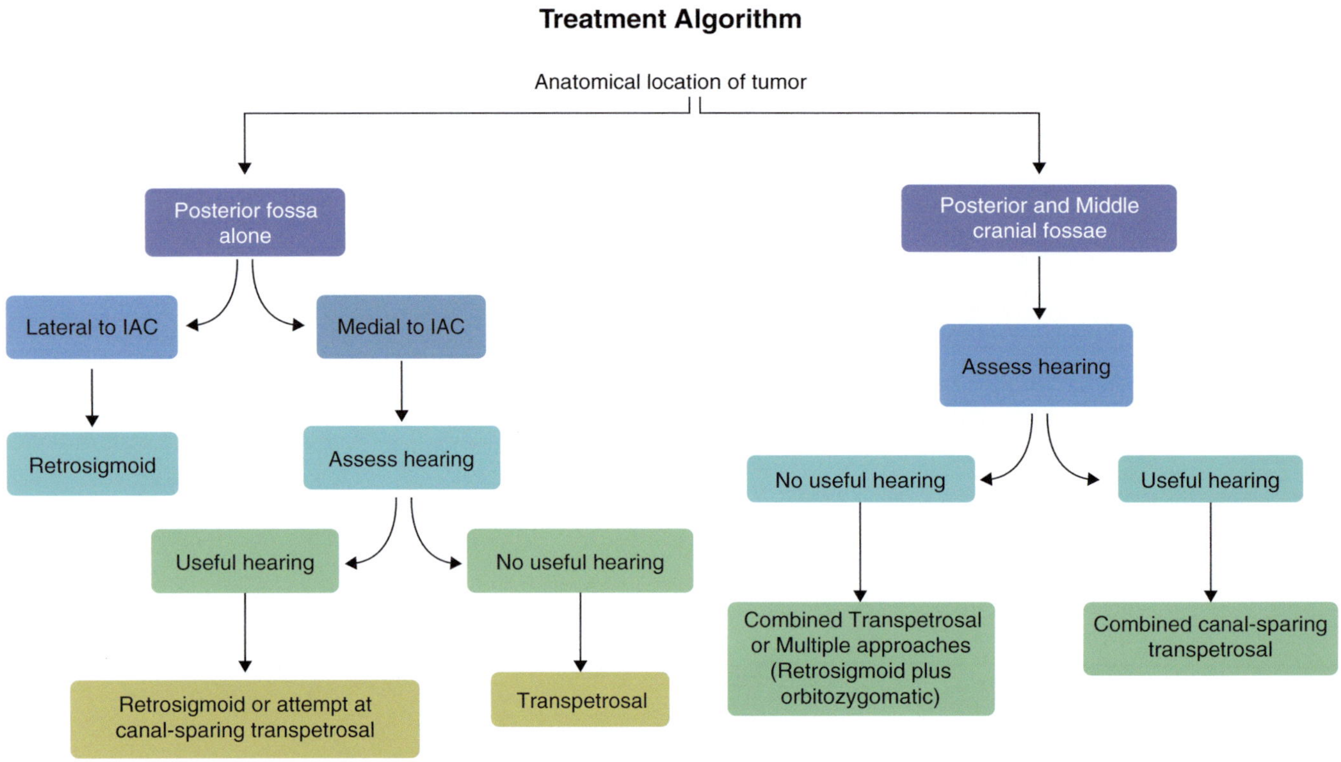

Fig. 23.6 Treatment algorithm based on anatomical location of the tumor [1]

Outcome

The patient had a good recovery, though she did develop a partial CN IV palsy due to manipulation of the nerve during tumor resection, requiring prism glasses for symptomatic management. At 3 years post-op, there was a small amount of recurrent tumor progression along the tentorium treated with gamma knife radiosurgery.

Pearls and Pitfalls

- Tumors extending both infratentorially and supratentorially as well as medial to the internal auditory canal (IAC) are well approached with a transpetrosal craniectomy.
- Hearing preservation is possible and should be considered when practical.
- Alternatively, a staged craniotomy from supratentorial (orbitozygomatic) and infratentorial (retrosigmoid) approach can be performed.

Discussion

It is important to combine skull base approaches to achieve the required exposure. In this case, a subtemporal approach allowed for resection of the supratentorial component, and a transpetrosal approach allowed for resection of the middle/posterior fossae component. Either approach alone would be insufficient to resect a tumor in this location.

An algorithm may be used to choose the surgical approach based on anatomical location of the tumor (Fig. 23.6). The best surgical approach provides the greatest degree of exposure to maximize the resection while minimizing the risk of surgical morbidity. Carefully consider the anatomical relationships of the tumor, particularly to the IAC and extent of tumor above or below the tentorium. Hearing preservation should also guide surgical decision making.

Video used with permission from the Congress of Neurological Surgeons, CNS Nexus Cases. 2018. https://www.cns.org/nexus/cases

Reference

1. Xu F, Karampelas I, Megerian CA, Selman WR, Bambakidis NC. Petroclival meningiomas: an update on surgical approaches, decision making, and treatment results. Neurosurg Focus. 2013;35(6):E11.

Case 3: Far-Lateral Approach for a Foramen Magnum Meningioma

24

Simone E. Dekker and Nicholas C. Bambakidis

Summary

This case illustrates issues surrounding a far-lateral approach for the resection of a foramen magnum meningioma.

Case Presentation

A 50-year-old female presented with progressive ataxia and weakness. Figure 24.1 shows the preoperative images of this patient.

Supplementary Information The online version contains supplementary material available at [https://doi.org/10.1007/978-3-031-12507-2_24].

S. E. Dekker
Department of Neurological Surgery, The Neurological Institute, University Hospitals Cleveland Medical Center, Case Western Reserve University, Cleveland, OH, USA

N. C. Bambakidis (✉)
Neurological Surgery, The Neurological Institute, University Hospitals of Cleveland, Case Western Reserve University School of Medicine, Cleveland, OH, USA
e-mail: Nicholas.Bambakidis2@UHhospitals.org

N. C. Bambakidis et al. (eds.), *Surgery of the Cerebellopontine Angle*, https://doi.org/10.1007/978-3-031-12507-2_24

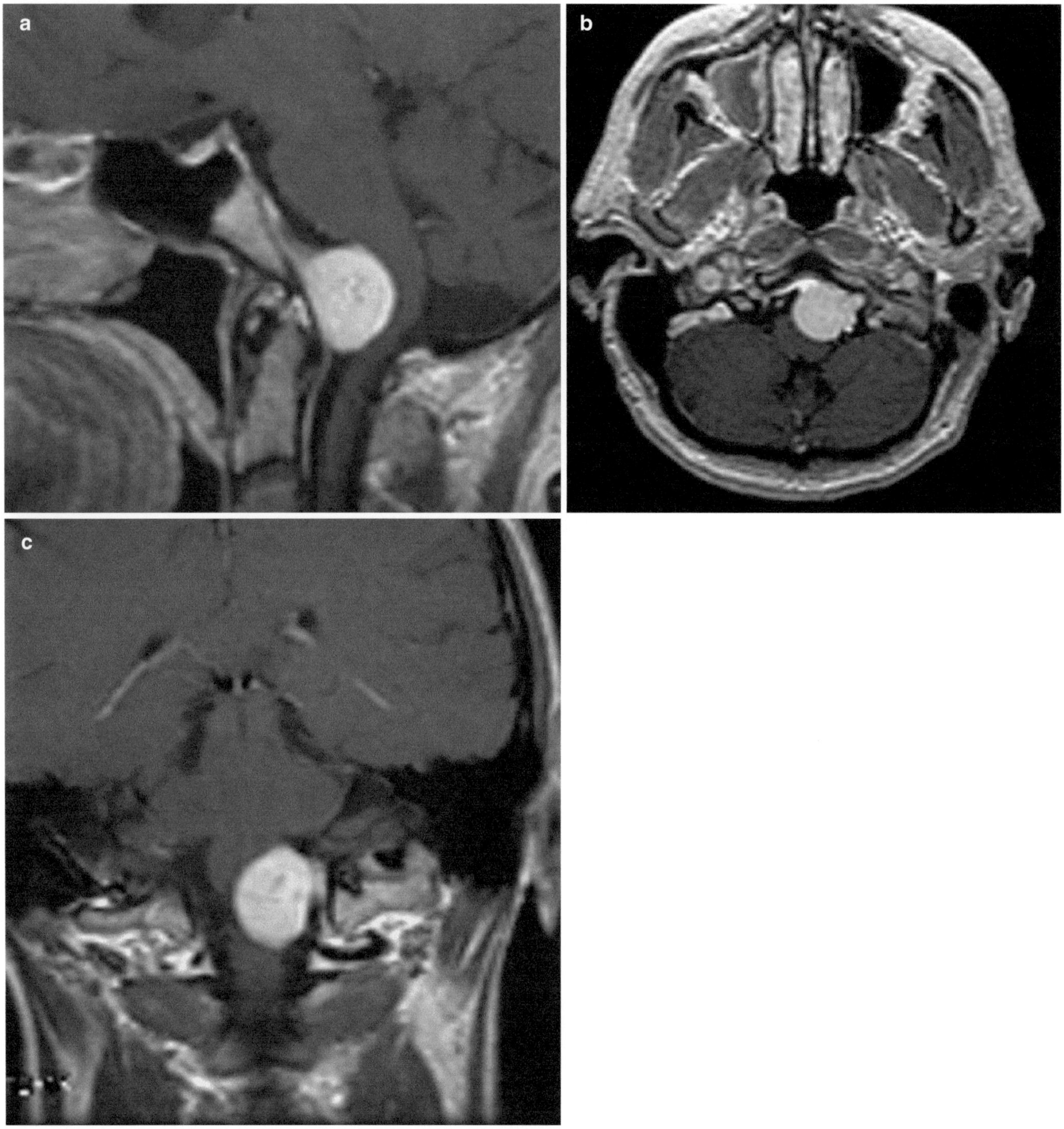

Fig. 24.1 Preoperative imaging: (**a**) sagittal, (**b**) axial, and (**c**) coronal

Approach

We used a far-lateral approach to resect this tumor (Fig. 24.2). An inverted hockey stick incision was used for both the far-lateral and extended far-lateral approaches. The burr hole was lateral to the sigmoid sinus, and a craniotomy was made back to the lip of the foramen magnum. Removal of the C1 posterior arch improves exposure. The suboccipital triangle was opened to expose the C1 posterior arch, vertebral artery, and posterior condylar vein. Spinal muscles were stripped laterally off the C1 posterior arch with subperiosteal dissection.

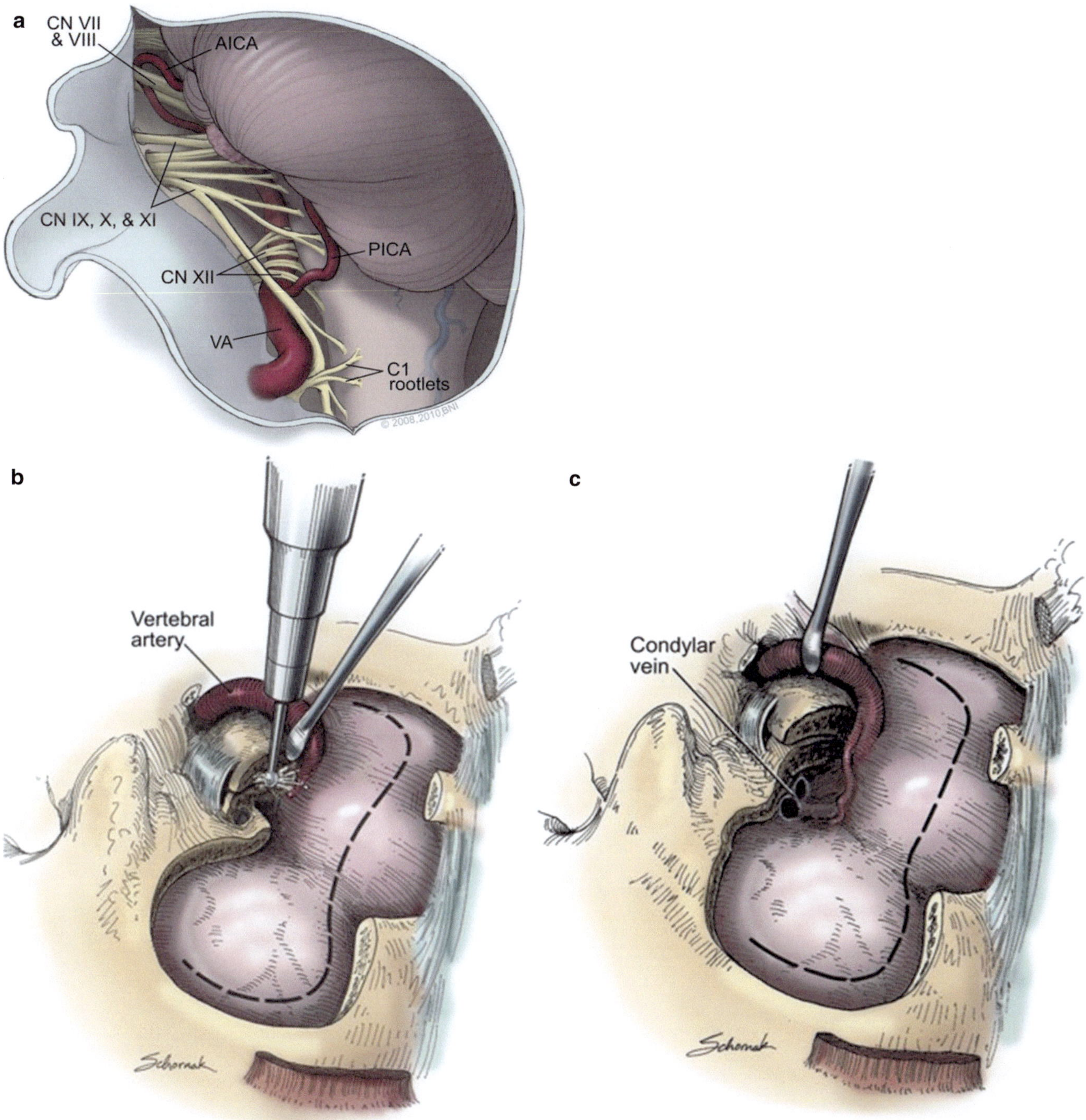

Fig. 24.2 Illustration of a far-lateral approach: (**a**) Intraoperative view following dural opening. (**b**) Approximately one-third of the condyle may be safely removed without jeopardizing the hypoglossal canal, the advent of which is noted by a change from cancellous to cortical bone to the condyle. The condylar vein is a helpful landmark; continued drilling beyond it is seldom helpful. (**c**) The dura is opened and based laterally, allowing visualization of the intradural anatomy. *AICA* anterior inferior cerebellar artery, *CN* cranial nerve, *PICA* posterior inferior cerebellar artery, *VA* vertebral artery

Alternatives

Alternatives for surgical treatment are conservative medical management with serial observation or stereotactic radiosurgery.

Positioning

The patient was placed in the park-bench position (Fig. 24.3).

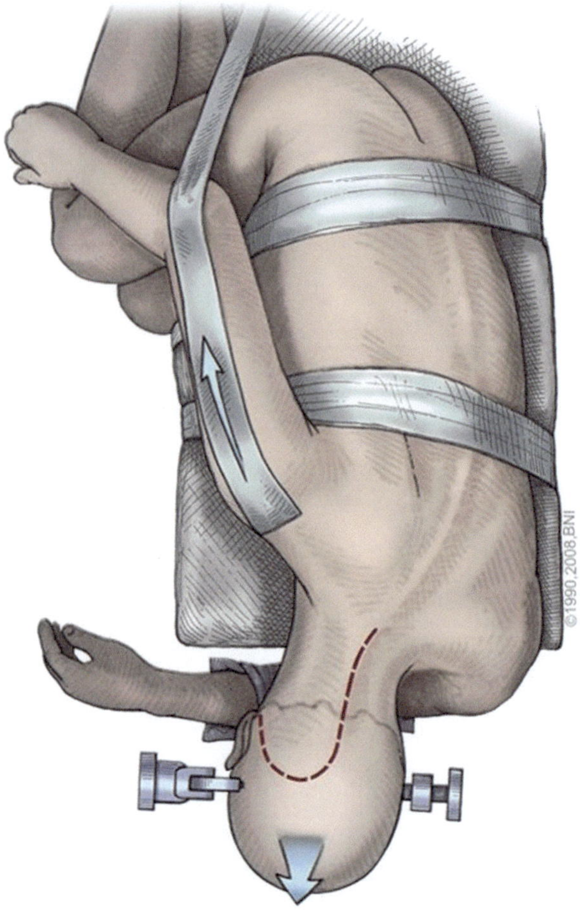

Fig. 24.3 Park-bench position

Incision

The incision extended from the midline level of C3 or C4 along the nuchal line, ending at the mastoid tip (Fig. 24.4).

Operation

The surgical video demonstrates the resection of a foramen magnum meningioma using a far-lateral approach (See Video 24.1).

Post-op

Postoperative recovery was uneventful, with discharge on postoperative day 5.

Outcome

The patient developed dysphagia and mild tongue weakness, which resolved over several weeks.

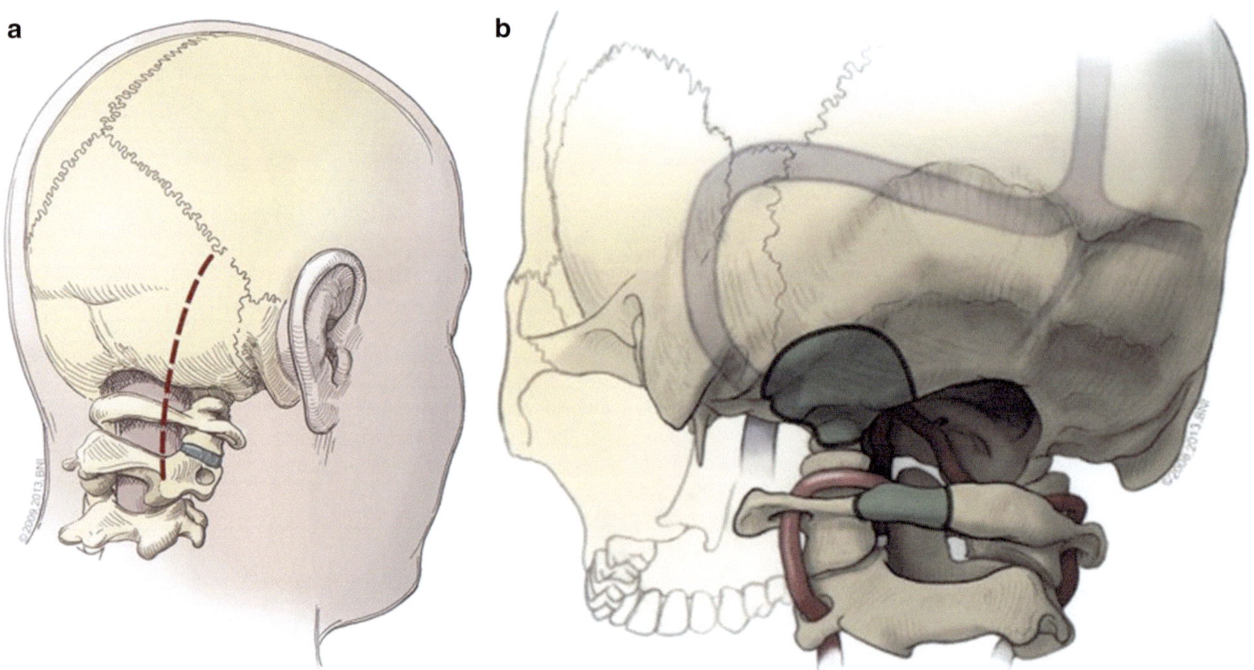

Fig. 24.4 Representation of surgical incision: (**a**) A linear incision is usually adequate for exposure. (**b**) The craniotomy extends to the level of the foramen magnum. The occipital condyle may then be partially removed to increase access to the intradural anatomy

Pearls and Pitfalls

- Foramen magnum meningiomas are typically extremely fibrous and difficult to remove without piecemeal resection.
- Because much of the dissection is tumor-related, condylar drilling is not typically helpful in increasing exposure.

Discussion

As with other procedures in the posterior fossa, a watertight closure is the goal to prevent postoperative spinal fluid leakage. Graft material may be liberally utilized in closing the dura, and the suboccipital bone and C1 lamina are replaced using bone plates and screws. If a cuff of muscle is preserved, it can be used in helping achieve a watertight closure as well.

Video used with permission from the Congress of Neurological Surgeons, CNS Nexus Cases. 2018. https://www.cns.org/nexus/cases

25 Case 4: Resection of an Acoustic Schwannoma Complicated by Tumor Encasement of the Anterior Inferior Cerebellar Artery Using a Translabyrinthine Approach

Simone E. Dekker, Chad A. Glenn, Kevin K. Yoo, Thomas Ostergard, Maroun T. Semaan, and Nicholas C. Bambakidis

Case Presentation

A 69-year-old male presented with hearing loss, ear fullness, and mild disequilibrium. Magnetic resonance imaging (MRI) demonstrated a contrast-enhancing mass within the right cerebellopontine angle cistern with extension into the internal auditory canal (Fig. 25.1a, b).

Supplementary Information The online version contains supplementary material available at [https://doi.org/10.1007/978-3-031-12507-2_25].

S. E. Dekker
Department of Neurological Surgery, The Neurological Institute, University Hospitals Cleveland Medical Center, Case Western Reserve University, Cleveland, OH, USA

C. A. Glenn
Comprehensive Brain Tumor Program, Neurosurgery, Stephenson Cancer Center, University of Oklahoma School of Medicine, Oklahoma City, OK, USA

K. K. Yoo
Alvarado Hospital Medical Center and Paradise Valley Hospital, Scripps Memorial Hospital Encinitas, San Diego, CA, USA

T. Ostergard
Carolina Neurosurgery and Spine Associates, Greensboro, NC, USA

M. T. Semaan
Otolaryngology—Otology, University Hospitals Cleveland Medical Center, Cleveland, OH, USA

N. C. Bambakidis (✉)
Neurological Surgery, The Neurological Institute, University Hospitals of Cleveland, Case Western Reserve University School of Medicine, Cleveland, OH, USA
e-mail: Nicholas.Bambakidis2@UHhospitals.org

N. C. Bambakidis et al. (eds.), *Surgery of the Cerebellopontine Angle*, https://doi.org/10.1007/978-3-031-12507-2_25

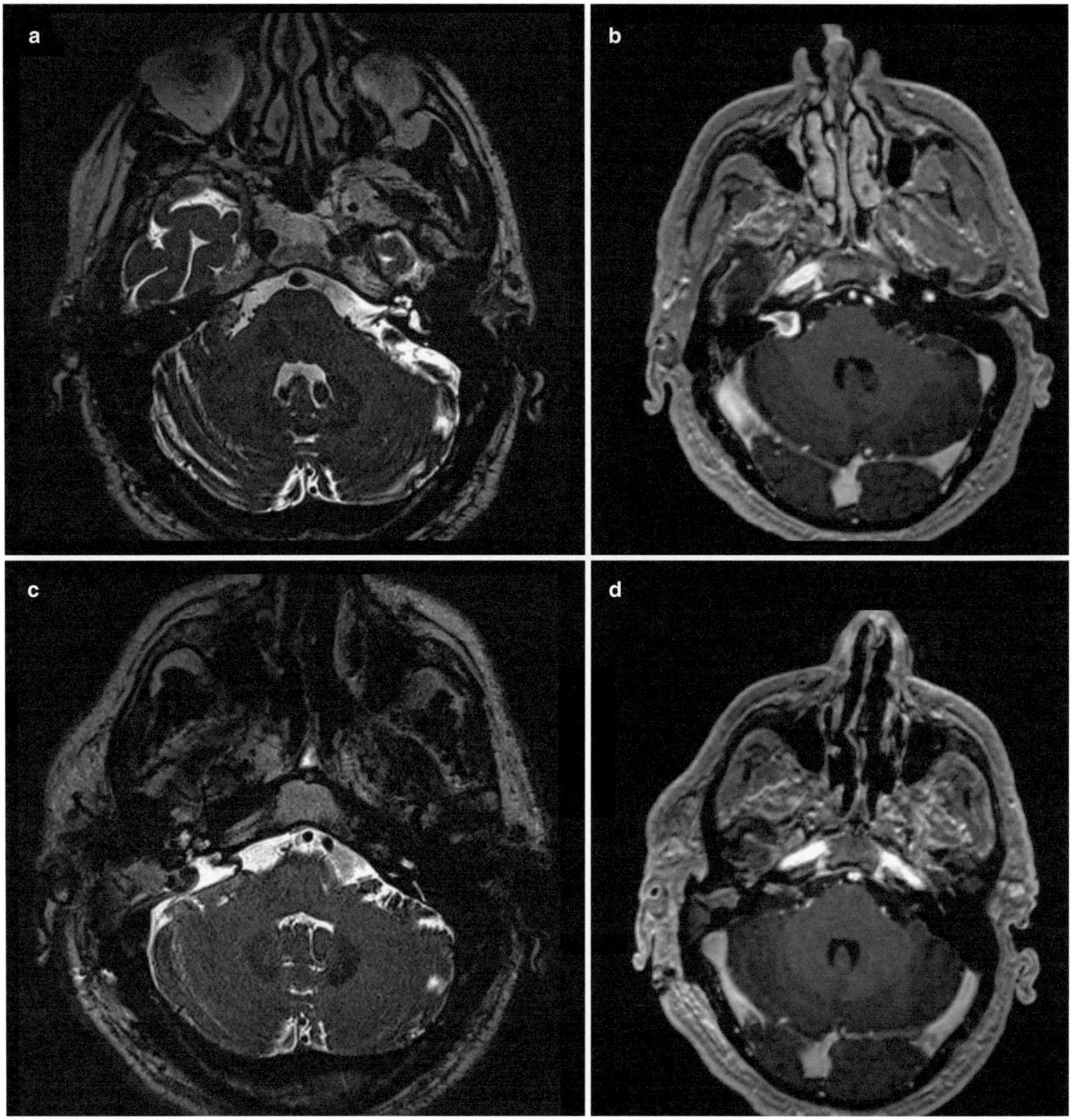

Fig. 25.1 Image shows (**a**) preoperative T2-weighted and (**b**) postcontrast T1-weighted MRI demonstrating a contrast-enhancing mass within the right cerebellopontine angle cistern with extension into the internal auditory canal. (**c**) Postoperative T2-weighted and (**d**) postcontrast T1-weighted MRI demonstrated gross total resection

Approach

Given the poorly serviceable hearing, a translabyrinthine approach was recommended.

Alternatives

- Radiotherapy.
- Observation.

Surgery

After the induction of anesthesia, a C-shaped curvilinear incision situated behind the postauricular sulcus was carried out. Next, a wide mastoidectomy was performed using a combination of cutting and diamond burs. Microsurgical resection utilizing the operative microscope and facial nerve monitoring was performed. Interestingly, the anterior inferior cerebellar artery (AICA) was identified anterior to the facial nerve and encased within the inferior pole of the tumor (Fig. 25.2). Gross tumor removal was completed with a small adherent residual remaining on the facial nerve. There were no complications (See Video 25.1).

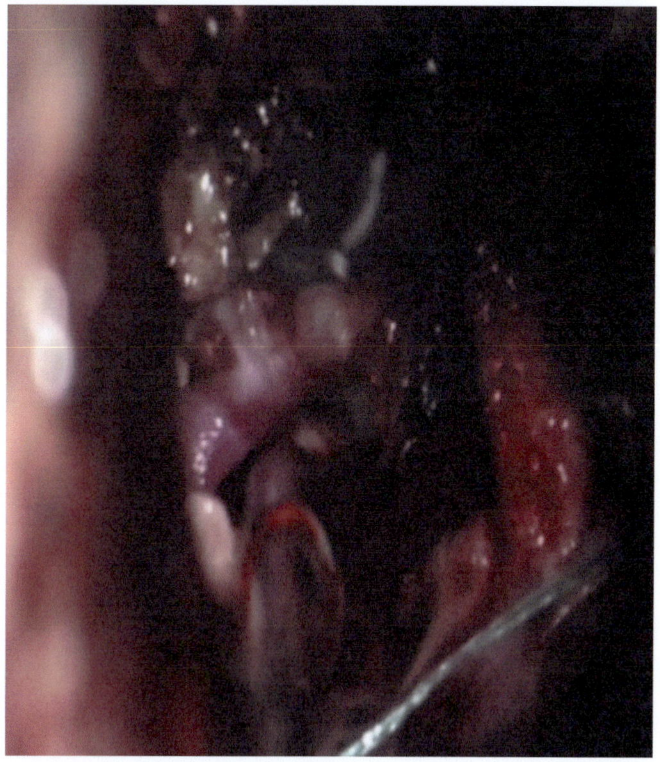

Fig. 25.2 Intraoperative still image illustrates the vestibular schwannoma in which the AICA was encased

Outcome

Postoperative MRI demonstrated gross total resection (Fig. 25.1c, d). The patient was discharged on postoperative day 3 with intact facial function. However, at his 2-week postoperative visit, he developed delayed facial weakness. After 2 months, the patient's facial weakness had gradually improved.

Case 5: Transcondylar Approach for Giant Aneurysm with Posterior Inferior Cerebellar Artery Bypass

26

Simone E. Dekker, Kevin K. Yoo, Anisha Garg, Wenceslas Krakowiecki, and Nicholas C. Bambakidis

Summary

This case illustrates a posterior inferior cerebellar artery (PICA) bypass surgery.

Supplementary Information The online version contains supplementary material available at [https://doi.org/10.1007/978-3-031-12507-2_26].

S. E. Dekker
Department of Neurological Surgery, The Neurological Institute, University Hospitals Cleveland Medical Center, Case Western Reserve University, Cleveland, OH, USA

K. K. Yoo
Alvarado Hospital Medical Center and Paradise Valley Hospital, Scripps Memorial Hospital Encinitas, San Diego, CA, USA

A. Garg
Yale New Haven Hospital, New Haven, CT, USA

W. Krakowiecki
School of Medicine and Dentistry, University of Rochester, Rochester, NY, USA

N. C. Bambakidis (✉)
Neurological Surgery, The Neurological Institute, University Hospitals of Cleveland, Case Western Reserve University School of Medicine, Cleveland, OH, USA
e-mail: Nicholas.Bambakidis2@UHhospitals.org

Case Presentation

A 76-year-old man presented with a history of hypertension, recent dysphagia, and vertigo. A 1.1-cm right PICA aneurysm was incidentally found (Figs. 26.1, 26.2, and 26.3). The patient experienced continued weight loss despite supplements and nutrition consultation.

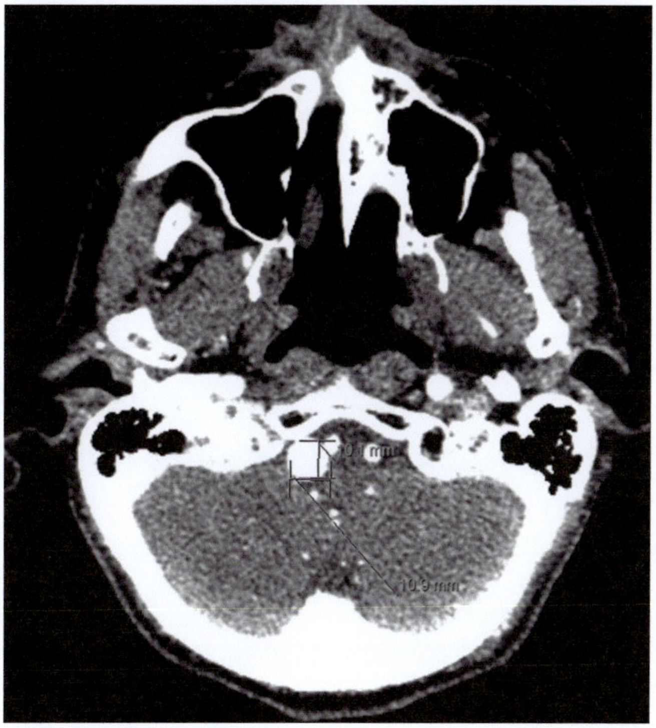

Fig. 26.1 Preoperative CT scan, axial

N. C. Bambakidis et al. (eds.), *Surgery of the Cerebellopontine Angle*, https://doi.org/10.1007/978-3-031-12507-2_26

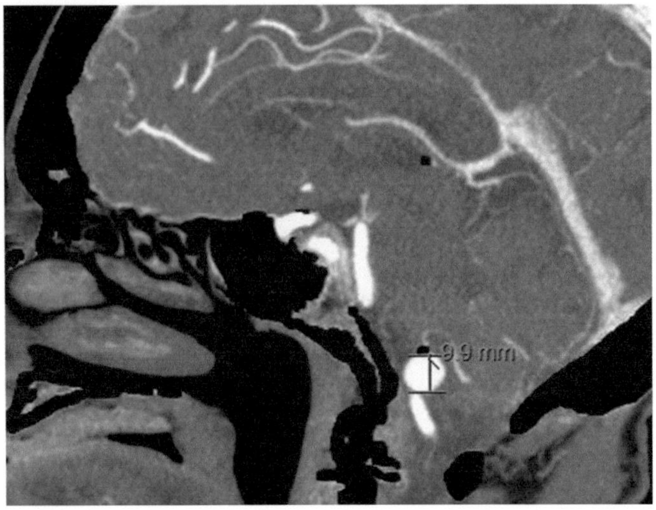

Fig. 26.2 Preoperative CT scan, sagittal

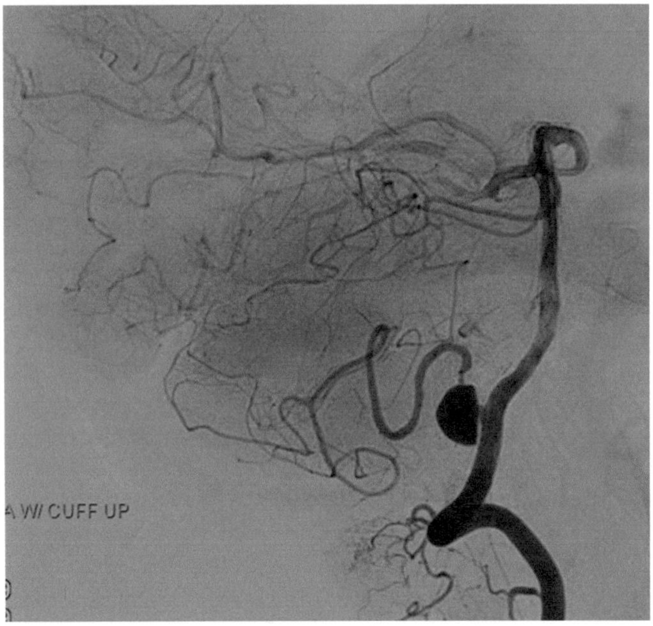

Fig. 26.3 Preoperative digital subtraction angiography

Approach

A far lateral transcondylar approach for a PICA-PICA bypass was planned [1].

Alternatives

Conservative medical management with serial observation is one alternative as is interventional radiology for coiling.

Positioning

The patient was put in a neutral, prone/flat position.

Incision

A posterior midline skin incision was made for sufficient exposure.

Surgery

A posterior midline skin incision was made. The scalp and temporalis muscle were reflected. The posterior lateral skull base bone was identified. The posterior fossa bone in the arch of C1 was then removed bilaterally exposing posterior fossa dura. A right-sided transcondylar approach was performed with a high-speed drill, removing portions of the occipital condyle to allow for a transcondylar approach of the posterior cranial skull base. Following removal of the condyle using drilling with separate different drill bits and the skull base approach, the dura was opened widely. The operating microscope was brought into position using stereotactic computer-assisted navigation to help in identifying the patient's giant right PICA origin aneurysm, which was found to be fusiform encompassing the PICA completely. Distal trapping was then performed with titanium aneurysm clips occluding outflow from the aneurysm. However, prior to this experience, attention was turned to the midline in order to enable adequate circulation and flow to the distal plaque. A separate PICA-PICA side-by-side anastomosis, with temporary clips placed in the PICA bilaterally in the midline with arteriotomy, was then performed. The side-to-side intracranial-to-intracranial anastomosis was completed with microdissection using 10–0 running and interrupted nylon sutures. There was excellent flow in the proximal and distal PICA branches bilaterally filling the PICA on the right side back to the level of the aneurysm (See Video 26.1).

Post-op

A postoperative computed tomography angiogram showed a patent PICA-PICA bypass (Fig. 26.4).

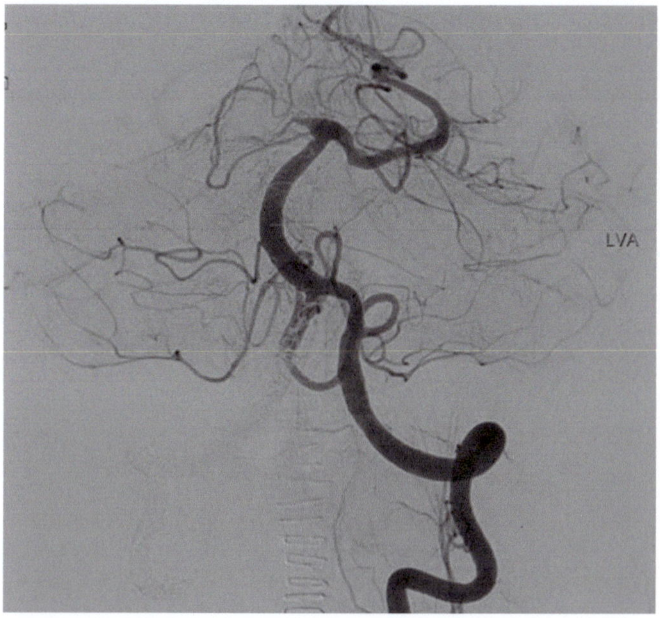

Fig. 26.4 Postoperative digital subtraction angiography, left vertebral artery injection

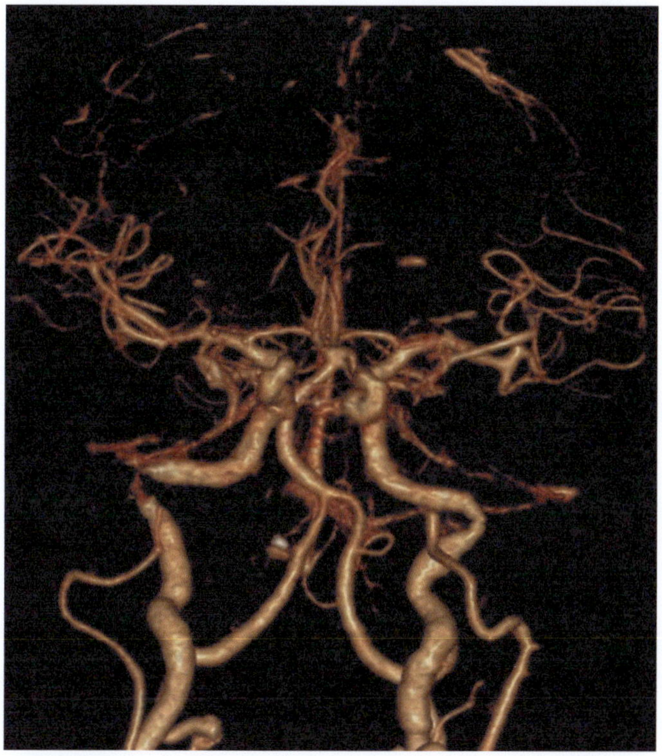

Fig. 26.5 Postoperative digital subtraction angiography, 3D reconstruction

Outcomes

No new neurologic deficits. Digital subtraction angiography shows patent bypass (Figs. 26.5 and 26.6).

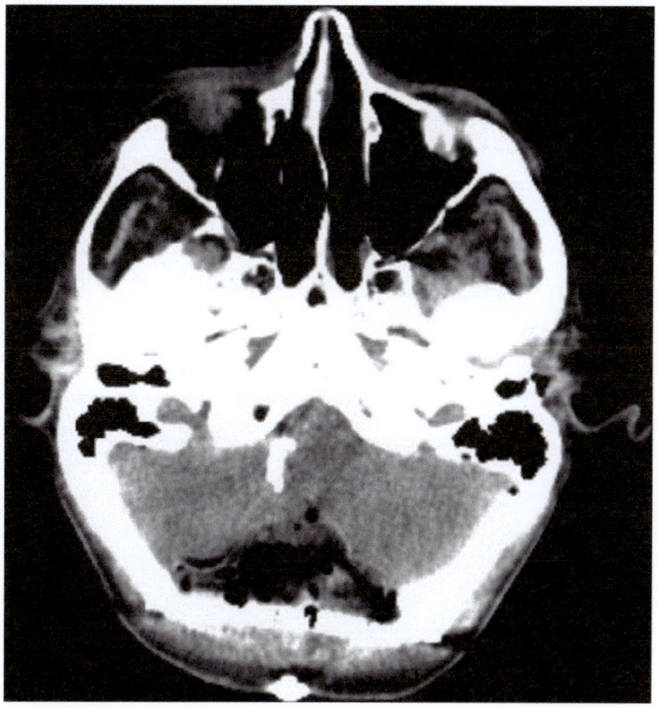

Fig. 26.6 Postoperative CT

Pearls and Pitfalls

- The decision for open surgery rather than endovascular treatment was based on the size of the aneurysm, symptoms of mass effect, and morphology incorporating the PICA.
- Distal clip occlusion was anticipated to cause thrombosis given the lack of outflow.
- However, the presence of brainstem perforators maintained aneurysm patency and caused delayed rupture due to the change in flow dynamics.
- Proximal trapping could have prevented delayed rupture but would have brought a high risk of brainstem stroke due to perforator occlusion.

Video used with permission from the Congress of Neurological Surgeons, CNS Nexus Cases. 2018. https://www.cns.org/nexus/cases

Reference

1. Bambakidis NC, Nakaji P, Amin-Hanjani S, Spetzler RF. Cerebrovascular surgery: an interactive video atlas. Shelton, CT: PMPH-USA; 2015.

Case 6: Far-Lateral Approach for a Posterior Inferior Cerebellar Artery Aneurysm Clipping

27

Simone E. Dekker, Kevin K. Yoo, Jeffrey T. Nelson, Wenceslas Krakowiecki, and Nicholas C. Bambakidis

Summary

This case illustrates the potential issues in a posterior inferior cerebellar artery (PICA) aneurysm clipping.

Case Presentation

A 71-year-old male presented with an incidental finding of a PICA aneurysm on a workup for progressive swallowing trouble and weight loss (Fig. 27.1). Past medical history was significant for stroke and transient ischemic attack, likely due to chronic small vessel ischemic disease. Exam revealed lower cranial nerve dysfunction and partial tongue weakness on left.

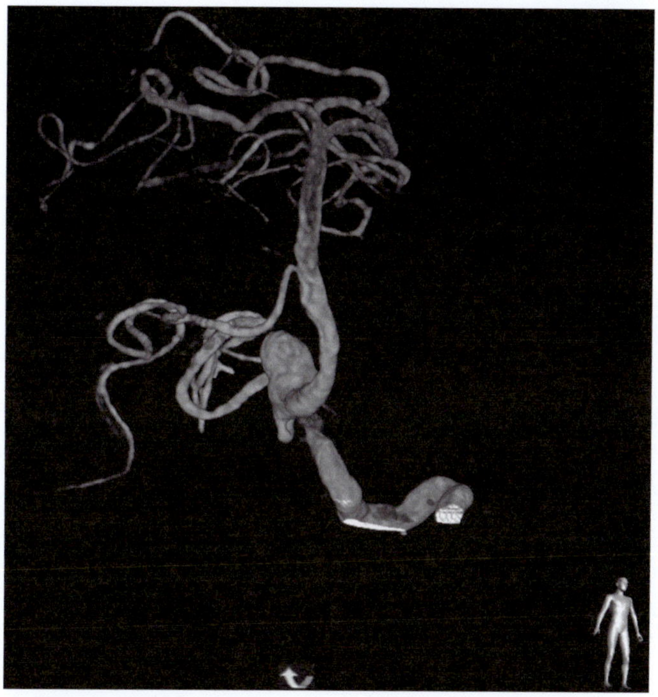

Fig. 27.1 Preoperative digital subtraction angiography, 3D reconstruction

Supplementary Information The online version contains supplementary material available at [https://doi.org/10.1007/978-3-031-12507-2_27].

S. E. Dekker
Department of Neurological Surgery, The Neurological Institute, University Hospitals Cleveland Medical Center, Case Western Reserve University, Cleveland, OH, USA

K. K. Yoo
Alvarado Hospital Medical Center and Paradise Valley Hospital, Scripps Memorial Hospital Encinitas, San Diego, CA, USA

J. T. Nelson
Case Western Reserve University School of Medicine, University Hospitals Cleveland Medical Center, Cleveland, OH, USA

W. Krakowiecki
School of Medicine and Dentistry, University of Rochester, Rochester, NY, USA

N. C. Bambakidis (✉)
Neurological Surgery, The Neurological Institute, University Hospitals of Cleveland, Case Western Reserve University School of Medicine, Cleveland, OH, USA
e-mail: Nicholas.Bambakidis2@UHhospitals.org

N. C. Bambakidis et al. (eds.), *Surgery of the Cerebellopontine Angle*, https://doi.org/10.1007/978-3-031-12507-2_27

Approach

A right-sided Clipping, using a far lateral approach was planned [1].

Alternatives

Conservative medical management with serial observation is one alternative as is interventional radiology for coiling.

Positioning

The patient was put in a neutral, right lateral position.

Incision

The previous surgery incision was reopened to avoid ischemic skin necrosis (Fig. 27.2).

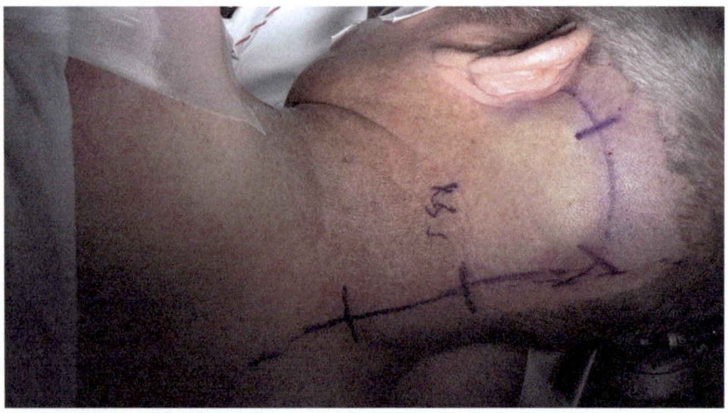

Fig. 27.2 Incision

Operation

After induction of general anesthesia, a lumbar drain was placed at the L3-L4 interspace through a percutaneous catheter with clear spinal fluid. Normal pressure was obtained, and the fluid was allowed to drain intermittently throughout the procedure. Postoperatively, the drain was tunneled and secured. A left-sided craniectomy was then performed as well as a hemilaminectomy at C1, exposing the left lateral skull base with additional drilling of the occipital condyle using a high-speed drill to allow access through the skull-base approach. A very large multilobulated, wide-necked, partially calcified posterior circulation PICA aneurysm was identified intradurally and addressed with intermittent temporary clip occlusion. Clip reconstruction of the PICA vertebral artery was then performed using a fenestrated clip, after intraoperative rupture and difficulty with control, which required sacrifice of intervening rootlets of cranial nerve XII. Complete occlusion of the aneurysm was confirmed with indocyanine green, video angiography, and microvascular Doppler. The wound was then copiously irrigated (See Video 27.1).

Post-op

Computed tomography of the head showed post-op changes (Fig. 27.3). The patient experienced difficulty swallowing. He was discharged to rehab on postoperative day 5.

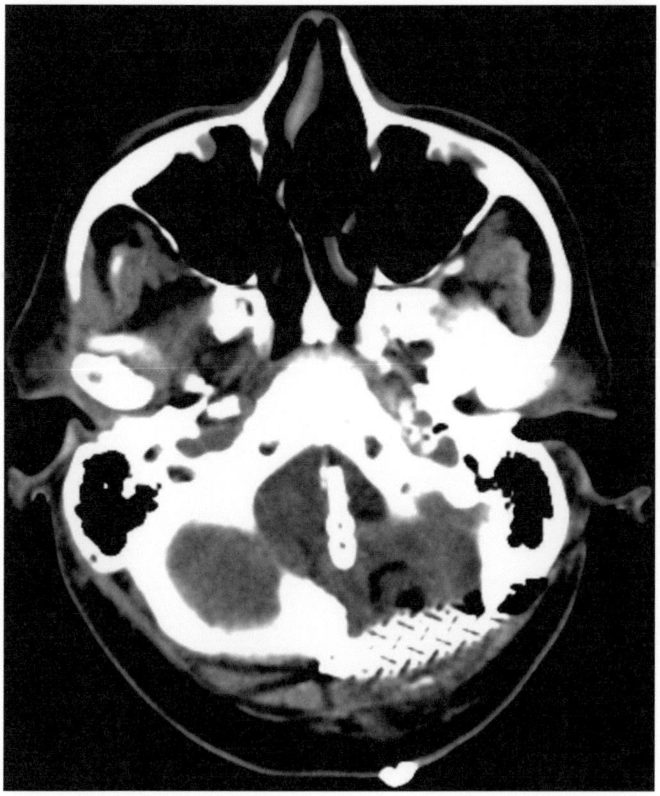

Fig. 27.3 Postoperative CT

Outcome

The patient was doing well at his 6-week follow-up. Cranial nerves were intact with mild left tongue deviation. His difficulty swallowing had resolved. Per the patient's wife, he had been refusing to eat and, therefore, was referred to a dietician for his weight loss and taste changes.

Discussion

There are few data on the incidence of postoperative dysphagia after PICA aneurysm clipping. Nelson and colleagues demonstrated that postoperative dysphagia occurred in the majority of patients undergoing craniotomy for trapping and bypass of a PICA aneurysm, with half requiring placement of a percutaneous endoscopic gastrostomy tube [2]. However, by the 6-week follow-up examination, all surviving patients had recovered normal swallowing function.

Pearls and Pitfalls

- This case illustrates clipping of a PICA aneurysm with postoperative dysphagia.
- The decision for open surgery versus endovascular treatment was made because of a wide aneurysm neck and presumed mass effect causing symptoms.
- Due to the location of the PICA in the posterior fossa, lower cranial nerve dysfunction is of particular concern.

Video used with permission from the Congress of Neurological Surgeons, CNS Nexus Cases. 2018. https://www.cns.org/nexus/cases

References

1. Bambakidis NC, Nakaji P, Amin-Hanjani S, Spetzler RF. Cerebrovascular surgery: an interactive video atlas. Shelton, CT: PMPH-USA; 2015.
2. Nelson J, Bambakidis NC. The incidence of post-operative dysphagia and gastrostomy tube placement in a series of six patients with posterior inferior cerebellar artery aneurysms treated by cerebrovascular bypass and aneurysm trapping. CNS Annual meeting 2016. San Diego, CA.

28 Case 7: Right Retrosigmoid Craniotomy for Microvascular Decompression for Trigeminal Neuralgia (Endoscope-Assisted)

Peter Nakaji, Rami Almefty, Brandon Liebelt, Michaela Lee, and Xiaochun Zhao

Summary

This case illustrates endoscope-assisted microvascular decompression for trigeminal neuralgia (Figs. 28.1, 28.2, and 28.3).

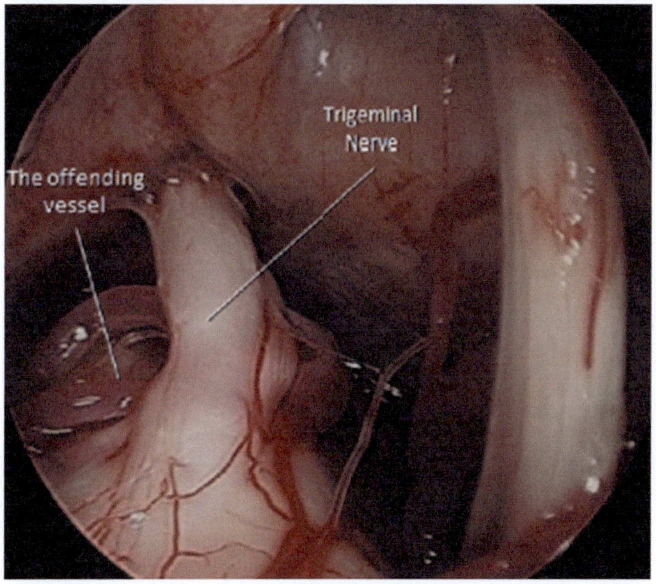

Fig. 28.1 An endoscopic view of the right cerebellopontine angle shows trigeminal nerves and the loop of offending superior cerebellar artery impacting it

Supplementary Information The online version contains supplementary material available at [https://doi.org/10.1007/978-3-031-12507-2_28].

P. Nakaji (✉)
Department of Neurosurgery, University of Arizona College of Medicine—Banner, Phoenix, AZ, USA

Surgery, University of Arizona College of Medicine—Phoenix, Phoenix, AZ, USA

Neurosurgery, Neuroscience Institute, Phoenix, AZ, USA
e-mail: Peter.Nakaji@bannerhealth.com

R. Almefty
Department of Neurosurgery, Temple University, Lewis Katz School of Medicine, Philadelphia, PA, USA

B. Liebelt
Larner College of Medicine, University of Vermont Medical Center, Burlington, VT, USA

M. Lee
University of Arizona College of Medicine, Banner—University Medical Center Phoenix, Phoenix, AZ, USA

X. Zhao
Department of Neurosurgery, University of Oklahoma Health Sciences Center, Oklahoma City, OK, USA

N. C. Bambakidis et al. (eds.), *Surgery of the Cerebellopontine Angle*, https://doi.org/10.1007/978-3-031-12507-2_28

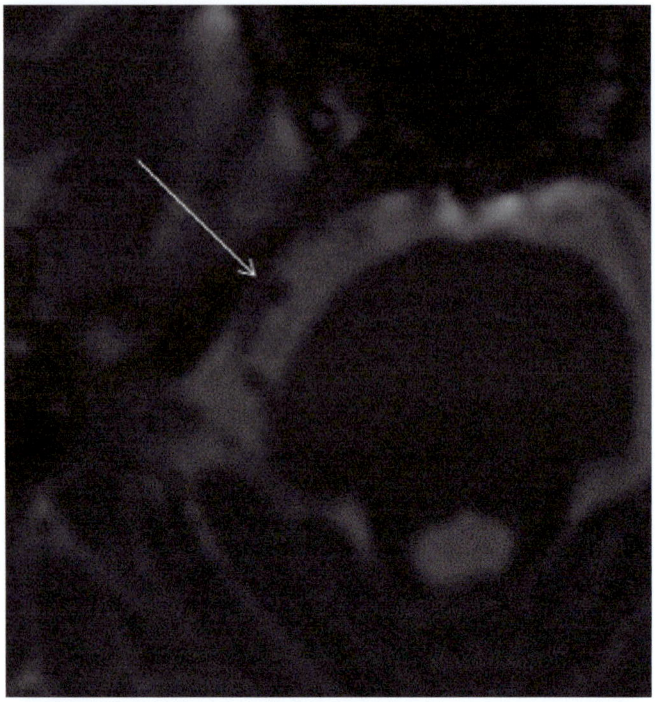

Fig. 28.2 An axial T2-weighted MRI shows the flow void of the vessel, which contacts the nerve both distally (arrow) and at the brainstem

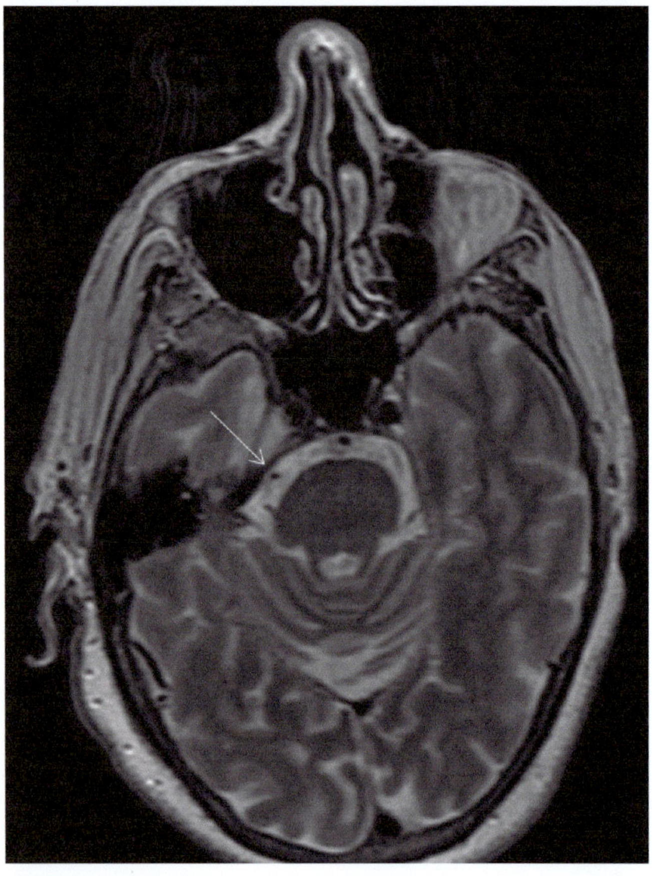

Fig. 28.3 A zoomed-out view of the vessel at the right cerebellopontine angle shows how deep the typical impact point is in the head

Case Presentation

An 85-year-old female with right-sided trigeminal neuralgia for 11 years presented with what she described as shock-like pains distributed in the V1 and V2 regions.

Approach

A right-sided keyhole retrosigmoid approach was planned (Fig. 28.4).

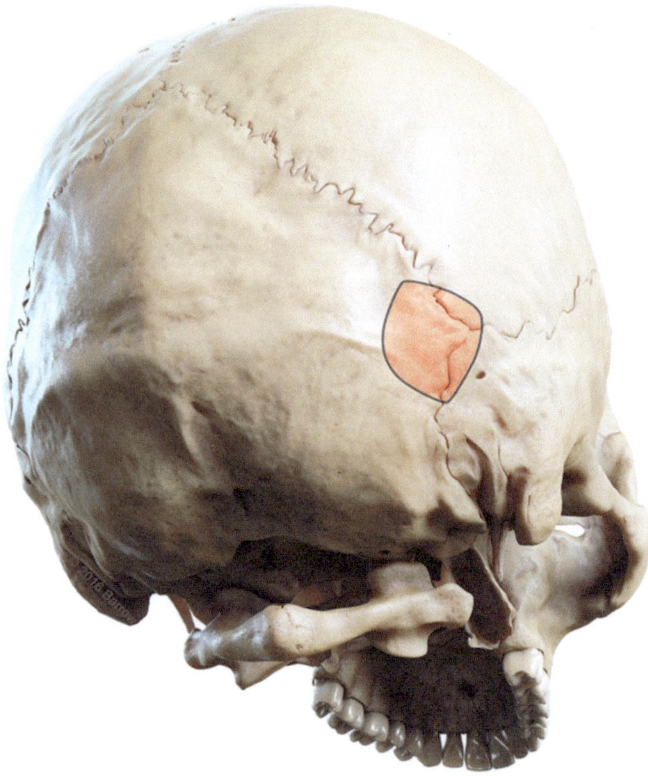

Fig. 28.4 The cranial figure shows the location of the planned craniotomy on the skull, which is typically up to the level of the asterion, just under the transverse sinus and immediately posterior to the sigmoid sinus

Alternatives

Anticonvulsants such as carbamazepine are usually the initial treatment. Other surgical treatments such as Gamma knife or cranial nerve (CN) V rhizotomy would affect normal sensation and chewing muscle; these surgical approaches carry less risk and may be appropriate for some older patients [1].

Anatomy

A representation of the surgical view is shown (Fig. 28.5).

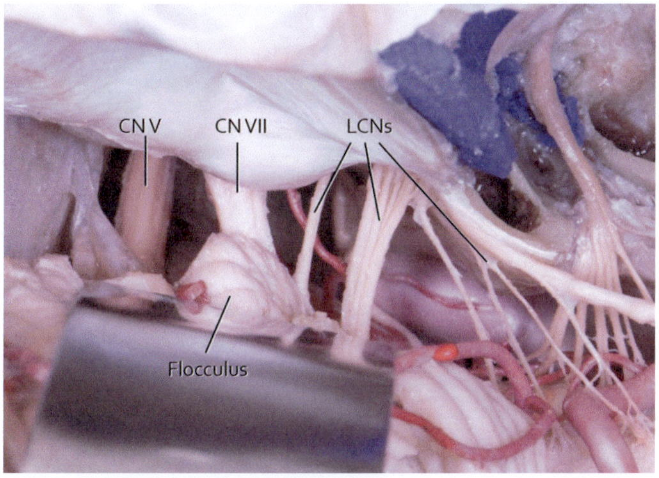

Fig. 28.5 A cadaveric anatomical dissection of the right cerebellopontine angle shows the cranial nerves from V to XII. Although the exposure shown is retrocerebellar, the corridor for microvascular decompression for CN V is high, at the petro-tentorial junction, and usually proceeds above the cerebellar hemisphere

Positioning

The patient was positioned supine with head turned to the left to expose the right retrosigmoid region. The shoulder should not be allowed to rise into the way. Some chin flexion may improve the angle to the trigeminal nerve (Fig. 28.6).

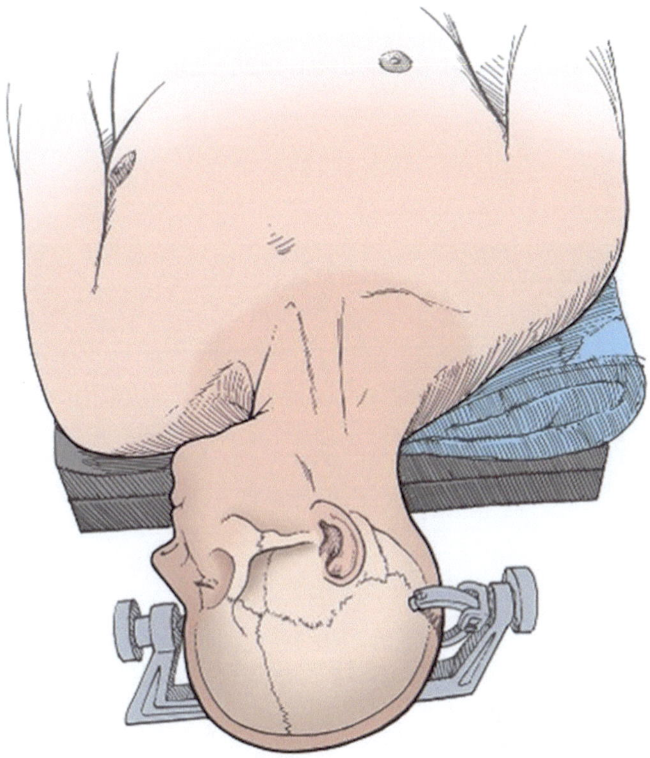

Fig. 28.6 The patient is positioned in the supine position with the head turned to the left, exposing the right retrosigmoid area. It is helpful to tip the bed up to relax the field and promote cerebrospinal fluid drainage and to flex the neck allowing a view up as high as possible

Incision

A horizontal incision over the transverse-sigmoid sinus junction was made.

Operation

A horizontal incision was this surgeon's choice; the standard is vertical (See Video 28.1). A small craniotomy over the transverse-sigmoid junction was made. Dura was opened and tacked up. The arachnoid membrane was opened, cerebrospinal fluid (CSF) released, and CN V exposed. The endoscope should be consulted. The vessel loop was freed and dissected away from CN V. A Teflon™ sponge was inserted and held in place with Evicel® glue. A watertight closure was achieved.

Post-Op

Figures 28.7, and 28.8.

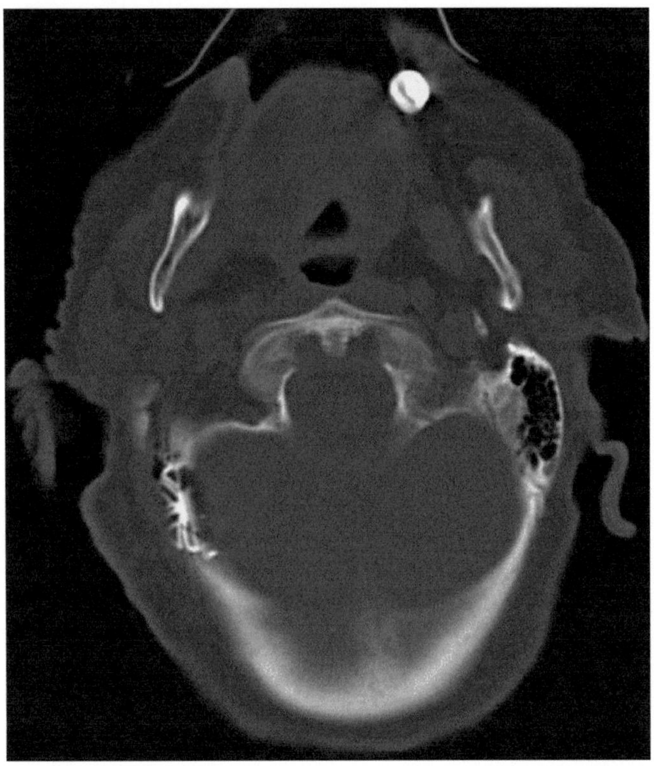

Fig. 28.7 An axial CT of the head without contrast with bone windowing shows the small craniectomy with an overlying burr hole cover for reconstruction

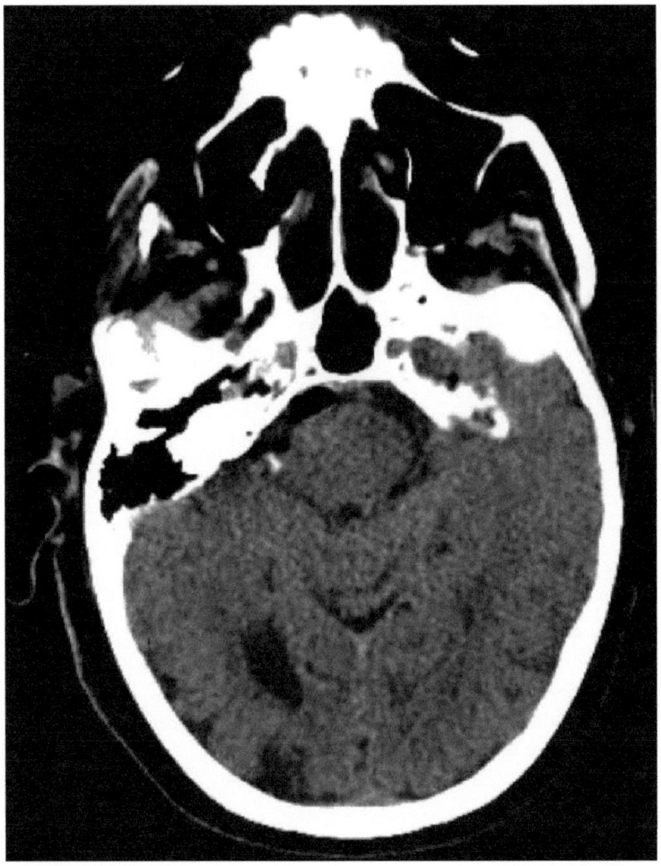

Fig. 28.8 An axial CT of the head performed without contrast shows a bright spot along the right brainstem where the Teflon sponge and fibrin glue were applied

Outcome

The patient's pain was relieved postoperatively and has not returned.

Pearls and Pitfalls

- The most common offending vessel for trigeminal neuralgia is the superior cerebellar artery.
- The entire length of the nerve must be examined, but compression is usually at the nerve root entry zone.
- Exposure of the root entry zone can be challenging, and inadequate exposure could cause failure of decompression.
- Injury to the labyrinthine artery should be avoided as it could cause postoperative hearing loss.
- Watertight dural closure and waxing of mastoid air cells are required to prevent CSF leakage.

Discussion

Anticonvulsants are the starting treatment, with surgical decompression an option for patients who can tolerate surgery and who fail medical treatment. Surgery is the most effective treatment. The entire length of the nerve, including the ventral side of the root entry zone, must be examined meticulously. Endoscopy can be helpful.

Video used with permission from the Congress of Neurological Surgeons, CNS Nexus Cases. 2018. https://www.cns.org/nexus/cases

Reference

1. Zakrzewska JM, Coakham HB. Microvascular decompression for trigeminal neuralgia: update. Curr Opin Neurol. 2012;25(3):296–301.

29 Case 8: Right Retrosigmoid Craniotomy for Microvascular Decompression of Hemifacial Spasm

Peter Nakaji, Rami Almefty, Brandon Liebelt, Michaela Lee, and Xiaochun Zhao

Summary

This case illustrates endoscope-assisted microvascular decompression for hemifacial spasm (Fig. 29.1).

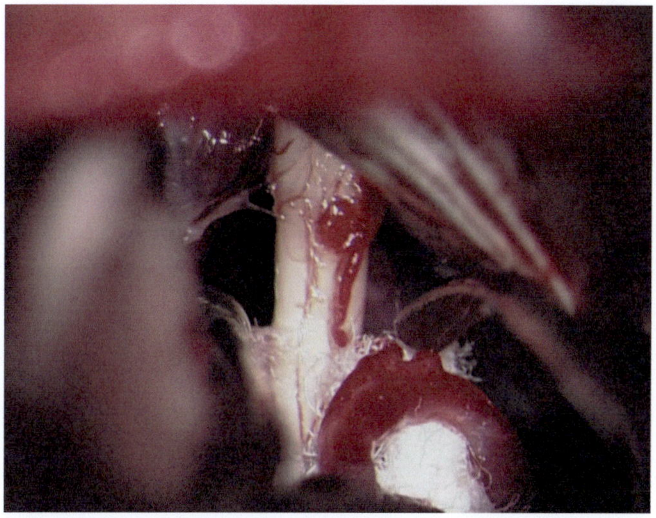

Fig. 29.1 An intraoperative view of the right cerebellopontine angle shows a pledget separating a loop of vessel away from CN VII

Supplementary Information The online version contains supplementary material available at [https://doi.org/10.1007/978-3-031-12507-2_29].

P. Nakaji (✉)
Department of Neurosurgery, University of Arizona College of Medicine—Banner, Phoenix, AZ, USA

Surgery, University of Arizona College of Medicine—Phoenix, Phoenix, AZ, USA

Neurosurgery, Neuroscience Institute, Phoenix, AZ, USA
e-mail: Peter.Nakaji@bannerhealth.com

R. Almefty
Department of Neurosurgery, Temple University, Lewis Katz School of Medicine, Philadelphia, PA, USA

B. Liebelt
Larner College of Medicine, University of Vermont Medical Center, Burlington, VT, USA

M. Lee
University of Arizona College of Medicine, Banner—University Medical Center Phoenix, Phoenix, AZ, USA

X. Zhao
Department of Neurosurgery, University of Oklahoma Health Sciences Center, Oklahoma City, OK, USA

N. C. Bambakidis et al. (eds.), *Surgery of the Cerebellopontine Angle*, https://doi.org/10.1007/978-3-031-12507-2_29

Case Presentation

A 69-year-old female presented with right-sided hemifacial spasm for 7 years (Fig. 29.2). She had a history of failed microvascular decompression complicated by a sigmoid sinus injury and occipital hemorrhagic stroke.

Approach

A right-sided retrosigmoid approach was planned (Fig. 29.3).

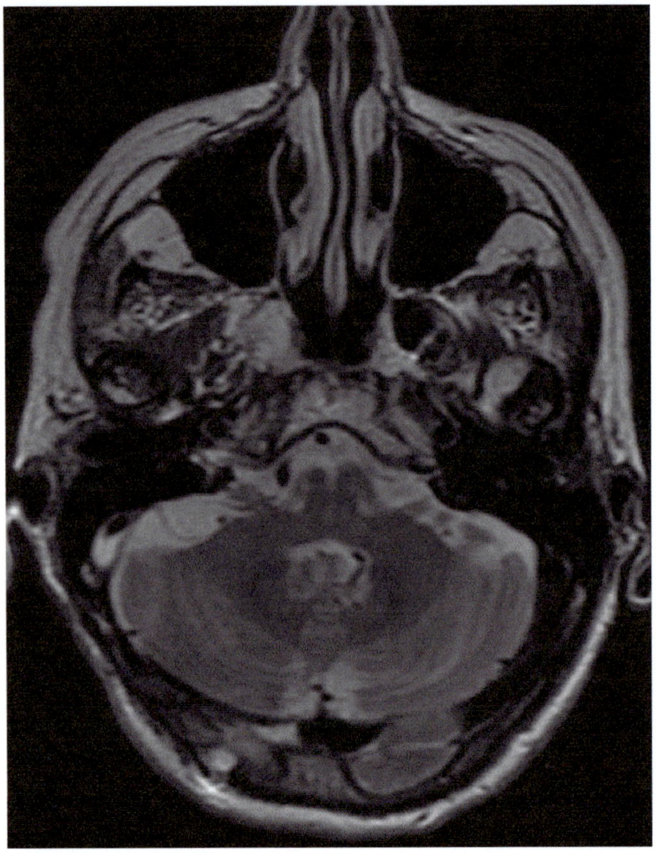

Fig. 29.2 The T2-weighted MRI shows a flow void on the right side of the brainstem

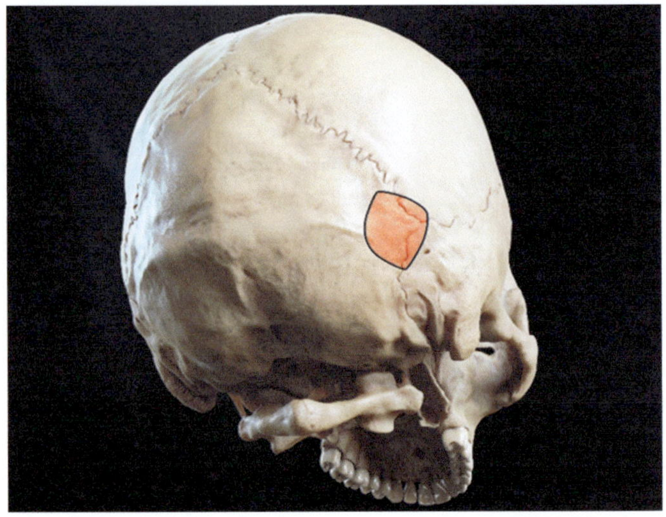

Fig. 29.3 A right-sided retrosigmoid craniotomy is shown

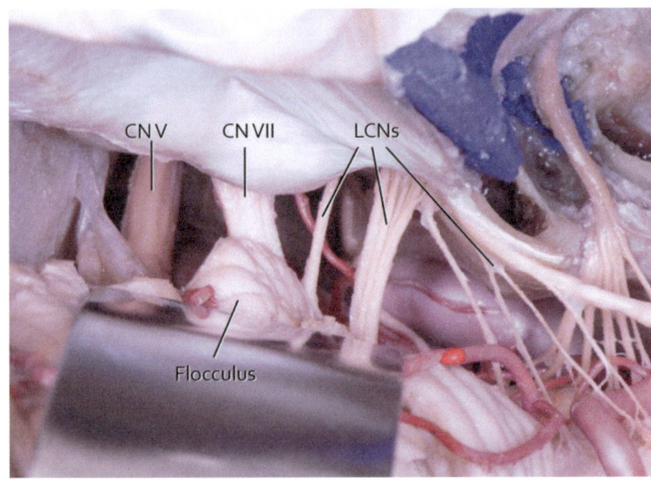

Fig. 29.4 An anatomical dissection shows a right-sided exposure of the cerebellopontine angle, with the right vertebral artery deep to the cranial nerve IX/X complex and below the CN VII/VIII complex, where compression in hemifacial spasm most often occurs

Alternatives

Medical treatments such as anticonvulsants, botulinum toxin injection, and baclofen are usually the initial treatment.

Anatomy

See Fig. 29.4.

Positioning

The patient was positioned supine with head turned to the left to expose the right retrosigmoid region (Fig. 29.5). The shoulder should not be allowed to rise into the way.

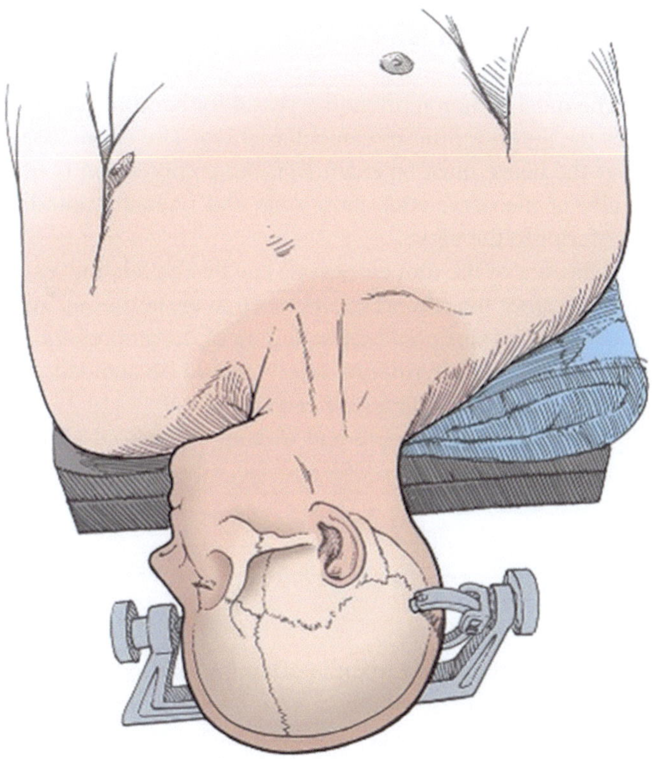

Fig. 29.5 Positioning for retrosigmoid craniotomy in most patients with a supple neck is straight supine with the neck turned. If the neck will tolerate it, this can be done without a shoulder bump. Elevating the head will lower venous pressure and relax the field some. Mildly flexing the neck will improve the approach angle

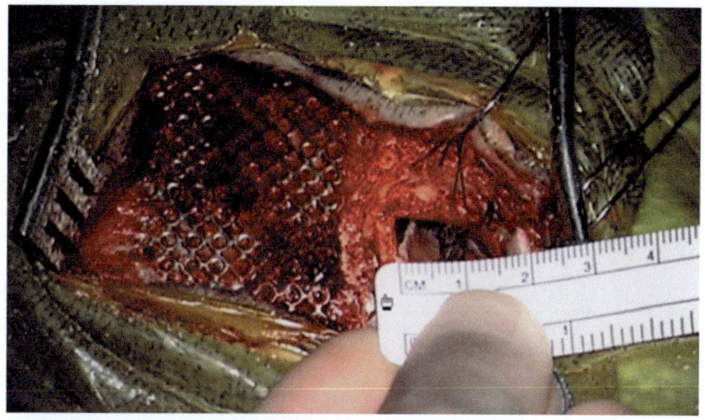

Fig. 29.6 A large exposure is shown due to the need to reuse the patient's prior incision. The prior titanium cranioplasty can be seen, with the new smaller craniotomy below

Incision

The previous surgery incision was reopened to avoid ischemic skin necrosis (Fig. 29.6).

Operation

A small craniotomy 1 cm below the transverse-sigmoid junction was made. Dura was opened in a triangular shape and tacked forward toward the sigmoid sinus. Arachnoid membranes were opened to release cerebrospinal fluid (CSF) and expose cranial nerve V. The endoscope should be consulted. The offending artery was identified and mobilized off the nerve. The endoscope brought reassurance that there were no other offending vessels. A Teflon™ sponge was inserted and secured with fibrin glue to keep the packing in place. A watertight closure was achieved (see Video 29.1).

Post-op

See Figs. 29.7 and 29.8.

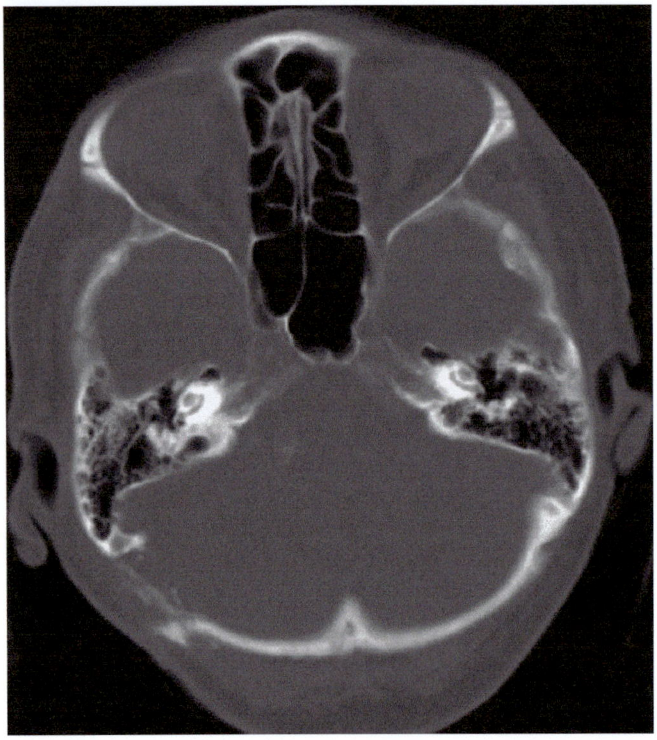

Fig. 29.7 Axial CT of the head without contrast with bone windowing shows the craniectomy in the right retrosigmoid area

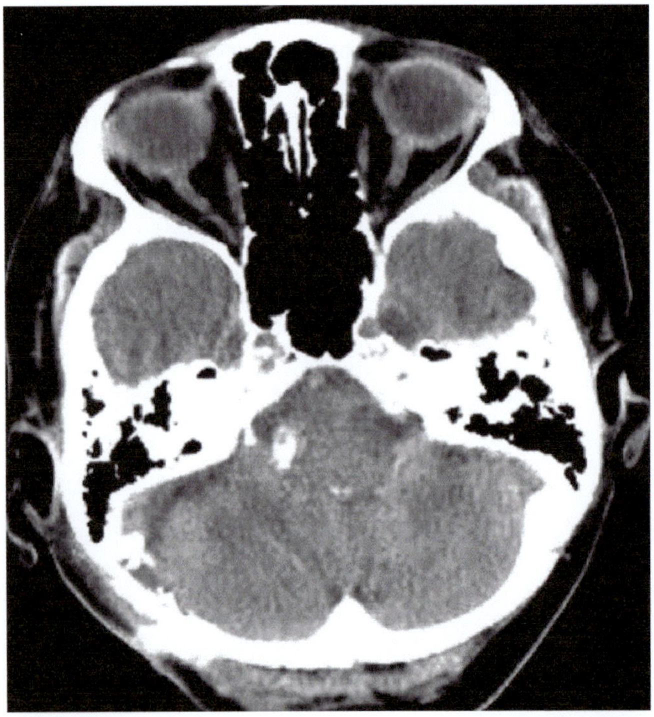

Fig. 29.8 An axial CT of the head without contrast shows a bright spot where the pledget and fibrin glue are

Outcome

The patient was discharged on postoperative day 3. Her hemifacial spasm improved after surgery and gradually resolved.

Pearls and Pitfalls

- The most common offending vessel for hemifacial spasm is the anterior inferior cerebellar artery. The entire length of the nerve must be examined, but compression is usually at the nerve root entry zone and typically anterior-inferior to the nerve.
- Exposure of the root entry zone can be challenging, especially since the compression is deep to the nerve and inadequate exposure could cause failure of decompression.
- Injury of the labyrinthine artery should be avoided as it could cause postoperative hearing loss.
- Watertight dural closure and waxing of mastoid air cells are required to prevent CSF leakage, especially in the case or reoperation.

Discussion

Baclofen or botulinum toxin is often the starting treatment. However, surgery is highly appropriate and effective for patients who can tolerate surgery. The entire length of the nerve, including the ventral side of the root entry zone, must be examined meticulously. The angled views provided by the endoscope can be helpful to see ventral to the cranial nerve VII/VIII and IX/X complexes where the offending most often contacts the nerve root entry zone [1].

Video used with permission from the Congress of Neurological Surgeons, CNS Nexus Cases. 2018. https://www.cns.org/nexus/cases

Reference

1. Lu AY, Yeung JT, Gerrard JL, Michaelides EM, Sekula RF, Bulsara KR. Hemifacial spasm and neurovascular compression. Sci World J. 2014;2014:349319.

Case 9: Left Retrosigmoid Craniotomy for Microvascular Decompression of Glossopharyngeal Neuralgia

30

Peter Nakaji, David Fusco, Brandon Liebelt, Michaela Lee, and Xiaochun Zhao

Summary

This case illustrates microvascular decompression for glossopharyngeal neuralgia (Fig. 30.1).

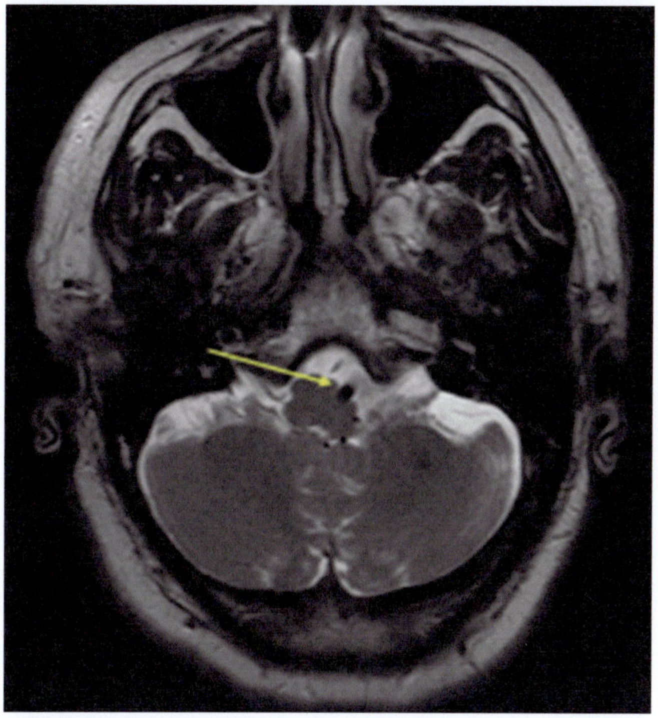

Fig. 30.1 Axial T2-weighted MRI shows the flow void of the vertebral artery impacting the brainstem at the facial nerve origin

Supplementary Information The online version contains supplementary material available at [https://doi.org/10.1007/978-3-031-12507-2_30].

P. Nakaji (✉)
Department of Neurosurgery, University of Arizona College of Medicine—Banner, Phoenix, AZ, USA

Surgery, University of Arizona College of Medicine—Phoenix, Phoenix, AZ, USA

Neurosurgery, Neuroscience Institute, Phoenix, AZ, USA
e-mail: Peter.Nakaji@bannerhealth.com

D. Fusco
Inpatient Neurosurgical Care, Chandler Regional Hospital, Phoenix, AZ, USA

B. Liebelt
Larner College of Medicine, University of Vermont Medical Center, Burlington, VT, USA

M. Lee
University of Arizona College of Medicine, Banner—University Medical Center Phoenix, Phoenix, AZ, USA

X. Zhao
Department of Neurosurgery, University of Oklahoma Health Sciences Center, Oklahoma City, OK, USA

N. C. Bambakidis et al. (eds.), *Surgery of the Cerebellopontine Angle*, https://doi.org/10.1007/978-3-031-12507-2_30

Case Presentation

A 75-year-old male presented with intermittent bilateral facial and neck pains for 12 years, triggered by speaking and swallowing (Figs. 30.2, 30.3, and 30.4).

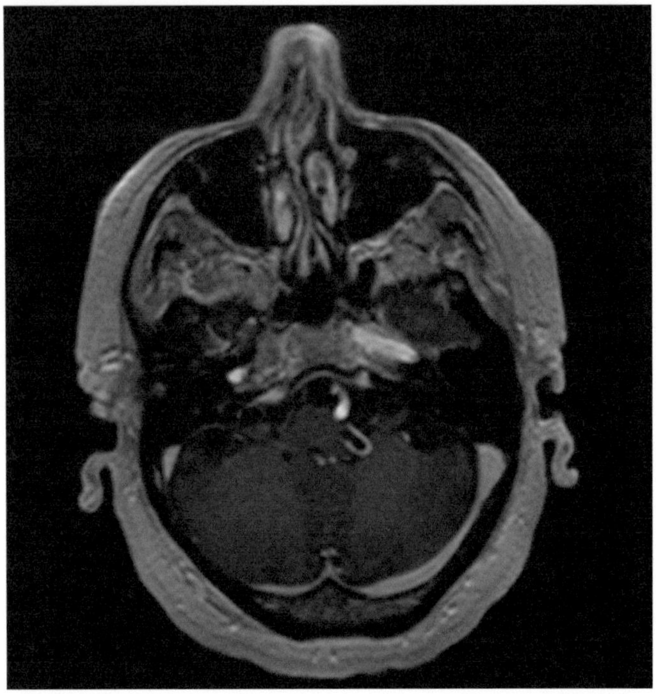

Fig. 30.2 The corresponding axial T1-weighted MRI with gadolinium also shows the vertebral artery impacting the brainstem at the facial nerve origin as well as a segment of the posterior inferior cerebellar artery immediately posterior to this, which is likely contributing to the compression

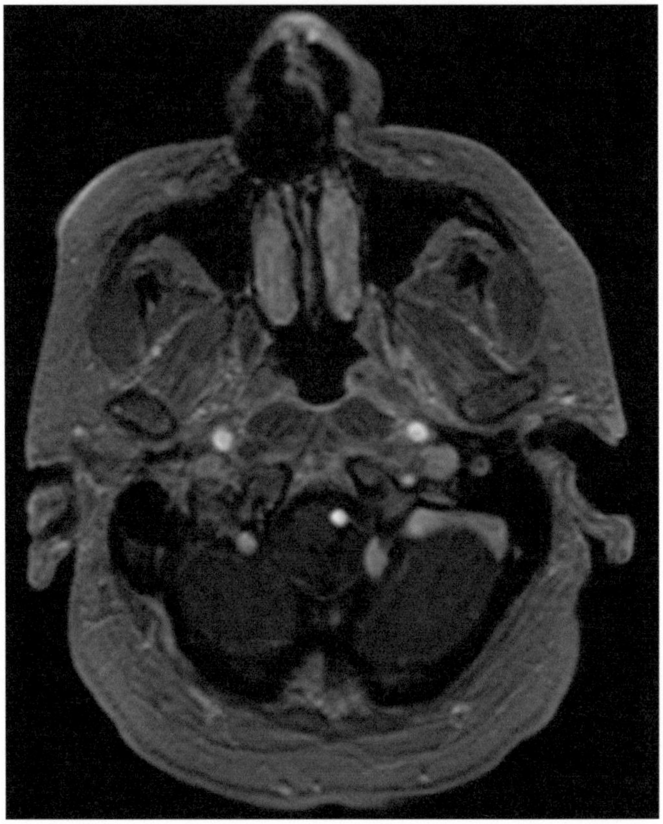

Fig. 30.3 Additional axial T1-weighted MRI with gadolinium also shows the vertebral artery impacting the brainstem even lower, which shows that a long segment of vessel will need decompression

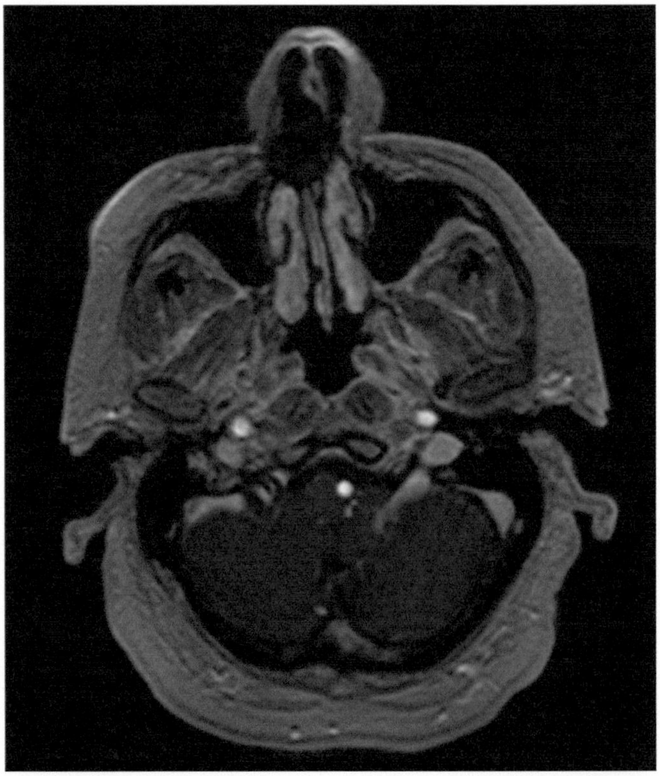

Fig. 30.4 The slice just above the one shown in Fig. 30.3 demonstrates more of the compression

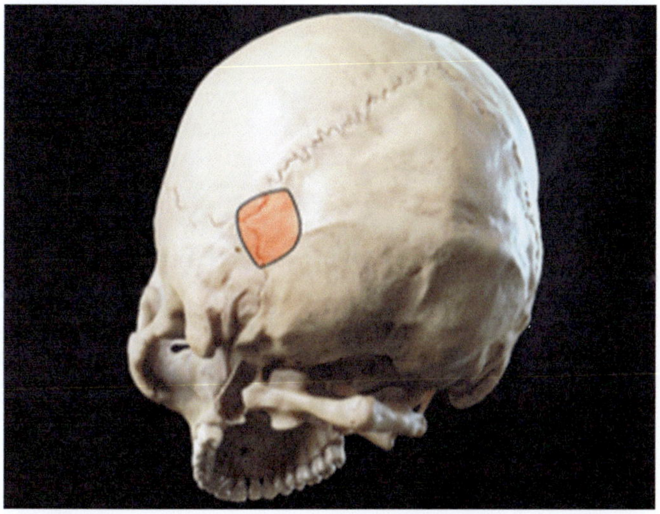

Fig. 30.5 A low retrosigmoid craniotomy provides access to the vertebral artery and the underside of the cranial nerve VII/VIII complex

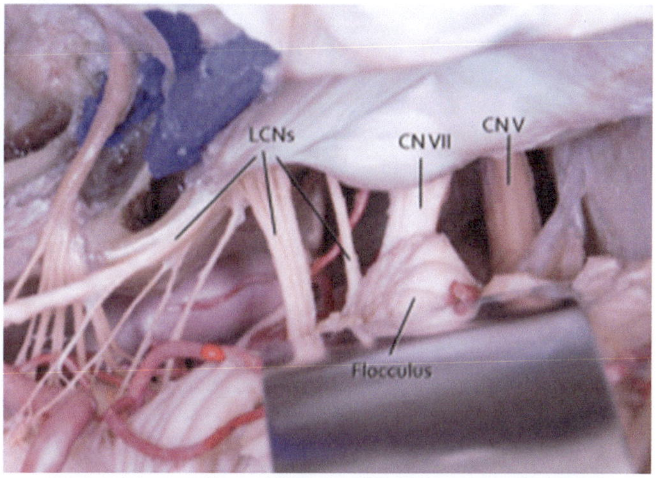

Fig. 30.6 An anatomical dissection of the left cerebellopontine angle shows the vertebral artery below the cranial nerve VII complex where it usually impacts the brainstem in hemifacial spasm

Approach

A left-sided retrosigmoid approach was planned (Fig. 30.5).

Alternatives

Anticonvulsants are the initial medical treatment for glossopharyngeal neuralgia. Radiosurgery such as Gamma knife may be appropriate for some older patients. Rhizotomy for cranial nerve (CN) IX and upper rootlets of CN X can be an alternative if no offending vessels are found, but it is associated with a high risk of permanent lower cranial nerve dysfunction such as dysphagia and vocal cord paralysis [1–3].

Anatomy

See Fig. 30.6.

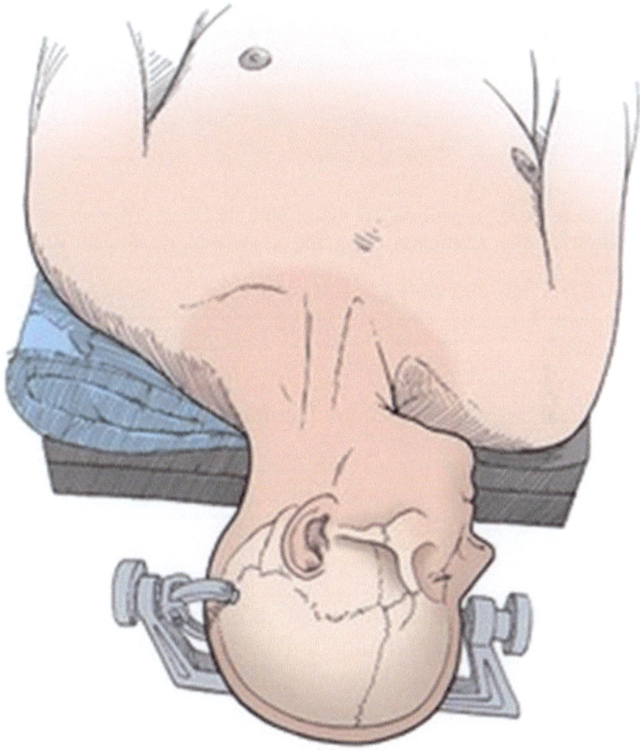

Fig. 30.7 Positioning for a retrosigmoid craniotomy in most patients with a supple neck is straight supine with the neck turned. If the neck will tolerate it, this can be done without a shoulder bump. Elevating the head will lower venous pressure and relax the field some. Mildly flexing the neck will improve the approach angle

Positioning

The patient was positioned supine with his head turned to the right to expose the left retrosigmoid region (Fig. 30.7). The shoulder should not be allowed to rise into the way.

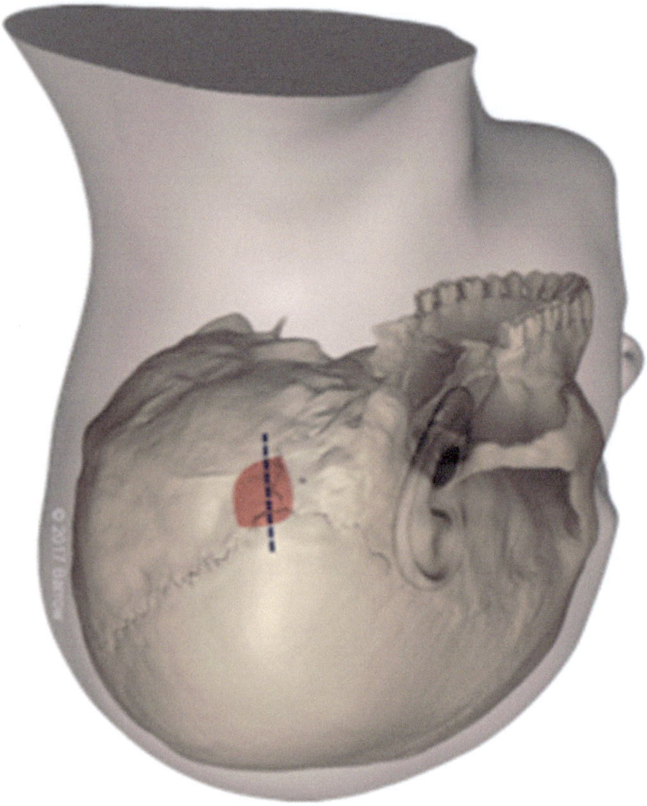

Fig. 30.8 A 3D reconstructed figure with the head down shows the location of the craniotomy and the associated traditional vertical incision

Incision

A vertical curvilinear incision behind the sigmoid sinus was made (Fig. 30.8).

Operation

A small retrosigmoid craniotomy posterior and inferior to the transverse-sigmoid junction was pursued. Dura was opened in a C-shaped fashion and tacked forward toward the sigmoid sinus. The arachnoid membrane was opened, cerebrospinal fluid (CSF) released, and CN IX exposed. The vertebral artery and loops from the posterior inferior cerebellar artery that were wedged into the brainstem were identified and dissected away. A 30-degree endoscope was brought into the surgical field to maximize the visualization. A Teflon™ sponge was inserted and held in place with Evicel® glue. A watertight closure was achieved (see Video 30.1).

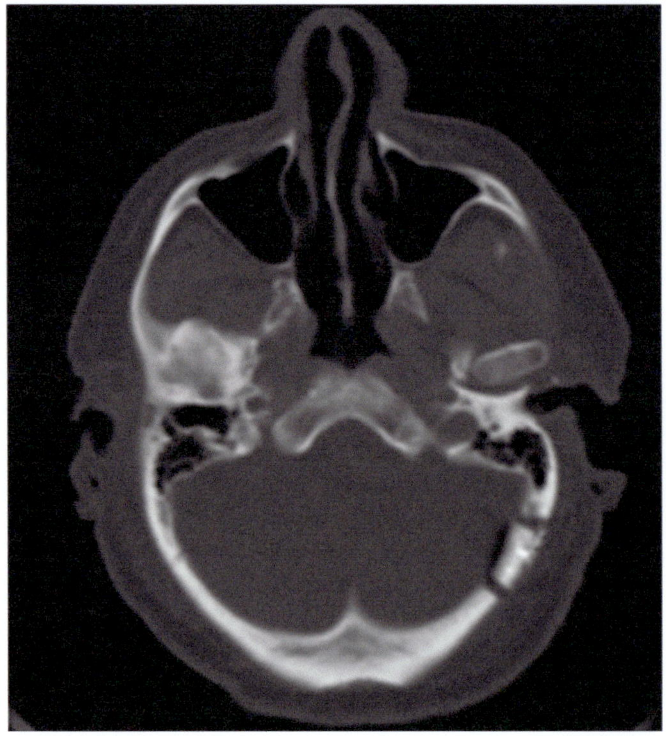

Fig. 30.9 An axial CT of the head without contrast shows the small left retrosigmoid craniotomy through which microvascular decompression is performed

Post-op

See Fig. 30.9.

Outcome

The pain was relieved postoperatively and did not return. The patient initially developed difficulty swallowing, though it resolved in the early postoperative period.

Pearls and Pitfalls

- Common offending vessels for glossopharyngeal neuralgia are the posterior inferior cerebellar artery and vertebral artery.
- The entire length of the nerve (particularly the root entry zone) must be examined.
- A watertight dural closure and waxing of mastoid air cells are required to prevent CSF leakage.

Discussion

Glossopharyngeal neuralgia is a disorder of CN IX, characterized with episodic pain at the posterior tongue, tonsil, throat, or external ear canal, which can be triggered by eating, swallowing, and speaking. Anticonvulsants are the starting treatment, with surgical decompression an option for patients who can tolerate surgery and who fail medical treatment. The entire length of the nerve, including the ventral side of the root entry zone, must be examined meticulously. Endoscopy can be helpful.

Video used with permission from the Congress of Neurological Surgeons, CNS Nexus Cases. 2018. https://www.cns.org/nexus/cases

References

1. Martinez-Alvarez R, Martinez-Moreno N, Kusak ME, Rey-Portoles G. Glossopharyngeal neuralgia and radiosurgery. J Neurosurg. 2014;121(Suppl 2):222–5.
2. Blumenfeld A, Nikolskaya G. Glossopharyngeal neuralgia. Curr Pain Head Reports. 2013;17(7):343.
3. Chen J, Sindou M. Vago-glossopharyngeal neuralgia: a literature review of neurosurgical experience. Acta neurochir. 2015;157(2):311–21.

Case 10: Anterior Transpetrosal Approach for Resection of Petroclival Meningioma

31

João Paulo Almeida, Sacit B. Omay, Theodore H. Schwartz, and Rohan Ramakrishna

Summary

True petroclival meningiomas are lesions originating medial to the porus trigeminalis. Different approaches can be used for resection of those lesions, including anterior or posterior petrosectomies and retrosigmoid approaches. This case illustrates the surgical nuances of the anterior petrosectomy approach (Kawase approach) for resection of petroclival meningiomas.

Case Presentation

A 68-year-old woman presented with a growing lesion, radiographically, diagnosed as a meningioma (Fig. 31.1). She exhibited gait instability and partial cranial nerve (CN) III palsy. Neuro exam revealed the following: intact, apart from trace left-sided weakness 4+, mild ptosis, and intermittent diplopia on medial/superior gaze.

Supplementary Information The online version contains supplementary material available at [https://doi.org/10.1007/978-3-031-12507-2_31].

J. P. Almeida
Department of Neurosurgery, Cleveland Clinic, Cleveland, OH, USA

S. B. Omay (✉)
Department of Neurosurgery, Yale School of Medicine, New Haven, CT, USA
e-mail: sacit.omay@yale.edu

T. H. Schwartz
Departments of Neurological Surgery, Otolaryngology and Neuroscience, Weill Cornell Medicine, New York, NY, USA

R. Ramakrishna
Department of Neurological Surgery and Neuro-oncology, New York–Presbyterian Brooklyn Methodist Hospital, Weill Cornell Medicine, New York, NY, USA

N. C. Bambakidis et al. (eds.), *Surgery of the Cerebellopontine Angle*, https://doi.org/10.1007/978-3-031-12507-2_31

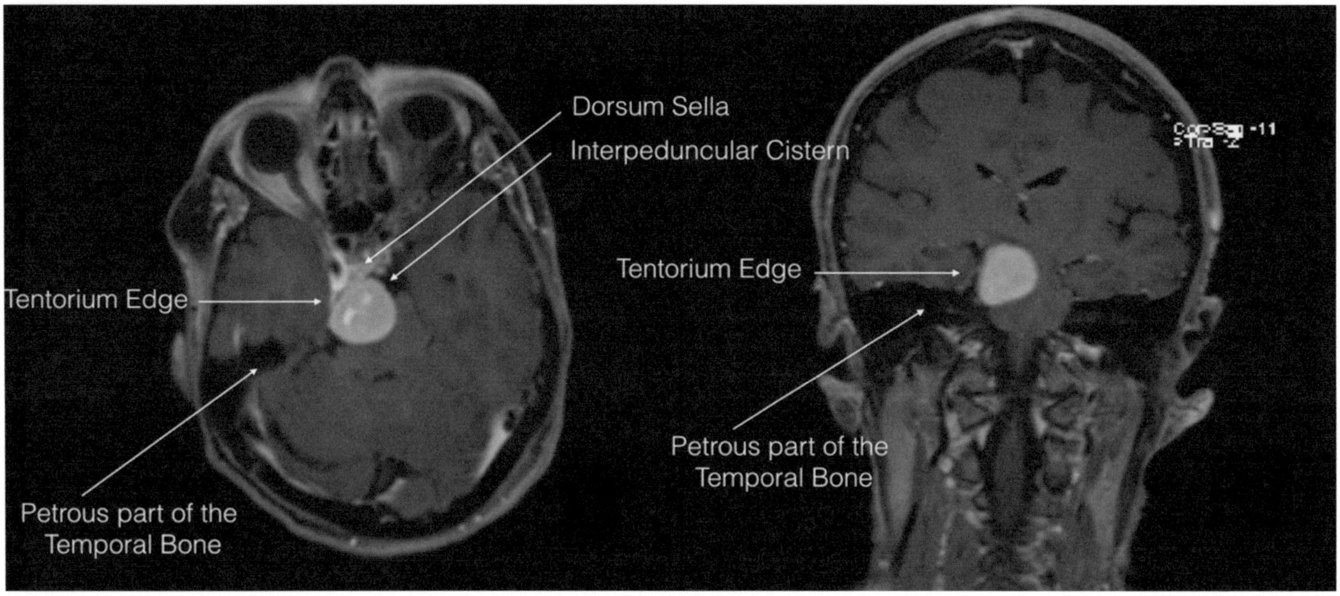

Fig. 31.1 Gadolinium-enhanced T1-weighted MRI demonstrating a right petroclival meningioma, arising medial to the porus trigeminus, posterior to the dorsum sellae, and closely related to the tentorial edge

Approach

An anterior petrosal approach (Kawase approach) was planned.

Alternatives

For petroclival meningiomas, observe the relation of the tumor with the tentorium and CNs V, VII, and VIII (internal auditory canal [IAC]) and extensions into the cavernous sinus/middle fossa. Lesions with significant supratentorial extension are good candidates for anterior petrosectomy. If the lesion is inferior to the IAC (VII/VIII), consider a posterior petrosectomy/retrosigmoid approach; if the lesion is superior to the IAC, consider an anterior petrosectomy. If the lesion extends into the middle fossa/cavernous sinus, an extended anterior petrosectomy (Dolenc-Kawase approach) may be preferred. A suprameatal retrosigmoid approach allows resection of middle fossa extensions. Combined approaches, such as pretemporal and retrosigmoid approaches, are also useful.

A middle fossa approach is an option for resection of lesions in the upper clivus, interpeduncular fossa, and prepontine cistern (above the level of the IAC). Attention should be given to the petrous internal carotid artery (ICA), V3, superior petrous sinus, and IAC.

Anatomy

Posterior medial (Kawase) triangle—quadrangular space (Fig. 31.2) [1]:

- Anterior limit of V3
- Lateral limit of the petrous ICA
- Posterior limit of the IAC
- Medial limit of the petrous apex/tentorial edge

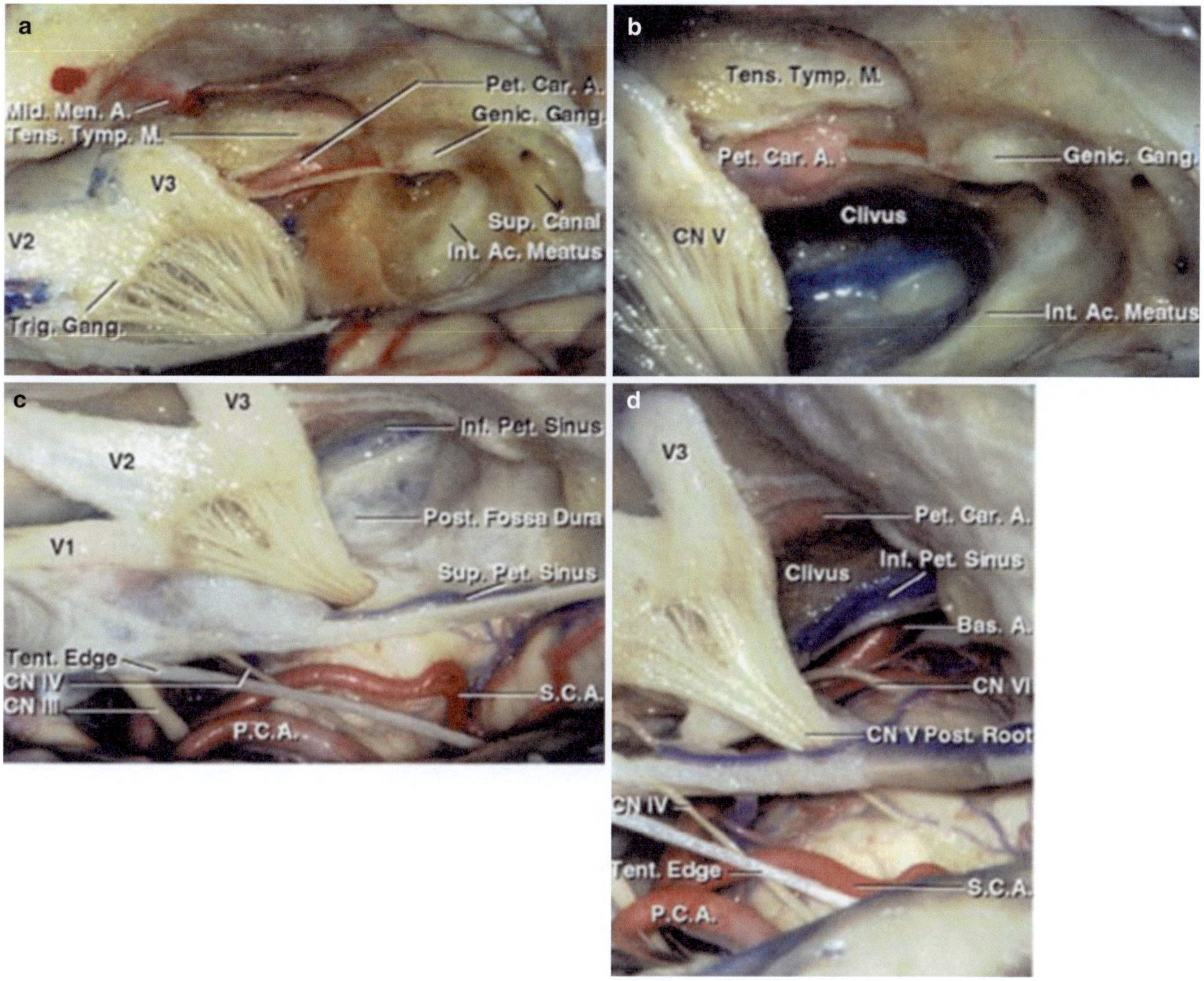

Fig. 31.2 (**a**) Exposure of the middle fossa after peeling is completed. The Kawase space is observed in the figure, located medial to the petrous carotid and GSPN, posterior to V3, anterior to the internal acoustic canal, and lateral to the petrous apex/tentorial edge. The geniculate ganglion, superior semicircular canal, and internal acoustic canal are visualized after partial drilling of the middle fossa. V2: maxillary segment of the trigeminal nerve; V3: mandibullary segment of the trigeminal nerve. (**b**) Drilling of the middle fossa/Kawase space is completed and the dura of the posterior fossa is observed. The limits of the Kawase space are easily identified in this figure and consist of: anterior limit—posterior aspect of V3; posterior limit—internal acoustic canal; medial limit—petrous apex/tentorial edge; lateral limit—petrous segment of the internal carotid artery. (**c**) The relationship of the tentorium and middle fossa is demonstrated in this figure. The trigeminal nerve crosses from the posterior fossa into the middle fossa through the porus trigeminus. The IV cranial nerve pierces the tentorial edge and runs anteriorly into the posterior aspect of the lateral wall of the cavernous sinus. When performing an anterior petrosctomy, the correct identification of the IV nerve, medial to the tentorium, is paramount for preservation of the trochlear nerve. (**d**) The inferior petrosal sinus represents the inferior limit of the Kawase/anterior petrosectomy. After such extensive drilling of the middle fossa, the VI nerve/abducens nerve is visualized, located lateral to the basilar trunk, running anteriorly towards Dorello's canal. Adapted from Rhoton AL. Overview of temporal bone. Neurosurgery. 2007;61(Suppl 4):S47–S460. Neurosurgery. Copyright © 2007 by the Congress of Neurological Surgeons

Positioning

The patient should be positioned supine, with her or his head rotated to the contralateral side (sagittal suture parallel to the floor). A shoulder roll should be placed under the ipsilateral shoulder. Secure the patient to allow for rotation, if needed.

Incision

A curvilinear, frontotemporal, or linear incision, from the root of the zygoma to the superior temporal line, was made.

Operation

A lumbar drain was placed after general anesthesia, followed by a temporal craniotomy (with or without supplementary removal of the zygomatic arch if needed for adequate exposure of the middle fossa) (Fig. 31.3) [2] (see Video 31.1).

Extradural Dissection: Subtemporal Corridor

The middle meningeal artery was identified and ligated, and the V3 and greater superficial petrosal nerve (GSPN) were

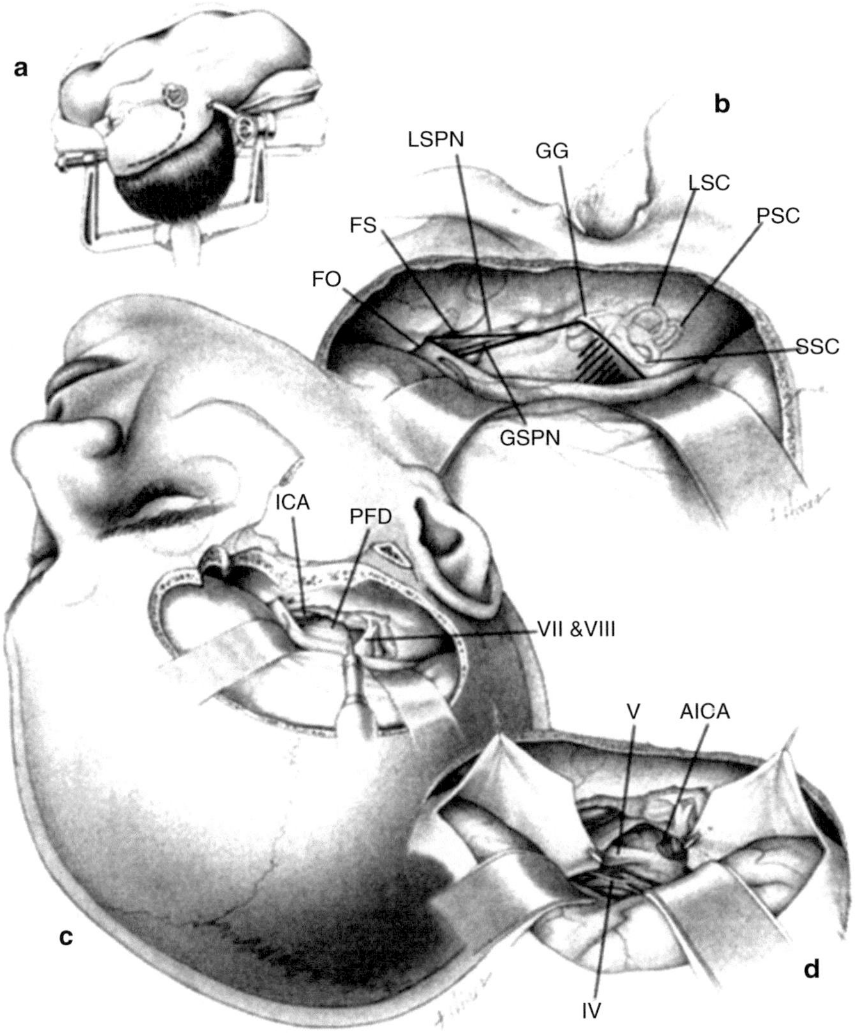

Fig. 31.3 Anterior petrosectomy: positioning and landmarks. (**a**) Patient is placed in supine positioned with head extended and rotated to the contralateral side, and fixed with use of a Mayfield headholder. (**b**) The middle fossa bone landmarks are exposed after the temporal craniotomy and peeling of the middle fossa. Drilling of the Kawase space is performed after identification of anatomical landmarks. (**c**) The posterior fossa dura (PFD) is exposed once middle fossa drilling is completed. (**d**) The tentorium and posterior fossa dura are cut and IV and V cranial nerves are identified as well as AICA , in close relationship with the VII–VIII complex. *FO* foramen ovale, *FS* foramen spinosum, *LSPN* lesser petrosal superficial nerve, *GG* geniculate ganglion, *LSC* lateral semicircular canal, *PSC* posterior semicircular canal, *SSC* superior semicircular canal, *GSPN* greater petrosal superficial nerve, *ICA* internal carotid artery, *PFD* posterior fossa dura, *AICA* anterior inferior cerebellar artery. Adapted from Aziz KM, van Loveren HR, Tew JM Jr, Chicoine MR. The Kawase approach to retrosellar and upper clival basilar aneurysms. Neurosurgery. 1999;44(6):1225–1234. Copyright © 1999, Neurosurgery, by the Congress of Neurological Surgeons

exposed. We identified the Kawase triangle/quadrangular space (V3, petrous ICA, petrous apex/tentorial edge, and arcuate eminence/IAC) [3]. The Kawase space was drilled with a diamond bit drill to expose the posterior fossa dura.

Dura Opening

Temporal dura was opened in a U-shaped fashion. The superior petrosal sinus was identified and coagulated, and CN IV was identified. The tentorium and posterior fossa dura were opened.

Tumor Resection

After coagulation of the dural insertion of the tumor, an ultrasonic aspirator was used for internal bulking. The tumor margins (brainstem, CN IV, CN V, tentorium edge) were dissected. After tumor resection, the surrounding dura was coagulated and resected. Meticulous hemostasis should be maintained.

Closure

Fat tissue and dural sealant were used for closure. Bone flap was replaced.

Post-op

The patient was discharged to rehab on postoperative day 4, neurologically intact apart from palsy of CN IV. Preoperative palsy of CN III resolved at 3-month follow-up.

Pearls and Pitfalls

- Use of neuronavigation and Doppler ultrasound facilitates identification of petrous ICA and bone landmarks.
- In the middle fossa, perform posterior to anterior dissection to avoid injury to the GSPN, which is connected to the geniculate ganglion posteriorly.
- Prior to cutting the tentorium, identify CN IV to avoid postoperative diplopia.
- Postoperative leak of cerebrospinal fluid (CSF) is a potential complication. The use of fat tissue for closure and postoperative lumbar drain for 48 to 72 h improves postoperative result. Be sure to wax any air cells that are opened during drilling process. Placing dural substitute along the middle fossa floor is also useful to cover small bony dehiscences exposed during initial exposure.
- Temporal lobe retraction can cause significant contusion/hematoma. Remove plenty of CSF and gravity assist (vertex down) to reduce the amount of retraction. Minimize the use of fixed retractors; they often can be removed after the tentorium has been cut. Make the craniotomy sufficiently large so that the temporal lobe is not retracted against the superior bone edge.
- CN IV is at high risk, particularly with meningiomas; counsel patients about possible CN IV palsy.
- Identify the vein of Labbé on preoperative imaging and preserve it during the operation.
- The tumor should not be chased into the cavernous sinus for benign lesions; radiosurgery is extremely effective for residual tumor in these areas.
- Neurophysiologic monitoring is key; CNs V, VII, VIII should be monitored. CNs III and VI can also be monitored but may be less useful. Somatosensory evoked potentials (SSEP)/motor evoked potentials (MEPs) are also useful.

Video used with permission from the Congress of Neurological Surgeons, CNS Nexus Cases. 2018. https://www.cns.org/nexus/cases

References

1. Rhoton AL. Overview of temporal bone. Neurosurgery. 2007;61(Suppl_4):S47–S460.
2. Aziz KM, van Loveren HR, Tew JM Jr, Chicoine MR. The Kawase approach to retrosellar and upper clival basilar aneurysms. Neurosurgery. 1999;44(6):1225–34.
3. Borghei-Razavi H, Tomio R, Fereshtehnejad SM, Shibao S, Schick U, Toda M, Kawase T, Yoshida K. Anterior petrosal approach: the safety of Kawase triangle as an anatomical landmark for anterior petrosectomy in petroclival meningiomas. Clin Neurol Neurosurg. 2015;139:282–7. Epub 2015 Oct 28

32 Case 11: Vestibular Schwannoma Resection with Facial Nerve Displaced Dorsally

Jacob Cherian, Alex D. Sweeney, and Akash J. Patel

Summary

Preservation of facial nerve function is critical during resections of vestibular schwannomas. In rare instances, the facial nerve can be displaced dorsally by a vestibular schwannoma, making its removal challenging [1, 2]. This case and accompanying video (Video 32.1) illustrate preoperative workup, surgically relevant anatomic variation, intraoperative decision making, and postoperative management.

Case Presentation

A 62-year-old woman presented with right-sided nonpulsatile tinnitus for 1 year, with progressive hearing loss and long standing episodic positional vertigo. On exam, she was awake, alert, and oriented. Hearing loss was worse on her right side. Facial function was symmetrical. MRI (T1 with contrast) was performed (Figs. 32.1 and 32.2).

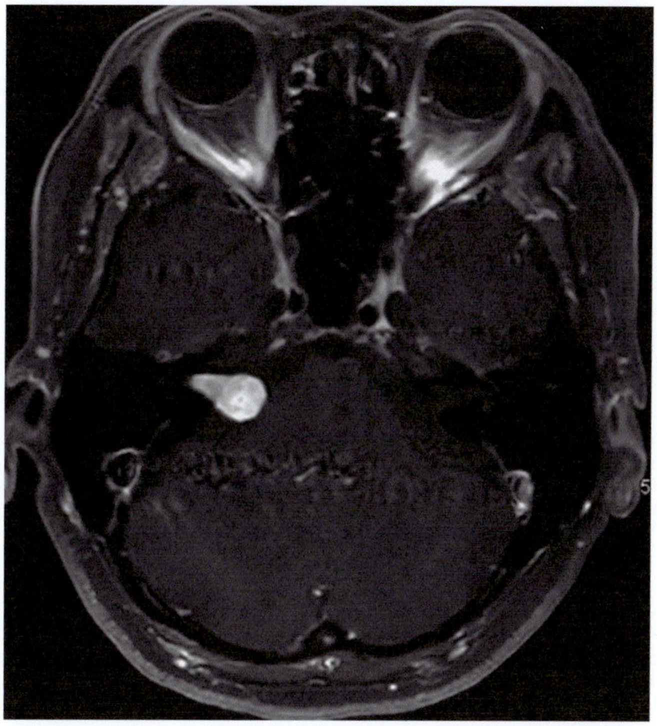

Fig. 32.1 Preoperative axial T1-weighted MRI with contrast demonstrates right sided vestibular schwannoma in the internal auditory canal and cerebellopontine angle cistern

Supplementary Information The online version contains supplementary material available at [https://doi.org/10.1007/978-3-031-12507-2_32].

J. Cherian (✉)
University of Maryland School of Medicine, Baltimore, MD, USA
e-mail: JCherian@som.umaryland.edu

A. D. Sweeney · A. J. Patel
Baylor College of Medicine, Houston, TX, USA

N. C. Bambakidis et al. (eds.), *Surgery of the Cerebellopontine Angle*, https://doi.org/10.1007/978-3-031-12507-2_32

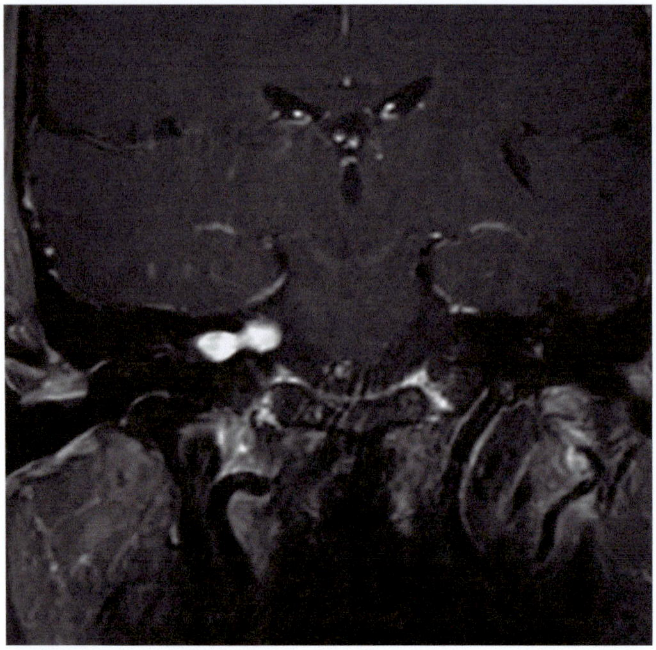

Fig. 32.2 Preoperative coronal T1-weighted MRI with contrast demonstrates right sided vestibular schwannoma

Approach

A retrosigmoid approach was planned. The surgical corridor was accessed through the space posterior and inferior to the transverse-sigmoid sinus junction. We opened the cisterna magna and cerebellopontine angle (CPA) cistern, providing brain relaxation.

Alternatives

Continued observation, a translabyrinthine approach, and radiosurgery are alternatives.

Positioning

The patient was put into park-bench position, with the affected side up. The patient should be secured to allow for rotation if needed.

Incision

A linear incision was made.

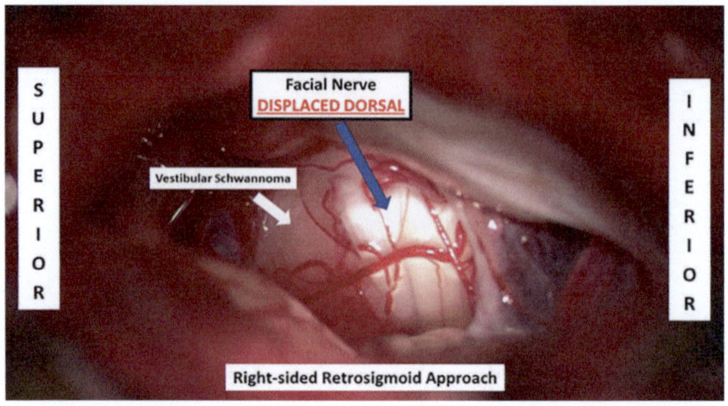

Fig. 32.3 Operative video demonstrated complete resection of vestibular schwannoma

Operation

We performed a craniotomy. The transverse-sigmoid junction was located using neuronavigation. Dura was opened in a linear fashion, with extension toward the sinus junction. The cisterna magna was opened, and the CPA cistern was dissected. Neuromonitoring was used to identify the course of the facial nerve (Fig. 32.3). The tumor was debulked and dissected away from the brainstem. The porus was drilled, and the intracanalicular tumor was removed, followed by the removal of the final tumor and then closure (Video 32.1).

Anatomy

- Transverse and sigmoid sinuses
- Cranial nerves V, VII, IX, and X
- Porus acousticus
- Anterior inferior cerebellar artery

Post-op

The patient had an uneventful recovery, with an overnight stay in the ICU. She was discharged home on post-op day 3 with a House-Brackmann score of 1. MRI demonstrated gross total resection (Fig. 32.4). Pathology revealed a schwannoma.

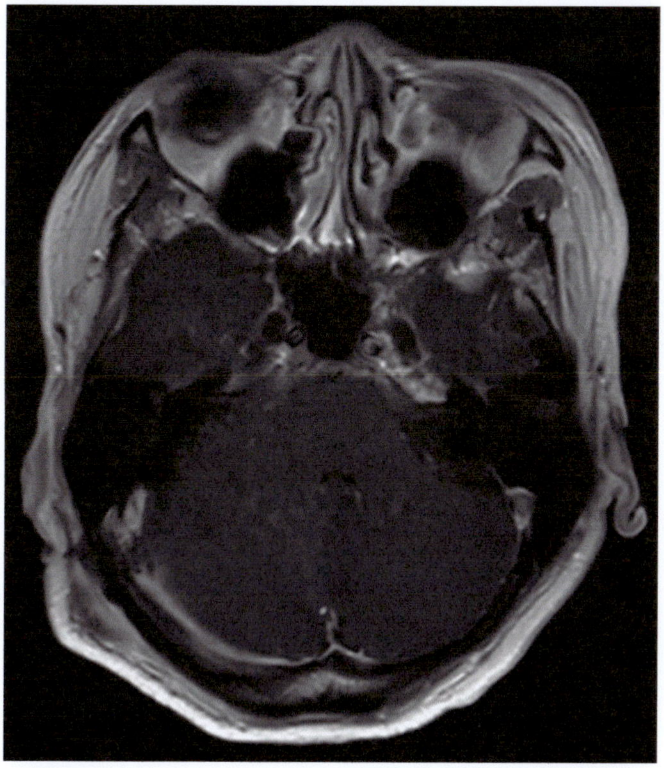

Fig. 32.4 Postoperative axial T1-weighted MRI with contrast demonstrates complete resection of right sided vestibular schwannoma

Pearls and Pitfalls

- Neuromonitoring with direct stimulation can identify an unexpected position of the facial nerve and maintain the nerve boundary during dissection.
- Debulking followed by sharp dissection and gentle mobilization allows for preservation of facial nerve function.
- Tumor dissection toward the porus acousticus is simplified after the medial boundary with the brainstem and the lateral boundary in the canal are identified.

Video used with permission from the Congress of Neurological Surgeons, CNS Nexus Cases. 2018. https://www.cns.org/nexus/cases, https://cnsnexus.crowdwisdomhq.net/nexus/article/13909

References

1. Mastronardi L, Cacciotti G, Roperto R, Di Scipio E, Tonelli MP, Carpineta E. Position and course of facial nerve and postoperative facial nerve results in vestibular schwannoma microsurgery. World Neurosurg. 2016;94:174–80.
2. Nejo T, Kohno M, Nagata O, Sora S, Sato H. Dorsal displacement of the facial nerve in acoustic neuroma surgery: clinical features and surgical outcomes of 21 consecutive dorsal pattern cases. Neurosurg Rev. 2016;39:277–88.

Case 12: Right Retrosigmoid Craniotomy for Pontine Cavernous Malformation

33

Xiaochun Zhao, Nikolay Martirosyan, Yashar Kalani, and Peter Nakaji

Summary

This case illustrates the resection of a pontine cavernous malformation via a retrosigmoid approach (Fig. 33.1).

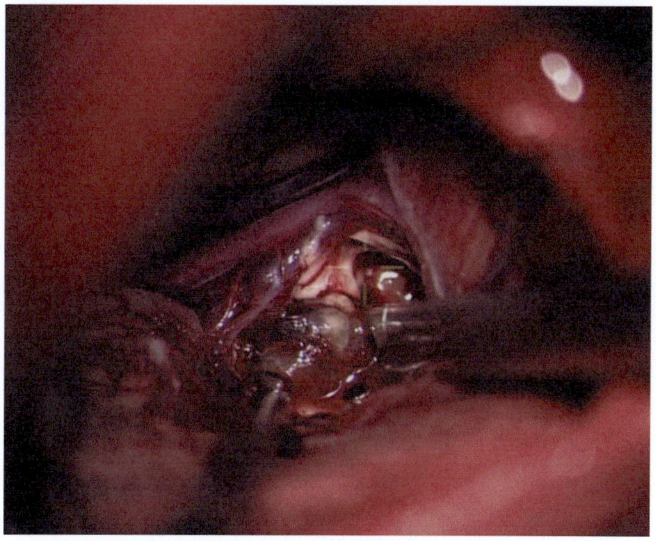

Fig. 33.1 Microscopic view of the cavernous malformation exposed through a pontine window via the right retrosigmoid approach

Supplementary Information The online version contains supplementary material available at [https://doi.org/10.1007/978-3-031-12507-2_33].

X. Zhao
Department of Neurosurgery, University of Oklahoma Health Sciences Center, Oklahoma City, OK, USA

N. Martirosyan
Unity Point Health, Allen Memorial Hospital, Waterloo, IA, USA

Y. Kalani
Department of Surgery, University of Oklahoma School of Medicine, Tulsa, OK, USA

P. Nakaji (✉)
Department of Neurosurgery, University of Arizona College of Medicine—Banner, Phoenix, AZ, USA

Surgery, University of Arizona College of Medicine—Phoenix, Phoenix, AZ, USA

Neurosurgery, Neuroscience Institute, Phoenix, AZ, USA
e-mail: Peter.Nakaji@bannerhealth.com

N. C. Bambakidis et al. (eds.), *Surgery of the Cerebellopontine Angle*, https://doi.org/10.1007/978-3-031-12507-2_33

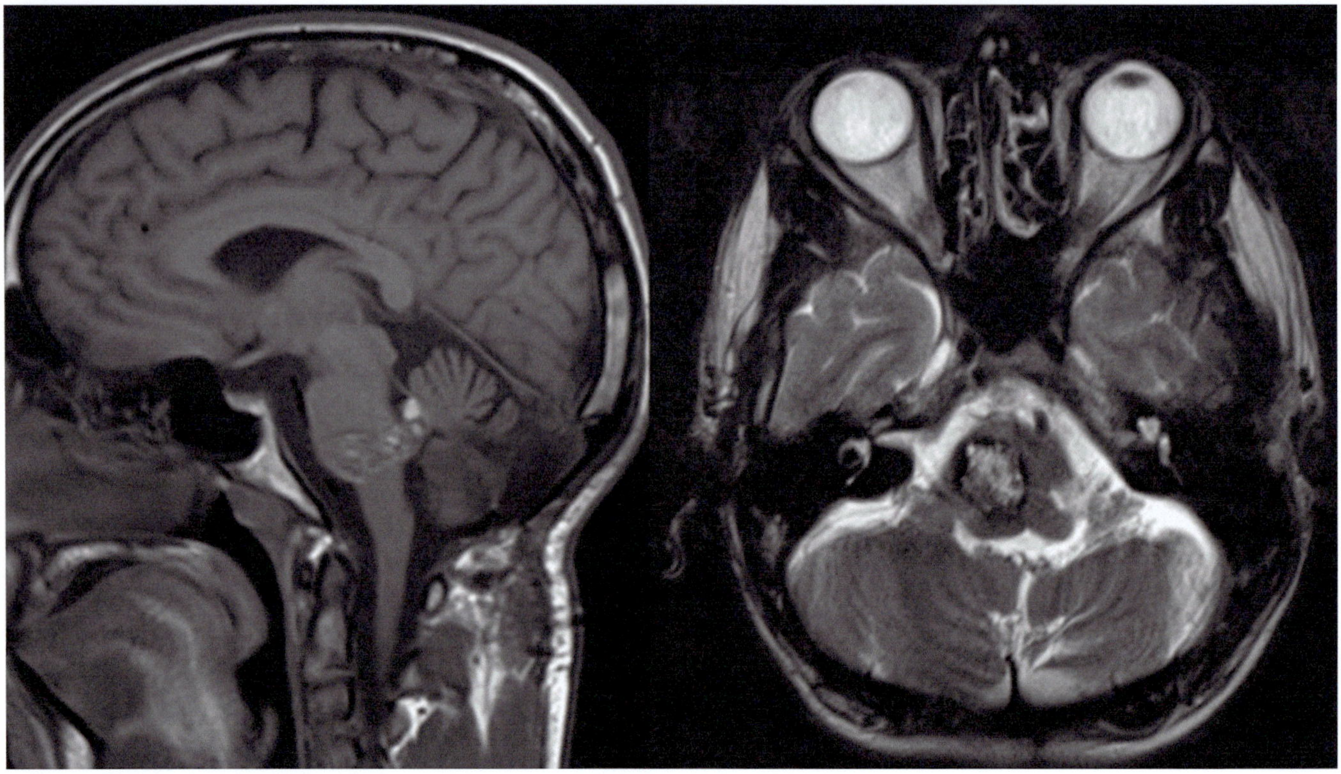

Fig. 33.2 Sagittal T1 and axial T2 MRI show the right pontine cavernous malformation

Case Presentation

A 28-year-old male presented with left side weakness, dysphagia, gait difficulties, and seizure (Fig. 33.2).

Approach

A right retrosigmoid approach was planned. This approach requires a trajectory through the middle cerebellar peduncle; any deficits can be expected to recover (Fig. 33.3) [1–3].

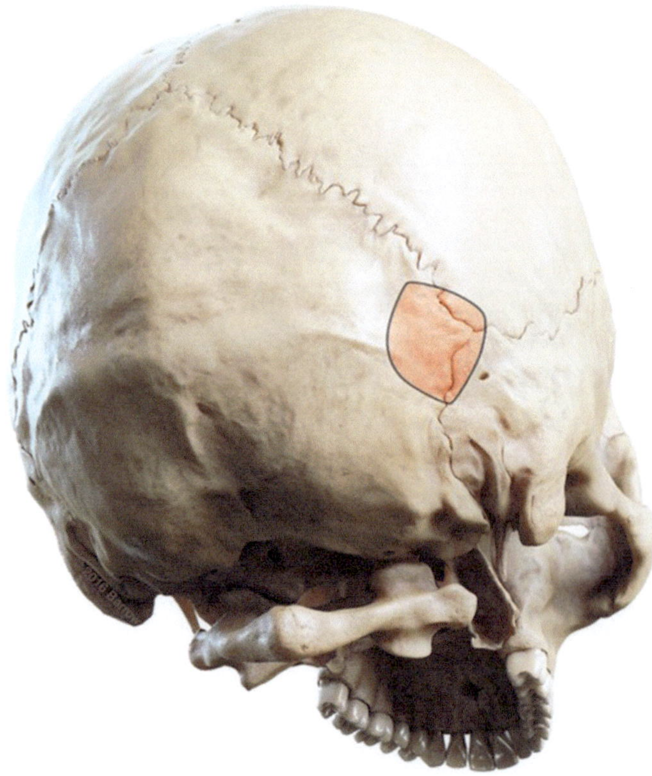

Fig. 33.3 The location of the right retrosigmoid craniotomy is shown in orange

Alternatives

The telovelar approach can be an alternative because of its proximity to the floor of the 4th ventricle (suprafacial/infrafacial collicular triangle). However, the peritrigeminal zone is more appropriate based on the two-point method and is usually better tolerated (Fig. 33.4) [2].

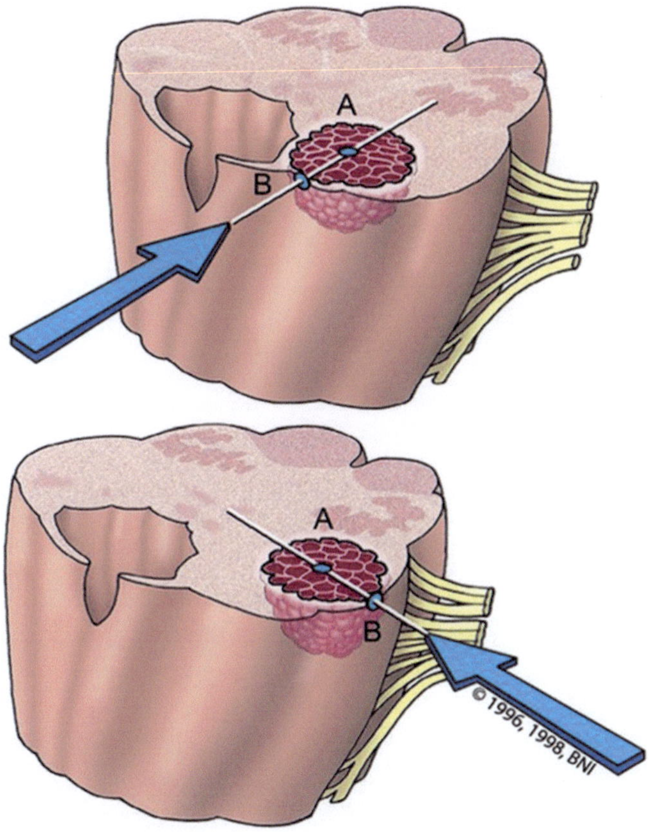

Fig. 33.4 A simple method for determining the trajectory to a brainstem lesion is to draw a straight line from the center of the lesion to the surface — the "two-point method"

Anatomy

A retrosigmoid craniotomy takes a posterior approach past the cranial nerves. The preferred entry zones into the pons are shown; in this case, the inferior entry below the trigeminal nerve and above the facial-vestibular complex was used. The cerebellum should be walked back to expose the lateral cerebellar peduncle (Figs. 33.5, 33.6, and 33.7).

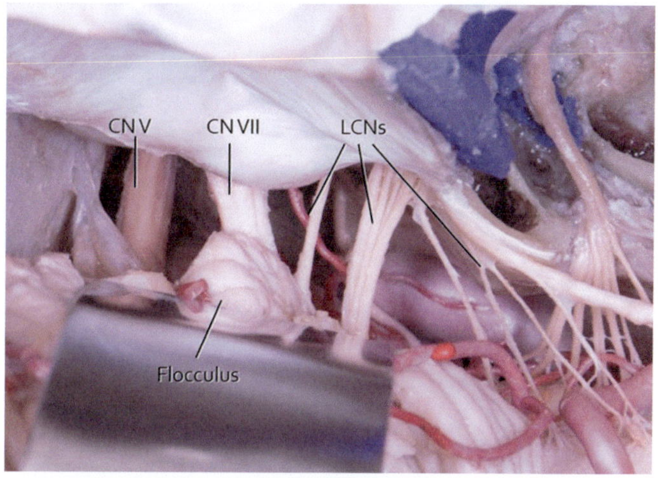

Fig. 33.5 A cadaveric view of the right lateral pons shows the anatomy of the right retrosigmoid space. Access to the pons would be through the window between CN V and CN VII, under the tip of the retractor blade (which would not be used in actual surgery)

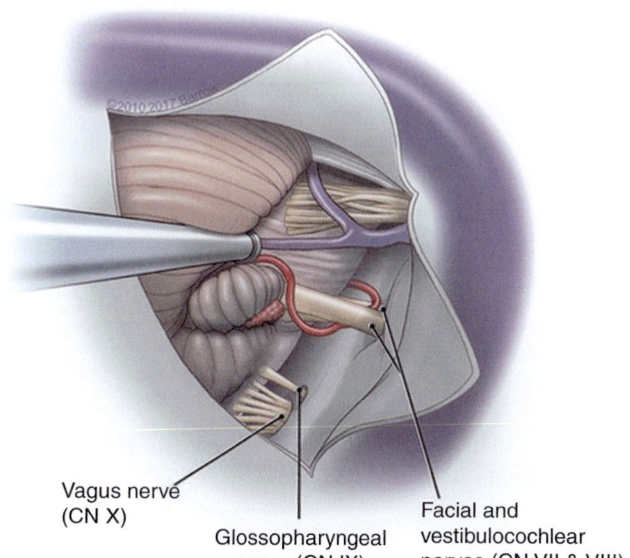

Fig. 33.6 Retrosigmoid craniotomy with cranial nerves indicated

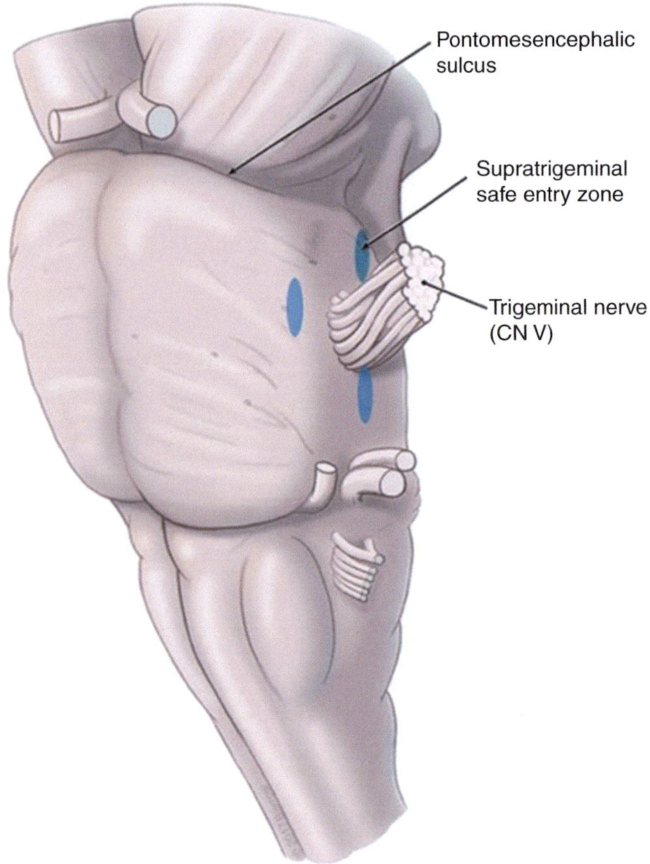

Fig. 33.7 Safe entry zones into the pons. There are a number of safe entry zones into the pons, especially including the zones just above and below the trigeminal nerve and just in front of it, in addition to entering from the middle cerebellar peduncle (not shown in this figure)

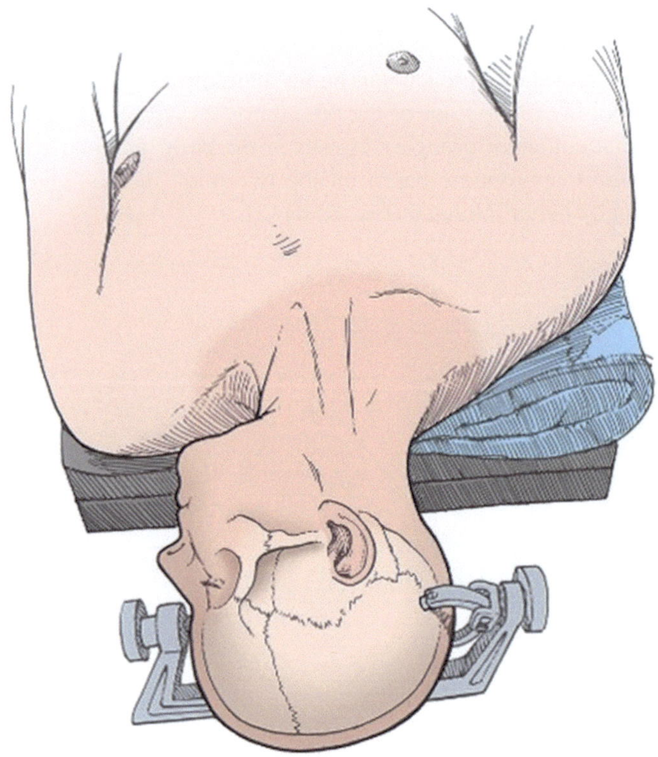

Fig. 33.8 Supine position with head turned to the left. For the retrosigmoid position, the head should be turned away to the opposite side as far as can safely be managed. Occasionally a bump is placed under the ipsilateral shoulder, though doing so should be avoided if possible. The chin should be tucked in some degree of flexion to decrease the steepness of the tentorium

Positioning

The patient was positioned supine with his head turned left to expose the right retrosigmoid region. The shoulder should not be allowed to rise into the way. Some chin flexion may improve the angle to the trigeminal nerve (Fig. 33.8).

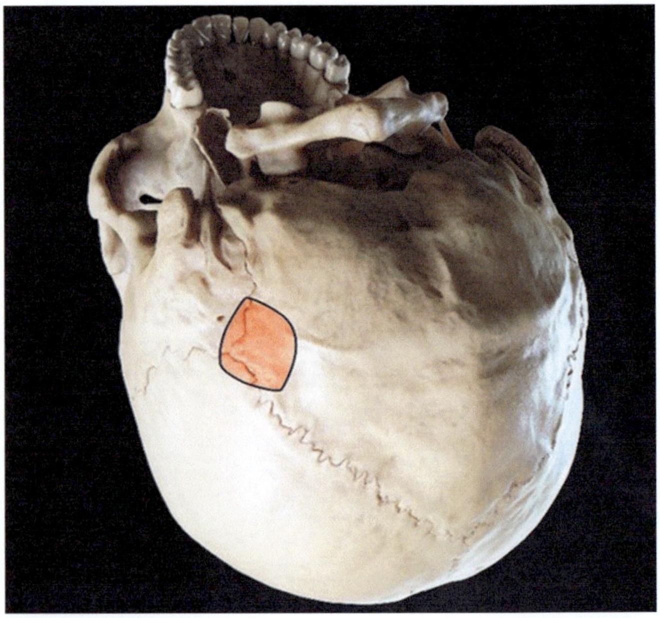

Fig. 33.9 Location of craniotomy. The craniotomy is located with the anterior-superior edge near the asterion, bordering the transverse and sigmoid sinuses

Incision

A vertical incision over the transverse-sigmoid sinus junction was made (Fig. 33.9).

Operation

As seen in Video 33.1, we made a vertical incision for a craniotomy below and behind the transverse sigmoid junction. The sigmoid sinus was fully exposed to increase the angle of the view. Dura was opened and tacked up. The arachnoid membrane was opened to release cerebrospinal fluid. The

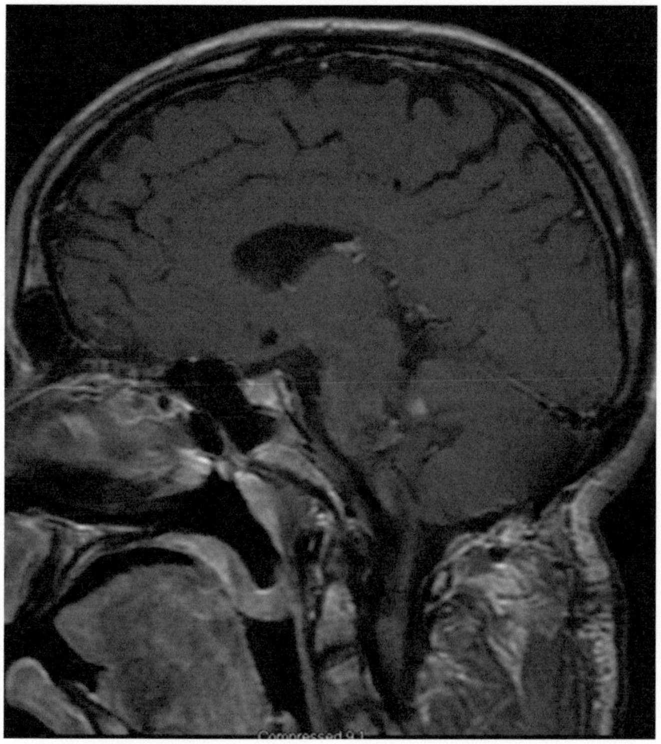

Fig. 33.10 Postoperative image. Sagittal MRI with gadolinium shows good resection of the lesion

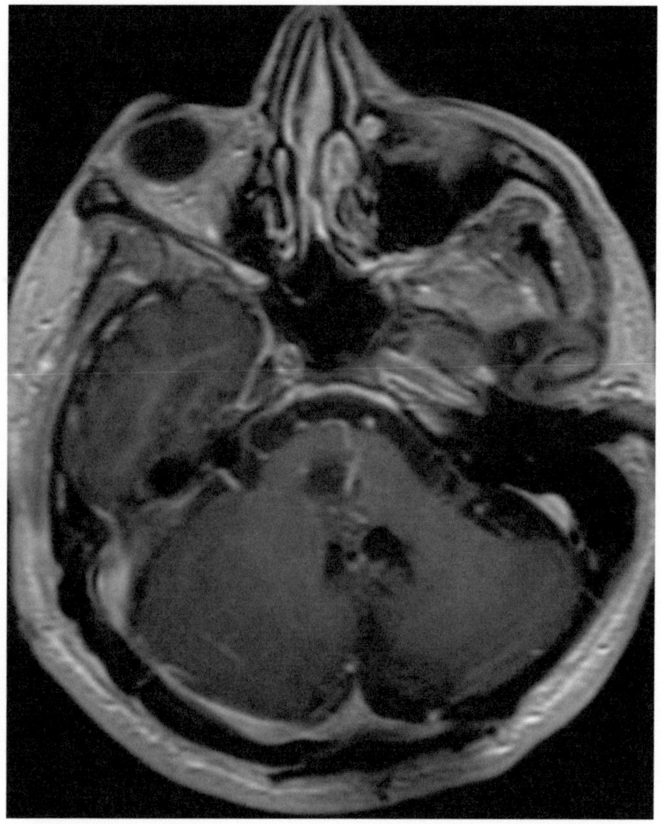

Fig. 33.11 Postoperative image. Axial MRI with gadolinium image shows good resection of the lesion with preservation of the developmental venous anomaly

flocculus was retracted to expose the middle cerebellar peduncle. The exact entry site was selected with the assistance of neuronavigation. Pursue minimal cauterization of the entry site and transgression of the parenchyma. The cavernous malformation was encountered, freed up circumferentially with dissectors, and taken out piecemeal. The cavity was inspected, and hemostasis was maintained. A watertight dural closure was achieved (see Video 33.1).

Post-op

Post-operative MRI demonstrates good resection of the cavernous malformation (Figs. 33.10 and 33.11). Note that the surrounding hemosiderin-stained brain is not cavernous malformation and is preserved.

Outcome

No new neurological deficits were observed. The patient was discharged on postoperative day 8.

Discussion

The parenchyma needs to be entered incising parallel to fiber tracts to decrease the risk of neurological deficits. The two-point method helps to evaluate and select the right surgical approach. A hemorrhagic cavernous malformation has a superior outcome if it is operated on within 6 weeks.

Pearls and Pitfalls

- The retrosigmoid approach is a quick and straightforward approach.
- A large petrosal vein (vein of Dandy) may affect the surgical exposure and manipulation.
- Use lateral pontomesencephalic fissure.

- For ventrally positioned lesions where a retrosigmoid approach is too oblique, an anterior/posterior petrosectomy or transclinoidal or endonasal approach may be more appropriate.

Video used with permission from the Congress of Neurological Surgeons, CNS Nexus Cases. 2018. https://www.cns.org/nexus/cases

References

1. Zaidi Mooney MA, Levitt MR, Dru AB, Abla AA, Spetzler RF. Impact of timing of intervention among 397 consecutively treated brainstem cavernous malformations. Neurosurgery. 2017;81(4):620–6.
2. Abla AA, Turner JD, Mitha AP, Lekovic G, Spetzler RF. Surgical approaches to brainstem cavernous malformations. Neurosurg Focus. 2010;29(3):E8.
3. Abla AA, Lekovic GP, Turner JD, de Oliveira JG, Porter R, Spetzler RF. Advances in the treatment and outcome of brainstem cavernous malformation surgery: a single-center case series of 300 surgically treated patients. Neurosurgery. 2011;68(2):403–15.

Case 13: Lateral Transcondylar Craniotomy for PICA Aneurysm

34

Anisha Garg, Kevin K. Yoo, Simone E. Dekker,
and Nicholas C. Bambakidis

Summary

This case illustrates issues in clipping a large left posterior inferior cerebellar artery (PICA) aneurysm in a 53-year-old male (Fig. 34.1).

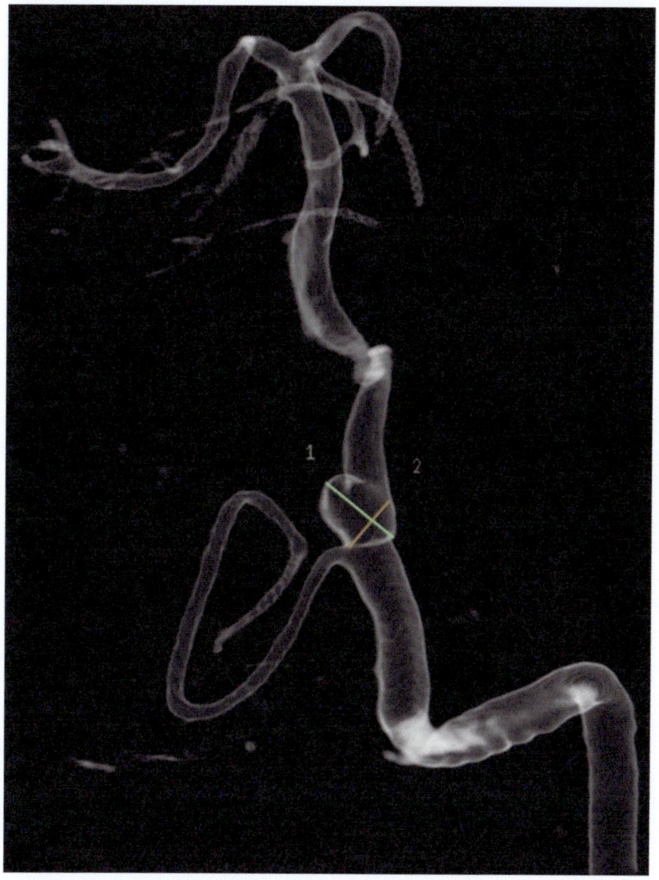

Fig. 34.1 Preoperative digital subtraction angiography

Case Presentation

The patient presented with 2 years of worsening headache and recent onset of left facial numbness. Imaging demonstrated a large left vertebral aneurysm distal to the take-off from PICA. He had a medical history of aneurysm, hypertension, and stroke (Figs. 34.2 and 34.3).

Supplementary Information The online version contains supplementary material available at [https://doi.org/10.1007/978-3-031-12507-2_34].

A. Garg
Yale New Haven Hospital, New Haven, CT, USA

K. K. Yoo
Alvarado Hospital Medical Center and Paradise Valley Hospital, Scripps Memorial Hospital Encinitas, San Diego, CA, USA

S. E. Dekker
Department of Neurological Surgery, The Neurological Institute, University Hospitals Cleveland Medical Center, Case Western Reserve University, Cleveland, OH, USA

N. C. Bambakidis (✉)
Neurological Surgery, The Neurological Institute, University Hospitals of Cleveland, Case Western Reserve University School of Medicine, Cleveland, OH, USA
e-mail: Nicholas.Bambakidis2@UHhospitals.org

N. C. Bambakidis et al. (eds.), *Surgery of the Cerebellopontine Angle*, https://doi.org/10.1007/978-3-031-12507-2_34

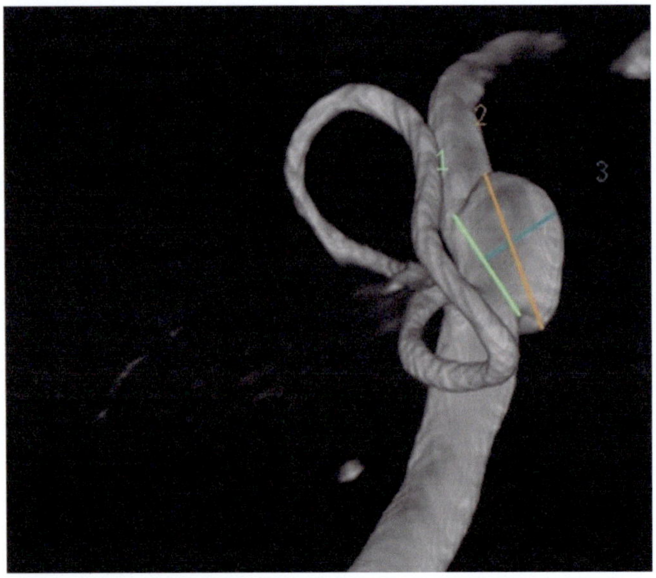

Fig. 34.2 Preoperative digital subtraction angiography

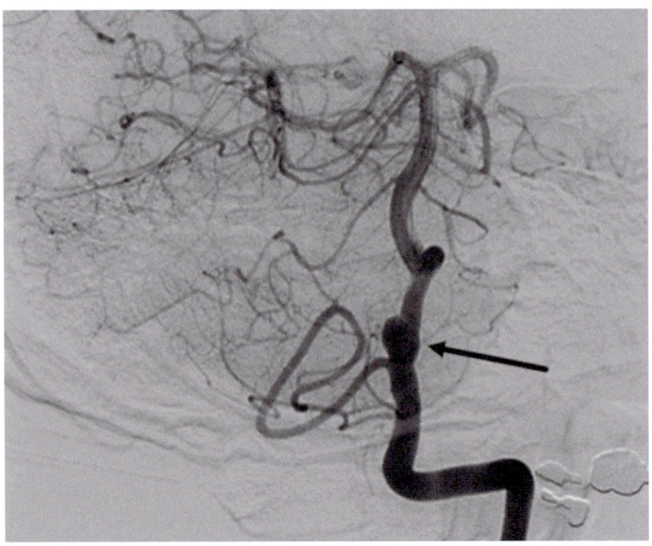

Fig. 34.3 Preoperative digital subtraction angiography

Approach

Lateral transcodylar craniotomy for clipping (Figs. 34.4, 34.5, and 34.6) [1–5].

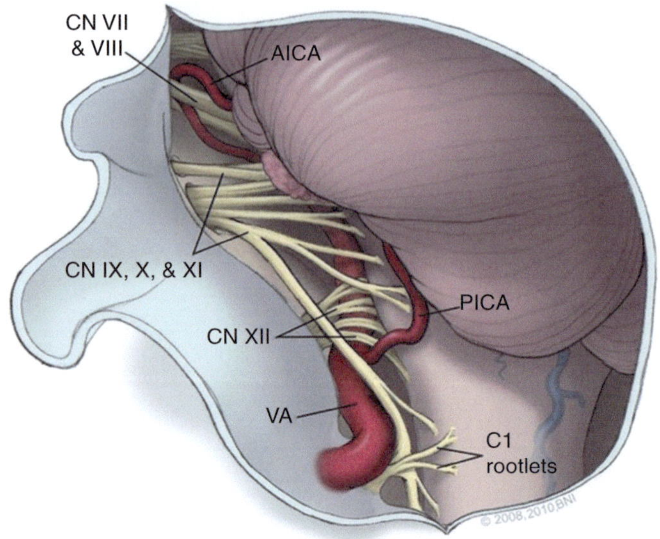

Fig. 34.4 Illustrative diagram demonstrates a left far lateral approach with intradural exposure. Lower cranial nerve origins from the brainstem with their respective relationships to PICA and VA are shown. Used with permission from Barrow Neurological Institute, Phoenix, Arizona

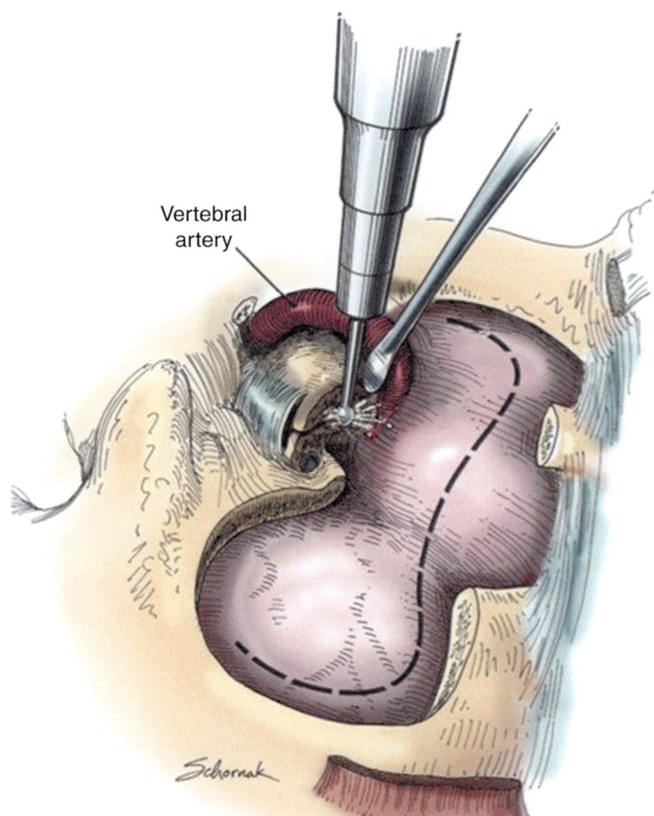

Fig. 34.5 Illustrative diagram demonstrates bony exposure of left far lateral approach. A C1 hemilaminectomy has been performed along with a suboccipital craniotomy and partial removal of the occipital condyle. A C-shaped incision with anterior projections at inferior and superior poles is marked (hashed lines). Used with permission from Barrow Neurological Institute, Phoenix, Arizona

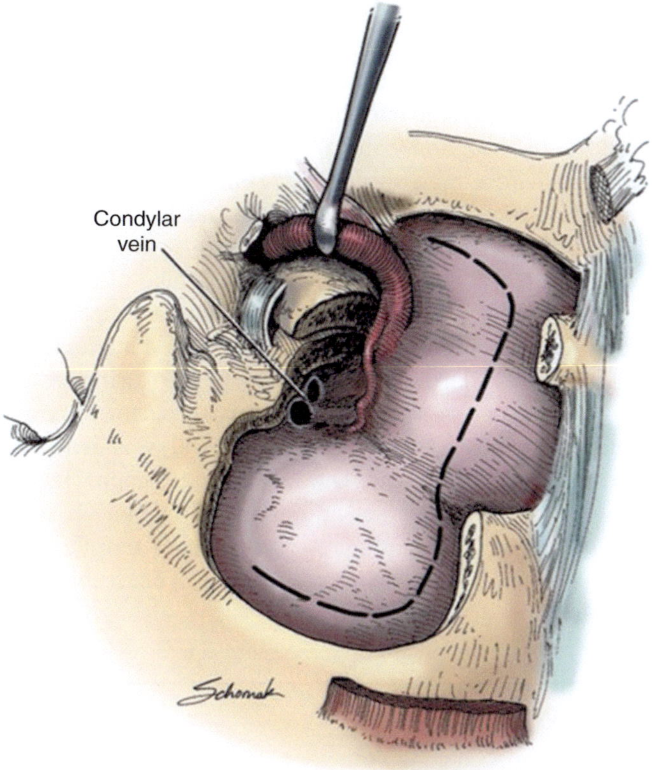

Fig. 34.6 Illustrative diagram demonstrates bony exposure of left far lateral approach. The occipital condyle is reduced until the dural entry of the vertebral artery is visualized. The condylar emissary vein depicted in the figure is often encountered with reduction of the condyle. Early skeletonization followed by cauterization is essential to minimize venous bleeding. Used with permission from Barrow Neurological Institute, Phoenix, Arizona

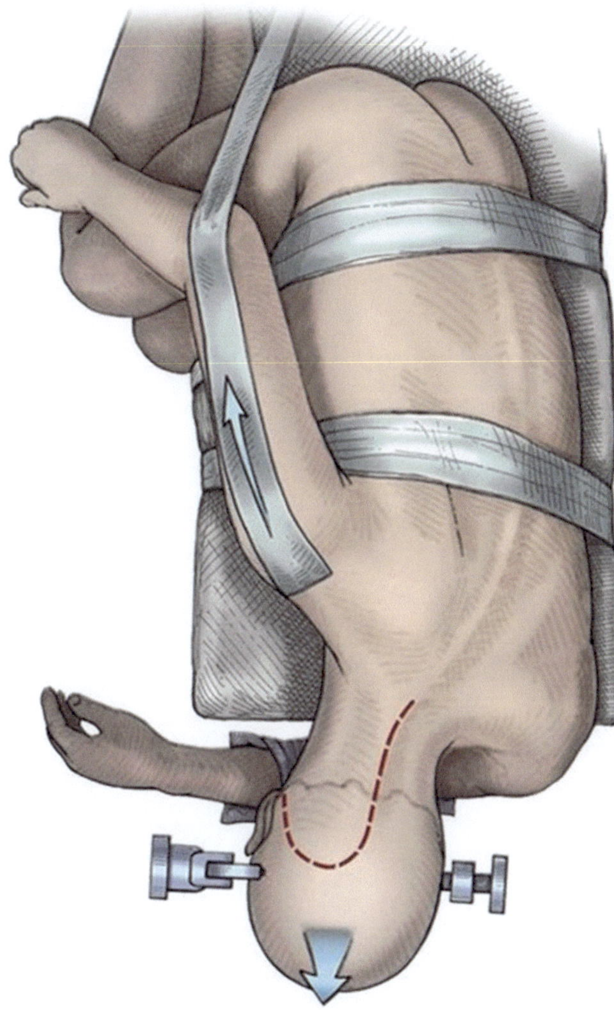

Fig. 34.7 Illustrative diagram demonstrates park-bench positioning. A hockey stick incision is planned (red hashed line) from the midline of the C2 spinous process to the inion, curving to the middle of the mastoid tip. Used with permission from Barrow Neurological Institute, Phoenix, Arizona

Alternatives

Conservative medical management with serial observation is one alternative. Interventional radiology for coiling may also be considered.

Positioning

The patient was placed in the park-bench position (Fig. 34.7).

Incision

The incision started at the external acoustic meatus and descended to the C2 level by passing posterior to the dorsal margin of the sternocleidomastoid muscle (SCM). A hockey-stick incision over the mastoid ascended to the superior nuchal line and descended to the C2 level midline (Figs. 34.8 and 34.9).

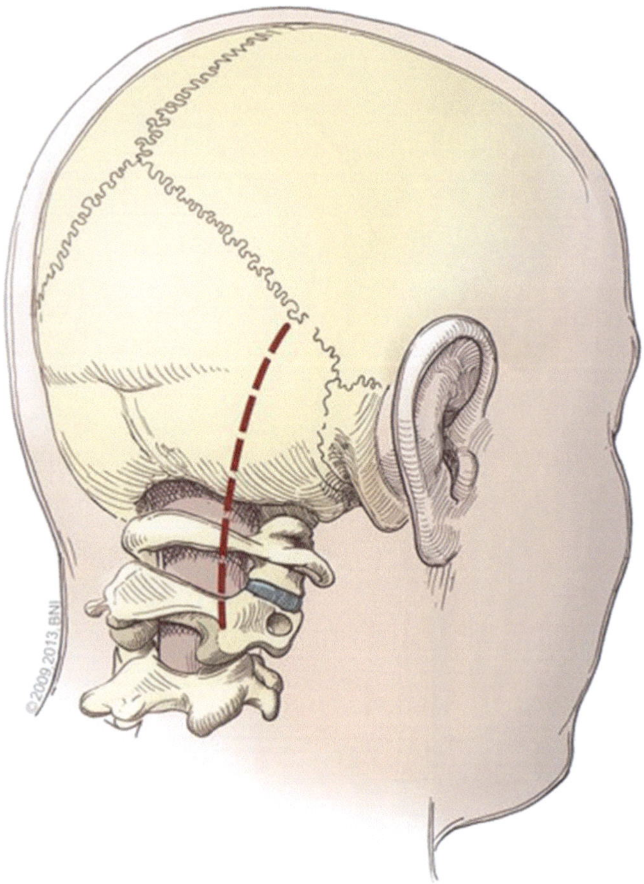

Fig. 34.8 Illustrative diagram demonstrates alternative curvilinear incision (red hashed lines) through lateral aspects of posterior elements of C1 and C2. Used with permission from Barrow Neurological Institute, Phoenix, Arizona

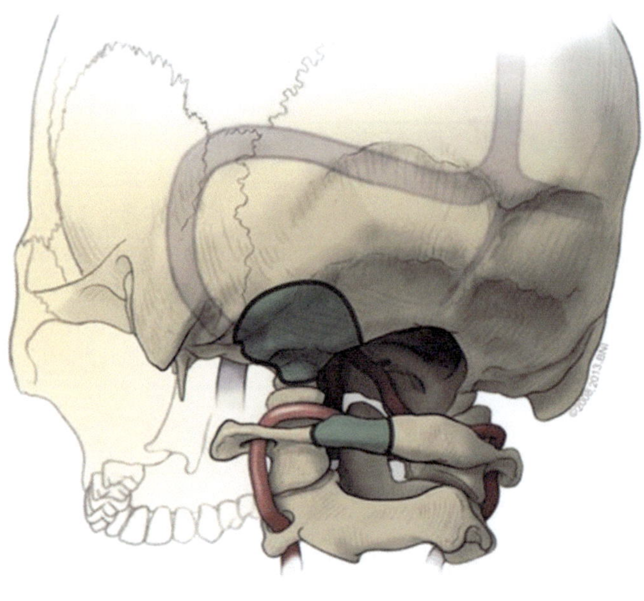

Fig. 34.9 Illustrative diagram demonstrates planned bony removal for adequate exposure for far lateral, transcondylar approach (green circles). Used with permission from Barrow Neurological Institute, Phoenix, Arizona

Operation

We used the left-sided transcondylar posterior cranial fossa approach with a large curvilinear skin incision in the retromastoid region. Bone and the lateral arch of C1 were removed with a high-speed drill. Dura was opened. With microdissection, the vertebral artery and PICA origin on the left side were exposed. The aneurysm was present on the left vertebral artery, distal to the PICA take-off, and was successfully occluded with titanium aneurysm clips. Initial intraoperative indocyanine green (ICG) video angiography and microvascular Doppler confirmed narrowing at the PICA origin; clips were rearranged with patent proximal vertebral and PICA arteries. The wound was irrigated. Hemostasis was excellent. Dura was loosely approximated and covered with a synthetic dural graft. Bone was covered with titanium mesh and screws. Scalp and muscle were reapproximated and closed with sutures. There were no complications (see Video 34.1).

Post-op

The patient was discharged to home with rehab on postoperative day 3, with continuing headaches and occasional left facial numbness (Fig. 34.10).

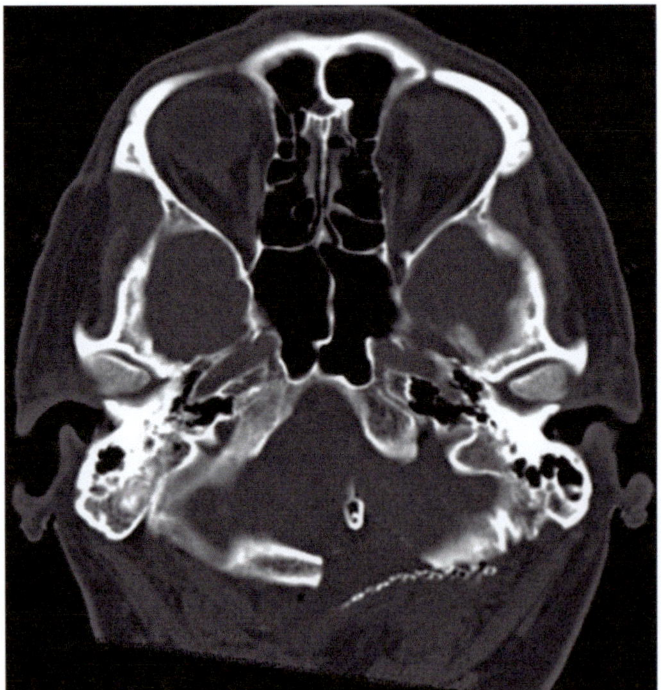

Fig. 34.10 Axial postoperative CT with bone window showing titanium mesh reconstruction of occipital bone along with aneurysm clip

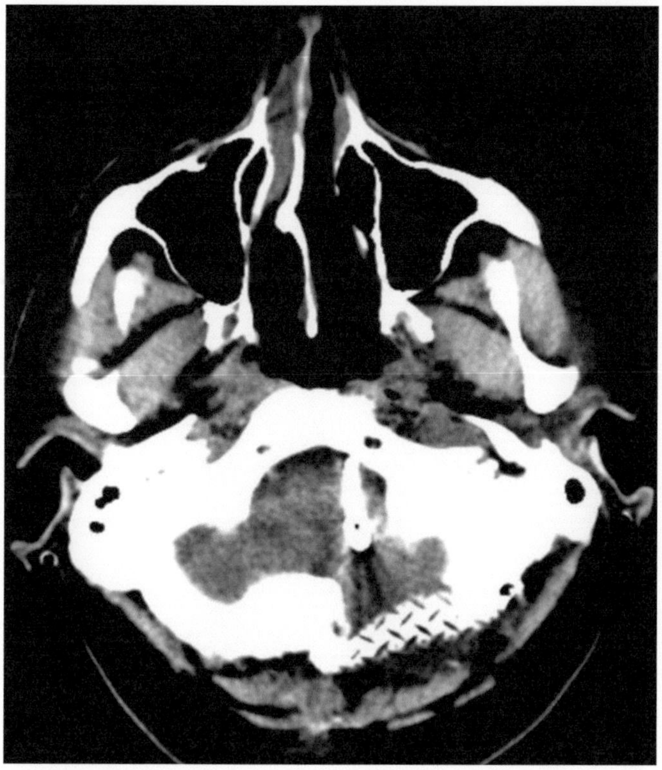

Fig. 34.11 Axial postoperative CT with soft tissue window showing titanium mesh reconstruction of occipital bone along with aneurysm clip

Outcome

The patient presented 5 months later with shooting "nerve" pain on the contralateral posterior scalp. Pain was determined to be present prior to the craniotomy and well controlled with injections. No further complications were reported (Fig. 34.11).

Discussion

Vertebrobasilar junction aneurysms are rare and often uncovered once the aneurysm begins dissecting. Vertebral aneurysms report an institutional incidence of 0.5% with most patients presenting with subarachnoid hemorrhages. Access to vertebrobasilar junction aneurysms is complicated due to the brainstem perforators and lower cranial nerves located in the same region. PICA aneurysms have an incidence of 2.8% with only 21% presenting unruptured.

The far lateral approach is used to approach lesions located ventral or ventrolateral to the brainstem. Compared to the retrosigmoid approach, it permits a better inferior-to-superior view and access anterior to the brainstem. It is particularly useful for access to the following:

- Vertebral artery and PICA, especially PICA aneurysms
- Upper cervical cord and medulla, especially anterolaterally
- Foramen magnum
- Caudal segment of the clivus
- Jugular foramen

Video used with permission from the Congress of Neurological Surgeons, CNS Nexus Cases. 2018. https://www.cns.org/nexus/cases

References

1. Balik V, Yamada Y, Talari S, Yamashiro K, Rile W, Suyama D, Kawase T, Takagi K, Takizawa K, Kato Y. Surgical treatment of unruptured dissecting intracranial aneurysms of vertebral-posterior inferior cerebellar artery region and review of the literature. J Neurosurg Sci. 2017;61(6):640–51.
2. Peluso JP, van Rooij WJ, Sluzewski M, Beute GN. Aneurysms of the vertebrobasilar junction: incidence, clinical presentation, and outcome of endovascular treatment. Am J Neurorad. 2007;28:1747–51.
3. Peluso JP, van Rooij WJ, Sluzewski M, Beute GN, Marjoie CB. Posterior inferior cerebellar artery aneurysms: incidence, clinical presentation, and outcome of endovascular treatment. Am J Neurorad. 2008;29:86–90.
4. Rhoton AL. Anatomy and surgical approaches of the temporal bone and adjacent areas. Neurosurgery. 2007;61(4):S4–1.
5. Bambakidis NC, Nakaji P, Amin-Hanjani S, Spetzler RF. Cerebrovascular surgery: an interactive video atlas. Shelton, CT: PMPH-USA; 2015.

Case 14: Left Retrosigmoid Approach in Large Vestibular Schwannoma in Patient with NF2

35

Marte van Keulen, Jeffrey T. Nelson, Sarah Mowry, and Nicholas C. Bambakidis

Summary

This case demonstrates the resection of a large left-sided vestibular schwannoma in a 25-year-old patient with a history of neurofibromatosis type 2 (NF2).

Case Presentation

A 25-year-old man with a history of NF2 presented with 2 months of progressive vision loss. The patient also reported 1 year of hearing loss in his left ear. A neurologic exam revealed the following:

- OD detects shapes/motion only, OS 20/200
- L PPRF/CN VI nuclear palsy
- L House-Brackmann 4
- Bilateral papilledema

MRI showed a large left-sided vestibular schwannoma (Fig. 35.1).

About 1.5 months prior to tumor resection, a ventriculoperitoneal (VP) shunt was placed for obstruction hydrocephalus. Despite slit ventricles on a CT scan and shunt tap 12 mmHg, OS visual acuity worsened. The patient underwent left optic fenestration 6 days prior to tumor resection because of the progressive nature of his vision problems and objectified papilledema.

A right-sided small vestibular schwannoma was visible (Fig. 35.2).

Supplementary Information The online version contains supplementary material available at [https://doi.org/10.1007/978-3-031-12507-2_35].

M. van Keulen · J. T. Nelson
Case Western Reserve University School of Medicine, University Hospitals Cleveland Medical Center, Cleveland, OH, USA

S. Mowry
Division of Otology/Neurotology, Department of Otolaryngology—Head and Neck Surgery, University Hospitals Cleveland Medical Center, Case Western Reserve University, Cleveland, OH, USA

N. C. Bambakidis (✉)
Neurological Surgery, The Neurological Institute, University Hospitals of Cleveland, Case Western Reserve University School of Medicine, Cleveland, OH, USA
e-mail: Nicholas.Bambakidis2@UHhospitals.org

N. C. Bambakidis et al. (eds.), *Surgery of the Cerebellopontine Angle*, https://doi.org/10.1007/978-3-031-12507-2_35

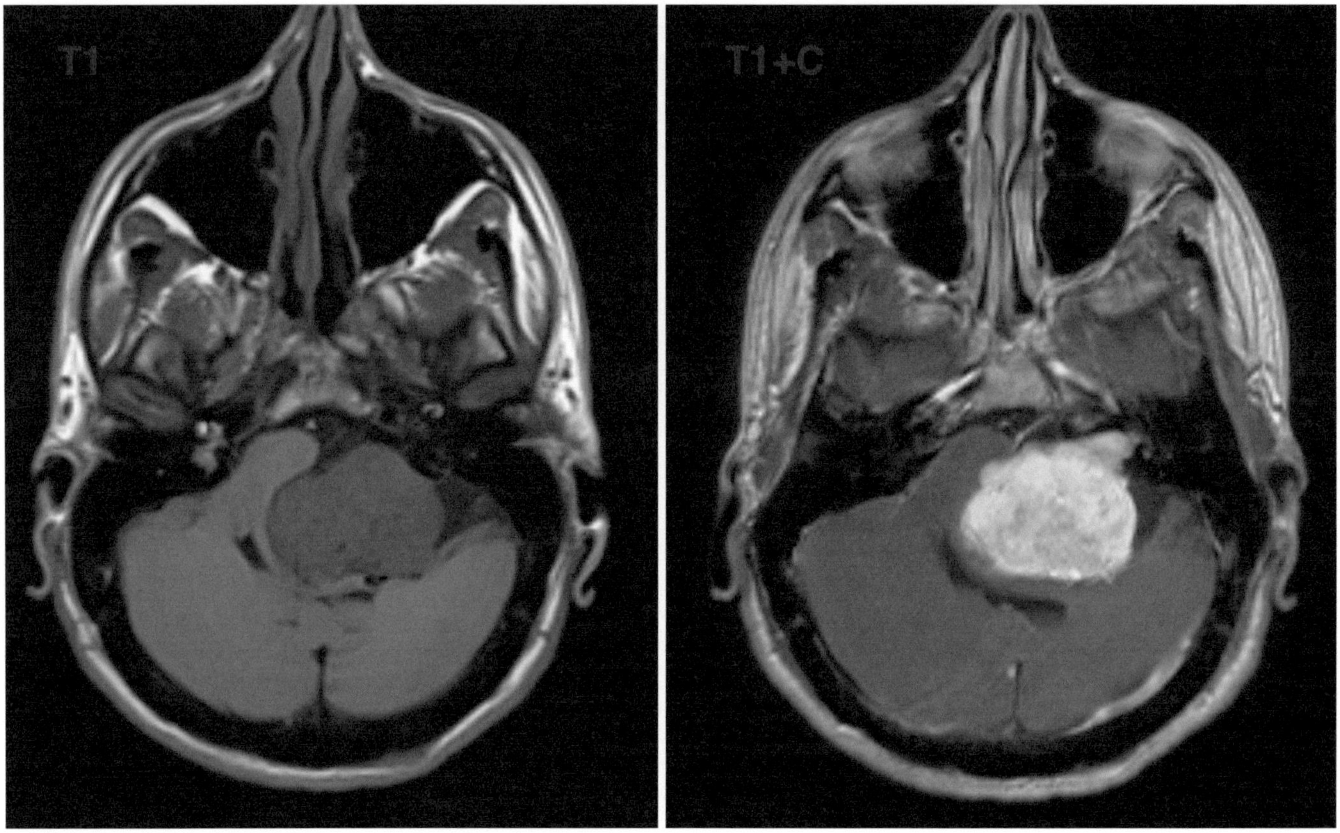

Fig. 35.1 Preoperative MRI, axial

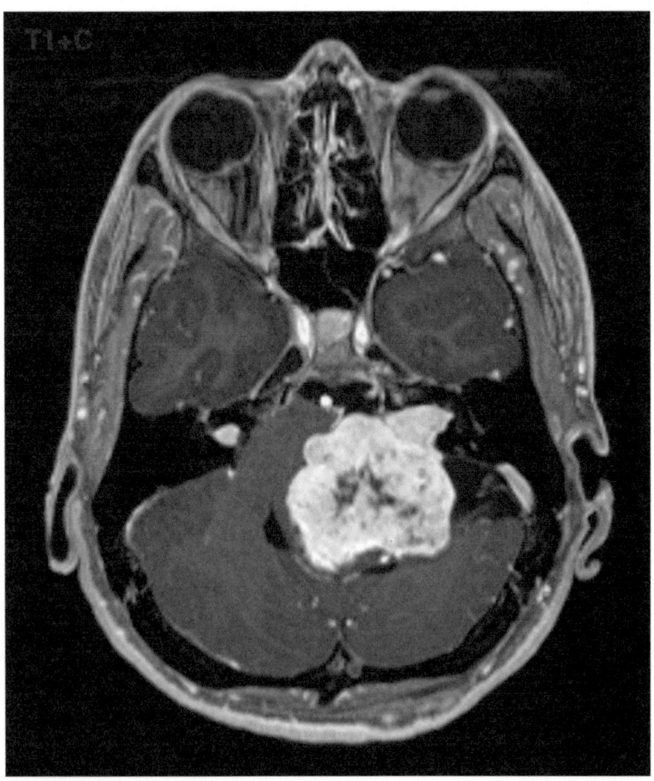

Fig. 35.2 Preoperative MRI, axial

Approach

A left retrosigmoid approach was chosen, in collaboration with otolaryngology surgery.

Alternatives

Nonoperative strategies were not a viable option due to the size of the tumor, pressure on the brainstem, and hydrocephalus. However, a translabyrinthine approach and an extended translabyrinthine approach were options. These were considered, but the surgical team opted for a retrosigmoid approach due to the size of the tumor and to restrict the length of surgery.

Positioning

The patient was positioned supine, with his head turned to the right, his left shoulder elevated, and the bed in a slight reverse Trendelenburg position (Fig. 35.3).

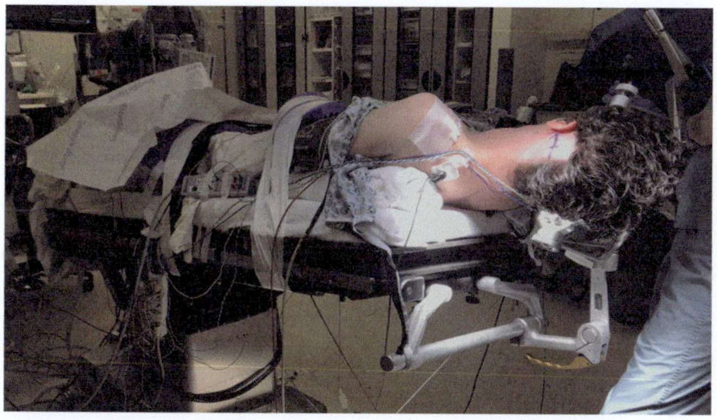

Fig. 35.3 Positioning

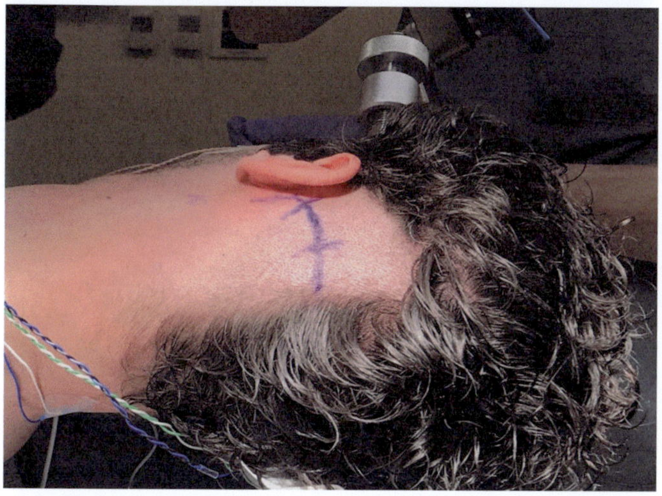

Fig. 35.4 Incision

Incision

A left-sided retromastoid postauricular skin incision was made to expose the mastoid process and the posterior fossa bone (Fig. 35.4).

Operation

The operation began with a craniotomy over the cerebellar hemisphere as well as skeletonization of the transverse sigmoid sinus and a partial mastoidectomy. Air cells were carefully waxed. Dura was opened widely. Additional intradural drilling of the internal auditory canal was performed by a neuro-otolaryngology surgeon. A gigantic acoustic tumor was encountered with significant vascularity around the circumference of the lesion, necessitating microdissection and stereotactic navigation to allow for removal of the very large vascular mass severely compressing the brainstem. Hemostasis was achieved, with closure. Dura was loosely approximated and covered with a synthetic dural graft. The bony defect was covered with titanium mesh, and the wound was closed in multiple layers using sutures (see Video 35.1).

Post-op

The patient was discharged to physical rehab on postoperative day 7 and readmitted with the complication of a VP shunt infection requiring externalization and eventual replacement (Fig. 35.5).

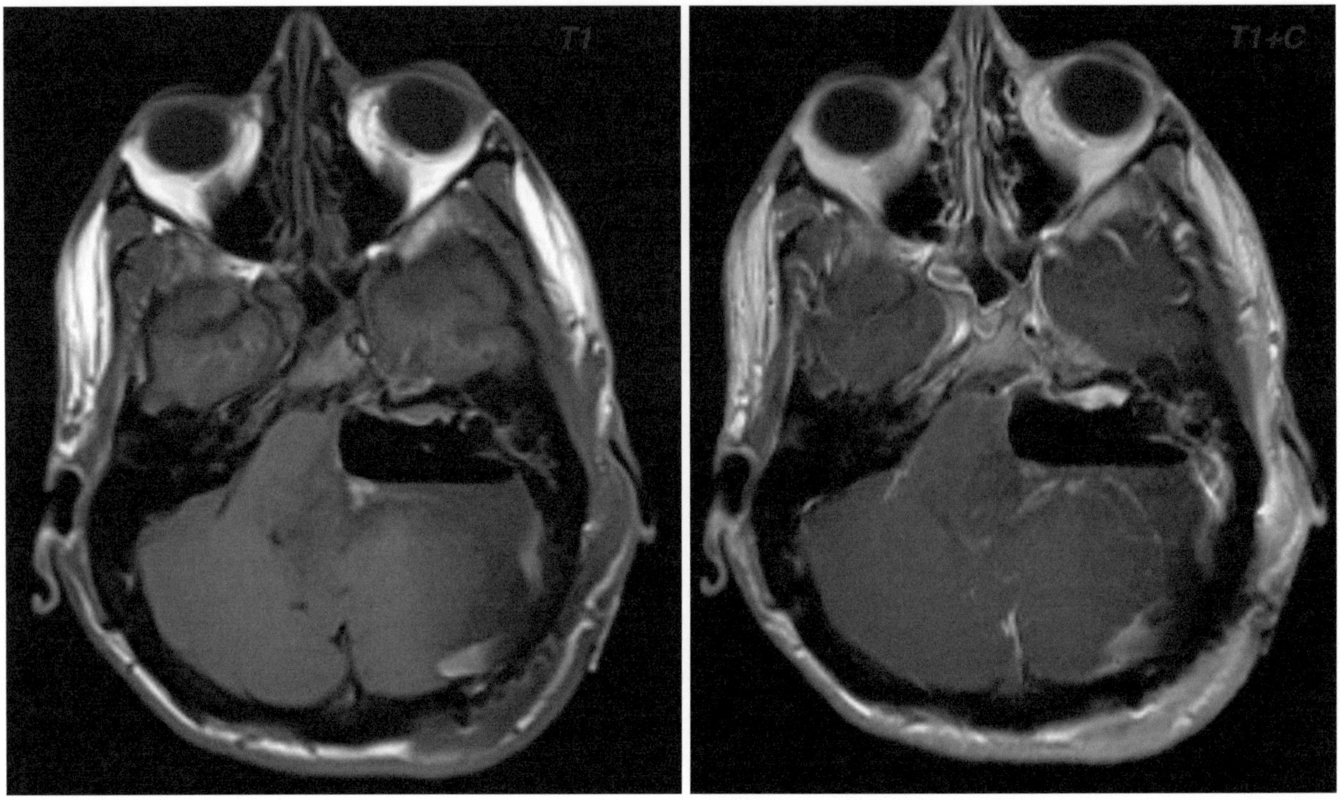

Fig. 35.5 Postoperative MRI

Outcome

Prior to surgery, the patient had bilateral vision loss (CN II) and peripheral facial palsy (CN VII) as well as hearing loss (CN VIII) and abducens palsy (CN VI) on his left side. These symptoms remained.

Discussion

This particular case shows a patient with an exceptionally large vestibular schwannoma, with numerous subsequent problems including hydrocephalus, progressive visual problems, and brainstem compression.

Pearls and Pitfalls

- No adequate stimulation of the facial nerve was identified during the procedure, which correlated with the patient's severe preoperative facial nerve palsy.
- The retrosigmoid approach provided an adequate and relatively rapid view of a tumor of this size in the cerebellopontine angle.

36 Case 15: Retrosigmoid Approach for a Left-Sided Trigeminal Schwannoma

Marte van Keulen, Jeffrey T. Nelson, and Nicholas C. Bambakidis

Summary

This case illustrates the resection of a trigeminal schwannoma in a patient presenting with trigeminal and brainstem compression symptoms.

Case Presentation

An 82-year-old male was active and healthy about 6 months ago (Figs. 36.1, 36.2, and 36.3). The patient presented with progressive left facial numbness and pain as well as double vision. He had experienced falls for the past 6 months as well as difficulty with gait and with eating; he failed a swallowing test. He was on a soft diet but had recently lost 10 pounds.

Supplementary Information The online version contains supplementary material available at [https://doi.org/10.1007/978-3-031-12507-2_36].

M. van Keulen · J. T. Nelson
Case Western Reserve University School of Medicine, University Hospitals Cleveland Medical Center, Cleveland, OH, USA

N. C. Bambakidis (✉)
Neurological Surgery, The Neurological Institute, University Hospitals of Cleveland, Case Western Reserve University School of Medicine, Cleveland, OH, USA
e-mail: Nicholas.Bambakidis2@UHhospitals.org

N. C. Bambakidis et al. (eds.), *Surgery of the Cerebellopontine Angle*, https://doi.org/10.1007/978-3-031-12507-2_36

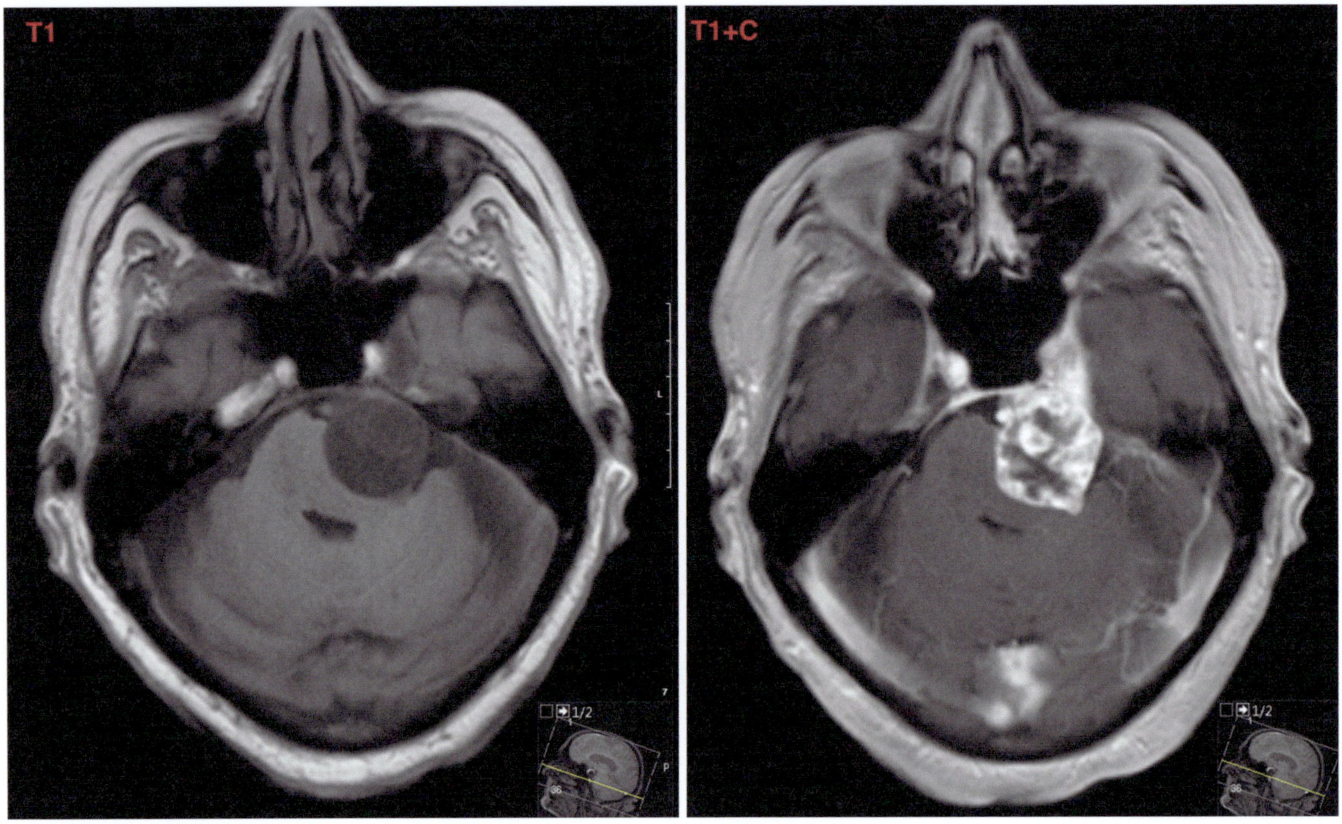

Fig. 36.1 Preoperative MRI, axial

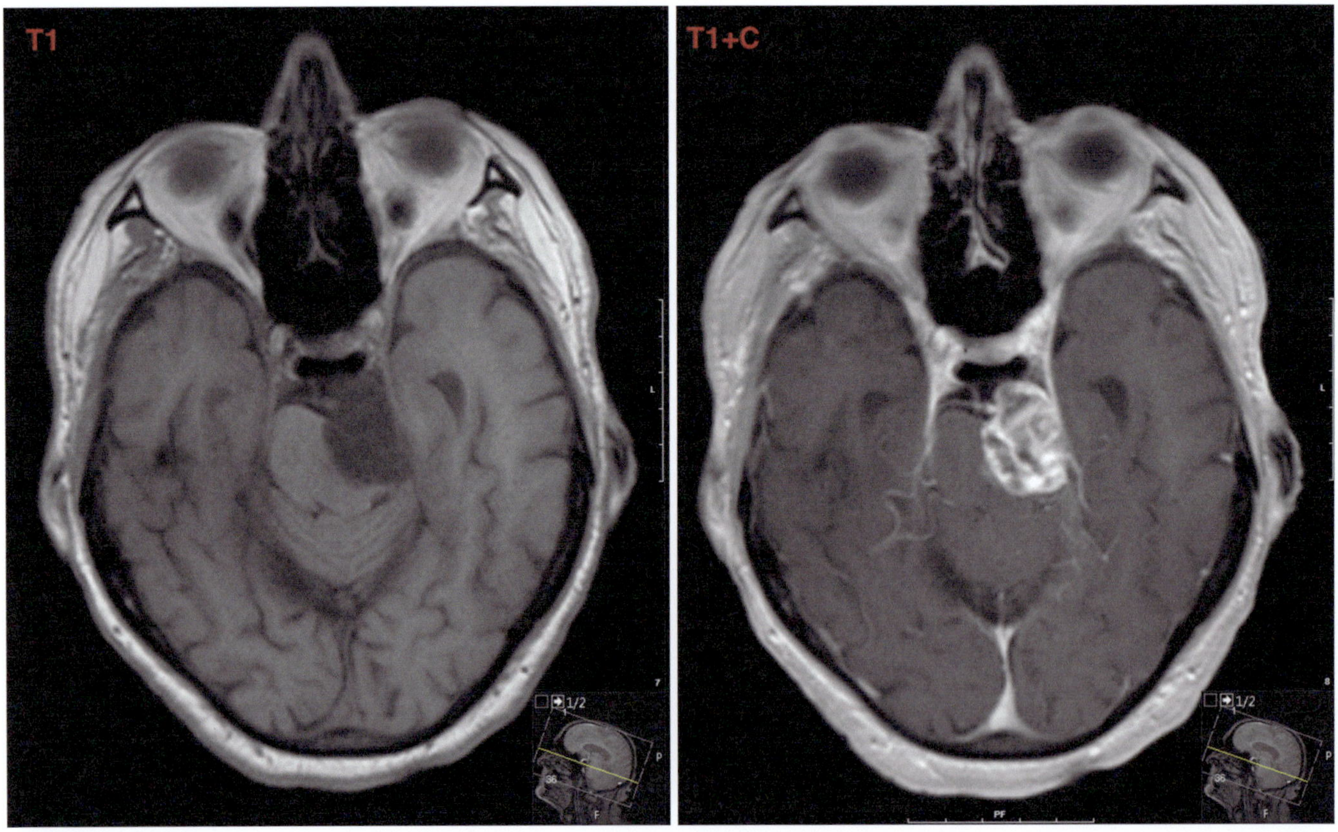

Fig. 36.2 Preoperative MRI, axial

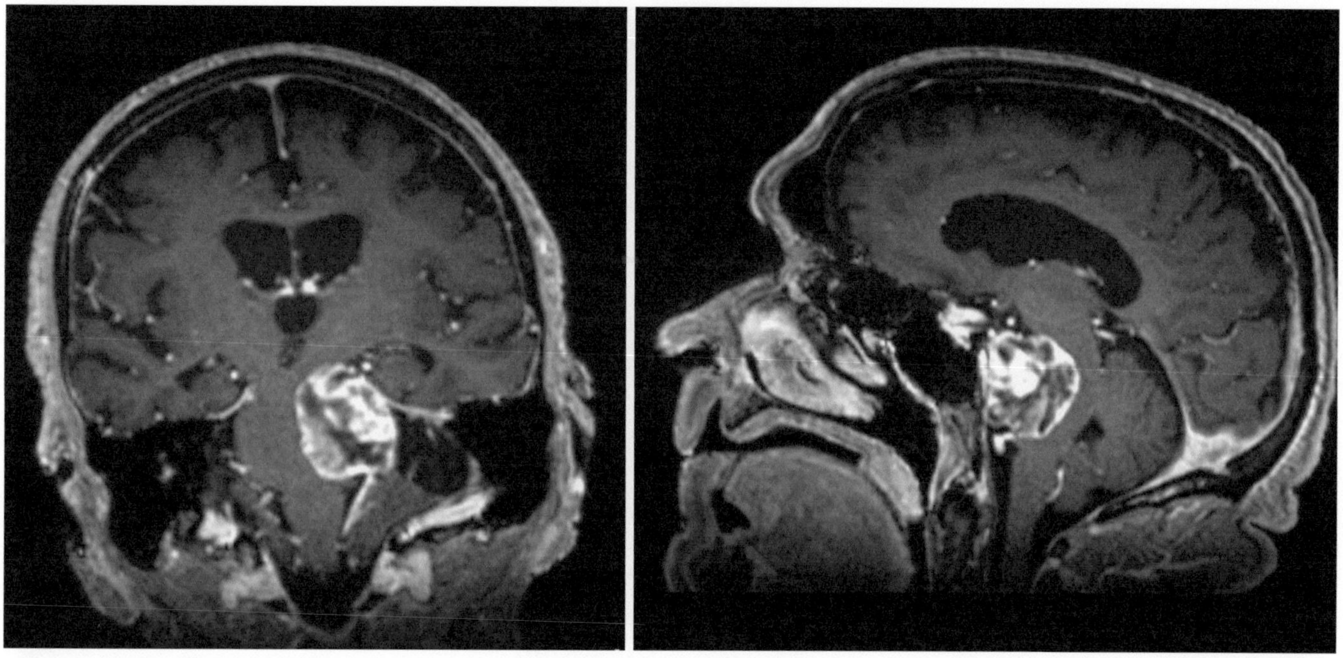

Fig. 36.3 Preoperative MRI, coronal and sagittal

Neurologic Exam

The patient was awake and alert and in a wheelchair, with fluent speech. The following was noted:

- Cranial nerves: L absent corneal reflex; L facial numbness; extraocular movement (EOM) full, tongue midline and face symmetric.
- Motor: extremity strength normal.
- Sensation: intact.
- Walking: gait limited due to imbalance and risk of falls.

MRI showed a left-sided 3-cm trigeminal schwannoma with extension into the cavernous sinus, Meckel's cave, and foramen ovale. It compressed the left middle cerebellar peduncle, anterior left cerebellum, and left aspect of the pons.

Approach

A retrosigmoid approach was planned.

Alternatives

Conservative measures were not an option due to the size and compression and subsequent symptoms. Surgical alternatives included a middle fossa approach, though it would not have provided the optimal view of the posterior components. The retrosigmoid approach achieved sufficient tumor view in this case and, therefore, was preferable over a translabyrinthine approach as well because it would not require hearing to be sacrificed.

Positioning

The patient was positioned supine, with head turned to the right (Figs. 36.4, and 36.5).

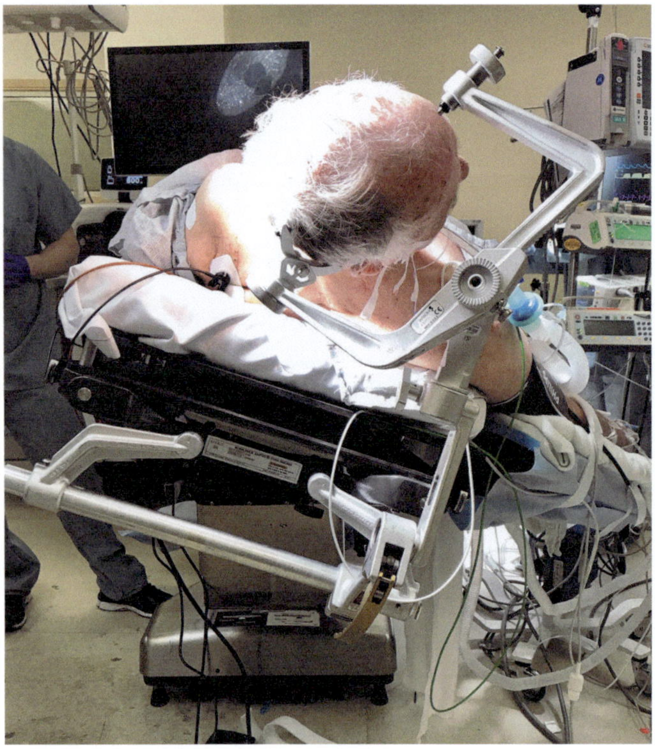

Fig. 36.4 Positioning

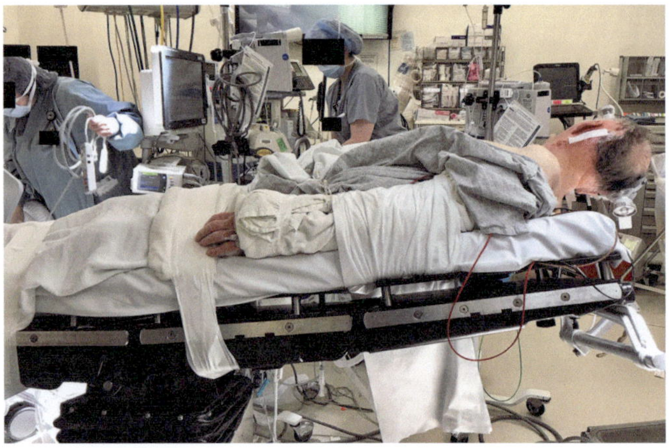

Fig. 36.5 Positioning

Incision

A retromastoid skin incision was made exposing posterior fossa bone (Fig. 36.6).

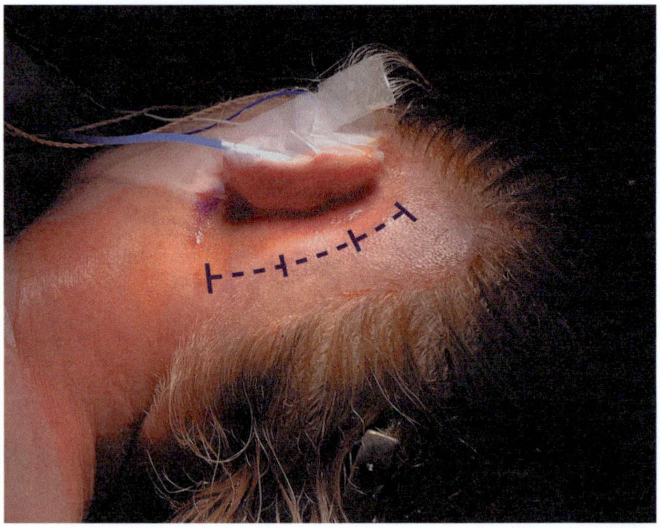

Fig. 36.6 Incision

Operation

Stereotaxis was used. The procedure was carried out under monitoring of the facial nerve, which was identified and preserved throughout this operation. Posterior fossa bone was removed with a high-speed drill. Dura was opened, widely allowing access to the cerebellopontine angle on the left side. Using microdissection stereotactic navigation, a trigeminal nerve schwannoma was encountered and internal resection and decompression of the tumor was accomplished with gross total resection of the intracranial components of the tumor portion of the tumor extending into Meckel's cave. The wound was copiously irrigated, and hemostasis was excellent. Dura was loosely approximated and covered with synthetic dural graft. The bone defect was covered with titanium mesh and closed in multiple layers using sutures (see Video 36.1).

Post-op

The following was noted postoperatively:

- House Brackmann (HB) 2, which had spontaneously resolved by his visit 6 weeks postoperatively (Figs. 36.7, and 36.8).
- L face numbness, bilateral upper extremity (UE) dysmetria.
- Discharge on postoperative day 3 (POD 3).

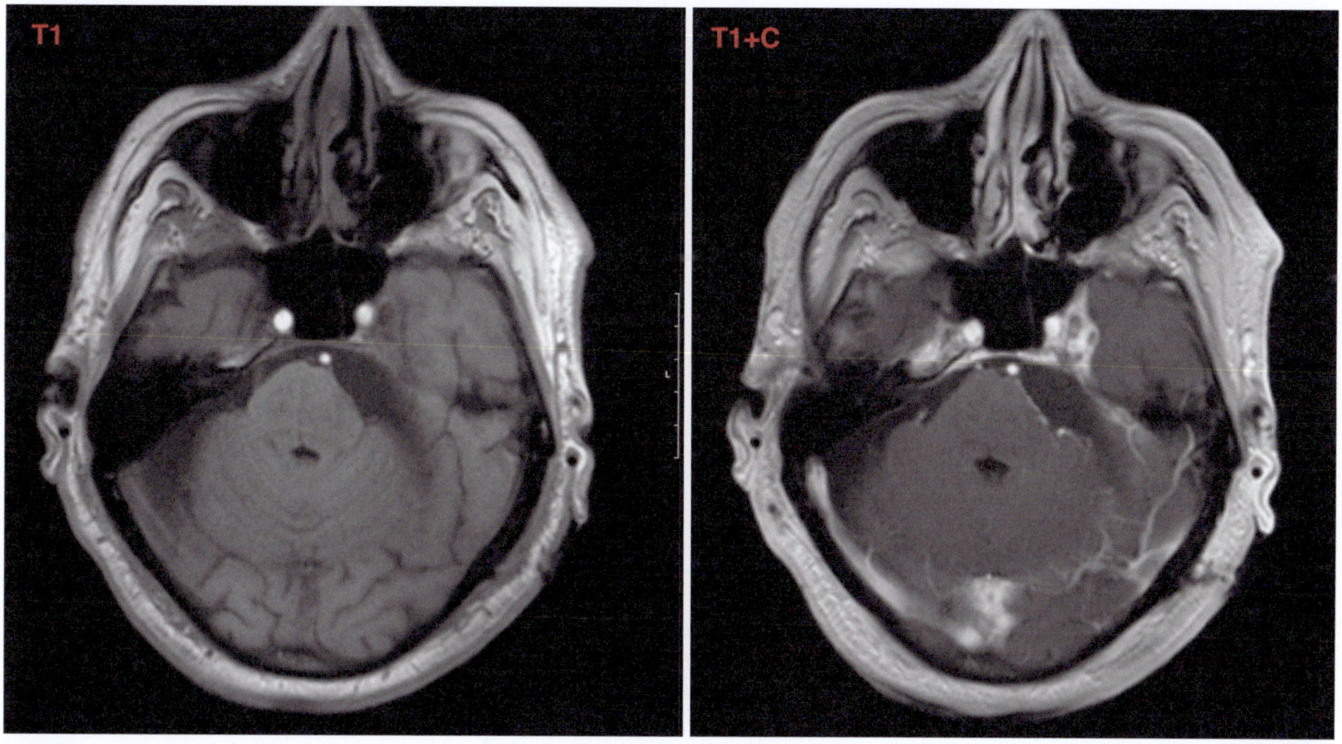

Fig. 36.7 Postoperative MRI, axial

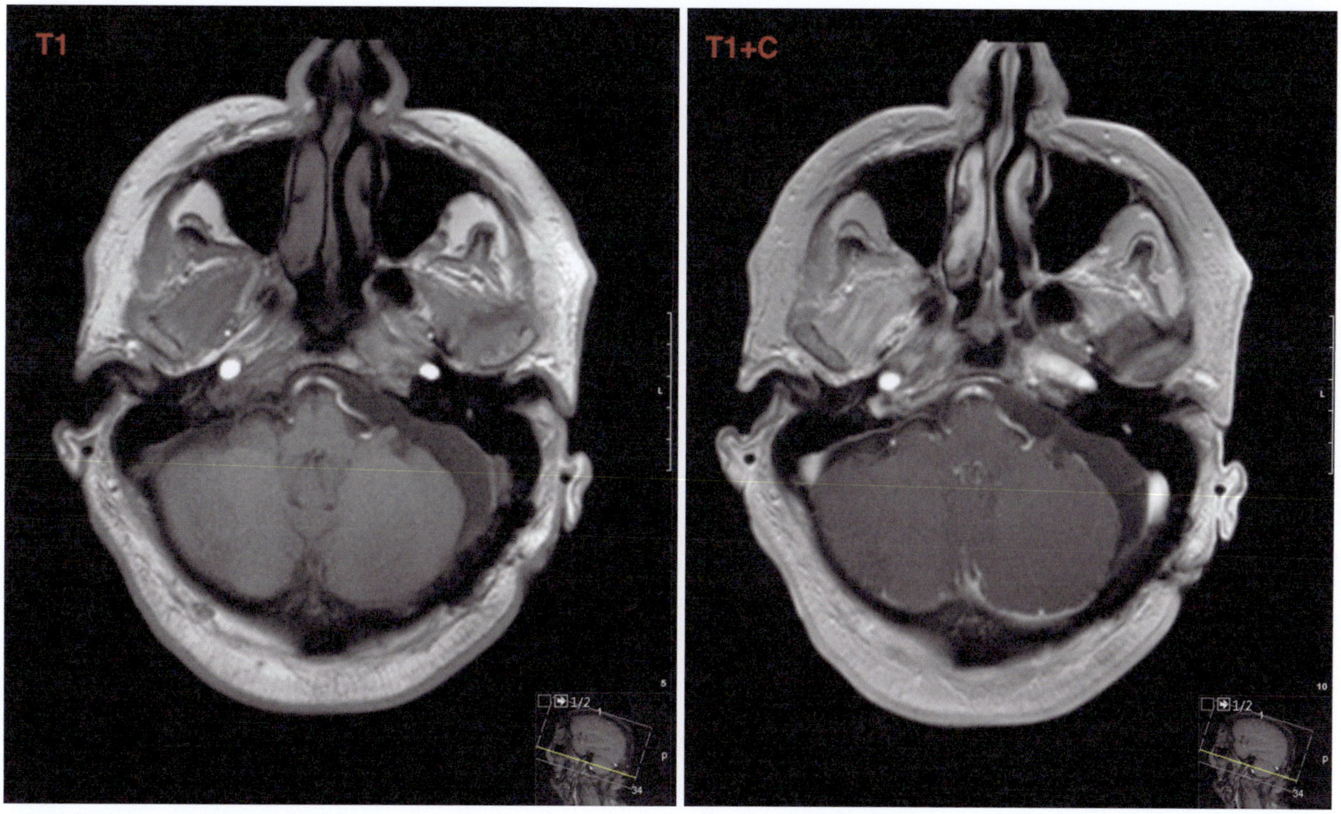

Fig. 36.8 Postoperative MRI, axial

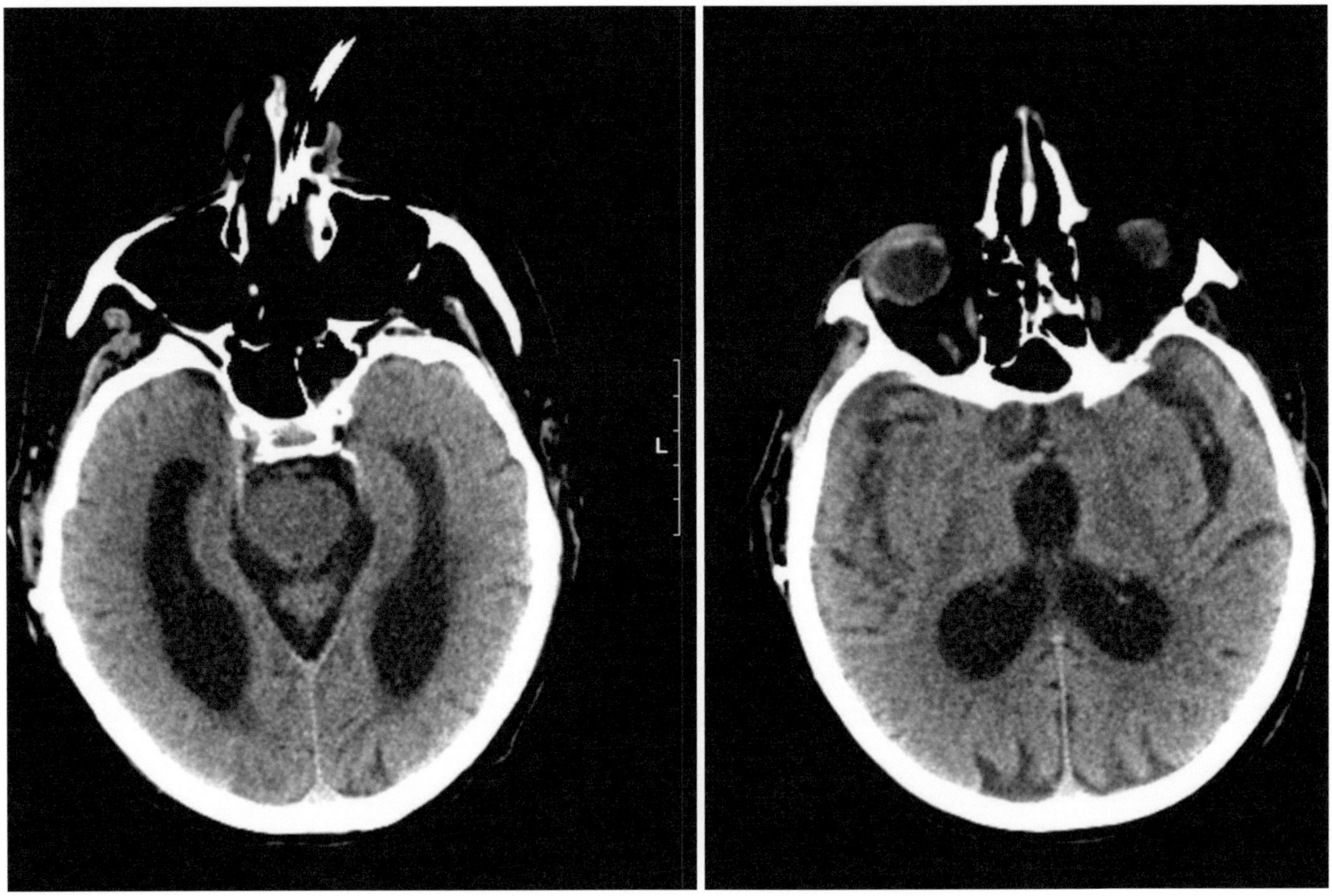

Fig. 36.9 Postoperative CT, axial

Outcome

The patient initially did well but presented 6 weeks postoperatively with gait difficulty and confusion. Imaging demonstrated hydrocephalus and pseudomeningocele, which were treated with a ventriculoperitoneal (VP) shunt, followed by a subsequent resolution of symptoms (Fig. 36.9).

Pearls and Pitfalls

- Facial and auditory nerve monitoring and early identification are vital in the attempt to preserve both nerves as dissection occurs deep to their anatomic location.
- The superior cerebellar artery is located immediately superior to the tumor location, and care must be taken to avoid vascular injury.

Case 16: Retrosigmoid Approach to Right-Sided Epidermoid Cyst

37

Marte van Keulen and Nicholas C. Bambakidis

Summary

This case illustrates the resection on a right-sided epidermoid cyst in a 55-year-old male, presenting with unilateral hearing loss and tinnitus.

Case Presentation

A 55-year-old male presented with progressive right-sided partial hearing loss and tinnitus for 1 to 2 years. Neurologic exam revealed objectifiable right partial hearing loss (otherwise intact), and MRI revealed a lesion in the right cerebellopontine angle (CPA) (30 × 23 mm), which was thought to be an epidermoid cyst (Figs. 37.1, and 37.2).

Supplementary Information The online version contains supplementary material available at [https://doi.org/10.1007/978-3-031-12507-2_37].

M. van Keulen
Case Western Reserve University School of Medicine, University Hospitals Cleveland Medical Center, Cleveland, OH, USA

N. C. Bambakidis (✉)
Neurological Surgery, The Neurological Institute, University Hospitals of Cleveland, Case Western Reserve University School of Medicine, Cleveland, OH, USA
e-mail: Nicholas.Bambakidis2@UHhospitals.org

N. C. Bambakidis et al. (eds.), *Surgery of the Cerebellopontine Angle*, https://doi.org/10.1007/978-3-031-12507-2_37

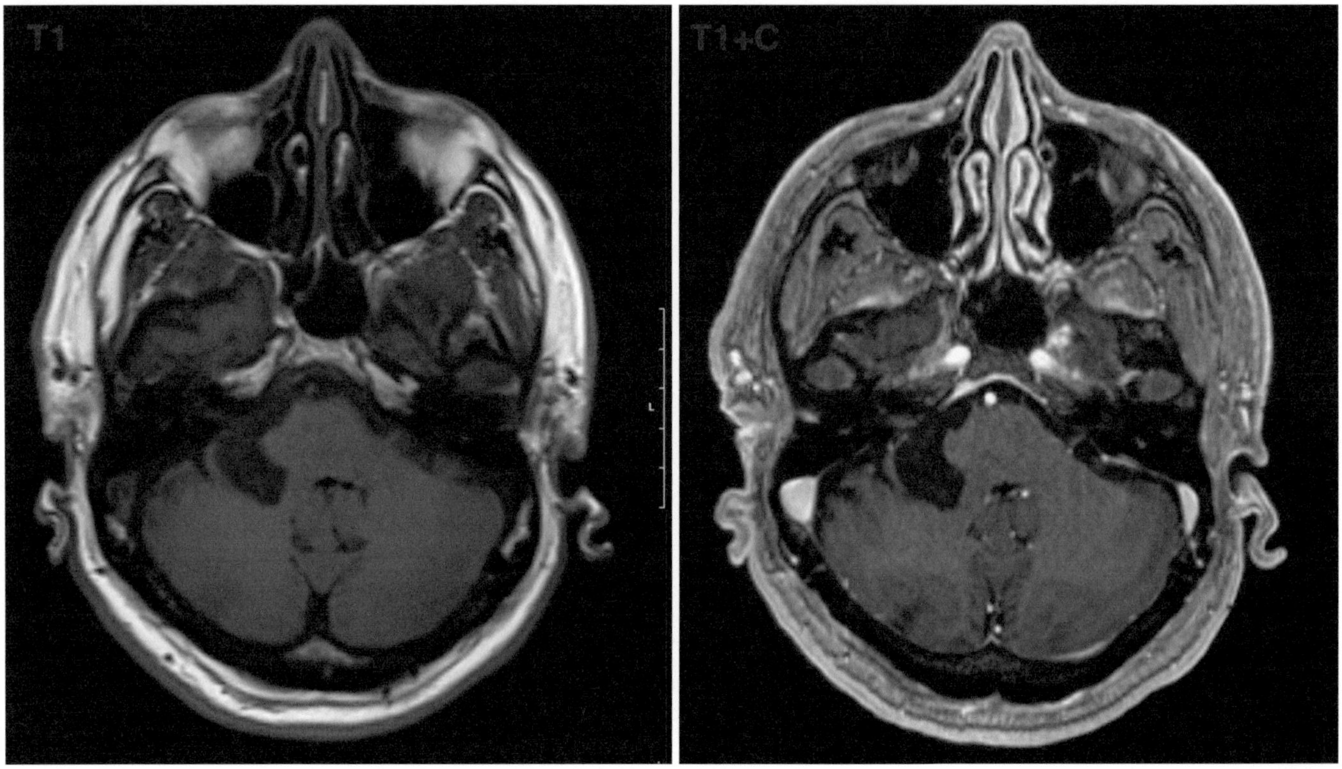

Fig. 37.1 Preoperative MRI, axial

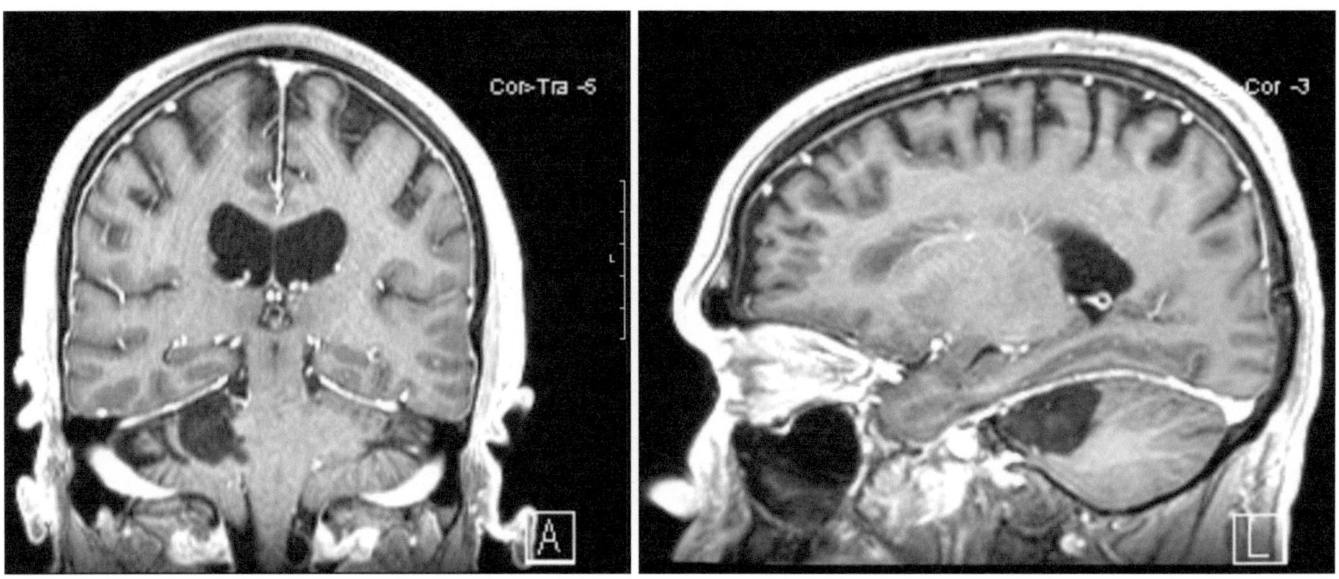

Fig. 37.2 Preoperative MRI, coronal and sagittal

Approach

A right-sided retrosigmoid approach allows for hearing preservation and resection of lesions with significant extension into the CPA. It does require cerebellar retraction and offers limited access to the fundus of the internal auditory canal (IAC).

Alternatives

A middle fossa approach was not chosen because this tumor did not enter the IAC and had a large posterior fossa component; therefore, this approach did not generate an optimal view to this tumor. A translabyrinthine approach was not chosen in attempt to preserve the patient's residual hearing.

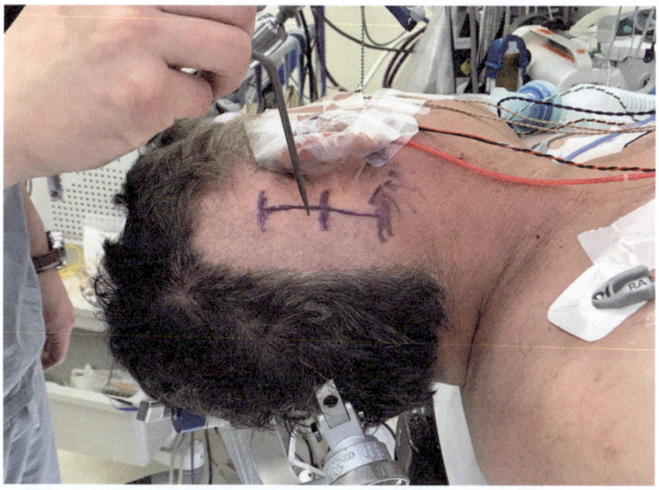

Fig. 37.3 Positioning and incision

Positioning

The patient was positioned supine, with his head turned to the left (Fig. 37.3).

Incision

A right-sided incision was made behind the ear, in the retrosigmoid region.

Operation

Stereotactic navigation was utilized (Fig. 37.4). Before the procedure, a lumbar drain catheter was placed to allow intermittent drainage throughout the procedure. A retromastoid

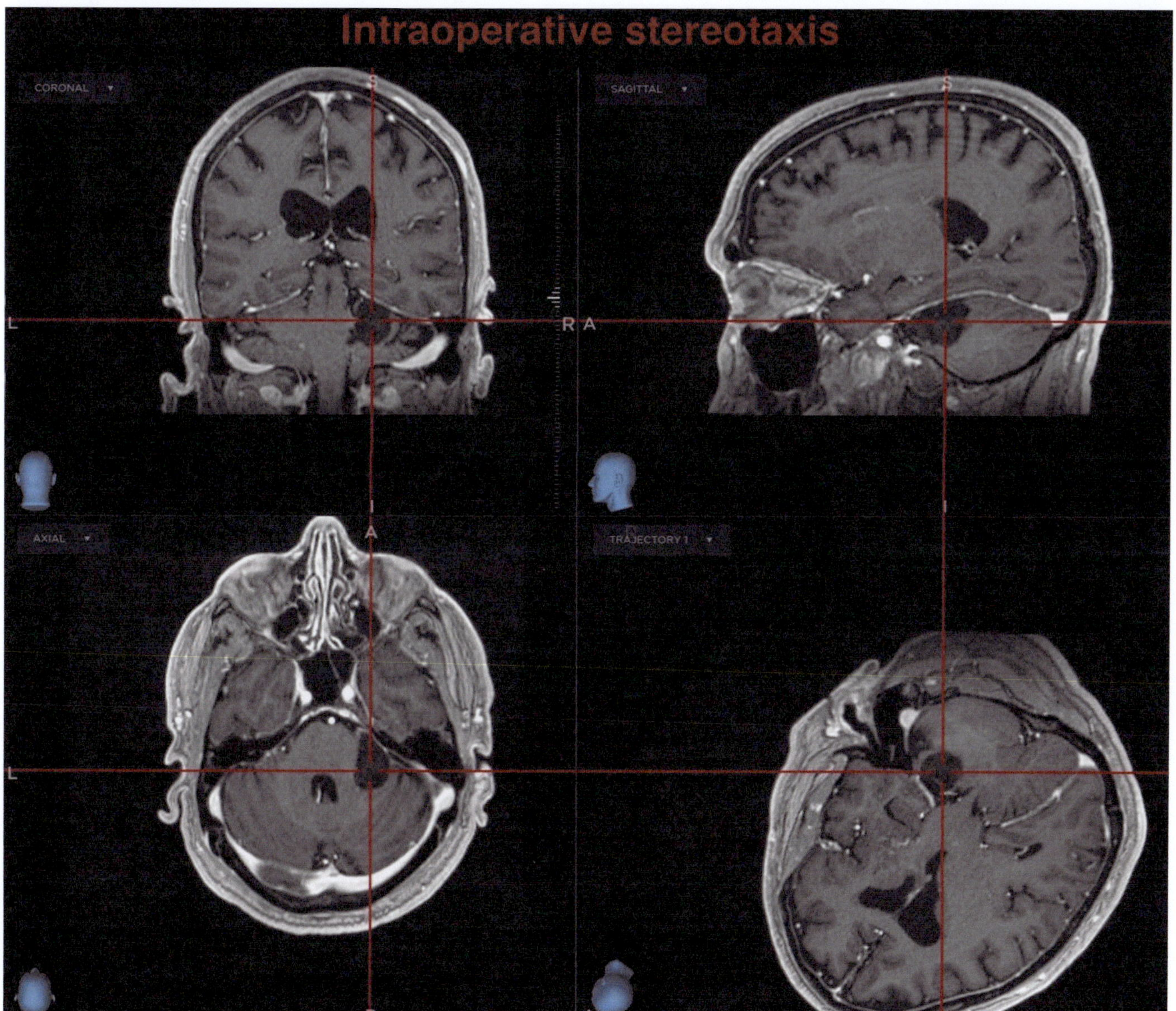

Fig. 37.4 Intraoperative stereotaxis

craniotomy was performed. Posterior fossa dura was opened widely. An epidermoid cyst neoplasm in the CPA was internally debulked, with careful preservation of the cranial nerve 7/8 complex as well as the other cranial nerves and brainstem. Gross total resection was achieved. The wound was copiously irrigated. Hemostasis was maintained. Dura was loosely approximated and covered with a synthetic dural graft. The bony defect was covered with titanium mesh (see Video 37.1).

Post-op

The patient's neurologic exam was the same as it was preoperatively (Figs. 37.5, and 37.6). He was discharged on postoperative day 3.

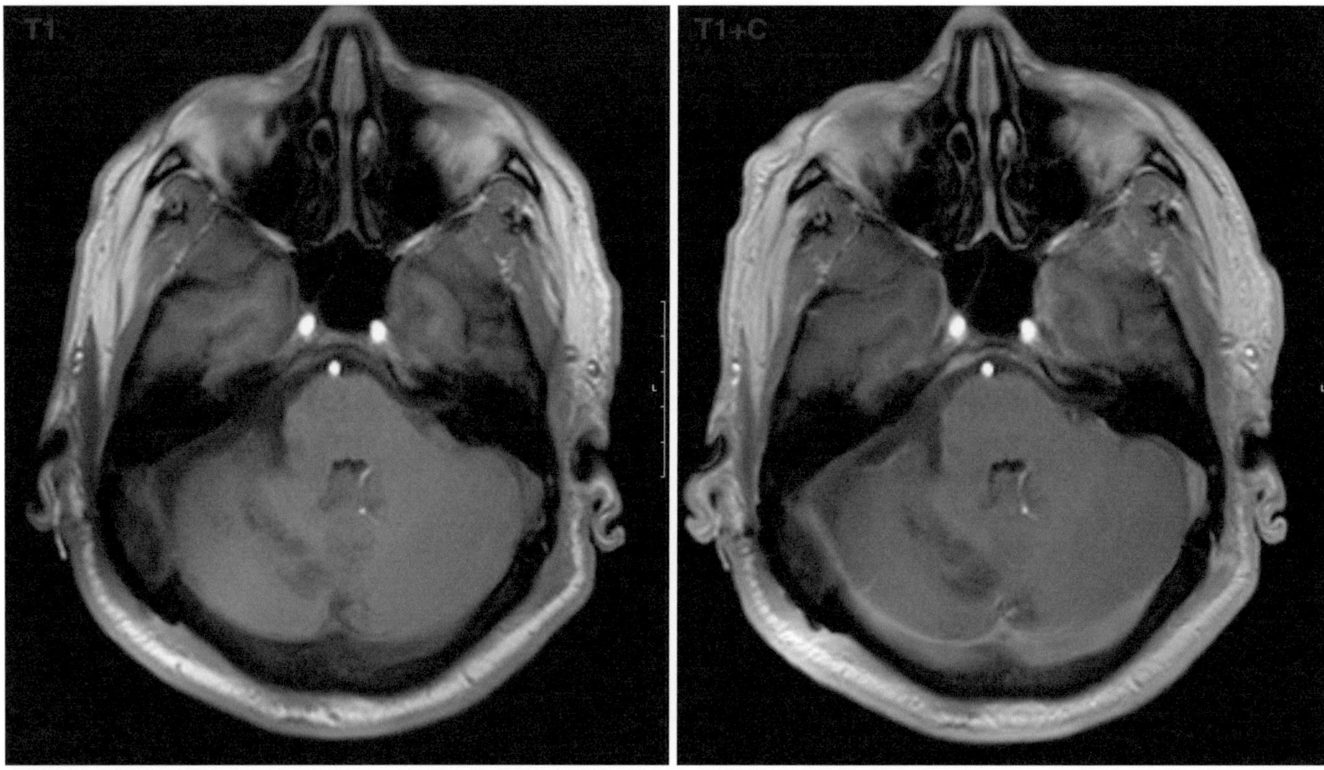

Fig. 37.5 Postoperative MRI, axial

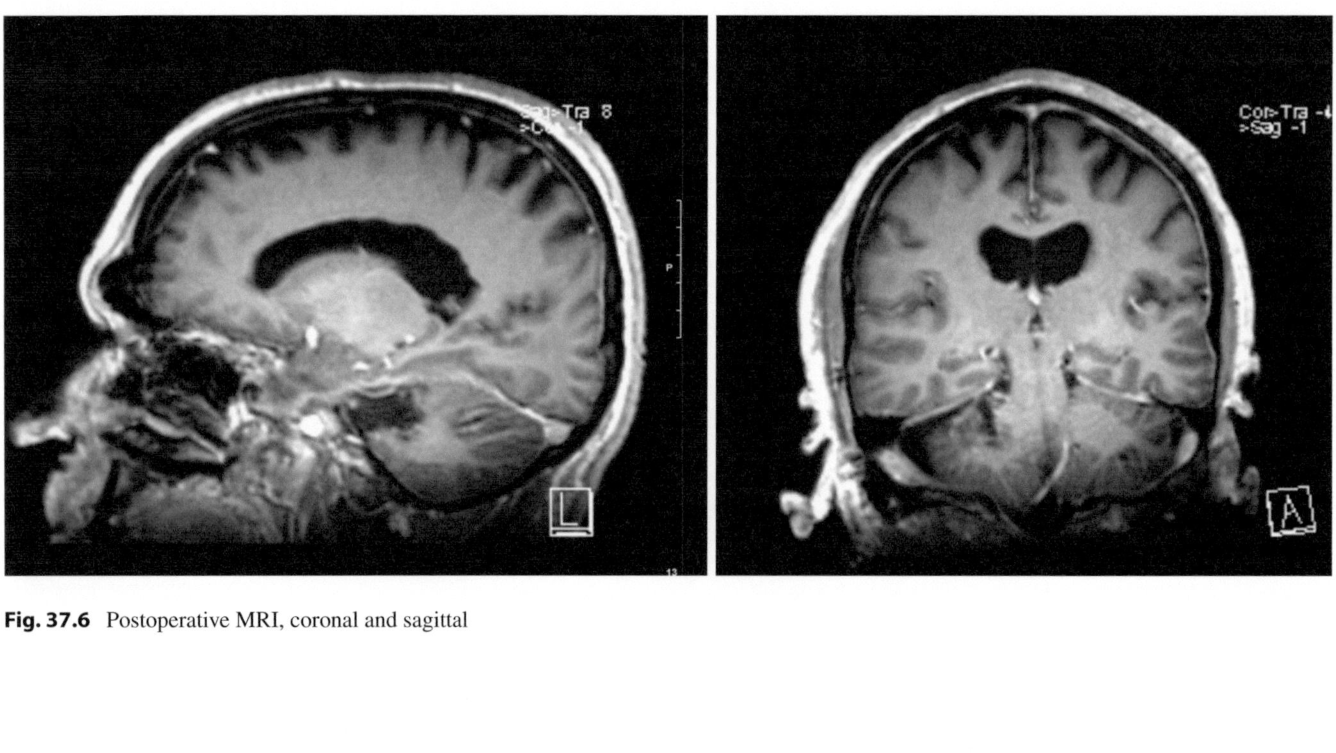

Fig. 37.6 Postoperative MRI, coronal and sagittal

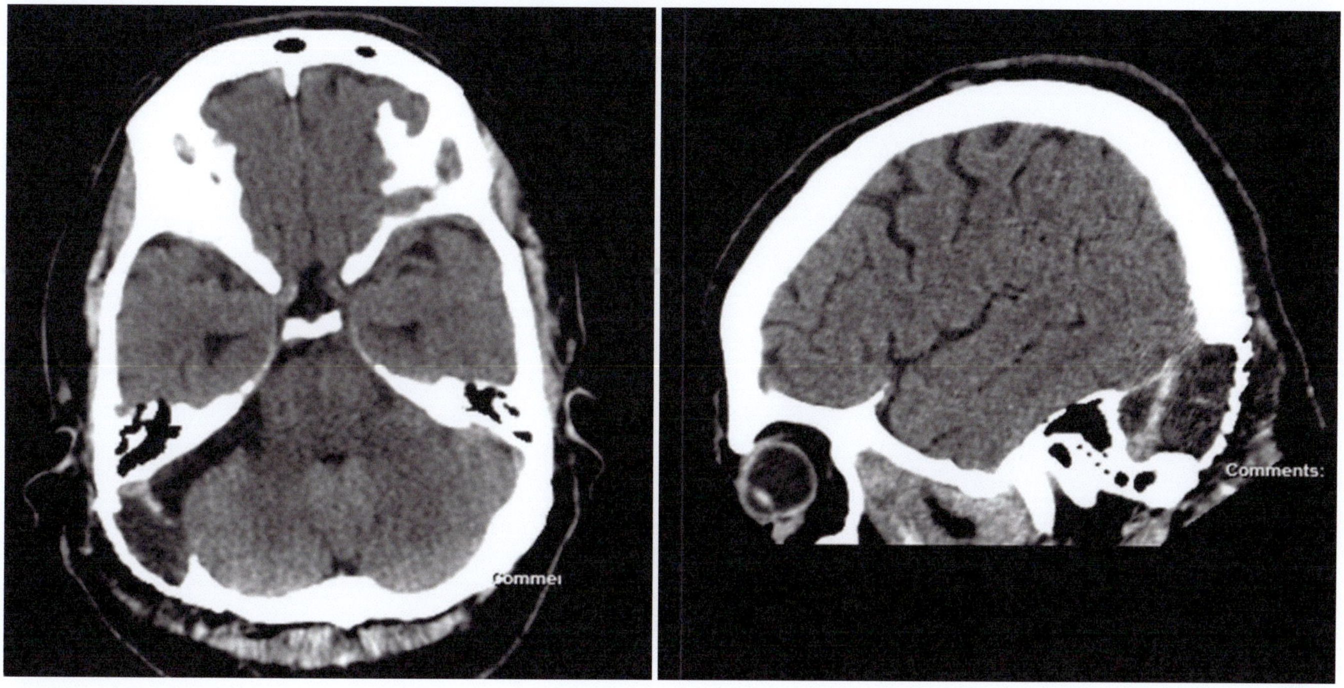

Fig. 37.7 Postoperative CT, axial and sagittal

Outcome

The patient was briefly readmitted with a cerebrospinal fluid (CSF) leak, based on a pseudomeningocele (Fig. 37.7). It was resolved with acetazolamide. No new neurological deficits were observed. In a follow-up exam, right-sided hearing was unchanged and tinnitus was gone.

Pearls and Pitfalls

- Preservation of the facial nerve and the vestibulocochlear nerve (auditory evoked potential monitoring) is an important and attainable goal.
- When these nerves cannot be properly visualized, intraoperative nerve monitoring should be considered.
- Epidermoid cyst contents are prone to causing a postoperative inflammatory reaction, which can result in aseptic meningitis and CSF resorption problems.
- As a result, temporary postoperative steroid treatment is usually utilized.

Case 17: Translabyrinthine Transtemporal Approach for Left Vestibular Schwannoma

38

Marte van Keulen, Sarah Mowry, and Nicholas C. Bambakidis

Summary

A 47-year-old woman presented with left facial twitching based on a known radiographically growing left-sided vestibular schwannoma, which was resected using a translabyrinthine approach.

Case Presentation

A 47-year-old woman with a known history of left-sided vestibular schwannoma for which she received fractionated stereotactic radiosurgery 8 years prior presented to our hospital. Repeat MRI scans revealed progressive growth of the tumor (Fig. 38.1). Over the past 6 months, she developed left facial twitching. Her neurologic exam showed Romberg to the left and left eyelid twitching.

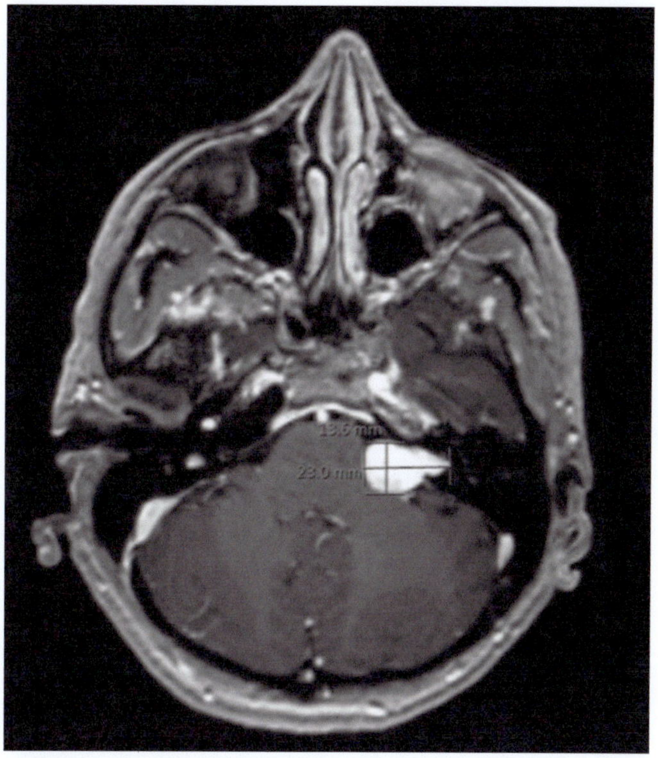

Fig. 38.1 Preoperative MRI, axial

Imaging

- Audiogram: deaf L ear.
- MRI showed a 2.2-cm acoustic tumor with intracanalicular component as well as a component within the cerebellopontine angle (CPA) (Figs. 38.2 and 38.3).

Supplementary Information The online version contains supplementary material available at [https://doi.org/10.1007/978-3-031-12507-2_38].

M. van Keulen
Case Western Reserve University School of Medicine, University Hospitals Cleveland Medical Center, Cleveland, OH, USA

S. Mowry
Division of Otology/Neurotology, Department of Otolaryngology—Head and Neck Surgery, University Hospitals Cleveland Medical Center, Case Western Reserve University, Cleveland, OH, USA

N. C. Bambakidis (✉)
Neurological Surgery, The Neurological Institute, University Hospitals of Cleveland, Case Western Reserve University School of Medicine, Cleveland, OH, USA
e-mail: Nicholas.Bambakidis2@UHhospitals.org

N. C. Bambakidis et al. (eds.), *Surgery of the Cerebellopontine Angle*, https://doi.org/10.1007/978-3-031-12507-2_38

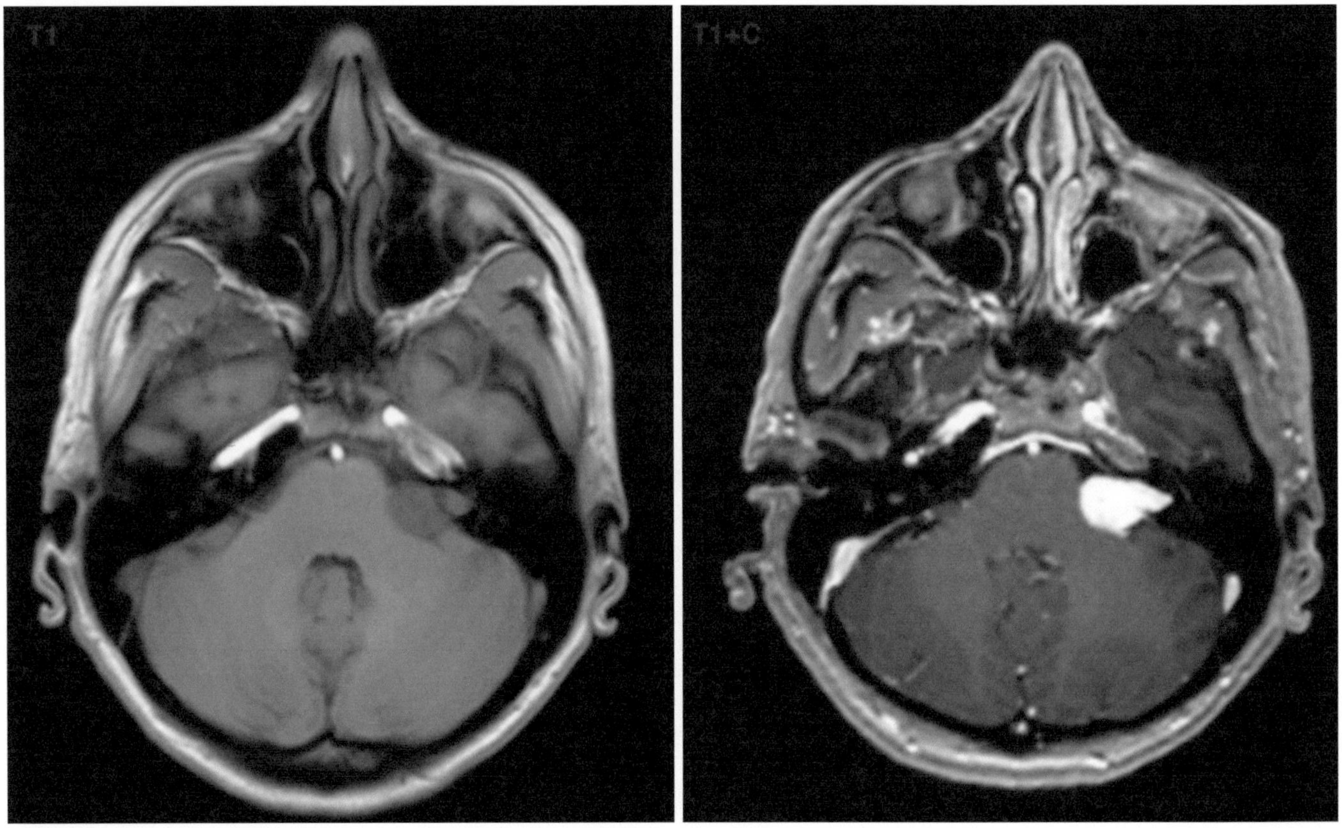

Fig. 38.2 Preoperative MRI, axial

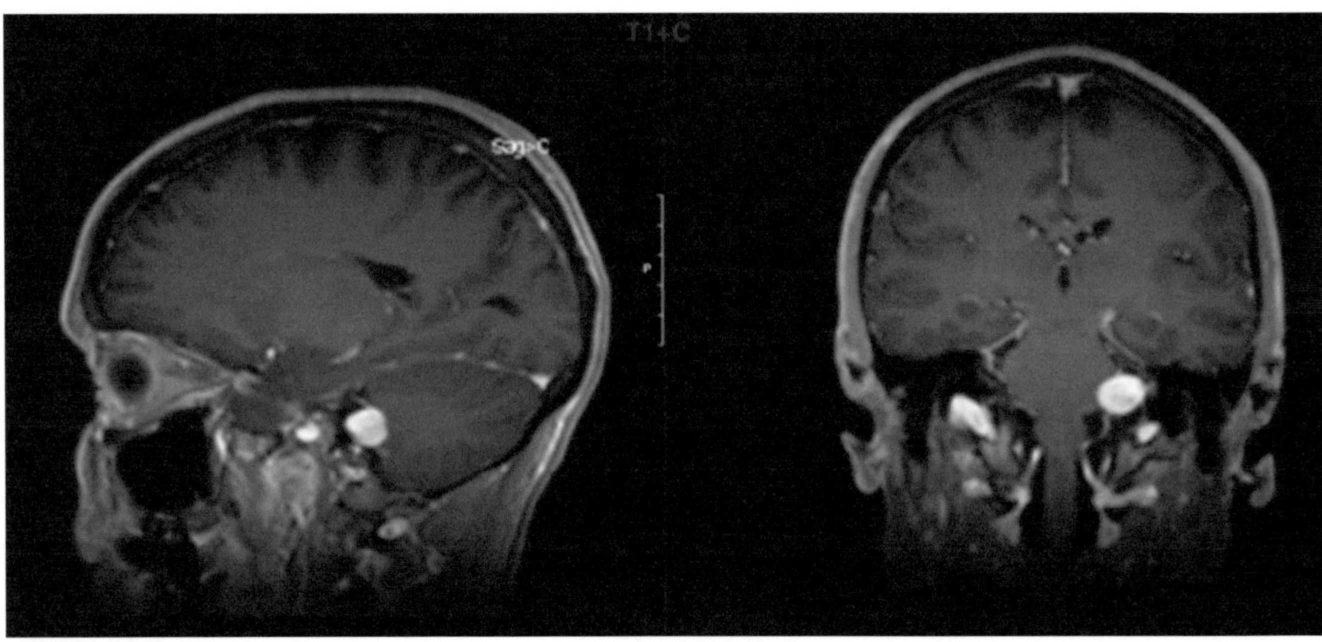

Fig. 38.3 Preoperative MRI, coronal and sagittal

Approach

A translabyrinthine approach was planned. The patient had no hearing in her left ear; therefore, hearing preservation did not have to be considered. The schwannoma had a relatively large component in the internal auditory canal (IAC).

Alternatives

- **Watchful waiting**. The tumor was growing, and the patient was experiencing symptoms.
- **Gamma knife therapy**. The patient had already received radiation that generally was not effective in subsequent treatments. The tumor was growing and causing symptoms, calling for a faster therapy than radiation.
- **Surgery: retrosigmoid approach**. This approach would have been more appropriate if the tumor had a smaller IAC component, left-sided hearing was sufficient, or comorbidities/age warranted a faster approach.

Positioning

The patient was positioned supine, turned 180° toward the surgeon.

Incision

A postauricular incision was made (Fig. 38.4).

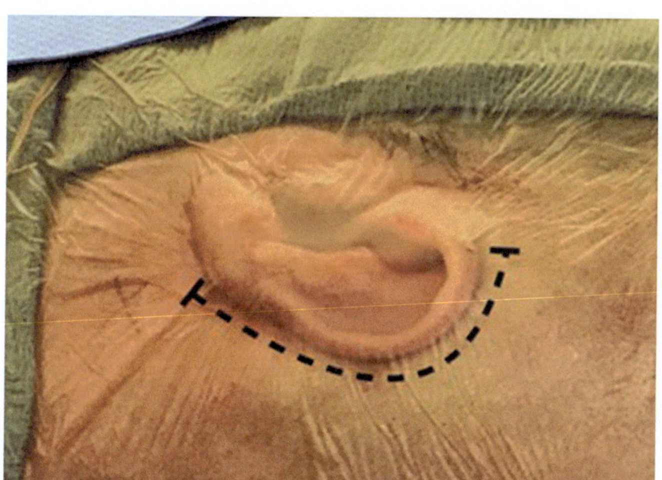

Fig. 38.4 Incision

Operation

Temporalis fascia was harvested and set aside for later use. The periosteum was incised with an anteriorly based Palva flap (see Video 38.1).

Mastoidectomy

On entering the antrum, the incus was removed. The horizontal canal was identified, followed by the identification of the descending segment of facial nerve. The retro-fascial air cells were drilled out. The sigmoid sinus was identified and skeletonized. Approximately 1–1/2 cm of bone behind the sigmoid sinus was removed to facilitate compression of the dura later. The mastoid emissary vein was isolated and ligated. The tegmen mastoideum was skeletonized as well. At this point, the dura was decorticated off the tegmen and the posterior fossa plate.

Labyrinthectomy

The IAC was identified by dissecting down along the posterior fossa dura to the reflection point of the porus acusticus. The inferior and the superior troughs were drilled out, with the cochlear aqueduct as the inferior limit and the petrous apex the superior limit. The IAC was isolated in 270 degrees. The superior vestibular nerve was identified as traveling through the bone to the insulated end of the superior canal. Posterior to this area, Bill's bar was identified so that the labyrinthine segment of the facial nerve could then be identified.

Dura Opening

Dura of the internal auditory canal was opened. Dura was reflected superiorly and inferiorly and the tumor was gently dissected away from the roof and the anterior wall of the IAC. The facial nerve, coursing from the labyrinthine segment along the anterior wall of the IAC, was identified. The superior vestibular nerve was removed from its passageway.

Tumor Resection

Gross total resection was achieved with microdissection of a large multilobulated acoustic tumor arising from the vestibular nerve both within the IAC and the posterior fossa (Fig. 38.5).

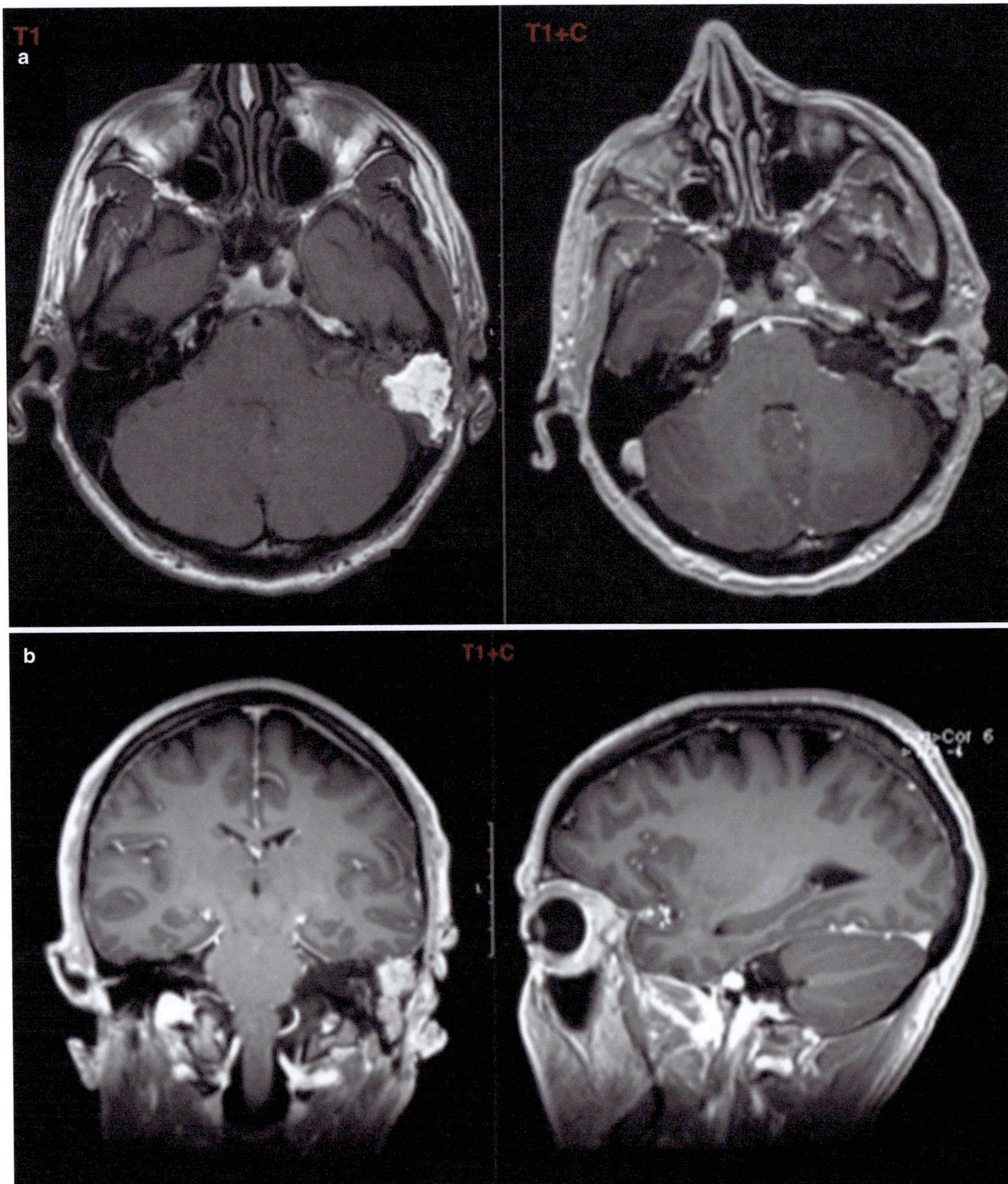

Fig. 38.5 Postoperative MRI, axial

Hemostasis and Closure

The dural defect was covered with synthetic dural graft, autologous fascia, and synthetic sealant. Preservation of the facial nerve was confirmed with a facial nerve monitor under direct visualization.

Post-op

No new neurologic deficits were noted. The patient was discharged home on postoperative day 4.

Outcome

Facial twitching disappeared. No new neurological deficits developed. The left ear remained deaf as it had been preoperatively.

Pearls and Pitfalls

- Injury to surrounding structures such as the sigmoid sinus, jugular bulb and the facial nerve should be avoided.
- Adequate bony drilling allows for adequate tumor access.
- Adipose tissue and synthetic dural sealant application minimize the risk of postoperative leak of cerebrospinal fluid.

Discussion

Important patient characteristics to consider in a vestibular schwannoma are location of the tumor (IAC and cerebellopontine angle component), hearing status, and comorbidities/age that would complicate the length of surgery and amount of anesthesia. We recommend a multidisciplinary process, combining the skills of otolaryngology and neurosurgery, from decision making to the actual surgery.

Case 18: Middle Cranial Fossa Craniotomy for a Left Petrous Apex Lesion

39

Marte van Keulen, Cliff A. Megerian, and Nicholas C. Bambakidis

Summary

This case illustrates a 61-year-old female with left-sided orbital pain and headaches that won't improve with conservative treatments. MRI and CT show a left petrous apex lesion.

Case Presentation

A 61-year-old female presented with left-sided orbital pain and bilateral headaches that have been present for 7 months. Symptoms did not improve after intravenous antibiotics and steroids, suggesting that this lesion was not infectious or inflammatory. Her pain was so severe and relentless that she could not perform her daily activities. Neurologic exam was intact.

Imaging

MRI showed a relatively poorly circumscribed left petrous apex lesion, isointense on T1, and hyperintense T2 lesion. Images showed a hypodense center with rim enhancement. There was no evidence of osteomyelitis or dural enhancement, or middle ear or mastoid enhancement (Fig. 39.1). The left petrous apex was not pneumatized. CT showed a lesion in the left petrous apex, with no destruction of surrounding bone. PET-CT showed no increased uptake in the left petrous apex lesion (Fig. 39.2).

Supplementary Information The online version contains supplementary material available at [https://doi.org/10.1007/978-3-031-12507-2_39].

M. van Keulen
Case Western Reserve University School of Medicine, University Hospitals Cleveland Medical Center, Cleveland, OH, USA

C. A. Megerian
University Hospitals Health System, Department of Otolaryngology-Head and Neck Surgery, Department of Neurological Surgery, Case Western Reserve University School of Medicine, Cleveland, OH, USA

N. C. Bambakidis (✉)
Neurological Surgery, The Neurological Institute, University Hospitals of Cleveland, Case Western Reserve University School of Medicine, Cleveland, OH, USA
e-mail: Nicholas.Bambakidis2@UHhospitals.org

N. C. Bambakidis et al. (eds.), *Surgery of the Cerebellopontine Angle*, https://doi.org/10.1007/978-3-031-12507-2_39

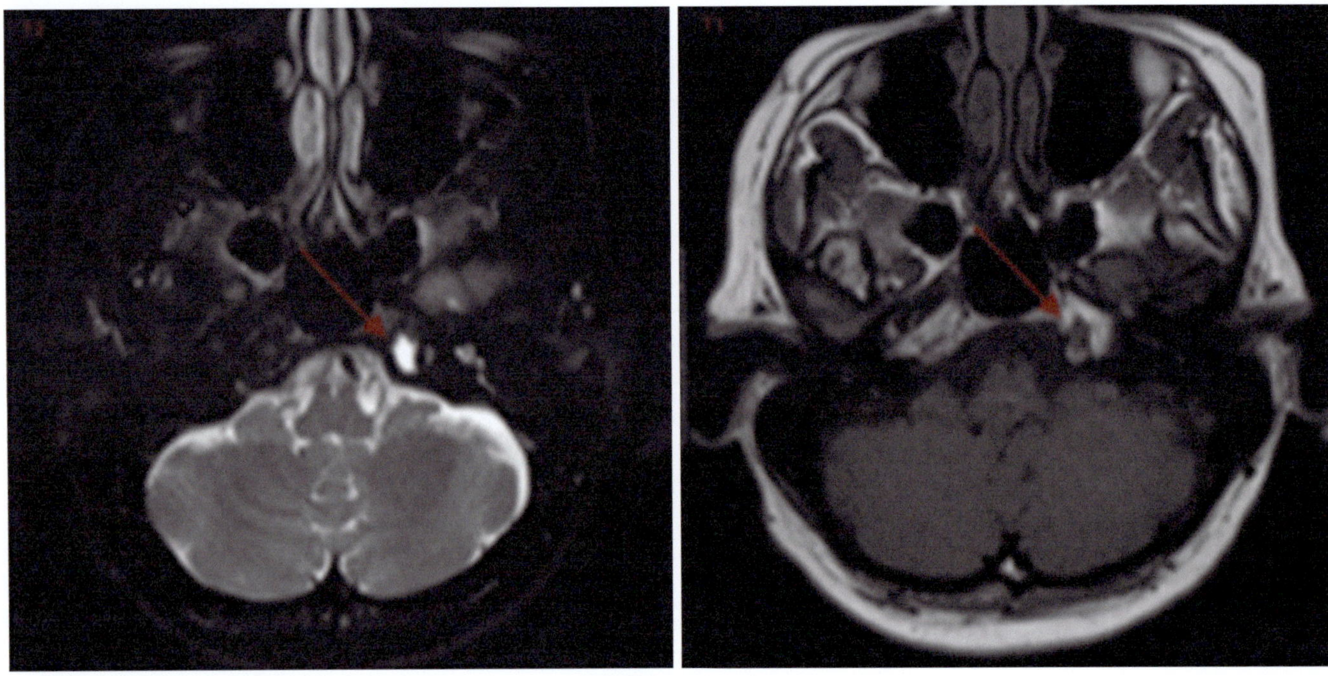

Fig. 39.1 Preoperative MRI, axial

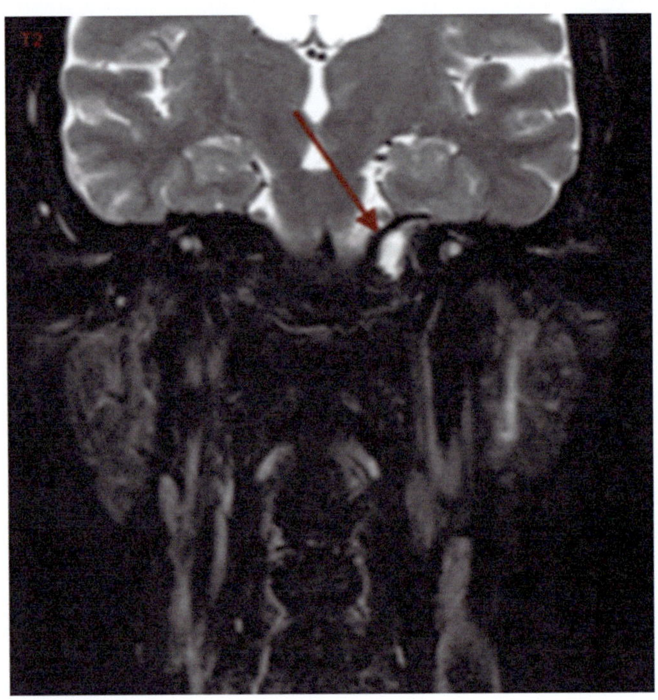

Fig. 39.2 Preoperative MRI, coronal

Approach

A middle cranial fossa approach was planned. This mostly extradural approach is ideal to reach the bony part of the middle cranial fossa floor.

Alternatives

A translabyrinthine approach would require sacrificing one-sided hearing in a healthy hearing individual. A retrosigmoid approach would not allow access to the petrous apex.

Positioning

The patient is positioned supine, with her head turned to the right 30°.

Incision

A reverse question mark incision, beginning in the preauricular crease and extending above the pinna approximately four fingerbreadths, was outlined (Fig. 39.3).

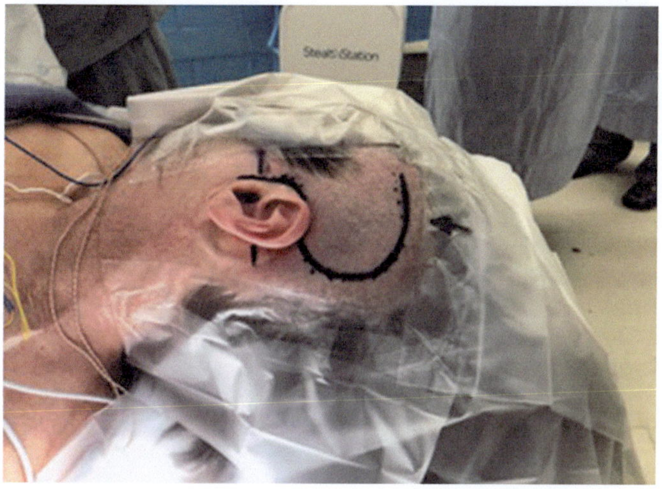

Fig. 39.3 Positioning and incision

Operation

A lumbar drain catheter was placed, allowing for intermittent release of cerebrospinal fluid (CSF) pressure to help facilitate temporal lobe relaxation and minimize retraction injury. The surgery was conducted under facial nerve monitoring (see Video 39.1).

Soft Tissue Dissection

A 5 × 5-cm craniotomy with additional drilling down to the middle cranial fossa floor exposed the internal auditory canal (IAC). The temporal lobe was elevated along the middle cranial fossa floor, exposing the typical landmarks.

Craniotomy

A middle cranial fossa retractor was secured in place with the lip just adjacent to the petrous ridge overlying the approximate location of the IAC. The middle meningeal artery was cauterized and closed. The trigeminal ganglion was visualized at the anterior aspect of the surgical field. The typical landmarks of the Kawase triangle were outlined with angle drills.

Lesion Removal

In the petrous apex, using stereotactic navigation and microdissection, an extradural intra bony lesion was encountered adjacent to the carotid artery. The roof of the petrous apex was removed. The lesion had the appearance of a soft benign neoplasm with fatty appearance. It was grossly removed down to the IAC inferiorly, anteriorly toward the petroclival junction, and laterally to the level of the internal carotid artery (ICA).

Hemostasis and Closure

Fascia was laid over the middle cranial fossa floor. Hemostasis was achieved. Bony defect was covered with locally harvested fascia. The bone was replaced using titanium plates and screws. The lumbar drain was removed.

Post-op

The patient's postoperative course was uncomplicated. CT of the head showed the expected postoperative changes. She was discharged home in stable condition on postoperative day 3.

Outcome

Pathology findings are insufficient for diagnosis. The patient reports improvement in the tension-like headaches, but the left-sided retro-orbital pain remains. Neurologic exam remains intact.

Pearls and Pitfalls

- Temporal lobe retraction should be minimized during the middle fossa approach.
- For lesions of the petrous apex, the course of the petrous ICA must be analyzed carefully.

Discussion

The middle fossa approach is an excellent choice for pathology of the bony floor of the middle cranial fossa. For this approach, hearing is preserved and the risk of CSF leak is very low.

Case 19: Extended Translabyrinthine Approach for Left-Sided Vestibular Schwannoma

40

Marte van Keulen, Sarah Mowry, and Nicholas C. Bambakidis

Summary

This case illustrates a 31-year-old woman presenting with progressive headaches, with MRI showing a large left-sided vestibular schwannoma. The tumor was removed via an extended translabyrinthine approach.

Case Presentation

A 31-year-old woman presented with progressive headaches for the past several years. Upon request, the patient reported some left-sided hearing loss and occasional tinnitus in both ears. Neurologic exam was intact.

Imaging

Audiogram shows normal hearing and normal tympanograms. MRI shows an approximately 3.5-cm left-sided lesion of the cerebellopontine angle, with cystic degeneration of the center of the tumor. There is flattening of the fourth ventricle, with partial compression of and deviation across the midline of the brainstem (Fig. 40.1).

Supplementary Information The online version contains supplementary material available at [https://doi.org/10.1007/978-3-031-12507-2_40].

M. van Keulen
Case Western Reserve University School of Medicine, University Hospitals Cleveland Medical Center, Cleveland, OH, USA

S. Mowry
Division of Otology/Neurotology, Department of Otolaryngology—Head and Neck Surgery, University Hospitals Cleveland Medical Center, Case Western Reserve University, Cleveland, OH, USA

N. C. Bambakidis (✉)
Neurological Surgery, The Neurological Institute, University Hospitals of Cleveland, Case Western Reserve University School of Medicine, Cleveland, OH, USA
e-mail: Nicholas.Bambakidis2@UHhospitals.org

N. C. Bambakidis et al. (eds.), *Surgery of the Cerebellopontine Angle*, https://doi.org/10.1007/978-3-031-12507-2_40

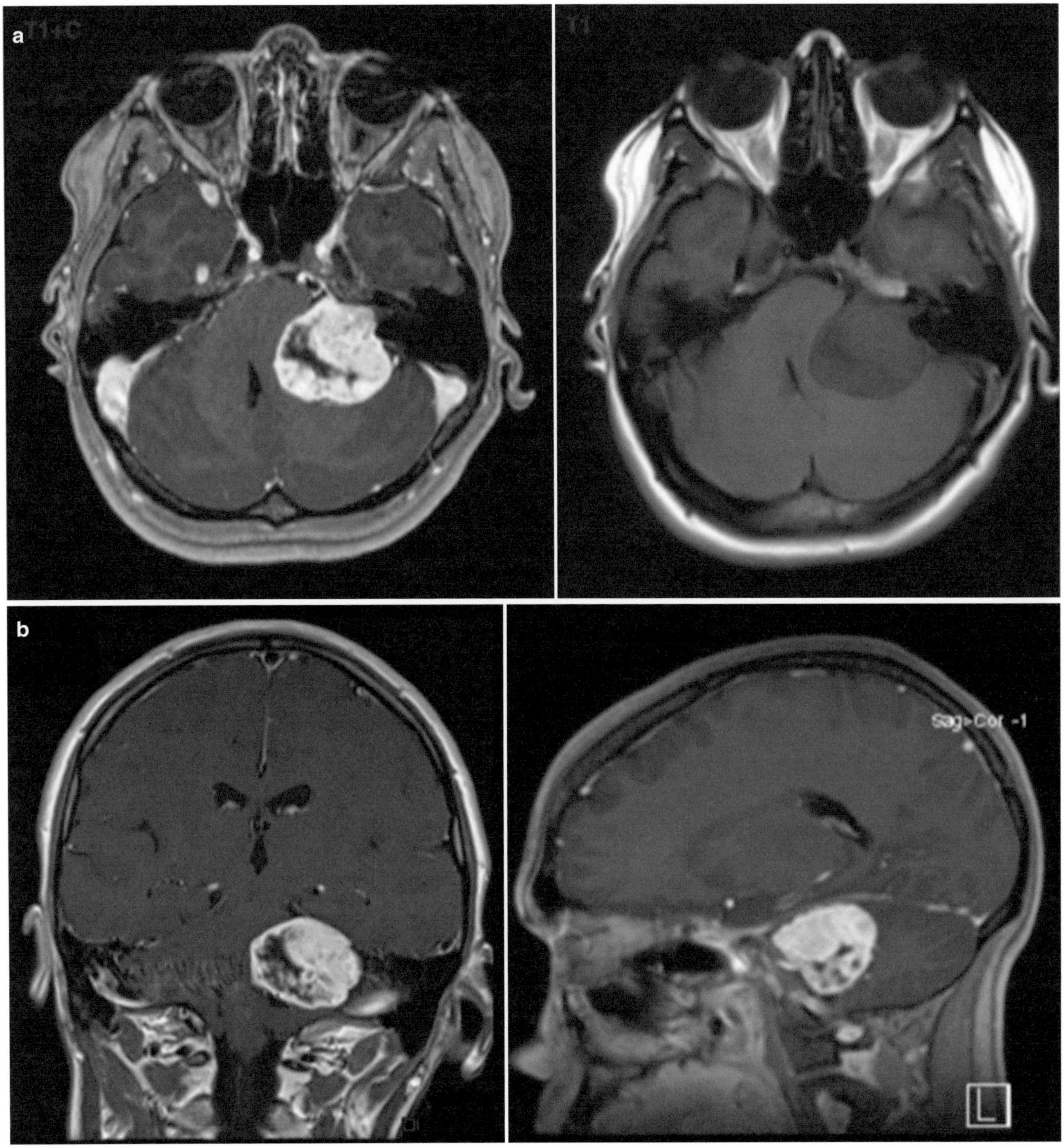

Fig. 40.1 (Left) Preoperative MRI, axial, (Right) Preoperative MRI, coronal and sagittal

Approach

An extended translabyrinthine approach was selected. For larger tumors, additional bony exposure with division of the tentorium allows for greater tumor access and minimal brain retraction.

Alternatives

While watchful waiting was an option, surgery was highly recommend based on the size of this lesion. Likewise, radiosurgery was not recommended because of tumor size. A retrosigmoid approach was a valid choice for this patient, but brain retraction would have been required.

Positioning

The patient is positioned supine, with her head turned to the right.

Incision

A postauricular curvilinear skin incision was made (Fig. 40.2).

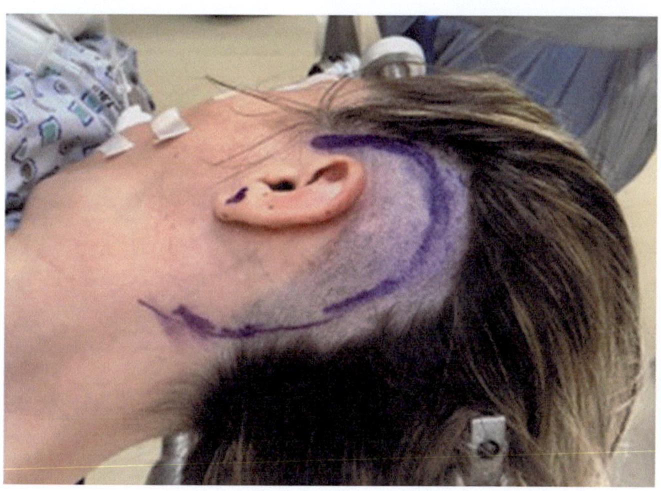

Fig. 40.2 Incision

Operation

A large piece of temporalis fascia was harvested and set aside for later use. An extended mastoidectomy/occipital/middle fossa bone flap exposed the transverse sinus, sigmoid sinus, retrosigmoid dura, and temporal lobe dura (see Video 40.1).

Mastoidectomy

On entering the antrum, the incus was removed. The horizontal canal was identified, and the descending segment of facial nerve was identified. The retro-fascial air cells were drilled out. The sigmoid sinus was skeletonized to the jugular bulb. The tegmen mastoideum was skeletonized and decorticated as well once the otic capsule bone was isolated.

Labyrinthectomy

The entirety of the labyrinth was removed. The internal auditory canal (IAC) was identified by dissecting down along the posterior fossa dura to the reflection point of the porus acusticus. The inferior and the superior troughs were then drilled out; the superior trough was very narrow, and the inferior trough was cleared to the jugular bulb. The inferior limit of the dissection was the cochlear aqueduct. Superiorly, we drilled down to the limit of the petrous apex. The IAC was isolated in 200°.

Opening Dura

The superior vestibular nerve was identified traveling through the bone to the ampullated end of the superior canal. Posterior to this area, Bill's bar and the labyrinthine segment of the facial nerve were identified. The dura of the IAC was opened and reflected superiorly and inferiorly. The tumor was then dissected away from the roof and the anterior wall of the IAC. The facial nerve was identified coursing from the labyrinthine segment along the anterior wall of the IAC. Once the nerve had been positively identified with the facial nerve stimulator, the superior vestibular nerve was removed from its passageway.

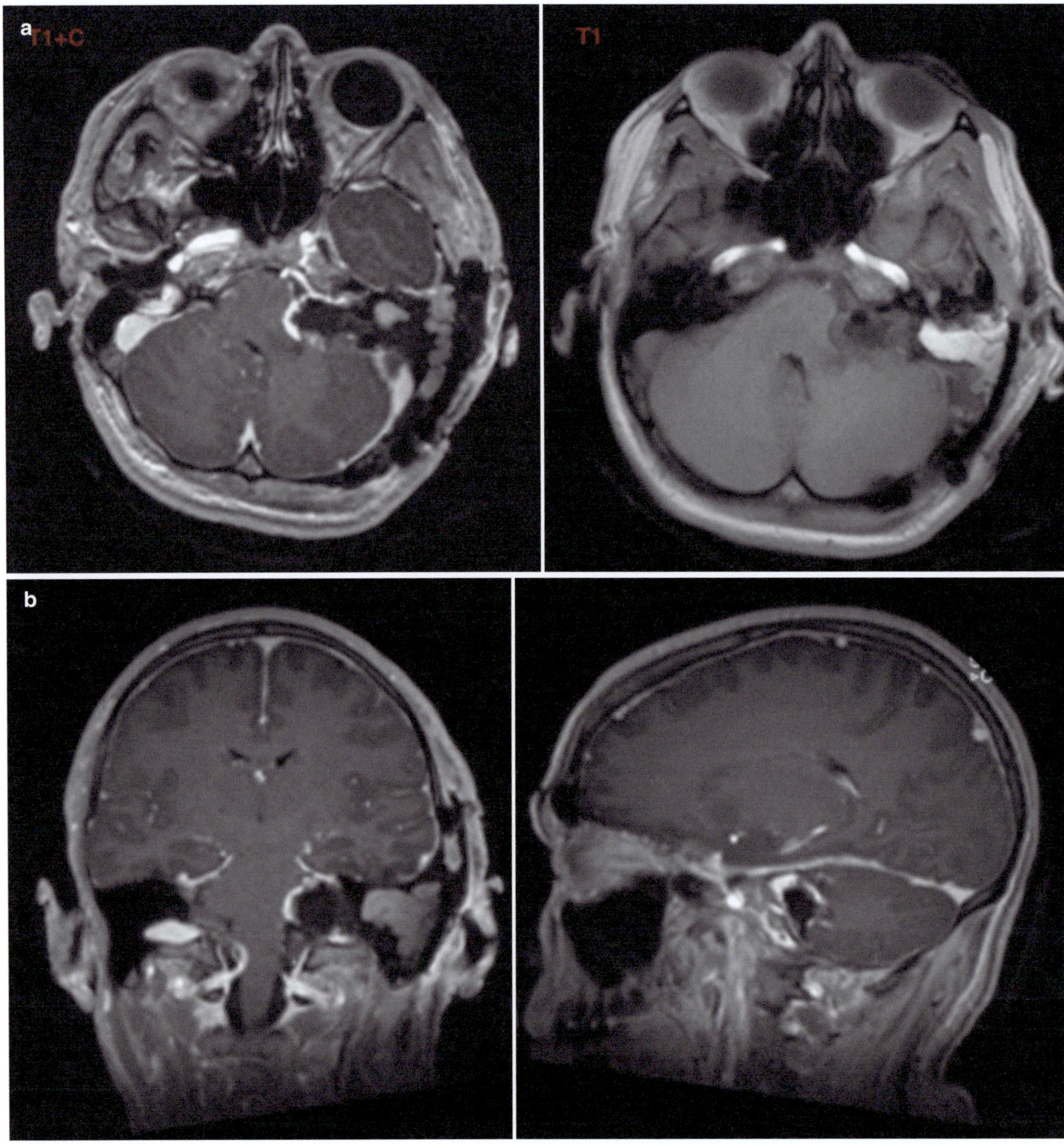

Fig. 40.3 (Left) Postoperative MRI, axial, (Right) Postoperative MRI, coronal and sagittal

Tumor Dissection

Following the skull-base approach, posterior cranial skull base presigmoid dura was opened widely as was the middle fossa dura, cutting tentorium to allow for exposure of a very large intradural acoustic tumor. Internal debulking of the acoustic tumor was completed, and the facial nerve was identified and preserved throughout the case. A small portion of the tumor was left adherent to the brainstem capsule and the facial nerve at the end of the procedure; however, the majority of the tumor was removed without complication (Fig. 40.3).

Closure

Irrigation and hemostasis were applied. Temporalis muscle was harvested, tensor tendon in the middle ear was cut, and the eustachian tube and the middle ear space were packed with muscle. A small piece of Surgicel® and bone wax was also pushed into the eustachian tube orifice. The durotomy was repaired using DuraGen®. The previously harvested piece of fascia was placed over the aditus ad antrum. DuraSeal® was then applied to the dural repair, and a lime-sized piece of fat (harvested from the abdomen) was placed over it. Bone was replaced with titanium plates and screws.

Post-op

No new neurologic deficits were observed. The patient was charged home on postoperative day 5.

Outcome

No new deficits were noted. Audiogram remains normal.

Pearls and Pitfalls

- Injury to surrounding structures such as the sigmoid sinus, jugular bulb, and the facial nerve should be carefully avoided.
- Adipose tissue and synthetic dural sealant application minimize the risk of postoperative leak of cerebrospinal fluid.
- When opening the tentorium to extend the translabyrinthine approach, the dural sinus anatomy must be carefully analyzed as well as the course of the vein of Labbé.
- In older patients, the dura is more adherent, which causes a greater risk of vessel rupture, making this exposure less desirable.

Discussion

For larger tumors, additional bony exposure with division of the tentorium allows for greater tumor access and minimal brain retraction.

41 Case 20: Right-Sided Retrosigmoid Approach to Small Vestibular Schwannoma

Marte van Keulen, Sarah Mowry, and Nicholas C. Bambakidis

Summary

This case illustrates a 61-year-old woman with progressive hearing loss, due to a growing vestibular schwannoma, undergoing a retrosigmoid resection.

Case Presentation

A 61-year-old woman presented to surgery 5 years prior with slowly progressive hearing loss in the right ear and mild vertigo, based on a small vestibular schwannoma. Her serial MRI showed tumor growth. Additionally, the patient reported increased hearing loss, which warranted treatment. An audiogram showed moderate right hearing loss with 72% word recognition (vs 96% contralateral). A planned serial MRI showed growth of the tumor from 11 × 11 × 16 mm to 14 × 12 × 19 in 3 months (Figs. 41.1 and 41.2).

Supplementary Information The online version contains supplementary material available at [https://doi.org/10.1007/978-3-031-12507-2_41].

M. van Keulen
Case Western Reserve University School of Medicine, University Hospitals Cleveland Medical Center, Cleveland, OH, USA

S. Mowry
Division of Otology/Neurotology, Department of Otolaryngology—Head and Neck Surgery, University Hospitals Cleveland Medical Center, Case Western Reserve University, Cleveland, OH, USA

N. C. Bambakidis (✉)
Neurological Surgery, The Neurological Institute, University Hospitals of Cleveland, Case Western Reserve University School of Medicine, Cleveland, OH, USA
e-mail: Nicholas.Bambakidis2@UHhospitals.org

N. C. Bambakidis et al. (eds.), *Surgery of the Cerebellopontine Angle*, https://doi.org/10.1007/978-3-031-12507-2_41

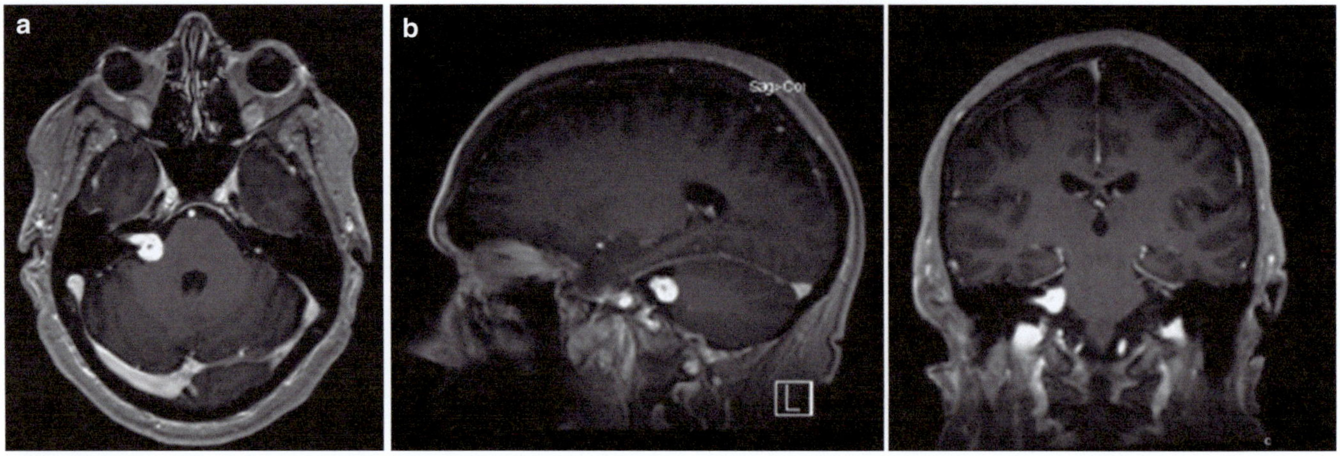

Fig. 41.1 (Left) Preoperative MRI, axial, (Center) Preoperative MRI, coronal and (Right) sagittal

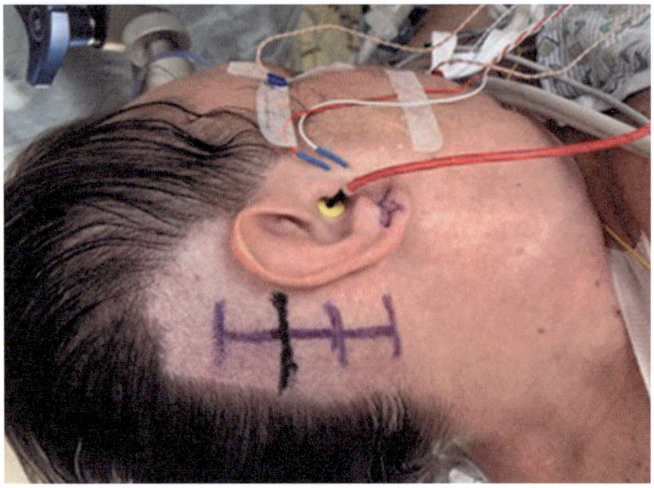

Fig. 41.2 Incision

Approach

A retrosigmoid craniotomy was an excellent choice for this small tumor but one that will require careful drilling out of the internal auditory canal (IAC) to reach the IAC component.

Alternatives

A translabyrinthine approach would have been a valid choice for this patient, but the relatively small size and therefore the accessibility to the IAC component via the retrosigmoid approach (with loss of hearing and increased length of surgery) made the retrosigmoid approach a wiser choice. A middle cranial fossa approach would have presented difficulties accessing the cerebellopontine angle component of the tumor. Given the size of the tumor, radiation could have been an option. However, because of the sudden growth and mild vertigo symptoms, which are better treated with surgery, we opted for surgery.

Positioning

The patient was positioned supine, with her head turned to the left.

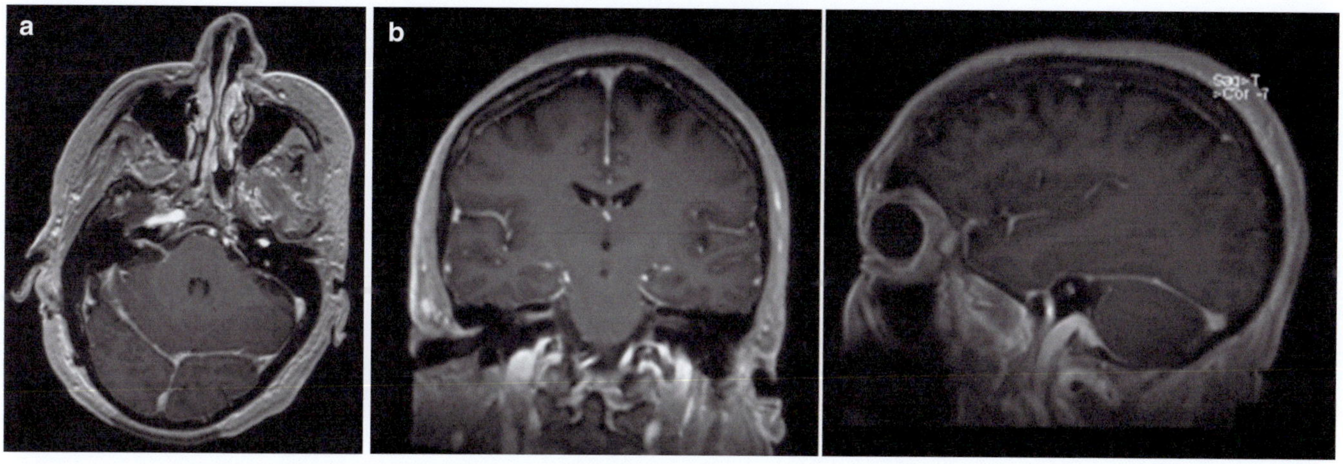

Fig. 41.3 (Left) Postoperative MRI, axial, (Center) Postoperative MRI, coronal and (Right) sagittal

Incision

A right-sided posterior retromastoid skin incision was made (Fig. 41.3).

Operation

A lumbar drain catheter was placed, allowing intermittent drainage throughout the procedure, followed by a retrosigmoid craniectomy and skeletonizing of the sigmoid sinus; a partial mastoidectomy, carefully waxing the mastoid air cells; and intradural drilling of the IAC. Despite continuity of the cochlear nerve, auditory brain wave responses were lost during the procedure. However, the facial nerve was carefully preserved using facial nerve monitor and stimulating well. The tumor was resected. Dura was loosely approximated and covered with synthetic dural graft. The bony defect was covered with titanium mesh (see Video 41.1).

Post-op

The patient lost all subjective hearing in her right ear. No other neurological deficits were noted. She was discharged home on postoperative day 3.

Outcome

The outcome is yet to be determined.

Pearls and Pitfalls

- We always recommend intraoperative electrophysiological monitoring for the facial nerve during this procedure as well as auditory evoked potentials for select cases.
- Despite careful preservation of the cochlear nerve during surgery, hearing preservation can be difficult for larger tumors likely secondary to vascular compromise of the nerve during microdissection.

Discussion

This retrosigmoid approach is a good choice for smaller vestibular schwannomas like this one. The approach requires a much shorter time, has a lower occurrence of cerebrospinal fluid leak, and usually preserves hearing.

Case 21: Transotic Approach to Left-Sided Jugular Paraganglioma/Glomus Tumor for Partial Debulking

42

Marte van Keulen, Nicholas C. Bambakidis, Maroun T. Semaan, and Sarah Mowry

Summary

This case illustrates a 64-year-old woman presenting with hearing loss and headaches, with a left jugular glomus tumor, which was resected using a transotic approach.

Case Presentation

A 64-year-old female presented with progressive left hearing loss and headaches and complaints of pounding headache, imbalance, progressive hearing loss, ear pain, and intermittent facial spasms and weakness that resolve spontaneously. She denied dysphagia and hoarseness. MRI showed a large 2.5 × 2.7 × 2.5 cm left petrous apex mass medial to jugular bulb, with paraganglioma rather than schwannoma (Figs. 42.1 and 42.2). A small extracranial extension was noted.

Supplementary Information The online version contains supplementary material available at https://doi.org/10.1007/978-3-031-12507-2_42.

M. van Keulen
Case Western Reserve University School of Medicine, University Hospitals Cleveland Medical Center, Cleveland, OH, USA

N. C. Bambakidis (✉)
Neurological Surgery, The Neurological Institute, University Hospitals of Cleveland, Case Western Reserve University School of Medicine, Cleveland, OH, USA
e-mail: Nicholas.Bambakidis2@UHhospitals.org

M. T. Semaan
Otolaryngology—Otology, University Hospitals Cleveland Medical Center, Cleveland, OH, USA

S. Mowry
Division of Otology/Neurotology, Department of Otolaryngology—Head and Neck Surgery, University Hospitals Cleveland Medical Center, Case Western Reserve University, Cleveland, OH, USA

N. C. Bambakidis et al. (eds.), *Surgery of the Cerebellopontine Angle*, https://doi.org/10.1007/978-3-031-12507-2_42

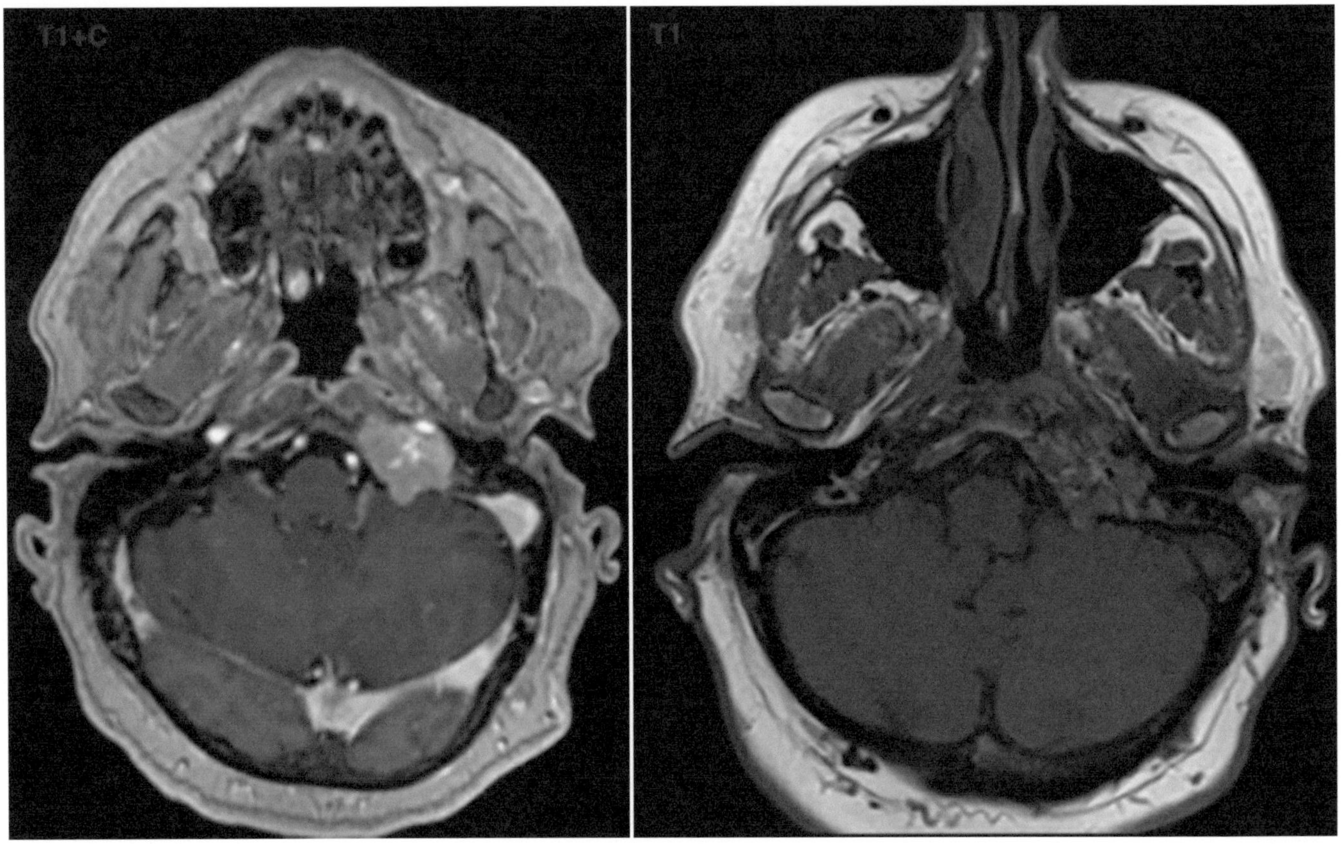

Fig. 42.1 Preoperative MRI, axial

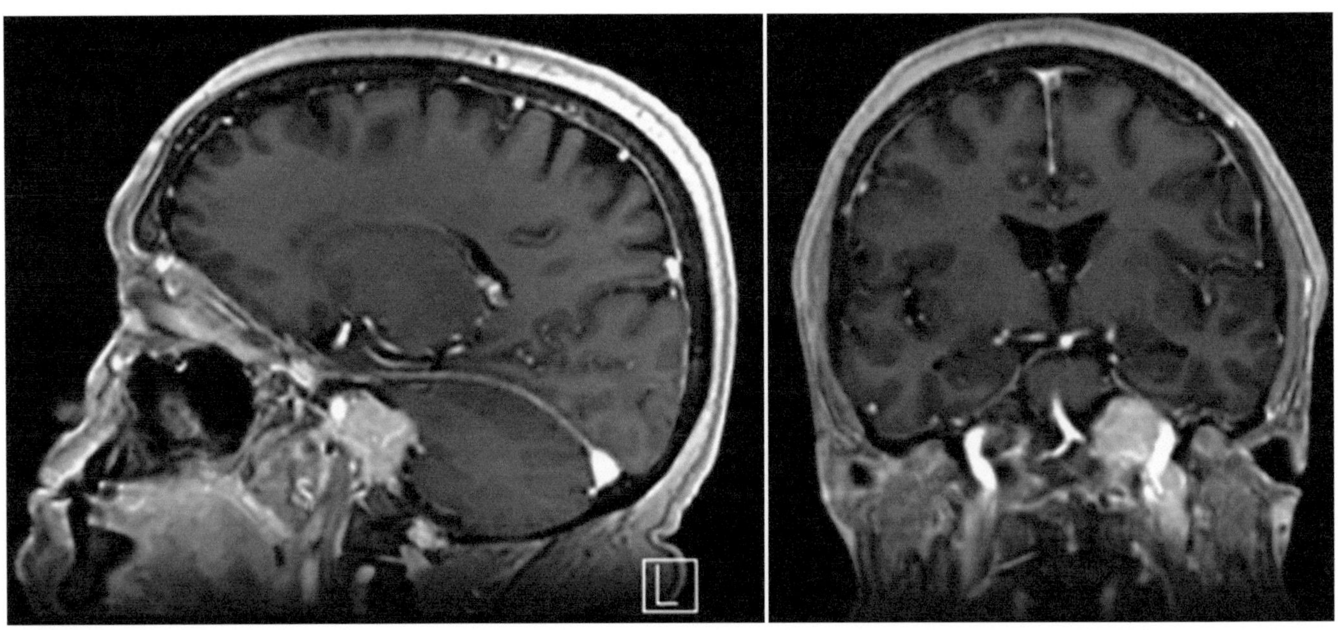

Fig. 42.2 Preoperative MRI, (Left) coronal and (Right) sagittal

Approach

A partial resection of the tumor utilizing a transotic approach, with adjuvant radiosurgery, was planned, given the anterior and inferior location of the tumor surrounding the jugular bulb and because the patient already had significant hearing loss on this side. This approach would create the biggest possible window to the tumor with the right angle.

Alternatives

This tumor would not be reached properly by a retrosigmoid approach because of its anterior and inferior localization. A translabyrinthine approach would create a window to the tumor possibly too small for proper debulking. A transcochlear approach, almost identical to the transotic approach, requires a full mobilization of the facial nerve and posterior translocation. Facial nerve function is usually compromised in the transcochlear approach due to loss of blood supply of the geniculate when the nerve is transposed.

Positioning

The patient was positioned supine, with her head turned to the right.

Incision

A left-sided horizontal cervical neck incision for vascular exploration was planned (Fig. 42.3). The postauricular incision was situated approximately two finger breadths behind the postauricular sulcus.

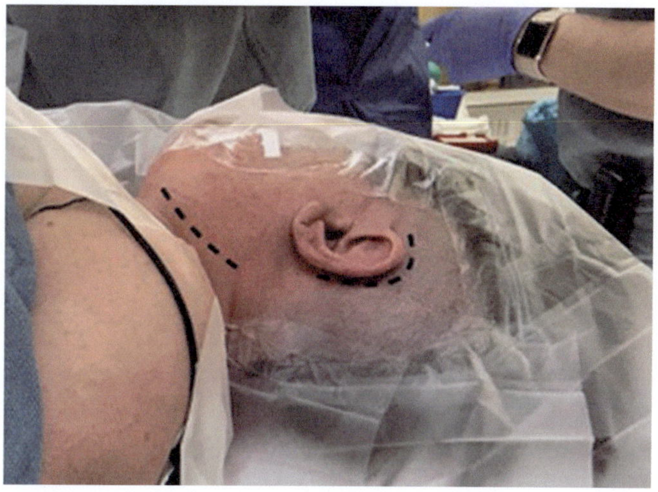

Fig. 42.3 Incision

Operation

A left-sided horizontal cervical neck incision was made. With dissection, the common carotid artery was identified medial to the sternocleidomastoid muscle. The artery was then isolated with vessel loops for proximal vascular control of the patient's skull-base tumor. The common carotid artery was isolated with vessel loops for proximal vascular control of the patient's skull-base tumor. The external auditory canal was transected at the bony cartilaginous junction circumferentially at 360°. Then the skin was elevated off the underlying cartilage, passed through the external auditory canal, and closed using 4–0 silk stitches to achieve a watertight closure in the event there would be a cerebrospinal fluid (CSF) leak.

Next, a wide mastoidectomy was performed using a combination of cutting and diamond burs. The mastoid was contracted, the tegmen was low, and the sigmoid was quite forward. Skeletonization and decompression of the tegmen and sigmoid were then performed, followed by identification of the descending segment of the facial nerve, which was traced down to the stylomastoid foramen. The facial recess was opened, and an extended facial recess approach was performed. The incudostapedial joint was separated, the incus was removed, and the tensor tympani tendon was sectioned. The ear canal skin including the tympanic annulus and the malleus were removed and discarded.

The canal wall was taken down, and bone along the hypotympanic ring was removed to expose the jugular bulb. There was obvious tumor extending through the promontory right below the round window niche involving the hypotympanic part to the middle ear.

A labyrinthectomy was then performed, and bone was removed down to the level of the internal auditory canal (IAC). Bone was also dissected in the retrofacial air cell tract all the way to the jugular bulb and sigmoid sinus. Once the bone was removed, the tumor was seen extending in that area beneath the IAC.

Surgical attention then turned back to performing the transcochlear approach by drilling off the cochlea. The ultrasound probe was used to identify the location of the internal carotid artery and the petrous bone. Stapes were removed, and the oval window that connected it to the round window niche was drilled. The cochlea was then removed by turning the basal turn followed by the middle turn and the apex. The tensor tympani muscle and its canal were maintained given our decision to use the transotic approach and avoid posterior routing of the facial nerve, which would have left the patient with complete facial paralysis. Furthermore, limited resection was the goal rather than complete resection. The bone was then skeletonized.

The bone around the facial canal was thinned all the way from the first genu to the stylomastoid foramen, and the bone lateral to the nerve along the lateral epitympanic recess was removed to better expose the entire temporal bone. After good exposure was acquired, bone medial to the nerve along the vestibule was removed to further improve the exposure around the nerve and facilitate tumor removal. Tumor was removed from around the nerve, posterior to the internal carotid artery and medial to it, and medial to the location of the cochlea and the jugular bulb as well.

Limited resection was performed, and hemostasis was achieved. The eustachian tube mucosa was everted, and free muscle grafting was placed to obliterate the eustachian tube. Bone wax was also placed. Abdominal fat was harvested for grafting, trimmed into strips, and placed into the mastoid defect to fill it. Titanium mesh was placed outside the filled defect for support and to recreate the contour of the mastoid (see Video 42.1).

Post-op

The postoperative course was uncomplicated, with no new deficits (Figs. 42.4, and 42.5).

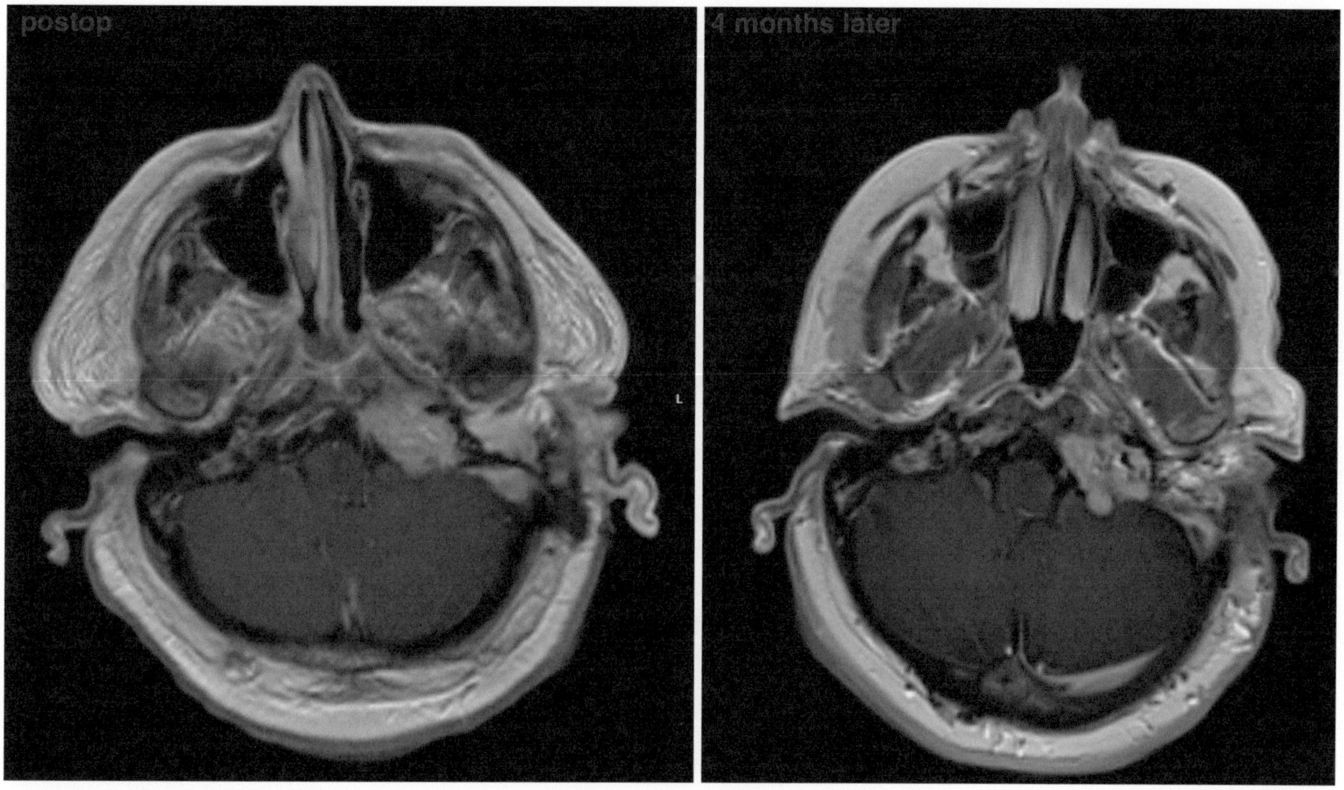

Fig. 42.4 Postoperative MRI, axial

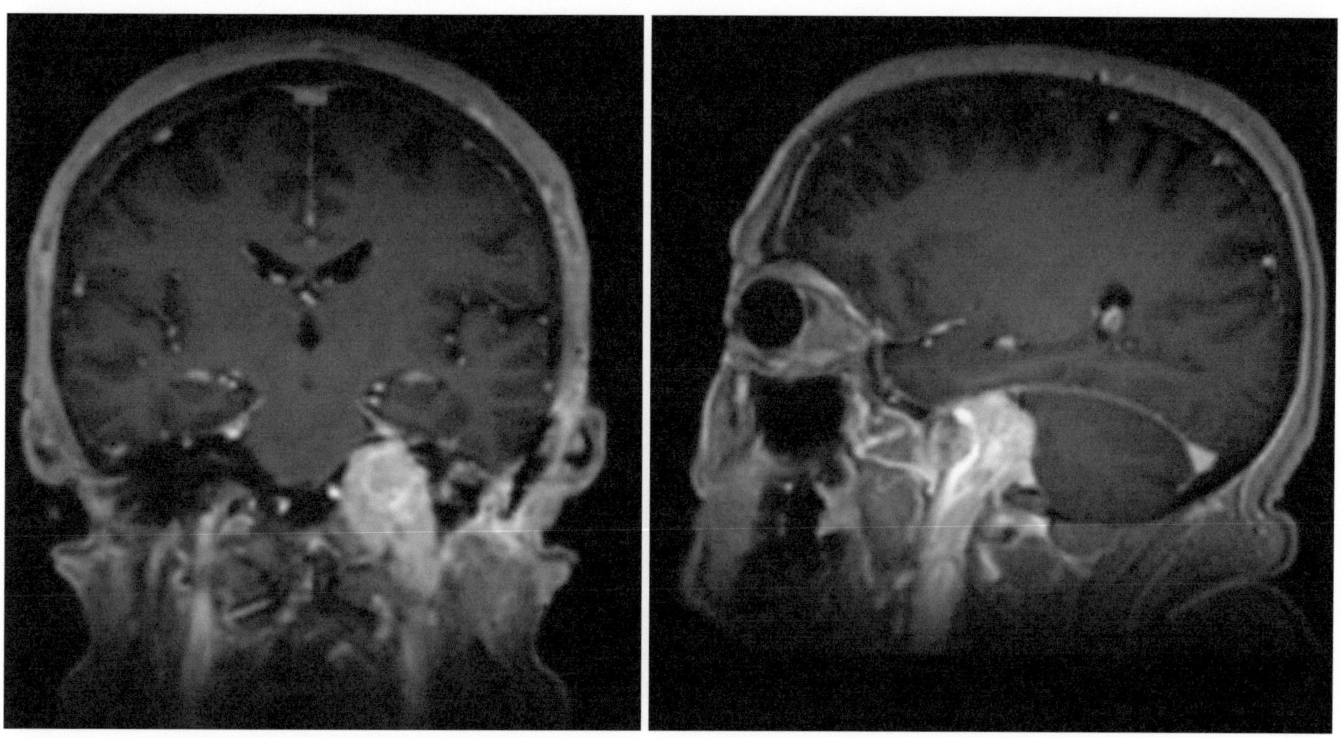

Fig. 42.5 Postoperative MRI, (Left) coronal and (Right) sagittal

Outcome

Pathology confirmed the diagnosis of a glomus tumor. The patient was scheduled to receive adjuvant gamma knife radiosurgery for the treatment of residual glomus jugular tumor. She was neurologically intact, besides the pre-existent loss of hearing in her left ear.

Pearls and Pitfalls

- Special care should be taken to preserve the facial nerve during multiple steps in this procedure.
- For example, when the cochlea is ready to be drilled out, the labyrinth segment of the facial nerve is located very close to the upper turn of the cochlea.
- When the facial nerve is skeletonized, care should be taken to protect the nerve from bone dust as the cochlea is drilled out; covering the nerve with Gelfoam is one option.
- Prevent CSF leaks by packing the middle ear and eustachian tube with fascia and by using a fat graft to obliterate the mastoid.

Discussion

We recommend a multidisciplinary approach for difficult cases like these. In this approach, a neuro-otolaryngologist who is qualified for such an extensive procedure is essential. The transotic approach provides a bigger window into the cerebellopontine angle but requires sacrifice of the labyrinth and the cochlea; its aim is to preserve facial function. Despite excellent exposure, glomus tumors can be very difficult to resect due to their hypervascular nature. Subtotal resection followed by radiation therapy is a reasonable treatment strategy.

Anatomic Dissection Appendix

Marte van Keulen, Biji Bahuleyan, Vasu Sidagam, Sarah Mowry, and Nicholas C. Bambakidis

This appendix illustrates the important surgical anatomy for a selection of the approaches to the cerebellopontine angle (CPA), using cadaver dissection images. We will discuss the transtemporal approaches (presigmoid/retrolabyrinthine, translabyrinthine, transcochlear) and the middle cranial fossa approach.

Translabyrinthine and Transcochlear Approaches

The translabyrinthine approach and the transcochlear approach contain similar steps early in the procedure, both starting with a mastoidectomy and labyrinthectomy. They are designed to work around the facial nerve in an attempt to preserve it in the resection of a vestibular tumor, most commonly. The transcochlear approach then diverges from the translabyrinthine approach by the removal of the cochlea, creating a more extensive view anteriorly into the CPA. By removal of vital auditory structures, both of these approaches require the sacrifice of a patient's hearing.

Mastoidectomy

Figure A.1 demonstrates the exposed mastoid bone, showing the important structures on the surface of the mastoid. Note MacEwan's triangle, bordered by the mastoid tip, root of the zygoma, and spine of Henle. The spine of Henle roughly overlies the mastoid antrum where the semicircular canals and facial nerve are located.

Mastoidectomy starts off with drilling of the mastoid cortex, exposing the mastoid air cells (Fig. A.2).

The mastoidectomy exposes vital structures residing in the mastoid bone, such as the sigmoid sinus, (part of) the facial nerve, and the labyrinth (Fig. A.3).

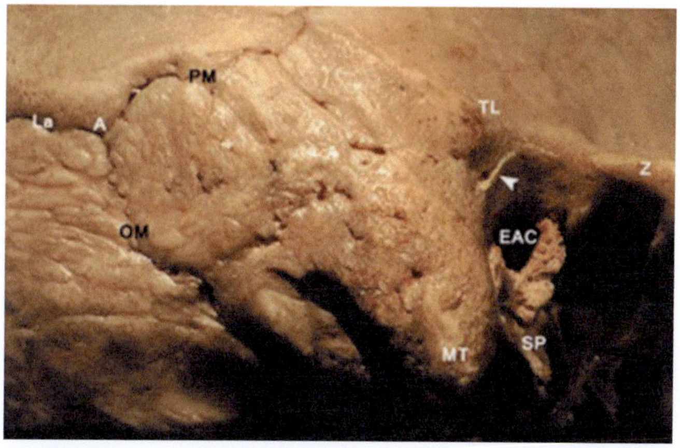

Fig. A.1 Lateral surface of the right mastoid bone and adjacent areas showing important structures pertaining to transtemporal approaches. La = lamdoid; A = asterion; PM = parietomastoid suture; OM = occipitomastoid suture; EAC = external auditory canal; TL = temporal line; MT = mastoid tip; SP = styloid process, Z = zygoma; Arrow = spine of Henle

M. van Keulen
University Hospitals Cleveland Medical Center, Case Western Reserve University School of Medicine, Cleveland, OH, USA

B. Bahuleyan
Lisie Hospital, Kaloor, Ernakulam, Kerala, India

V. Sidagam
University Hospitals Cleveland Medical Center, Cleveland, OH, USA

S. Mowry
Department of Otolaryngology—Head and Neck Surgery, University Hospitals Cleveland Medical Center, Case Western Reserve University, Cleveland, OH, USA

N. C. Bambakidis
Neurological Surgery, The Neurological Institute, University Hospitals of Cleveland, Case Western Reserve University School of Medicine, Cleveland, OH, USA

N. C. Bambakidis et al. (eds.), *Surgery of the Cerebellopontine Angle*, https://doi.org/10.1007/978-3-031-12507-2

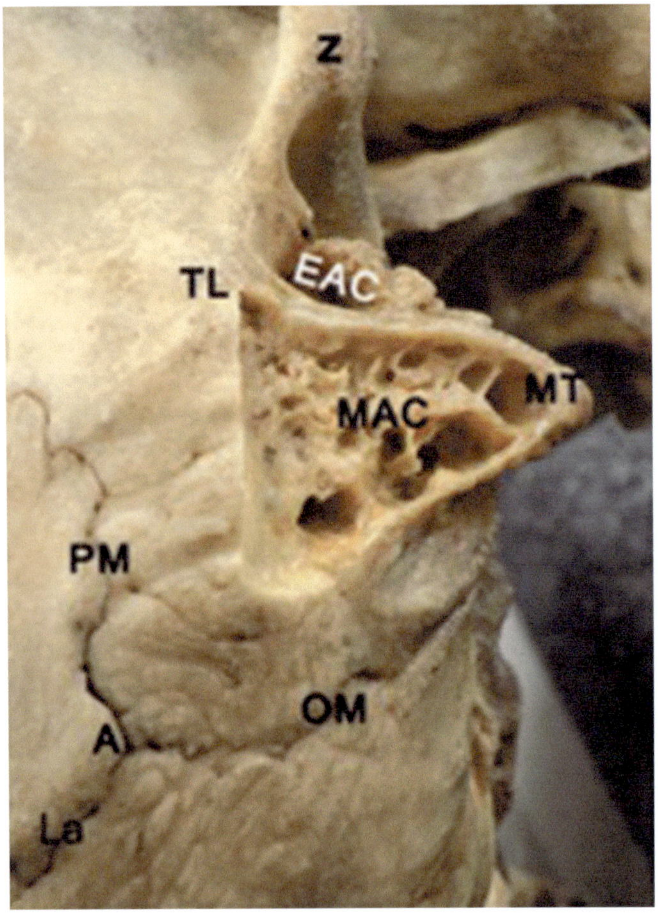

Fig. A.2 Right mastoid after drilling the mastoid cortex. *La* lamdoid, *A* asterion, *PM* parietomastoid suture, *OM* occipitomastoid suture, *EAC* external auditory canal, *TL* temporal line, *MT* mastoid tip, *MAC* mastoid air cells, *Z* zygoma

Translabyrinthine Approach

After the mastoidectomy, the translabyrinthine approach proceeds with a labyrinthectomy.

Labyrinthectomy

The labyrinthectomy starts with drilling out the three semicircular canals (Figs. A.4 and A.5) and then opening and removing the lateral, posterior, and superior canals. The ampullated end of the superior canal can be used as a land-

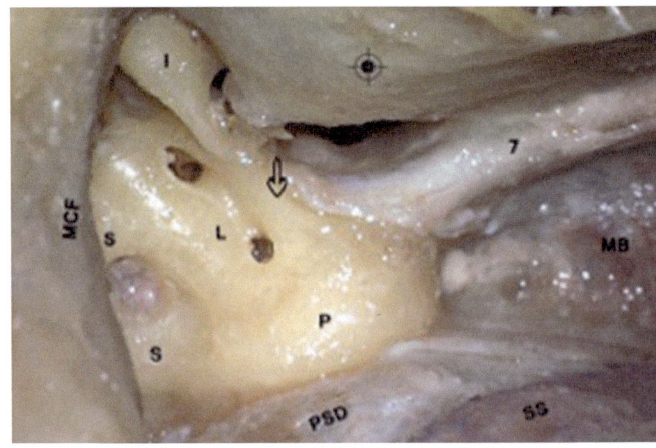

Fig. A.4 Right mastoid after simple mastoidectomy showing a view of the semicircular canals with drilling of the lateral semicircular canal. I = incus; MCF = middle cranial fossa floor; S = superior semicircular canal; L = lateral semicircular canal; P = posterior semicircular canal; SS = sigmoid sinus; PSD = presigmoid dura; 7 = facial nerve; DR = digastric ridge; MB = marrowbone deep to retrofacial air cells; Empty arrow = bone over second genu of facial nerve; Target sign = bony external auditory canal

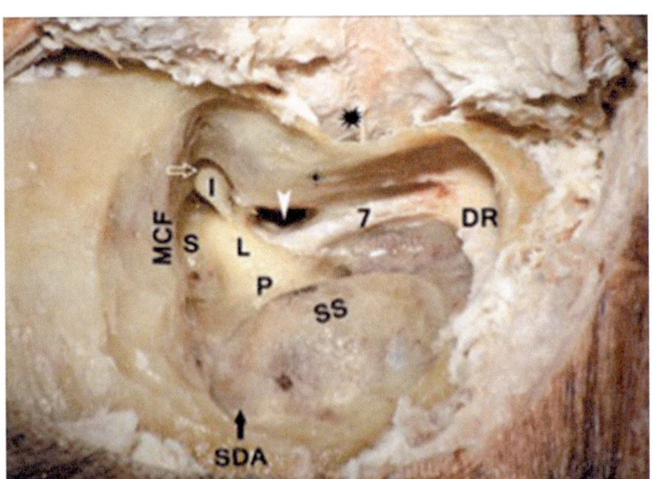

Fig. A.3 Right mastoid after simple mastoidectomy showing ventral surface of the dissection cavity. MCF = middle cranial fossa floor, I = incus; S = superior semicircular canal; L = lateral semicircular canal; P = posterior semicircular canal; SS = sigmoid sinus; SDA = sinodural angle; 7 = facial nerve; DR = digastric ridge; Target sign = posterior wall of external auditory canal; Asterisk = external auditory canal; Empty arrow = middle ear cavity; Arrow head = facial recess

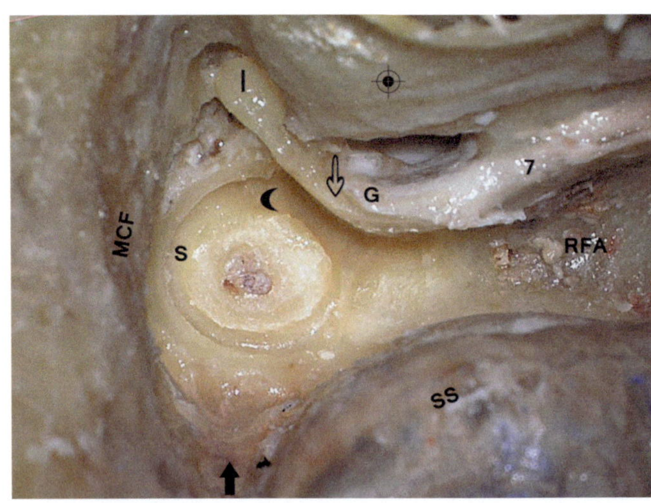

Fig. A.5 Right mastoid after simple mastoidectomy showing a view of the semicircular canals with drilling all semicircular canals. MCF = middle cranial fossa floor; S = superior semicircular canal; SS = sigmoid sinus; 7 = facial nerve; G = genu of facial nerve; DR = digastric ridge; RFA = retrofacial air cells; Empty arrow = bone over the seventh nerve; Target sign = bony external auditory canal; Moon = ampullated end of the superior canal mark for the labyrinthine segment of the facial nerve (Fig. A.5).

The next step in the translabyrinthine approach is exposing the internal auditory canal (IAC) and the facial nerve trajectory by drilling inferior and superior troughs (Figs. A.6 and A.7).

The dura is then opened along the IAC, presenting an unhindered view of cranial nerves 7 and 8 (Fig. A.8).

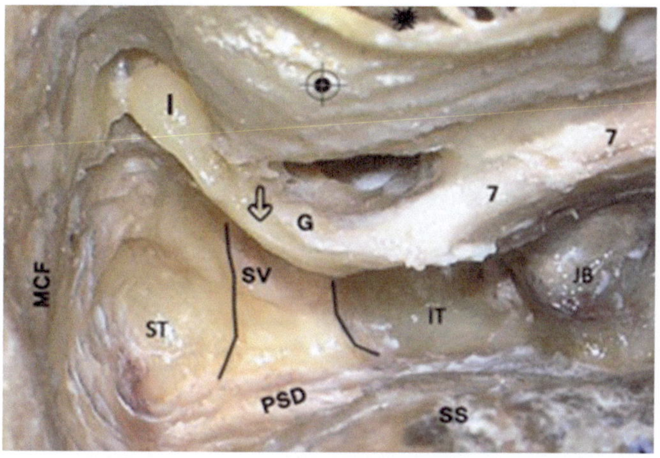

Fig. A.6 Right mastoid after simple mastoidectomy and drilling of all semicircular canals showing a closer view of the internal acoustic meatus with its contents. MCF = middle cranial fossa floor; SV = superior vestibular nerve; PSD = presigmoid dura; SS = sigmoid sinus; 7 = facial nerve; G = genu of facial nerve; Target sign = bony external auditory canal; Asterisk = external auditory canal; ST = superior trough; IT = inferior trough; JB = jugular bulb; Between the lines = IAC; Empty arrow = bone over the seventh nerve

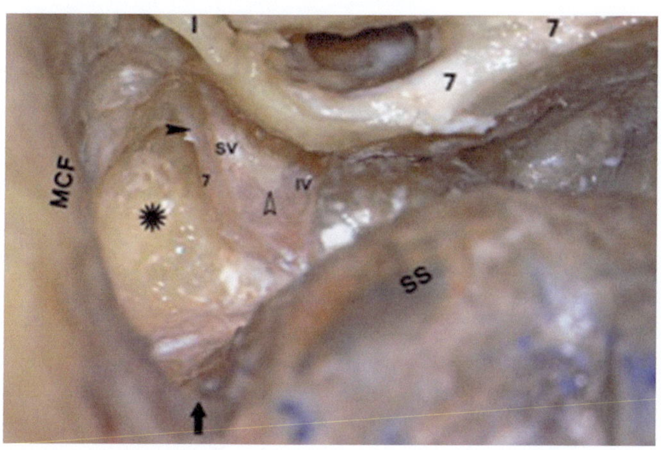

Fig. A.7 Right mastoid after simple mastoidectomy and drilling of all the semicircular canals showing a view of the internal acoustic meatus with its contents. MCF = middle cranial fossa floor; I = incus; Star = superior through; SV = superior vestibular nerve; IV = inferior vestibular nerve; Empty arrowhead = horizontal crest; Black arrowhead = Bill's bar; SS = sigmoid sinus; 7 = facial nerve; Black arrow = sinodural angle

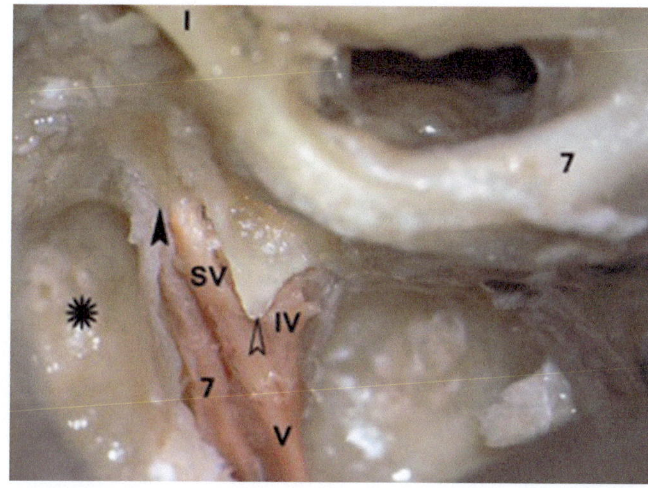

Fig. A.8 Right mastoid after simple mastoidectomy and drilling of all semicircular canals showing a view of the internal acoustic meatus with its contents. I = incus; Star = region after removal of semicircular canals; SV = superior vestibular nerve; IV = inferior vestibular nerve; V = vestibular nerve; Empty arrowhead = horizontal crest; Black arrowhead = Bill's bar; 7 = facial nerve

Transotic and Transcochlear Approach

After performing a mastoidectomy, labyrinthectomy, and skeletonizing the facial nerve (Fig. A.9), the transcochlear approach proceeds to remove the cochlea for a more extensive view into the CPA. This approach is similar to the transotic approach. The transcochlear approach requires a full mobilization of the facial nerve and posterior translocation. The transotic approach leaves the facial nerve in situ medially, and only the descending facial nerve is translocated anteriorly. Both procedures aim to preserve the facial nerve, but function is usually compromised in the transcochlear approach due to loss of blood supply of the geniculate when the nerve is transposed posteriorly (Fig. A.10).

The procedure then proceeds to fully skeletonize the facial nerve, exposing the labyrinthine segment, geniculate ganglion, and tympanic segment of the facial nerve (Fig. A.11).

Note the proximity of the labyrinth segment to the upper turn of the cochlea (Fig. A.12). The cochlea is then fully drilled out (Fig. A.13).

After removal of the cochlea (Fig. A.14), the facial nerve is skeletonized out further and soon to be transposed.

Figures A.15 and A.16 show further mobilization of the facial nerve and the transposition thereof. From this point on, the procedure is considered to be transcochlear and no longer transotic.

The dura can now be opened, exposing the CPA medial to the cochlea (Fig. A.17).

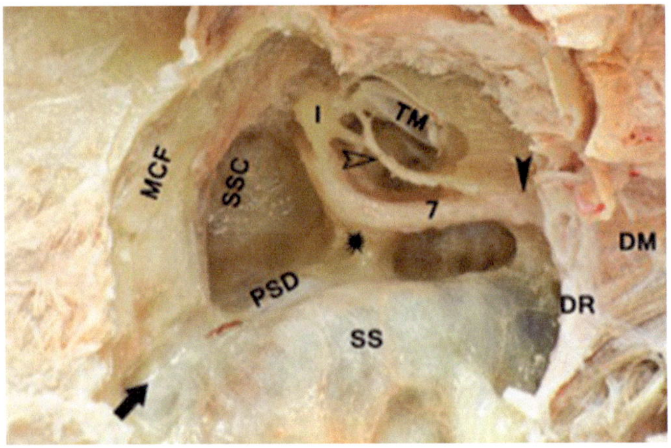

Fig. A.9 Right temporal bone after removal of all the semicircular canals and skeletonizing the facial nerve. MCF = middle cranial fossa floor; I = incus; SSC = region of superior semicircular canal after removal of the bone; Empty arrowhead = chorda tympani nerve; TM = tympanic membrane; PSD = presigmoid dura; SS = sigmoid sinus; 7 = facial nerve; Asterisk = internal auditory meatus; PSD = presigmoid dura; TM = tympanic membrane; DR = digastric ridge; DM = digastric muscle; Black arrowhead = facial nerve at stylomastoid foramen; Black arrow = sinodural angle

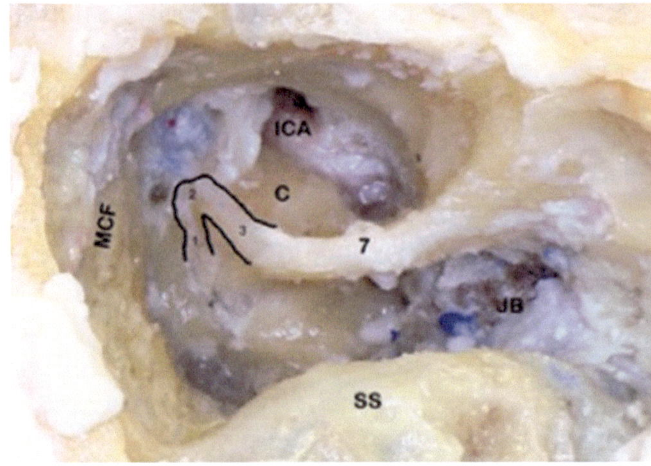

Fig. A.11 Right temporal bone after full skeletonization of the facial nerve from the IAC to the stylomastoid foramen. C = cochlea; MCF = middle cranial fossa dura; TM = tympanic membrane; SS = sigmoid sinus; JB = jugular bulb; ICA = internal carotid artery; 7 = facial nerve; 1 = labyrinthine segment; 2 = geniculate ganglion; 3 = tympanic segment

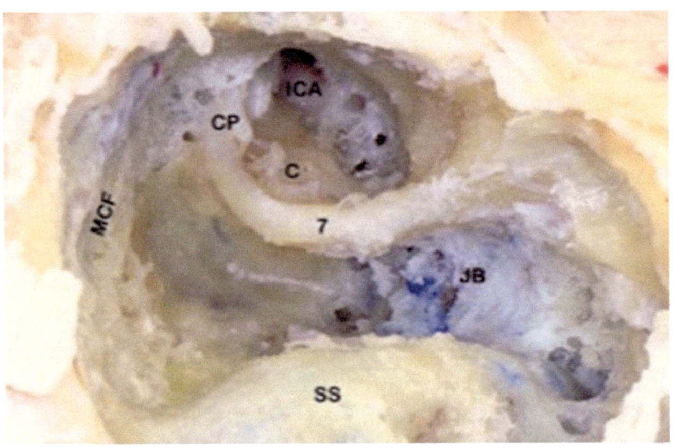

Fig. A.10 Right temporal bone, after performing mastoidectomy and labyrinthectomy and skeletonizing the facial nerve. The tympanic membrane, ossicular chain, and chorda tympani have been removed. C = cochlea; CP = cochleariform process; I = incus; MCF = middle cranial fossa dura; 7 = facial nerve; TM = tympanic membrane; SS = sigmoid sinus; ICA = internal carotid artery

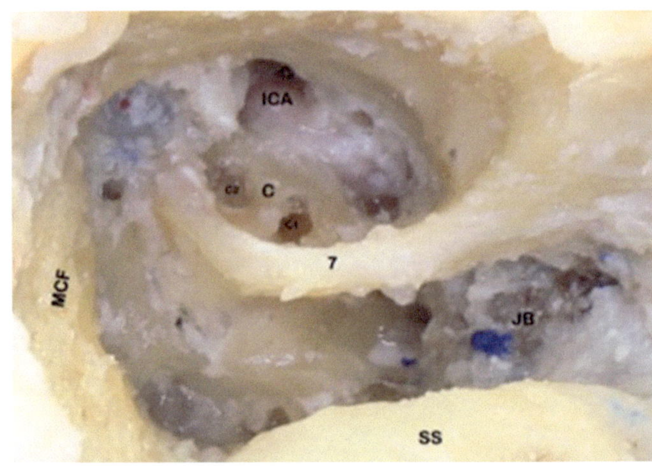

Fig. A.12 Right temporal bone after opening the cochlear duct. MCF = middle cranial fossa floor; 7 = facial nerve; SS = sigmoid sinus; JB = jugular bulb; ICA = internal carotid artery; C = cochlea; C_1 = basal turn; C_2 = upper hole of the cochlea

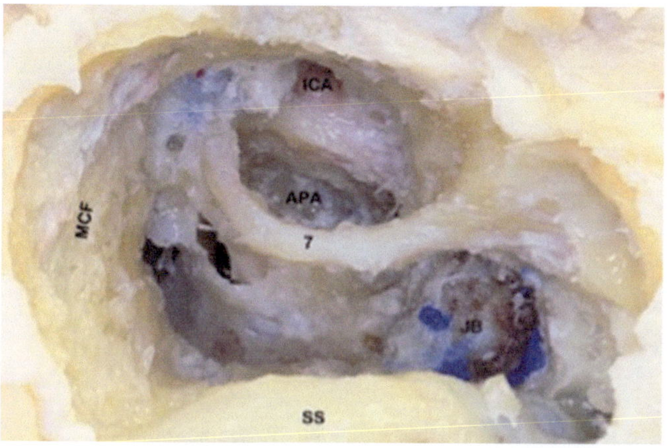

Fig. A.13 Right temporal bone, with the cochlea removed, exposing the anterior petrous apex prior to opening the dura and transposition of the facial nerve. MCF = middle cranial fossa floor; 7 = facial nerve; TM = tympanic membrane; SS = sigmoid sinus; JB = jugular bulb; ICA = internal carotid artery; APA = anterior petrous apex

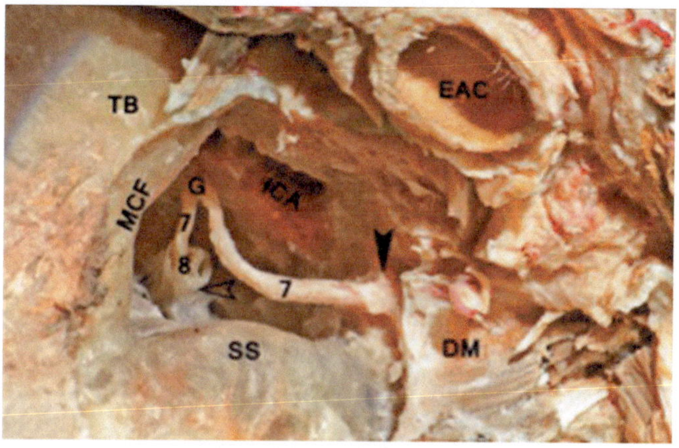

Fig. A.15 Ventral and deep view of the structures in the right temporal bone after transecting the external auditory canal. TB = temporal bone; MCF = middle cranial fossa floor; EAC = external auditory canal after transection; SS = sigmoid sinus 7 = facial nerve; G = Genu of facial nerve; 8 = vestibulocochlear nerve; ICA = internal carotid artery; DM = digastric muscle; Black arrowhead = facial nerve at stylomastoid foramen; Empty arrowhead = dura over the internal auditory meatus (IAM)

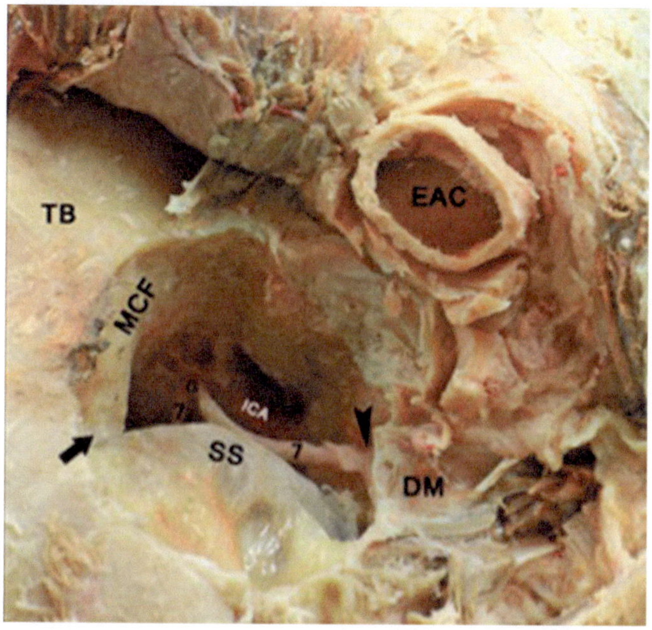

Fig. A.14 Ventral view of the deep structures in the right temporal bone after removal of all the semicircular canals, skeletonizing the facial nerve and transecting the external auditory canal. TB = temporal bone; MCF = middle cranial fossa floor; EAC = external auditory canal after transection; SS = sigmoid sinus; 7 = facial nerve; G = Genu of facial nerve; ICA = internal carotid artery; DM = digastric muscle; Black arrowhead = facial nerve at stylomastoid foramen; Black arrow = sinodural angle

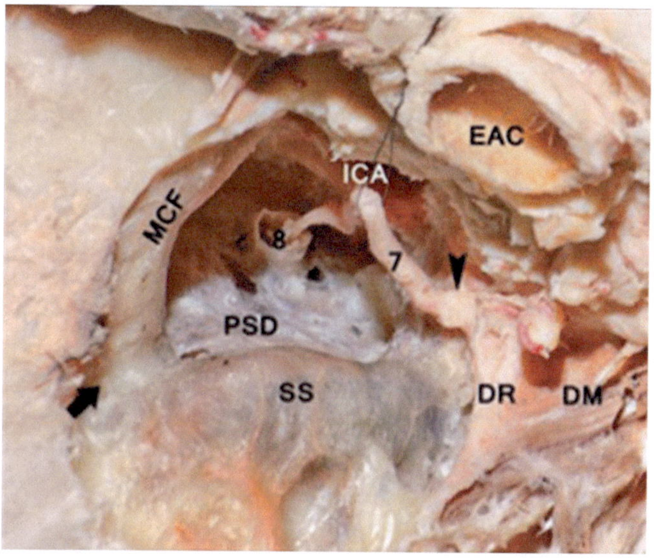

Fig. A.16 Posterior view of the dissection cavity of the right temporal bone after translocation of the facial nerve anteriorly. MCF = middle cranial fossa floor; EAC = external auditory canal after transection; SS = sigmoid sinus; 7 = facial nerve being transpositioned anteriorly; 8 = vestibulocochlear nerve; ICA = internal carotid artery; DR = digastric ridge; DM = digastric muscle; Black arrowhead = facial nerve at stylomastoid foramen; PSD = Presigmoid dura; Black arrow = sinodural angle

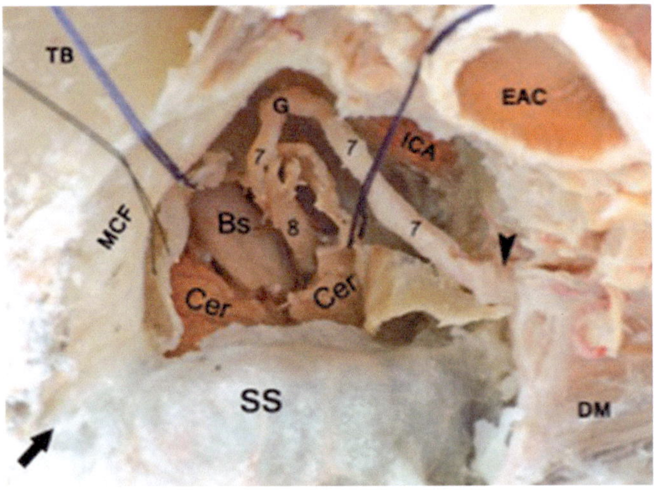

Fig. A.17 A view of the operative field of the right temporal bone after opening and retracting the dura in the presigmoid and adjacent areas, exposing the contents of the posterior fossa. TB = temporal bone; MCF = middle cranial fossa floor; EAC = external auditory canal after transection; SS = sigmoid sinus; 7 = facial nerve; 8 = vestibulocochlear nerve; ICA = internal carotid artery; DM = digastric muscle; Cer = cerebellum; Bs = brain stem; Black arrowhead = facial nerve at stylomastoid foramen; G = genu of seventh nerve; Black arrow = sinodural angle

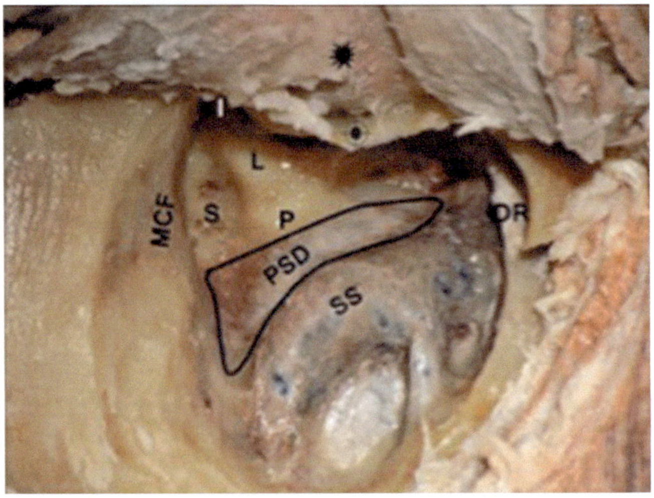

Fig. A.18 Right mastoid after simple mastoidectomy, showing posterior surface of the dissection cavity after drilling of the bone over the presigmoid area and over the retrofacial air cells. MCF = middle cranial fossa floor, I = incus; L = lateral semicircular canal; P = posterior semicircular canal; SS = sigmoid sinus; DR = digastric ridge; Target sign = posterior wall of external auditory canal; Asterisk = external auditory canal; PSD = presigmoid dura

Presigmoid/Retrolabyrinthine Approach

After a previously described mastoidectomy, the presigmoid approach proceeds with removal of the more posterior temporal bone. Bone posterior to the labyrinth is removed by drilling over the presigmoid area and retrofacial air cells until the presigmoid dura is completely exposed (Fig. A.18).

After the dura is incised, the endolymphatic sac is identified and included in the dural flap to preserve endolymphatic flow (Fig. A.19). Dural opening reveals the cerebellopontine cistern with its contents (Fig. A.20), creating a limited view of the 7–8 cranial nerve complex (Fig. A.21).

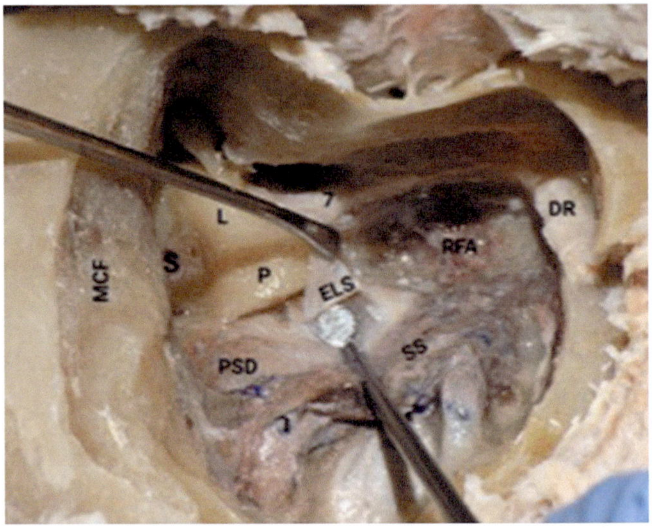

Fig. A.19 Right mastoid showing posterior surface of the dissection cavity after drilling of the bone over the presigmoid area and over the retrofacial air cells, showing the endolymphatic sac. MCF = middle cranial fossa floor; S = superior semicircular canal; I = incus; L = lateral semicircular canal; P = posterior semicircular canal; SS = sigmoid sinus; PSD = presigmoid dura; 7 = facial nerve; DR = digastric ridge; ELS = endolymphatic sac

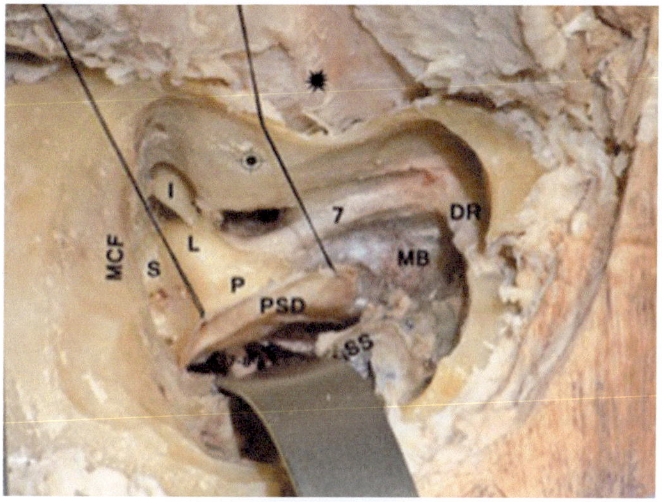

Fig. A.20 Right mastoid after simple mastoidectomy, exposure of the presigmoid area, and dural reflection ventrally to expose the cerebellopontine cistern with its contents after retraction of the cerebellum. MCF = middle cranial fossa floor; S = superior semicircular canal; L = lateral semicircular canal; P = posterior semicircular canal; SS = sigmoid sinus; PSD = presigmoid dura; DR = digastric ridge; MB = marrow bone deep to retrofacial air cells; Target sign = bony external auditory canal; Asterisk = external auditory canal; 7–8 = facial and vestibulocochlear nerve complex in the CPA seen after retraction of the cerebellum

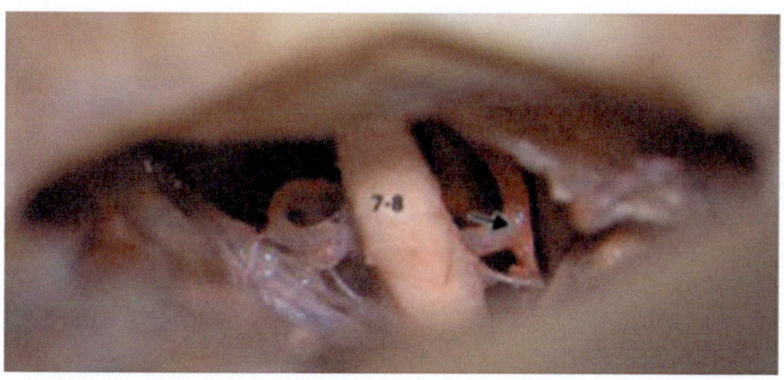

Fig. A.21 Right mastoid after simple mastoidectomy and reflection of the presigmoid dura ventrally, showing a close view of the contents of the cerebellopontine cistern after retraction of the cerebellum. 7–8 = facial and vestibulocochlear nerve complex seen after retraction of cerebellum; Empty arrow = anterior inferior cerebellar artery

Middle Cranial Fossa Approach

The middle cranial fossa approach provides a more lateral and superior trajectory of the CPA and the IAC. It does not provide a full view of the medial and inferior CPA. It does provide an early encounter of the facial nerve and an opportunity to spare hearing.

Craniotomy and Extradural Dissection

The procedure starts with a temporal bone craniotomy, followed with extradural dissection between the temporal bone and dura (Fig. A.22).

Figure A.23 demonstrates the placement of the MF retractor and the GSPN. The bone of the meatal plane (asterisk) is then removed over the superior IAC, and troughs are drilled on either side of the IAC from the porus laterally.

Care must be taken laterally; the distal IAC, the membranous labyrinth, and the cochlea are immediately adjacent to the IAC and are easily violated (Fig. A.24).

The dura over the superior aspect of the IAM is seen, opened from its medial to lateral end. The dura posterior to MMA is also opened.

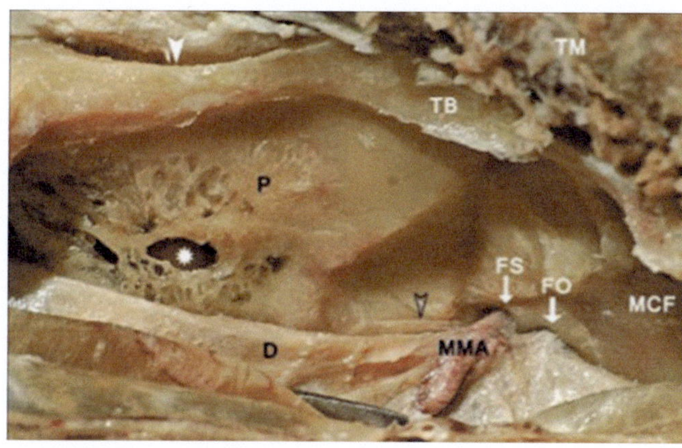

Fig. A.22 Extradural dissection of left temporal bone from lateral to medial, showing the initial important neurovascular structures encountered. White arrowhead = region of external auditory meatus; TB = temporal bone; TM = temporalis muscle; Empty arrowhead = GSPN; P = petrous temporal bone; White star = mastoid air cells; FS = foramen spinosum; MMA = middle meningeal artery; D = dura; FO = foramen ovale; MCF = middle cranial fossa floor

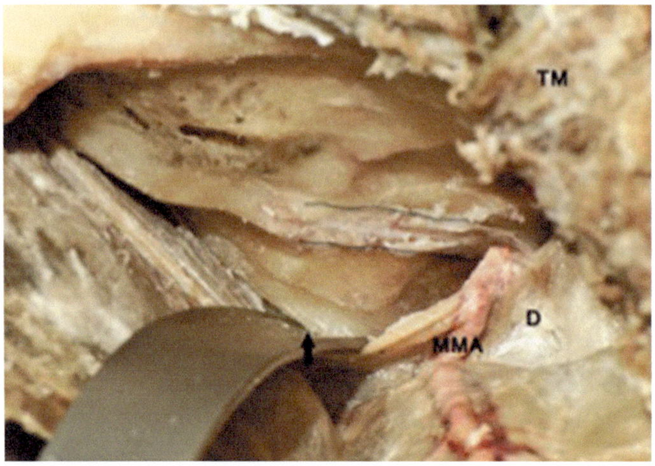

Fig. A.23 Extradural dissection of the left temporal bone from lateral to medial. TM = temporalis muscle; MMA = middle meningeal artery after transection; D = dura; Dark arrow = Petrous ridge; Between grey lines = GSPN

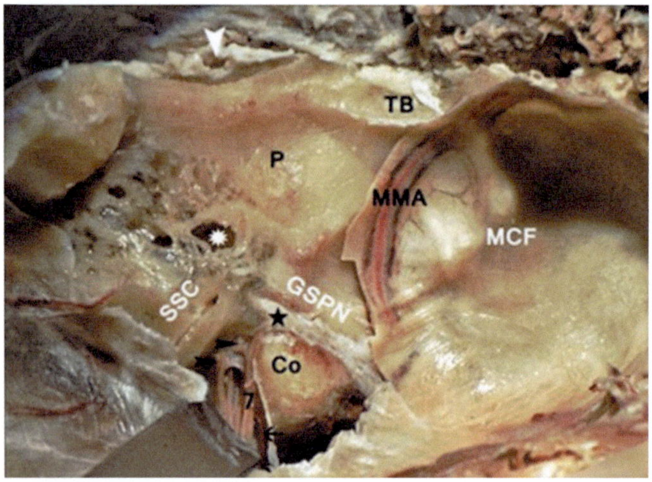

Fig. A.24 Superior view of left temporal bone over the IAM and after removal of bone at the petrous apex. White arrowhead = region of external auditory meatus; TB = temporal bone; GSPN = greater superficial petrosal nerve; MMA = middle meningeal artery; MCF = middle cranial fossa floor; White asterisk = mastoid air cell; P = petrous temporal bone; SSC = exposed superior semicircular canal after drilling the arcuate eminence; IAM = internal auditory meatus; 7 = facial nerve in internal auditory meatus; Black arrow = cochlear nerve in internal auditory meatus; Co = cochlea; Star = geniculate ganglion

Anterior Petrosectomy (Kawase Approach)

The approach then proceeds to the medial end of the petrous ridge after dissection of the middle meningeal artery near the foramen spinosum (Fig. A.25), remaining extradural. The anterior petrosectomy is performed in order to provide access to the pre-pontine cistern and anterior CPA and involves removing the bone at the petrous apex. The bone posterior to the horizontal portion of the petrous carotid, lateral to the Gasserian ganglion and anterior to the IAC, is removed to expose the dura of the posterior fossa anterior to the porus acusticus.

The superior vestibular nerve is excised at its lateral end to expose the inferior vestibular nerve.

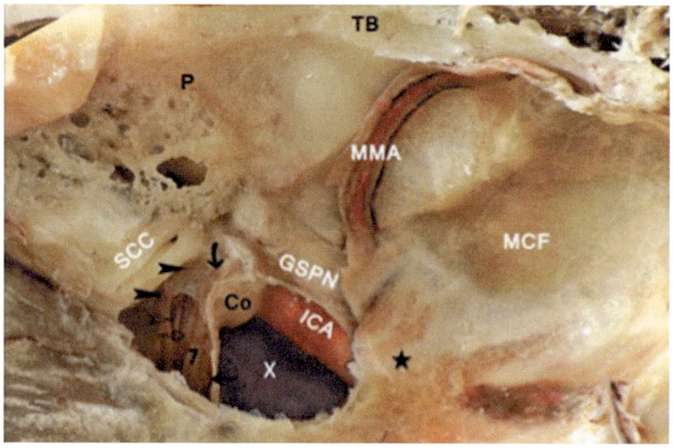

Fig. A.25 Superior view of left temporal bone. TB = temporal bone; GSPN = greater superficial petrosal nerve; MMA = middle meningeal artery; MCF = middle cranial fossa floor; P = petrous temporal bone; SSC = exposed superior semicircular canal after drilling the arcuate eminence; 7 = facial nerve in internal auditory meatus; Black arrow = ventral dura of IAM after its superior aspect is excised; Empty arrow = cochlear nerve; 7 = facial nerve; Empty arrow = cochlear nerve; Co = cochlea; Empty arrowhead = inferior vestibular nerve; Black arrowheads = ends of the superior vestibular nerve after its excision at its lateral end; ICA = internal carotid artery; Star = Gasserian ganglion; X = looking through Kawase triangle into the anterior CPA angle

Index

N. C. Bambakidis et al. (eds.), *Surgery of the Cerebellopontine Angle*, https://doi.org/10.1007/978-3-031-12507-2

D

FSC
www.fsc.org
MIX
Papier aus verantwortungsvollen Quellen
Paper from responsible sources
FSC® C105338

If you have any concerns about our products,
you can contact us on
ProductSafety@springernature.com

In case Publisher is established outside the EU,
the EU authorized representative is:
Springer Nature Customer Service Center GmbH
Europaplatz 3, 69115 Heidelberg, Germany

Printed by Libri Plureos GmbH
in Hamburg, Germany